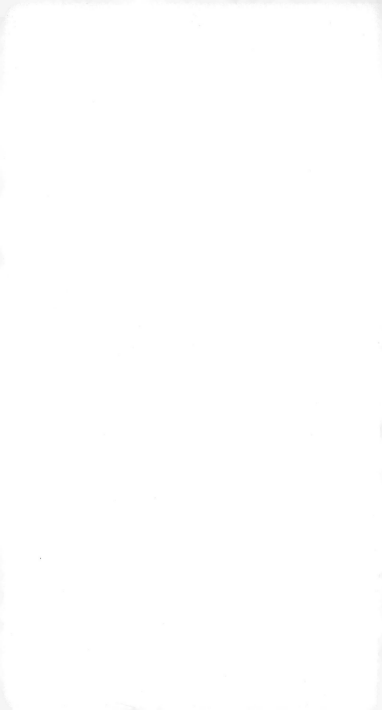

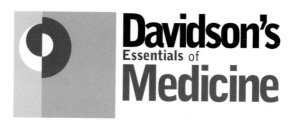

Davidson's
Essentials of

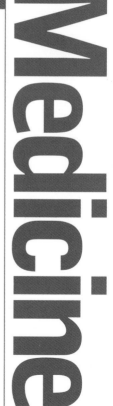

Medicine

2nd Edition

Edited by

J. Alastair Innes
PhD FRCP(Ed)

Consultant Physician and Honorary Reader in
Respiratory Medicine, Western General Hospital,
Edinburgh, UK

With a contribution by

Simon Maxwell
PhD FRCP FRCP(Ed) FBPharmacolS FHEA

Professor of Student Learning (Clinical Pharmacology
and Prescribing), University of Edinburgh; Honorary
Consultant Physician, Western General Hospital,
Edinburgh, UK

ELSEVIER

Edinburgh London New York Oxford Philadelphia St Louis Sydney Toronto 2016

ELSEVIER

First edition 2009
Second edition 2016

ISBN-13   978-0-7020-5592-8
International Edition ISBN-13   978-0-7020-5593-5
Ebook ISBN-13 978-0-7020-5595-9

ELSEVIER your source for books, journals and multimedia in the health sciences

www.elsevierhealth.com

Working together to grow libraries in developing countries

www.elsevier.com • www.bookaid.org

The publisher's policy is to use paper manufactured from sustainable forests

Content Strategist:
Laurence Hunter
Content Development Specialist:
Helen Leng
Project Manager:
Anne Collett
Designer:
Miles Hitchen
Illustration Manager:
Amy Faith Naylor
Illustrator:
TNQ

Printed in China

Contents

Sir Stanley Davidson (1894–1981)

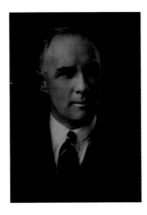

Davidson's Principles and Practice of Medicine was the brainchild of one of the great Professors of Medicine of the 20th century. Stanley Davidson was born in Sri Lanka and began his medical undergraduate training at Trinity College, Cambridge; this was interrupted by World War I and later resumed in Edinburgh. He was seriously wounded in battle, and the carnage and shocking waste of young life that he encountered at that time had a profound effect on his subsequent attitudes and values.

In 1930 Stanley Davidson was appointed Professor of Medicine at the University of Aberdeen, one of the first full-time Chairs of Medicine anywhere and the first in Scotland. In 1938 he took up the Chair of Medicine at Edinburgh and was to remain in this post until retirement in 1959. He was a renowned educator and a particularly gifted teacher at the bedside, where he taught that everything had to be questioned and explained. He himself gave most of the systematic lectures in Medicine, which were made available as typewritten notes that emphasised the essentials and far surpassed any textbook available at the time.

Principles and Practice of Medicine was conceived in the late 1940s with its origins in those lecture notes. The first edition, published in 1952, was a masterpiece of clarity and uniformity of style. It was of modest size and price, but sufficiently comprehensive and up to date to provide students with the main elements of sound medical practice. Although the format and presentation have seen many changes in 21 subsequent editions, Sir Stanley's original vision and objectives remain. More than half a century after its first publication, his book continues to inform and educate students, doctors and health professionals all over the world.

Preface

In the 63 years since *Davidson's Principles and Practice of Medicine* was first published, the rapid growth in the understanding of pathophysiology, in the variety of available diagnostic tests and in the range of possible treatments has posed an increasing challenge to those seeking to summarise clinical medicine in a single textbook. An inevitable consequence has been a parallel growth in the physical size of all the major textbooks, including *Davidson*. *Davidson's Essentials of Medicine* seeks to complement the parent volume by helping those who also need portable information to study on the move – whether commuting, travelling between training sites or during remote attachments and electives.

In this second edition, the entire content of *Essentials* has been comprehensively revised and updated to reflect the core content from *Davidson*, while retaining a size which can easily accompany readers on their travels. Although the text is concise, every effort has been made to maximise the readability and to avoid dry and unmemorable lists; the intention has been to produce a genuine miniature textbook. The text draws directly on the enormous depth and breadth of experience of the parent *Davidson* writing team and presents the essential elements in a format to suit hand luggage. Key *Davidson* illustrations have been adapted and retained, and 'added value' sections include a chapter on 'Interpreting key investigations' and a fully updated chapter on 'Therapeutics and prescribing' describing the typical clinical use of the major drug groups.

In an age when on-line information is ever more accessible to doctors in training, most still agree that there is no substitute for the physical page when systematic study is needed. With this book, we hope that the proven value of the parent *Davidson* can be augmented by making the essential elements accessible while on the move.

J.A.I.
Edinburgh

Acknowledgements

I am very grateful to the chapter authors of *Davidson's Principles and Practice of Medicine*, without whom this project would have been impossible. I would also like to acknowledge the invaluable contribution of the team of assistant editors who helped to sift and select the relevant information during preparation of the first edition: Kenneth Baillie, Sunil Adwani, Donald Noble, Sarah Walsh, Nazir Lone, Jehangir Din, Neeraj Dhaun and Alan Japp.

I remain indebted to Nicki Colledge and Brian Walker for inviting me to help create *Essentials* and for their support and guidance in the early stages. Thanks also to Laurence Hunter, Helen Leng, Ailsa Laing and Wendy Lee at Elsevier for their constant support and meticulous attention to detail.

Finally, I would like to thank Hester, Ailsa, Mairi and Hamish for their encouragement and support during the gestation of this book, and to dedicate it to the memory of my father, James Innes, who worked with Stanley Davidson on the early editions of *Davidson's Principles and Practice of Medicine*.

J.A.I.
Edinburgh

Contributors to *Davidson's Principles and Practice of Medicine*, 22nd Edition

The core of this book is based on the contents of *Davidson's Principles and Practice of Medicine*, with material extracted and re-edited to make a uniform presentation to suit the format of this book. Although some chapters and topics have, by necessity, been cut or substantially edited, contributors of all chapters drawn upon have been acknowledged here in recognition of their input into the totality of the parent textbook.

Albiruni Ryan Abdul Razak MRCPI
Consultant Medical Oncologist, Princess Margaret Cancer Centre, Toronto; Assistant Professor, University of Toronto, Canada

Brian J. Angus BSc DTM&H FRCP MD FFTM(Glas)
Reader in Infectious Diseases, Nuffield Department of Medicine, University of Oxford; Director, Oxford Centre for Tropical Medicine, UK

Quentin M. Anstee BSc MBBS PhD MRCP(UK)
Senior Lecturer, Institute of Cellular Medicine, Newcastle University, Newcastle upon Tyne; Honorary Consultant Hepatologist, Freeman Hospital, Newcastle upon Tyne, UK

Andrew W. Bradbury BSc MBChB(Hons) MD MBA FEBVS(Hon) FRCSE
Sampson Gamgee Professor of Vascular Surgery, Director of Quality Assurance and Enhancement, College of Medical and Dental Sciences, University of Birmingham, UK

Leslie Burnett MBBS PhD FRCPA FHGSA
Consultant Pathologist, NSW Health, PaLMS Pathology North, Royal North Shore Hospital, Sydney; Clinical Professor in Pathology and Genetic Medicine, Sydney Medical School, University of Sydney, Australia

Mark Byers *OBE* FRCGP MCEM MFSEM DA(UK)
General Practitioner, Ministry of Defence, UK

Jenny I.O. Craig MD FRCPE FRCPath
Consultant Haematologist, Addenbrooke's Hospital, Cambridge, UK

Allan D. Cumming BSc MD FRCPE
Dean of Students, College of Medicine and Veterinary Medicine, University of Edinburgh, UK

Graham Dark MBBS FRCP FHEA
Senior Lecturer in Cancer Education, Newcastle University; Consultant Medical Oncologist, Freeman Hospital, Newcastle upon Tyne, UK

Richard J. Davenport FRCPE DM
Consultant Neurologist, Royal
Infirmary of Edinburgh and
Western General Hospital,
Edinburgh; Honorary Senior
Lecturer, University of Edinburgh,
UK

Robert S. Dawe MD FRCPE
Consultant Dermatologist,
Ninewells Hospital and Medical
School, Dundee; Honorary Clinical
Reader, University of Dundee, UK

David Dockrell MD FRCPI
FRCPG FACP
Professor of Infectious Diseases,
University of Sheffield, UK

Michael J. Field AM MD FRACP
Emeritus Professor, Sydney Medical
School, University of Sydney,
Australia

David R. FitzPatrick MD FRCPE
Consultant in Clinical Genetics,
Royal Hospital for Sick Children,
Edinburgh; Professor, University
of Edinburgh, UK

Jane Goddard PhD FRCPE
Consultant Nephrologist, Royal
Infirmary of Edinburgh; Part-time
Senior Lecturer, University of
Edinburgh, UK

Neil R. Grubb MD FRCP
Consultant Cardiologist, Edinburgh
Heart Centre; Honorary Senior
Lecturer, University of Edinburgh,
UK

Phil Hanlon BSc MD MPH
Professor of Public Health,
University of Glasgow, UK

Richard P. Hobson PhD
MCRP(UK), FRCPath
Consultant Microbiologist, Leeds
Teaching Hospitals NHS Trust;
Honorary Senior Lecturer, Leeds
University, UK

Sally H. Ibbotson BSc(Hons)
MD FRCPE
Clinical Senior Lecturer in
Photobiology, University of
Dundee; Honorary Consultant
Dermatologist, Ninewells Hospital
and Medical School, Dundee, UK

J. Alastair Innes PhD FRCPE
Consultant Physician, Western
General Hospital, Edinburgh;
Honorary Reader in Respiratory
Medicine, University of Edinburgh,
UK

David E. Jones MA BM BCh PhD
FRCP
Professor of Liver Immunology,
Institute of Cellular Medicine,
Newcastle University, Newcastle
upon Tyne; Consultant
Hepatologist, Freeman Hospital,
Newcastle upon Tyne, UK

Peter Langhorne PhD FRCPG
Professor of Stroke Care, University
of Glasgow; Honorary Consultant,
Royal Infirmary, Glasgow, UK

Stephen M. Lawrie MD(Hons)
FRCPsych FRCPE(Hon)
Head, Division of Psychiatry,
School of Clinical Sciences,
University of Edinburgh; Honorary
Consultant Psychiatrist, Royal
Edinburgh Hospital, UK

John Paul Leach MD FRCPG
FRCPE
Consultant Neurologist, Institute of
Neuroscience, Southern General
Hospital, Glasgow; Honorary
Associate Clinical Professor,
University of Glasgow, UK

Charlie W. Lees MBBS
FRCPE PhD
Consultant Gastroenterologist,
Western General Hospital,
Edinburgh; Honorary Senior
Lecturer, University of Edinburgh,
UK

Gary Maartens MBChB MMed
Consultant Physician, Department of Medicine, Groote Schuur Hospital, Cape Town; Professor of Clinical Pharmacology, University of Cape Town, South Africa

Helen M. Macdonald BSc(Hons) PhD MSc RNutr(Public Health)
Chair in Nutrition and Musculoskeletal Health, University of Aberdeen, UK

Lynn M. Manson MD FRCPE FRCPath
Consultant Haematologist, Scottish National Blood Transfusion Service; Honorary Clinical Senior Lecturer, University of Edinburgh, UK

Sara E. Marshall FRCPE FRCPath PhD
Honorary Consultant Immunologist, NHS Tayside; Professor of Clinical Immunology, University of Dundee, UK

Simon Maxwell MD PhD FRCP FRCPE FBPharmacolS FHEA
Professor of Student Learning (Clinical Pharmacology and Prescribing), University of Edinburgh; Honorary Consultant Physician, Western General Hospital, Edinburgh, UK

Rory J. McCrimmon MD FRCPE
Professor of Experimental Diabetes and Metabolism, University of Dundee; Honorary Consultant, Ninewells Hospital and Medical School, Dundee, UK

Iain B. McInnes FRCP PhD FRSE FMedSci
Muirhead Professor of Medicine and Director of Institute of Infection, Immunity and Inflammation, College of Medical, Veterinary and Life Sciences, University of Glasgow, UK

David E. Newby FESC FACC FMedSci FRSE
British Heart Foundation John Wheatley Professor of Cardiology, University of Edinburgh; Consultant Cardiologist, Royal Infirmary of Edinburgh, UK

John D. Newell-Price MA PhD FRCP
Reader in Endocrinology and Honorary Consultant Endocrinologist, Department of Human Metabolism, School of Medicine and Biomedical Science, Sheffield, UK

Graham R. Nimmo MD FRCPE FFARCSI FFICM
Consultant Physician in Intensive Care Medicine and Clinical Education, Western General Hospital, Edinburgh, UK

Simon I.R. Noble MBBS MD FRCP Dip Pal Med PGCE
Clinical Senior Lecturer in Palliative Medicine, Cardiff University; Honorary Consultant, Palliative Medicine, Royal Gwent Hospital, Newport, UK

David R. Oxenham MRCP
Consultant in Palliative Care, Marie Curie Hospice, Edinburgh; Honorary Senior Lecturer, University of Edinburgh, UK

Ewan R. Pearson PhD FRCPE
Professor of Diabetic Medicine, University of Dundee; Honorary Consultant in Diabetes, Ninewells Hospital and Medical School, Dundee, UK

Ian D. Penman BSc MD FRCPE
Consultant Gastroenterologist, Royal Infirmary of Edinburgh; Honorary Senior Lecturer, University of Edinburgh, UK

Stuart H. Ralston MD FRCP FMedSci FRSE
Arthritis Research UK Professor of Rheumatology, University of Edinburgh; Honorary Consultant Rheumatologist, Western General Hospital, Edinburgh, UK

Peter T. Reid MD FRCPE
Consultant Physician, Western General Hospital, Edinburgh; Honorary Senior Lecturer in Respiratory Medicine, University of Edinburgh, UK

Gordon R. Scott BSc FRCP
Consultant in Genitourinary Medicine, Chalmers Sexual Health Centre, Edinburgh; Honorary Senior Lecturer, University of Edinburgh, UK

Jonathan R. Seckl BSc MBBS PhD FRCPE FMedSci FRSE
Professor of Molecular Medicine, Executive Dean (Medicine) and Vice-Principal (Research), University of Edinburgh; Honorary Consultant Physician, Royal Infirmary of Edinburgh, UK

Michael Sharpe MA MD FRCP FRCPE FRCPsych
Professor of Psychological Medicine, University of Oxford; Honorary Professor, University of Edinburgh; Honorary Consultant in Psychological Medicine, Oxford University Hospitals NHS Trust and Oxford Health NHS Foundation Trust, UK

Peter Stewart FRACP FRCPA MBA
Clinical Director, Sydney South West Pathology Service; Clinical Associate Professor, University of Sydney, Australia

Mark W.J. Strachan MD FRCPE
Consultant in Diabetes and Endocrinology, Western General Hospital, Edinburgh; Honorary Professor, University of Edinburgh, UK

David Sullivan FRACP FRCPA FCSANZ
Clinical Associate Professor, Central Clinical School, Sydney Medical School, University of Sydney, Australia

Shyam Sundar MD FRCP FNA
Professor of Medicine, Institute of Medical Sciences, Banaras Hindu University, Varanasi, India

Simon H.L. Thomas BSc MD FRCP FRCPE
Consultant Physician, Newcastle Hospitals NHS Foundation Trust; Professor of Clinical Pharmacology and Therapeutics, Newcastle University, Newcastle upon Tyne, UK

A. Neil Turner PhD FRCP
Professor of Nephrology, University of Edinburgh; Honorary Consultant Physician, Royal Infirmary of Edinburgh, UK

Simon W. Walker DM FRCPath FRCPE
Senior Lecturer in Clinical Biochemistry, University of Edinburgh; Honorary Consultant Clinical Biochemist, Royal Infirmary of Edinburgh, UK

Tim Walsh BSc(Hons) MBChB(Hons) FRCA FRCP FFICM MD MRes
Professor of Critical Care, University of Edinburgh; Honorary Consultant, Royal Infirmary of Edinburgh, UK

Henry Watson MD FRCPE FRCPath
Consultant Haematologist, Aberdeen Royal Infirmary; Honorary Senior Lecturer, University of Aberdeen, UK

Julian White MD FACTM
Consultant Clinical Toxicologist and Head of Toxinology, Women's and Children's Hospital, Adelaide; Associate Professor, Department of Paediatrics, University of Adelaide, Australia

John P.H. Wilding DM FRCP
Professor of Medicine, Head of
Department of Obesity and
Endocrinology, Institute of Ageing
and Chronic Disease, University of
Liverpool; Honorary Consultant
Physician, University Hospital
Aintree, Liverpool, UK

Miles D. Witham BM BCh PhD
FRCPE
Clinical Senior Lecturer in Ageing
and Health, University of Dundee;
Honorary Consultant Geriatrician,
NHS Tayside, Dundee, UK

List of abbreviations

ABGs	arterial blood gases
ACE	angiotensin-converting enzyme
ACTH	adrenocorticotrophic hormone
ADH	antidiuretic hormone
AIDS	acquired immunodeficiency syndrome
ANA	antinuclear antibody
ANCA	antineutrophil cytoplasmic autoantibody
ANF	antinuclear factor
APTT	activated partial thromboplastin time
ARDS	acute respiratory distress syndrome
ASO	antistreptolysin O
AST	aspartate aminotransferase
AXR	abdominal X-ray
BCG	Calmette–Guérin bacillus
BMI	body mass index
BP	blood pressure
CK	creatine kinase
CNS	central nervous system
CPAP	continuous positive airways pressure
CRP	C-reactive protein
CSF	cerebrospinal fluid
CT	computed tomography/tomogram
CVP	central venous pressure
CXR	chest X-ray
DEXA	dual-energy X-ray absorptiometry
DIC	disseminated intravascular coagulation
dsDNA	double-stranded deoxyribonucleic acid
DVT	deep venous thrombosis
ECG	electrocardiography/electrocardiogram
ELISA	enzyme-linked immunosorbent assay
ERCP	endoscopic retrograde cholangiopancreatography
ESR	erythrocyte sedimentation rate
FBC	full blood count
FDA	Food and Drug Administration
FEV$_1$/FVC	forced expiratory volume in 1 sec/forced vital capacity
FFP	fresh frozen plasma
5-HT	5-hydroxytryptamine; serotonin
FOB	faecal occult blood
GI	gastrointestinal
GMC	General Medical Council
GU	genitourinary
HDL	high-density lipoprotein
HDU	high-dependency unit
HIV	human immunodeficiency virus

HLA	human leucocyte antigen
HRT	hormone replacement therapy
ICU	intensive care unit
IL	interleukin
IM	intramuscular
INR	International Normalised Ratio
IV	intravenous
IVU	intravenous urogram/urography
JVP	jugular venous pressure
LDH	lactate dehydrogenase
LDL	low-density lipoprotein
LFTs	liver function tests
MRC	Medical Research Council
MRCP	magnetic resonance cholangiopancreatography
MRI	magnetic resonance imaging
MRSA	meticillin-resistant *Staphylococcus aureus*
MSU	mid-stream sample of urine
NG	nasogastric
NICE	National Institute for Health and Care Excellence
NIV	non-invasive ventilation
NSAID	non-steroidal anti-inflammatory drug
PA	postero-anterior
PCR	polymerase chain reaction
PE	pulmonary embolism
PET	positron emission tomography
PTH	parathyroid hormone
RBC	red blood count
RCT	randomised controlled clinical trial
SPECT	single-photon emission computed tomography
STI	sexually transmitted infection
TB	tuberculosis
TFTs	thyroid function tests
TNF	tumour necrosis factor
U&Es	urea and electrolytes
USS	ultrasound scan
VTE	venous thromboembolism
WBC/WCC	white blood/cell count
WHO	World Health Organisation

Picture credits

We are grateful to the following individuals and organisations for permission to reproduce the figures and boxes listed below.

Chapter 2
Comprehensive geriatric assessment (p. 10) Wasted hand and kyphosis insets: Afzal Mir M. Atlas of Clinical Diagnosis. 2nd edn. Edinburgh: Saunders; 2003. **Box 2.5** Hodkinson HM, Evaluation of a mental test score for assessment of mental impairment in the elderly Age and Ageing 1972; 1(4): 233–8

Chapter 5
Clinical examination of patients with infectious disease (p. 48) Splinter haemorrhages inset: Dr Nick Beeching, Royal Liverpool University; Roth's spots inset: Prof. Ian Rennie, Royal Hallamshire Hospital, Sheffield. **Fig. 5.11** Malaria retinopathy inset: Dr Nicholas Beare, Royal Liverpool University Hospital; blood films insets, *P. vivax* and *P. falciparum*: Dr Kamolrat Silamut, Mahidol Oxford Research Unit, Bangkok, Thailand. **Box 5.20** WHO. Severe falciparum malaria. In: Severe and complicated malaria. 3rd edn. Trans Roy Soc Trop Med Hyg 2000; 94 (suppl. 1): S1–41

Chapter 6
Fig. 6.3 Adapted from Flenley D. Lancet 1971; 1: 1921

Chapter 8
Clinical examination of the cardiovascular system (p. 202) Splinter haemorrhage, jugular venous pulse, malar flush and tendon xanthomas insets: Newby D, Grubb N. Cardiology: An Illustrated Colour Text. Edinburgh: Churchill Livingstone; 2005. **Fig. 8.4** Resuscitation Council (UK). **Fig. 8.18** NICE Clinical Guideline 127, Hypertension; August 2011) **Box 8.7** European Society of Cardiology Clinical Practice Guidelines: Atrial Fibrillation (Management of) 2010 and Focused Update (2012). Eur Heart J 2012; 33: 2719–2747

Chapter 9
Clinical examination of the respiratory system (p. 266) Idiopathic kyphoscoliosis inset: Dr I. Smith, Papworth Hospital, Cambridge. **Fig. 9.8** Adapted from Detterbeck FC, Boffa DJ, Tanoue LT. The new lung cancer staging system. Chest 2009; 136:260–271). **Fig. 9.9** Johnson N McL. Respiratory Medicine. Oxford: Blackwell Science; 1986

Chapter 10
Fig. 10.3 Toxic multinodular goitre inset: Dr P.L. Padfield, Western General Hospital, Edinburgh

Chapter 12
Fig. 12.3 Hayes P, Simpson K. Gastroenterology and Liver Disease. Edinburgh: Churchill Livingstone; 1995

Chapter 13
Clinical examination of the abdomen for liver and biliary disease (p. 476) Spider naevi inset: Hayes P, Simpson K. Gastroenterology and liver disease. Edinburgh: Churchill Livingstone; 1995. Aspiration inset: Strachan M. Davidson's clinical cases. Edinburgh: Churchill Livingstone; 2008 (Fig. 65.1). Palmar erythema inset: Martin P. Approach to the patient with liver disease. In: Gold L and Schafter AI. Goldman's Cecil Medicine. 24th edn. Philadelphia: WB Saunders; 2012 (Fig. 1148-2, p. 954)

Chapter 14
Blood disease Box 14.6 From Wells PS. New Engl J Med 2003; 349: 1227; copyright © 2003 Massachusetts Medical Society

Chapter 16
Fig. 16.7 Courtesy of Dr B Cullen. **Fig. 16.10** Courtesy of Dr A. Farrell and Professor J. Wardlaw

Chapter 17
Skin disease Fig. 17.13 White GM, Cox NH. Diseases of the skin. London: Mosby; 2000; copyright Elsevier

Good medical practice

1

Patients (and doctors) differ in their beliefs, attitudes and expectations. Good medical practice requires the ability to recognise and respect these individual differences. This chapter describes how to:

- Provide patients and their families with complex information.
- Discuss management options. • Reach appropriate ethical decisions within resource constraints.

THE DOCTOR–PATIENT RELATIONSHIP

While some medical knowledge is based on clear evidence, much reflects wisdom and understanding passed down generations of doctors over hundreds of years. This wisdom is central to how doctors and patients interact; it demands respect, and if combined with compassion, fosters the development of trust.

The doctor–patient relationship is itself therapeutic; a successful consultation with a trusted practitioner will have benefits irrespective of other therapies. It is also dynamic, bilateral, and influenced by differing attitudes and beliefs. Patients with chronic diseases increasingly interact with a multidisciplinary team of health professionals. The doctor usually leads in determining the overall direction of care but must also:

- Guide the patient through the unfamiliar language and customs of clinical care. • Interpret and convey complex information. • Help patient and family to participate in decision-making.

Regulatory bodies seek to define the duties of a doctor (e.g. Box 1.1), and many medical schools require students to sign an ethical code based on such statements. Difficulties arise if the patient perceives the doctor to have failed in one of these duties. Early recognition and open acknowledgement of patients' concerns are key to restoring trust.

1.1 The duties of a doctor registered with the UK GMC

- Make the care of your patient your first concern
- Protect and promote the health of patients and the public
- Provide a good standard of practice and care
    - Keep up to date
    - Recognise and work within the limits of your competence
    - Work with colleagues in the ways that best serve patients' interests
- Treat patients as individuals and respect their dignity
    - Be polite and considerate
    - Respect confidentiality
- Work in partnership with patients
    - Respect their concerns and preferences
    - Give them information in a way they can understand
    - Respect their right to reach decisions with you about their care
    - Support them so that they can care for themselves and improve their health
- Be honest and open
    - Act without delay if you believe patients are being put at risk by you or a colleague
    - Never discriminate unfairly against patients or colleagues
    - Never abuse your patients' trust in you or in the profession

1.2 Some barriers to good communication in health care

The clinician

- Authoritarian or dismissive attitude
- Hurried approach
- Use of jargon
- Inability to speak first language of patient
- No experience of patient's cultural background

The patient

- Anxiety
- Reluctance to discuss sensitive or seemingly trivial issues
- Misconceptions
- Conflicting sources of information
- Cognitive impairment
- Hearing/speech/visual impediment

COMMUNICATION AND OTHER CLINICAL SKILLS

Good communication is the single most important component of good practice. Failures in communication are common, and lead to poor health outcomes, strained working relations, dissatisfaction, anger and litigation among patients, their families and their carers. Some common barriers to good communication are listed in Box 1.2.

Doctors must first establish a good rapport, starting with a friendly and culturally appropriate greeting, looking at the patient, *not* the notes. They should start by outlining, in simple language, the contents and objectives of the consultation, while also checking the patient's prior knowledge and expectations.

The main aim of a consultation is to establish a factual account of the patient's illness. The clinician must allow the patient to describe the problems with appropriate questions, not leading or overbearing ones. In addition, the clinician must explore the patient's feelings, their interpretation of their symptoms, and their concerns and fears, before agreeing a plan. These goals will not be met unless clinicians demonstrate understanding and empathy. Many patients have multiple concerns and will not discuss these if they sense the clinician is uninterested, or likely to dismiss their complaints as irrational or trivial. Non-verbal cues and body language are important; communication will be impaired if the clinician appears indifferent, unsympathetic or short of time. The patient's facial expressions and body language may betray hidden fears. The clinician can help the patient to talk more freely by smiling or nodding appropriately.

Careful questioning and listening will usually yield a provisional diagnosis, establish rapport, and determine which investigations are appropriate. The doctor must always ensure that dignity is preserved and that the patient feels comfortable throughout the consultation. For clinical examination, this always requires advance explanation and may also entail the presence of a chaperone.

INVESTIGATIONS

Modern medical practice is dominated by investigations. Judicious use of these is crucially dependent on good clinical skills. Indeed, a test should only be ordered if the value of the result clearly justifies the discomfort, risk and cost incurred. Clinicians should therefore prepare a provisional management plan before requesting any investigations.

The 'normal' (or reference) range

Although some tests provide qualitative results (present or absent), most provide a quantitative value. To classify quantitative results as normal or abnormal, it is necessary to define a 'normal range'. Many biological measurements exhibit a bell-shaped, 'normal distribution', described statistically by the mean and the standard deviation (SD, which describes the spread of results). The 'normal range' or 'reference range' is conventionally defined as the range that includes 95% of the population, i.e. two SDs above and below the mean. Results more than two SDs from the mean occur either because the person is one of the 5% of the normal population whose result is outside the reference range, or because their disease is affecting the result.

It is also important to define results that correlate with biological disadvantage. In some diseases, there is no overlap between results from the normal and abnormal population (e.g. creatinine in renal failure). In many diseases, however, there is overlap with the reference range (e.g. thyroxine in toxic multinodular goitre). The greater the difference between the test result and the reference range, the higher the chance that disease is present, but normal results may be 'false negatives' and results outside the reference range may be 'false positives'. Similarly, for quantitative risk factors, the clinical decision may not depend on whether or not the result is 'normal'. For example, higher total cholesterol is associated with higher risk of myocardial infarction within the normal population, and cholesterol-lowering therapy may benefit people with normal cholesterol values. Similar arguments may apply for blood pressure, blood glucose, bone mineral density and so on.

Each test in a normal person carries a 5% (1 in 20) chance of a result outside the 'reference range'. Indiscriminate repeat testing increases the chance of such 'abnormal' results and should be avoided.

Reference ranges defined either by test manufacturers or local laboratories are often established in small numbers of young healthy people who are not necessarily representative of the patient population.

If a substantial proportion of the normal population have an unrecordably low result (e.g. serum troponin), the distribution cannot be described by mean and SD. In these circumstances, results from normal and abnormal people are used to identify 'cut-off' values associated with a certain risk of disease.

Sensitivity and specificity

All diagnostic tests can produce false positives (abnormal result in the absence of disease) and false negatives (normal test in a patient with disease). The diagnostic accuracy of a test can be expressed in terms of its sensitivity and its specificity (Box 1.3). In practice, there is a trade-off between sensitivity and specificity. For example, defining an exercise ECG as abnormal if there is ≥ 0.5 mm ST depression ensures that very little coronary disease is missed, but would generate many false-positive tests. Conversely, a cut-off of ≥ 2.0 mm ST depression will detect most important coronary disease with far fewer false-positive results.

1.3 The accuracy of diagnostic tests

	Affected	Unaffected
Positive test	True +ve (a)	False +ve (b)
Negative test	False −ve (c)	True −ve (d)
Sensitivity (%)		Specificity (%)
$= [a/(a + c)] \times 100$		$= [d/(b + d)] \times 100$
Positive predictive value		Negative predictive value
$= a/(a + b)$		$= d/(c + d)$

Predictive value

The value of a test is determined by the prevalence of the condition in the test population. Bayes' theorem allows the probability that a subject has a particular condition (the post-test probability) to be calculated if the pre-test probability and the sensitivity and specificity of the test are known. The positive predictive value (see Box 1.3) is the probability that a patient with a positive test has the condition. The negative predictive value is the probability that a patient with a negative test does not have the condition.

The interpretation of a test is critically dependent on clinical context. For example, 2 mm ST elevation in ECG leads V_2 and V_3 is likely to represent myocardial infarction in a 54-yr-old Caucasian male with multiple risk factors and typical chest pain, but will probably be a normal variant in an asymptomatic 18-yr-old Afro-Caribbean man.

Screening

While screening programmes may be useful in detecting early disease, they also raise anxiety by generating false positives. Screening should only be considered for diseases with high prevalence, where an affordable, sensitive and specific test exists and where effective treatment is available.

ESTIMATING AND COMMUNICATING RISK

Medical decisions are usually made by balancing the anticipated benefits of a procedure or treatment against the potential risks. Providing relevant facts is seldom sufficient to communicate risk because a patient's perception of risk is often coloured by emotional or irrational factors. Patients receive information from multiple, potentially conflicting sources (e.g. Internet, books, magazines, self-help groups, other health-care professionals, friends and family).

A key step in decision-making is to present the evidence base. Statistics and probabilities can be confusing and data can be presented in many ways (Box 1.4).

1.4 Explaining the risks and benefits of therapy

Would you take a drug once a day for a year to prevent stroke if:
- it reduced your risk of having a stroke by 47%?
- it reduced your chance of suffering a stroke from 0.26% to 0.14%?
- there was 1 chance in 850 that it would prevent you from having a stroke?
- 849 out of 850 patients derived no benefit from the treatment?
- there was a 99.7% chance that you would not have a stroke anyway?

All these statements are derived from the same data* and describe an equivalent effect.

*MRC trial of treatment of mild hypertension (bendroflumethiazide vs placebo). BMJ 1985; 291:97–104.

Relative risk describes the proportional increase in risk, while absolute risk describes the actual chance of an event, which is what matters to most patients. Whenever possible, clinicians should quote numerical information using consistent denominators (e.g. '90 of every 100 patients who have this operation feel much better, 1 will die at operation and 2 will suffer a stroke').

Uncertainty often remains where evidence is incomplete. Here, doctors should use their best judgement and discuss risk and management options openly with patients, guarding against bias.

CLINICAL ETHICS

The four key principles of clinical ethics are often abbreviated to:
• Autonomy. • Beneficence. • Non-maleficence. • Justice.

Respect for persons and their autonomy

Patients seek a physician in order to prevent disability or disease from limiting their autonomy (the power or right of self-determination). The physician must therefore respect the individual's autonomy, including the right to refuse therapy, while empowering the patient with information.

Truth-telling

Telling the truth is essential for doctor–patient trust. This includes providing information about the illness, prognosis and therapeutic alternatives, and answering questions honestly and with sensitivity to the patient's capacity to cope with bad news. There are two rare situations where the truth may sometimes be withheld:
• If it will cause real harm to patients (e.g. depressed patients likely to commit suicide if told they have cancer). • If patients make it clear that they do not want to hear the bad news (bearing in mind that this may be a stage in the patient's adjustment to the condition).

Informed consent

To facilitate an informed decision, the clinician must provide an adequate explanation, with details of the relevant risks, benefits and uncertainties of each option. The amount of information will depend on the patient's condition, the complexity of the proposed treatment, and the physician's assessment of the patient's understanding. Legally and ethically, the patient retains the right to decide what is in his or her best interests. If patients make choices that seem irrational or at variance with professional advice, that does not mean they lack capacity. In this context, capacity means the patient is able (with help) to understand the key information, consider the relevant options and communicate a decision.

When the patient does lack capacity, the clinician must always act in the patient's best interests. In an emergency, consent may be presumed for treatment that is immediately necessary to preserve life and health, provided there is no clear evidence that this would be against the patient's previous wishes when competent (e.g. blood transfusion in an adult Jehovah's Witness). If the patient has a legally entitled surrogate decision-maker, that person's consent should be sought wherever possible. It is good practice to involve close relatives in decision-making, depending on local laws and culture.

Confidentiality

Confidentiality concerning patient-specific information is important in maintaining trust between patients and doctors. Health-care teams must prevent unauthorised access to patient records, and may disclose information only when the patient has given consent or when required by law. Where such information is shared, it should be done on a strictly 'need-to-know' basis.

Beneficence

This is the principle of doing good, or acting in another person's best interests. It means considering patients' views of their own best interests, as well as their medical best interests. If there is a conflict between what is good for the individual and what is best for society, the traditional approach is that 'The health of my patient will be my first consideration.'

Non-maleficence

This is the principle of doing no harm: *primum non nocere*.

Justice

In order to distribute health resources justly, the concept of utility – 'the greatest good for the greatest number' – must be considered. In the case of individual patients, however, justice is also equated with being 'fair' and 'even-handed'. Three perspectives apply:

Respect for the needs of the individual: Health care is given first to those who need it most.

Respect for the rights of a person: Everyone who needs health care is entitled to a fair share of the available resources.

Respect for merit: Health care is delivered on the basis of financial, political or social value judgements relating to the value of the individual to society. In the health-care setting these value judgements are difficult to make and to defend ethically.

PERSONAL AND PROFESSIONAL DEVELOPMENT

Good doctors never stop learning. In the UK, the Royal Colleges monitor and regulate the learning activity of registered doctors as part of their continuous professional development (CPD), reviewed at annual appraisal. For trainees, satisfactory performance is judged against defined competencies based on the relevant undergraduate and postgraduate curricula.

COMPLEMENTARY AND ALTERNATIVE MEDICINE

Complementary and alternative medicine (CAM) refers to medical and health-care practices and products that are outside conventional medicine. It ranges from well-established physical therapies such as osteopathy to spiritual measures such as prayer specifically for health. Several complementary therapies (e.g. aromatherapy and massage) are inherently pleasurable, contributing to their therapeutic benefit. Proponents maintain that CAM focuses on the whole person as well as the physical complaints.

'Complementary medicine': Describes the use of these treatments in conjunction with conventional medicine (e.g. acupuncture to reduce post-operative pain).

'Alternative medicine': Describes their use in place of conventional medicine (e.g. reflexology instead of anti-inflammatory drugs for arthritis).

'Integrative medicine': Describes the use of conventional therapy together with complementary therapies for which there is evidence of efficacy and safety.

Evidence

Since the widespread acceptance of evidence-based medicine, advocates of CAM are increasingly challenged to justify these treatments through independent, well-conducted, randomised controlled clinical trials. In some cases this may be difficult (e.g. the placebo arm of a double-blind trial of acupuncture). The literature in this area is growing rapidly but, at present, only a small minority of CAM therapies, in a small subset of conditions, are supported by evidence of an acceptable standard for conventional medicine.

Regulation

Many CAM therapies have professional regulatory frameworks in place; some others are following suit. Nevertheless, for many CAM therapies, there is no established structure of training, certification and accreditation, and practice is effectively open to all. Set against the demanding training and lifelong CPD required in conventional medicine, this constitutes an important barrier to integrative medicine.

Ageing and disease

2

In the developed world, improvements in life expectancy have increased the proportion of older people in the population. For example, the UK population has grown by 11% in the past 30 yrs, but the number of those >65 yrs has risen by 24%. Although the proportion of the population aged >65 is greater in developed countries, most older people live in the developing world. Two-thirds of the world population aged >65 live in developing countries at present, and this is projected to rise to 75% in 2025.

Geriatric medicine is concerned mainly with frail older people, in whom reductions in physiological capacity increase susceptibility to disease and mortality. These patients frequently suffer from multiple comorbidities, and illness often presents in atypical ways with confusion, falls or loss of mobility and day-to-day functioning. Frail older people are also prone to adverse drug reactions, partly because of polypharmacy and partly because of age-related changes in responses to drugs and their elimination. Disability is common in old age but patients' function can often be improved by the interventions of the multidisciplinary team (Box 2.1), which includes nurses as well as physiotherapists, occupational therapists and speech therapists, and medical staff.

INVESTIGATION IN THE ELDERLY

Frailty makes investigation more taxing for patients, and a judgement must be made, often together with the family, about how much investigation is safe and appropriate in each case, taking care not to mistake disability caused by reversible disease for irreversible decline.

PRESENTING PROBLEMS IN GERIATRIC MEDICINE

Although the common presenting problems are described individually here, in reality older patients often present with several at the

COMPREHENSIVE GERIATRIC ASSESSMENT

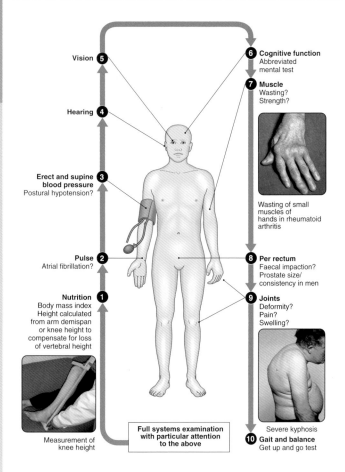

5 Vision

6 Cognitive function
Abbreviated mental test

7 Muscle
Wasting?
Strength?

4 Hearing

3 Erect and supine blood pressure
Postural hypotension?

Wasting of small muscles of hands in rheumatoid arthritis

2 Pulse
Atrial fibrillation?

8 Per rectum
Faecal impaction?
Prostate size/ consistency in men

1 Nutrition
Body mass index
Height calculated from arm demispan or knee height to compensate for loss of vertebral height

9 Joints
Deformity?
Pain?
Swelling?

Measurement of knee height

Full systems examination with particular attention to the above

Severe kyphosis

10 Gait and balance
Get up and go test

2.1 Multidisciplinary team (MDT) and functional assessment	
Team member	**Activity assessed and promoted**
Physiotherapist	Mobility, balance and upper limb function
Occupational therapist	Activities of daily living, e.g. dressing, cooking
	Assessment of home environment and care needs
Dietitian	Nutrition
Speech and language therapist	Communication and swallowing
Social worker	Care needs and discharge planning
Nurse	Motivation, initiation of activities, feeding, continence, skin care, communication with family and team
Doctor	Diagnosis and management of illness, team coordinator

2.2 Investigations to identify acute illness

- FBC
- U&Es, LFTs, calcium and glucose
- CXR
- ECG
- CRP: useful marker for occult infection or inflammation
- Blood and urine cultures if pyrexial

same time, particularly confusion, incontinence and falls. These share some underlying causes and may precipitate each other.

The approach to most presenting problems in old age can be summarised as follows:

Obtain a collateral history: Find out the patient's usual status (e.g. mobility, cognitive state) from a relative or carer.

Check medication: Have there been any recent changes?

Search for and treat any acute illness: See Box 2.2.

Identify and reverse predisposing risk factors: These depend on the presenting problem.

Falls

Falls are very common in older people, with 40% of those over 80 falling each year. Although only 10–15% of falls result in serious injury, they cause 90% of hip fractures in this age group. Falls also lead to loss of confidence and fear, and are frequently the 'final straw' that makes an older person decide to move to institutional care. The approach to the patient varies according to the underlying cause of falls, as follows.

Acute illness

Falling is one of the classical atypical presentations of acute illness in the frail. The reduced reserves in older people's integrative

> ### 2.3 Risk factors for falls
>
> - Muscle weakness
> - History of falls
> - Gait or balance abnormality
> - Use of a walking aid
> - Visual impairment
> - Arthritis
> - Impaired activities of daily living
> - Depression
> - Cognitive impairment
> - Age >80 yrs
> - Psychotropic medication

neurological function mean that they are less able to maintain their balance when challenged by an acute illness. Suspicion should be high when falls have occurred suddenly over a few days. Common underlying illnesses include infection, stroke, metabolic disturbance and heart failure. Thorough examination and investigation are required to identify these (see Box 2.2). Recently started psychotropic or hypotensive drugs may also cause falls. Once an underlying acute illness has been treated, falls may no longer be a problem.

Blackouts

A proportion of older people who 'fall' have, in fact, had a syncopal episode. It is important to ask about loss of consciousness and, if this is a possibility, to perform appropriate investigations (pp. 265 and 607).

Mechanical and recurrent falls

Those who have simply tripped once may not require detailed assessment but recurrent or unexplained falls should be investigated. Many such patients are frail with multiple medical problems and chronic disabilities. Their tendency to fall is associated with risk factors that have been well established from prospective studies (Box 2.3). The annual risk of falling increases linearly with the number of risk factors present. Although such patients may present with a fall resulting from an acute illness or syncope, as above, they will remain at risk of further falls even when the acute illness has resolved.

It has been shown that an effective way of preventing further falls in this group is multiple risk factor intervention. Examples of such interventions are shown in Box 2.4 and require a multidisciplinary approach. The most effective is balance and exercise training by physiotherapists. Rationalising medication may help to reduce sedation, although many older patients are reluctant to stop their hypnotic. It will also help reduce postural hypotension, defined as a drop in BP of >20 mmHg systolic or >10 mmHg diastolic pressure

2.4 Multifactorial interventions to prevent falls

- Balance and exercise training
- Rationalisation of medication, especially psychotropic drugs
- Correction of visual impairment (e.g. cataracts)
- Home environmental hazard assessment and safety education
- Calcium and vitamin D supplementation in institutional care

on standing from supine. Observation of gait may reveal other treatable underlying disease (e.g. Parkinson's disease) contributing to falls.

DEXA scanning to detect osteoporosis should be considered in all older patients who have recurrent falls, particularly if they have already sustained a fracture. Treatment is described on page 600.

Dizziness

Dizziness is very common, affecting at least 30% of those aged >65 yrs, according to community surveys. Acute dizziness is relatively straightforward and common causes include:

• Hypotension due to arrhythmia, acute myocardial infarction, gastrointestinal bleed or pulmonary embolism, etc. • Acute posterior fossa stroke. • Vestibular neuronitis.

Older people, however, more commonly present with recurrent dizzy spells. They often find it difficult to describe the sensation they experience, so assessment can be very frustrating. Nevertheless, the most effective way of establishing the cause(s) of the problem is to determine which of the following is the predominant symptom, even if more than one is present:

- Lightheadedness, suggestive of reduced cerebral perfusion.
- Vertigo, suggestive of labyrinthine or brainstem disease.
- Unsteadiness/poor balance, suggestive of joint or neurological disease.

In lightheaded patients, aortic stenosis, postural hypotension and arrhythmias should be considered and excluded. Vertigo is most often due to benign positional vertigo (p. 647) but with other neurological signs merits further brain imaging (e.g. MRI).

Delirium

Delirium is a transient reversible cognitive dysfunction. It affects up to 30% of older inpatients and is associated with increased mortality and longer hospital stays.

Clinical assessment should begin with routine cognitive testing, e.g. the Abbreviated Mental Test 10 (Box 2.5) or Mini-Mental State Examination (MMSE). In addition, a broader assessment of confusion, including conscious level, disorganised speech or thinking, and collateral history of the time course of confusion from an accompanying person, should be used to diagnose delirium and to differentiate it from dementia (though these may coexist).

2.5 Abbreviated Mental Test 10

Each correct answer scores 1 mark:
1. What age are you? (exact year)
2. What time is it? (to the nearest hour)
3. Please memorise the following address: 42 West Street – ask patient to repeat at end
4. What year is it?
5. What is the name of this place/hospital?
6. Can patient recognise two people? (e.g. relative in photograph, doctor, nurse)
7. What is your date of birth?
8. When did the First World War begin?
9. Who is the present monarch?
10. Please count backwards from 20 down to 1

The Mini-Mental State Examination (MMSE) is used for more detailed assessment.

The presentation, diagnosis and management of acute confusion are described on page 611. Almost any acute illness in the elderly may present with confusion, but the most common causes are infection, stroke or the recent addition of a drug. Predisposing factors in older people include visual or hearing impairment, underlying dementia, alcohol misuse and poor nutrition.

In addition to the investigations shown in Box 2.2, CT is indicated if there is a history of injury or focal neurological signs, and in those who fail to improve despite appropriate treatment of the underlying cause. If confusion puts patients or others at risk, sedation with low-dose haloperidol or a benzodiazepine may be required as a last resort.

Urinary incontinence

Urinary incontinence is defined as the involuntary loss of urine, sufficiently severe to cause a social or hygiene problem. It occurs in all age groups but becomes more prevalent in old age. While age-dependent changes in the lower urinary tract predispose older people to incontinence, it is not an inevitable consequence of ageing and always requires investigation. Urinary incontinence is frequently precipitated by acute illness in old age and is commonly multifactorial (Box 2.6; see also p. 161).

Adverse drug reactions

These cause up to 20% of admissions in people >65. Polypharmacy, defined as the use of four or more drugs, is common in old age. Older people receive many more prescribed drugs than younger people and this is increasing in the UK. Even when appropriate – many cardiovascular conditions such as hypertension, myocardial infarction and heart failure dictate the use of several drugs – multiple drugs put older patients at increased risk of adverse drug

2.6 Causes of transient incontinence

- Restricted mobility
- Acute confusional state
- Urinary tract infection
- Severe constipation
- Drugs, e.g. diuretics, sedatives
- Hyperglycaemia
- Hypercalcaemia

reactions and interactions, falls and acute confusion. Age-related changes in how drugs are absorbed and excreted can compound these problems. The clinical presentations of polypharmacy are extremely diverse, so for any presenting problem in old age, the possibility that the patient's medication is a contributory factor should always be considered.

Hypothermia

Hypothermia occurs when the body's core temperature falls below 35°C. The very young are susceptible because they have poor thermoregulation and a high body surface area-to-weight ratio, but the elderly are at highest risk.

Clinical assessment

Diagnosis is dependent on recognition of the environmental circumstances and measurement of core (rectal) body temperature. Measurement of tympanic membrane, cutaneous or oral temperatures can be misleading. Clinical features depend on the degree of hypothermia:

Mild hypothermia: Shivering, confusion, dehydration, ataxia.

Severe hypothermia: Depressed conscious level, muscle stiffness, failed vasoconstriction/shivering, bradycardia, hypotension, ECG J waves, dysrhythmias.

Below 28°C: Coma, absent pupillary reflexes, dead appearance, absent corneal reflex (<23°C), cardiac standstill.

It is very difficult to diagnose death reliably by clinical means in a cold patient. Resuscitative measures should continue until the core temperature is normal and only then should a diagnosis of brain death be considered.

Investigations

Haemoconcentration and metabolic acidosis are common. J waves, which occur at the junction of the QRS complex and the ST segment, may be seen on the ECG (Fig. 2.1). Cardiac dysrhythmias, including ventricular fibrillation, may occur. Serum aspartate aminotransferase and CK may be elevated secondary to muscle damage; serum

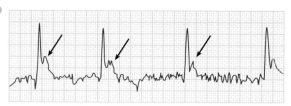

Fig. 2.1 ECG showing J waves (arrows) in a hypothermic patient.

amylase is often high due to subclinical pancreatitis. If the cause of hypothermia is not obvious, additional tests should identify thyroid and pituitary dysfunction, hypoglycaemia and the possibility of drug intoxication.

Management

Mild hypothermia (32–35°C): Patients should be maintained in a warm room, with additional thermal insulation (blankets and/or space film blanket) and heat packs placed in the abdomen and groin. They should be given warm fluids to drink and an adequate calorie intake. Rewarming at 1–2°C/hr is ideal, and underlying conditions should be treated.

Severe hypothermia (< 32°C): This is associated with metabolic disturbance and cardiac dysrhythmias. In the presence of cardio-pulmonary arrest, rapid rewarming (>2°C/hr) is needed to restore perfusion, and is best achieved by cardiopulmonary bypass or extra-corporeal membrane oxygenation. Pleural, peritoneal or bladder lavage with warmed fluids is an alternative if the former methods are not available. In addition to supplementary oxygen, warm IV fluids should be given and acidosis corrected. Monitoring of cardiac rhythm and ABGs is essential.

REHABILITATION

Acute illness in older people is often associated with loss of mobility and self-care skills. Rehabilitation aims to improve the ability of people of all ages to perform day-to-day activities and to restore their physical, mental and social capabilities as far as possible.

The process

Rehabilitation is a problem-solving process focused on improving a patient's physical, psychological and social function. It entails:

Assessment: The nature and extent of the patient's problems are identified from a comprehensive assessment using the framework in Box 2.7.

Goal-setting: Goals are specific to the patient's problems, realistic and agreed between the patient and the rehabilitation team.

2.7 International Classification of Functioning and Disability

Factor	Intervention required
Health condition	
The underlying disease, e.g. stroke, osteoarthritis	Medical or surgical treatment
Impairment	
The symptoms or signs of the condition, e.g. hemiparesis, visual loss	Medical or surgical treatment
Activity limitation	
The resultant loss of function, e.g. walking, dressing	Rehabilitation, assistance, aids
Participation restriction	
The resultant loss of social function, e.g. cooking, shopping	Adapted accommodation Social services

Intervention: This includes active treatments, individualised to the patient's circumstances, to achieve the set goals and to maintain the patient's health and quality of life.

Reassessment: There is ongoing re-evaluation of the patient's function and progress towards the set goals, with modification of the interventions if necessary. This requires regular review by all members of the rehabilitation team, the patient and the carer.

A critically ill patient is at imminent risk of death. The principle underpinning intensive care is the simultaneous assessment of illness severity and stabilisation of life-threatening physiological abnormalities. The goal is to prevent deterioration and improve the patient's condition as the diagnosis is established. Over-emphasis on either resuscitation or diagnosis, to the exclusion of the other, results in worse outcomes. Physiological monitoring is central to assessment and monitoring of progress in critical care medicine.

RECOGNISING THE CRITICALLY ILL PATIENT

Standardised Early Warning System (SEWS) charts (Fig. 3.1; Box 3.1) are used increasingly to detect deterioration in patients' condition. They provide a useful means of alerting staff who can escalate management appropriately.

MONITORING

Monitoring in intensive care requires a combination of clinical and automated recordings. ECG is continuously monitored and oxygen saturation, BP and usually central venous pressure (CVP) are measured hourly. Clinical monitoring of physical signs such as respiratory rate and conscious level is equally important.

Monitoring the circulation

ECG monitoring records changes in heart rate and rhythm. Arterial BP is measured continuously using an arterial line placed in the radial artery. CVP is monitored using a catheter placed in the right internal jugular vein or the subclavian vein with the distal end sited in the upper right atrium. If the CVP is low in the presence of a low BP, fluid resuscitation is necessary. However, a raised CVP does not necessarily mean that the patient is adequately volume-resuscitated, as pulmonary hypertension or right ventricular dysfunction can also

CLINICAL EXAMINATION OF THE CRITICALLY ILL PATIENT

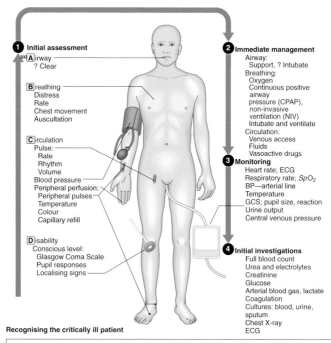

1 Initial assessment

Airway
  ? Clear

Breathing
  Distress
  Rate
  Chest movement
  Auscultation

Circulation
  Pulse:
    Rate
    Rhythm
    Volume
  Blood pressure
  Peripheral perfusion:
    Peripheral pulses
    Temperature
    Colour
    Capillary refill

Disability
  Conscious level:
    Glasgow Coma Scale
    Pupil responses
    Localising signs

2 Immediate management
  Airway:
    Support, ? Intubate
  Breathing:
    Oxygen
    Continuous positive
    airway
    pressure (CPAP),
    non-invasive
    ventilation (NIV)
    Intubate and ventilate
  Circulation:
    Venous access
    Fluids
    Vasoactive drugs

3 Monitoring
  Heart rate; ECG
  Respiratory rate; SpO_2
  BP—arterial line
  Temperature
  GCS; pupil size, reaction
  Urine output
  Central venous pressure

4 Initial investigations
  Full blood count
  Urea and electrolytes
  Creatinine
  Glucose
  Arterial blood gas, lactate
  Coagulation
  Cultures: blood, urine,
  sputum
  Chest X-ray
  ECG

Recognising the critically ill patient

Cardiovascular signs
- Cardiac arrest
- Pulse rate < 40 or > 140 bpm
- Systolic blood pressure (BP) < 100 mmHg
- Tissue hypoxia:
    Poor peripheral perfusion
    Metabolic acidosis
    Hyperlactataemia
- Poor response to volume resuscitation
- Oliguria: < 0.5 mL/kg/hr (check urea, creatinine, K^+)

Respiratory signs
- Threatened or obstructed airway
- Stridor, intercostal recession
- Respiratory arrest
- Respiratory rate < 8 or > 35/min
- Respiratory 'distress': use of accessory muscles; unable to speak in complete sentences
- SpO_2 < 90% on high-flow O_2
- Rising $PaCO_2$ > 8 kPa (> 60 mmHg), or > 2 kPa (> 15 mmHg) above 'normal' with acidosis

Neurological signs
- Threatened or obstructed airway
- Absent gag or cough reflex
- Failure to maintain normal PaO_2 and $PaCO_2$
- Failure to obey commands
- Glasgow Coma Scale (GCS) < 10
- Sudden fall in level of consciousness (GCS fall > 2 points)
- Repeated or prolonged seizures

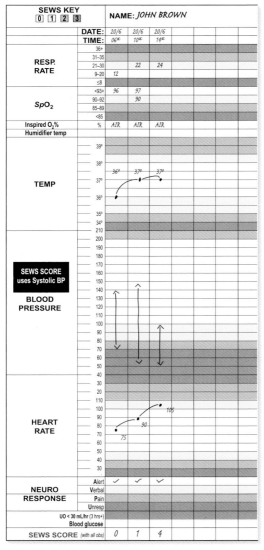

Fig. 3-1 Standard Early Warning System (SEWS) scoring sheet.

3.1 Recognition of critical illness: Standardised Early Warning System (SEWS)

- Record standard observations on the SEWS chart: respiratory rate, SpO_2, temperature, BP, heart rate, neurological response
- Note whether the observation falls in the shaded 'at-risk zone' and the corresponding points
- Add points for key observations and record the total on the SEWS chart
- If SEWS score ≥4, a doctor should assess the patient within 20 mins
- If SEWS score ≥6, a senior doctor should assess the patient within 10 mins

lead to a raised CVP. In pulmonary hypertension or right ventricular dysfunction, it may be appropriate to insert a pulmonary artery flotation catheter so that pulmonary artery pressure and pulmonary artery 'wedge' pressure (PAWP), which approximates to left atrial pressure, can be measured and used to guide fluid resuscitation. Cardiac output can be assessed with the thermodilution technique using a pulmonary artery catheter. Less invasive alternative methods include oesophageal Doppler USS. Bedside echocardiography is used increasingly to assess ventricular function. Urine output is a sensitive measure of renal perfusion, provided that the kidneys are not damaged (e.g. acute tubular necrosis) or affected by drugs (e.g. diuretics, dopamine), and can be monitored accurately if a urinary catheter is in place. A metabolic acidosis with base deficit >5 mmol/L often indicates increased lactic acid production in poorly perfused, hypoxic tissues. Serial lactate measurements may help in monitoring response to treatment.

Monitoring respiratory function

Oxygen saturation (SpO_2) is measured continuously. ABGs are measured several times a day in a ventilated patient so that inspired oxygen and minute volume can be adjusted to achieve the desired PaO_2 and $PaCO_2$. End-tidal CO_2 mirrors $PaCO_2$ in patients with healthy lungs, but is frequently lower than $PaCO_2$ in lung disease. Transcutaneous CO_2 can be measured continuously and approximates to $PaCO_2$.

GENERAL PRINCIPLES OF CRITICAL CARE MANAGEMENT

Assessment and initial resuscitation

Airway and breathing: If the patient is talking, the airway is clear. Check for abnormal breath sounds and tachypnoea, and use oximetry and blood gases to judge the need for supplemental oxygen.

Circulation: Feel a carotid pulse, then check peripheral pulses. Establish venous access and apply a cuff for BP monitoring.

Disability: Record conscious level using the Glasgow Coma Scale (GCS; Box 16.3).

Daily clinical management in the ICU

Key elements are:

Regular clinical examination.

Management of complications: Evidence-based measures should be rigorously applied to reduce complications. The mnemonic FAST HUG may be used, indicating the need to review:

• Feeding. • Analgesia. • Sedation. • Thromboprophylaxis. • Head-of-bed elevation. • Ulcer prophylaxis. • Glucose control.

Sedation and analgesia: ICU is very stressful for patients and adequate sedation is essential, but excessive sedation can cause delirium. Continuous infusions are usually used for sedatives and for analgesics like morphine, but care must be taken to avoid accumulation of drug or its metabolites and toxicity if renal or hepatic function is deranged.

Muscle relaxants: These promote critical illness neuropathy and myopathy and should be avoided, apart from specific indications, e.g. during intubation.

Delirium: This is a common problem. Management should include removal of reversible causes (p. 613), then treatment, if required, with haloperidol in 2.5 mg increments.

SPECIFIC PRESENTING PROBLEMS IN THE ICU

Circulatory failure: 'shock'

'Shock' exists when oxygen delivery fails to meet the metabolic requirements of the tissues. Shock is not synonymous with hypotension, although hypotension may be a late manifestation of circulatory failure. Clinical features of shock are shown in Box 3.2. The causes of shock may be classified into low stroke volume or vasodilatation.

Low stroke volume

Hypovolaemic: Any major reduction in blood volume, e.g. haemorrhage, severe burns, dehydration.

3.2 Clinical features of shock	
Rapid, shallow respiration Tachycardia (> 100/min) Hypotension (systolic BP < 100 mmHg) Drowsiness, confusion, irritability Oliguria (urine output < 0.5 mL/hr/kg) Multi-organ failure	
Vasodilated shock	**Hypovolaemic shock**
Warm peripheries Low diastolic BP	Cold, clammy skin

3.3 Systemic inflammatory response syndrome (SIRS)

Encompasses inflammatory response to both infective and non-infective causes such as pancreatitis, trauma, cardiopulmonary bypass, vasculitis, etc.

Defined by presence of two or more of:

Respiratory rate >20/min	$PaCO_2$ <4.3 kPa (<32 mmHg) or ventilated
Heart rate >90/min	Temperature >38.0°C or <36.0°C
WCC >12 × 10^9/L or <4 × 10^9/L	

Cardiogenic: Severe heart failure, e.g. myocardial infarction, acute mitral regurgitation.

Obstructive: Obstruction to blood flow around the circulation, e.g. major pulmonary embolism, cardiac tamponade, tension pneumothorax.

Vasodilatation

Sepsis: Infection or other causes of a systemic inflammatory response syndrome (SIRS, Box 3.3) that produce widespread endothelial damage with vasodilatation, arteriovenous shunting, microvascular occlusion and tissue oedema, resulting in organ failure.

Anaphylactic: Inappropriate vasodilatation triggered by an allergen (e.g. bee sting).

Neurogenic: Caused by major brain or spinal injury producing disruption of brainstem and neurogenic vasomotor control; may be associated with neurogenic pulmonary oedema.

Management

The primary goals of circulatory support are to:

• Restore global oxygen delivery by ensuring an adequate cardiac output. • Maintain a BP that ensures adequate perfusion of vital organs. • Avoid levels of left atrial pressure that produce pulmonary oedema.

The initial management of circulatory collapse is shown in Box 3.4. If cardiac output is poor despite an adequate preload, the therapeutic options are to provide inotropic support or reduce the afterload with vasoactive drugs (Box 3.5), or to control the heart rate and rhythm if this is abnormal.

Respiratory failure, including ARDS

Respiratory failure is classified by ABGs as either:

• Type 1 (hypoxia without hypercapnia, resulting from perfused but under-ventilated lung units). • Type 2 (hypoxia with hypercapnia, resulting from gross ventilation/perfusion mismatch or overall alveolar hypoventilation).

The mechanisms and underlying causes are covered elsewhere (p. 274). Hypoxaemia should always be assessed with reference to the inspired oxygen fraction; the lower the ratio of PaO_2 to inspired oxygen (FiO_2), the more severe the disease.

3.4 Initial management of circulatory collapse

Correct hypoxaemia: oxygen therapy
Consider ventilation:

Intractable hypoxaemia	Respiratory distress
Hypercapnia: $PaCO_2$ >6.7 kPa (50 mmHg)	Impaired conscious level

Assess circulation:

Heart rate	CVP
BP: direct arterial pressure	Peripheral perfusion

Optimise volume status: fluid challenge(s):
CVP <6 mmHg: 250 mL 0.9% saline or colloid
CVP >6 mmHg or poor ventricular function suspected: 100 mL boluses
Consider pulmonary artery catheter or oesophageal Doppler
Optimise Hb concentration: 70–90 g/L; 100 g/L if ischaemic heart disease. Red cells as required
Achieve target BP: use vasopressor/inotrope once hypovolaemia corrected
Achieve adequate CO and DO_2: inotropic agent if fluid alone inadequate
Monitor trend in haemodynamics, ABGs, H^+, base deficit, lactate

3.5 Actions of commonly used vasoactive drugs

Drug	Vasoconstrictor	Inotrope	Chronotrope
Adrenaline (epinephrine)	++	++	+
Noradrenaline (norepinephrine)	++++	+	(+)
Dobutamine	*	++++	++

*In most patients dobutamine acts as a vasodilator but in some it causes vasoconstriction.

Acute respiratory distress syndrome

Acute respiratory distress syndrome (ARDS) describes the acute, diffuse pulmonary inflammatory response to either direct (via airway or chest trauma) or indirect blood-borne insults from extrapulmonary pathology. It is characterised by:

• Neutrophil sequestration in pulmonary capillaries. • Increased capillary permeability. • Protein-rich pulmonary oedema.

If this early phase does not resolve with treatment of the underlying cause, a fibroproliferative phase ensues and causes pulmonary fibrosis. It is frequently associated with other organ dysfunction as part of multiple organ failure.

The term ARDS is often limited to patients requiring ventilatory support on the ICU, but less severe forms, conventionally referred to as acute lung injury (ALI) and having similar pathology, occur on acute medical and surgical wards. The clinical picture is non-specific and shares features with other conditions (diffuse bilateral shadowing on CXR in the absence of raised left atrial pressure, hypoxaemia, impaired lung compliance).

Management

Respiratory support is indicated to maintain the patency of the airway, correct hypoxaemia and hypercapnia, and reduce the work of breathing.

Oxygen therapy: Ensure adequate arterial oxygenation (SpO_2 >90%). If a patient remains hypoxaemic on high-flow oxygen, other measures are required.

Non-invasive respiratory support: If the patient has respiratory failure associated with decreased lung volume, application of continuous positive airway pressure (CPAP) will improve oxygenation by recruitment of under-ventilated alveoli and reduce the work of breathing. CPAP is most successful when alveoli are readily recruited (e.g. pulmonary oedema, post-operative atelectasis). Patients should be cooperative, be able to protect their airway and have the strength to breathe spontaneously and cough effectively. In non-invasive positive pressure ventilation (NIV), the patient's spontaneous breathing is supported by increased inspiratory and expiratory pressures delivered using a bi-level ventilator (BiPAP). For NIV to succeed, the patient's spontaneous breathing must be sufficient to trigger the machine and they must be able to tolerate a tight-fitting facemask. NIV reduces the work of breathing, relieves breathlessness and is proven to reduce the need for endotracheal intubation in patients with type 2 respiratory failure (e.g. exacerbations of COPD; p. 285). It is also used during weaning from conventional ventilation.

Endotracheal intubation and mechanical ventilation: Many patients admitted to ICU require intubation and mechanical ventilation. Indications for intubation are summarised in Box 3.6. The various types of invasive ventilatory support are summarised in Box 3.7.

In the conscious patient, intubation requires induction of anaesthesia and muscle relaxation, while in more obtunded patients sedation alone may be adequate. Hypotension commonly follows sedation or anaesthesia because of direct cardiovascular effects of the drugs and loss of sympathetic drive; positive pressure ventila-

---

3.6 Indications for tracheal intubation and mechanical ventilation

Protection of airway
Respiratory arrest or rate <8/min
Inability to tolerate necessary oxygen therapy (mask/CPAP/NIV)
Removal of secretions
Hypoxaemia (PaO_2 <8 kPa (<60 mmHg); SpO_2 <90%) despite CPAP with FiO_2 >0.6
Worsening hypercapnia or respiratory acidosis
Vital capacity <1.2 L in neuromuscular disease
Removing the work of breathing in exhausted patients

3.7 Modes of invasive ventilatory support

Volume-controlled	
Synchronised intermittent mandatory ventilation (SIMV)	Pre-set rate and V_T of mandatory breaths. Allows spontaneous breaths (may be pressure-supported) between mandatory breaths. Risk of excess pressure (barotrauma)
Pressure-controlled	
Pressure-controlled ventilation (PCV)	Pre-set rate and inspiratory pressure; used in acute respiratory failure to avoid high airway pressure
Bi-level positive airway pressure (BiPAP)	Two levels of positive airway pressure (higher level in inspiration); in fully ventilated patients
Pressure support ventilation (PSV)	Provides positive pressure to augment patient's spontaneous breaths; useful for weaning
Positive end-expiratory pressure (PEEP)	Applied during expiration; improves oxygenation by recruiting atelectatic or oedematous lung; may reduce cardiac output
Advanced modes	
High-frequency oscillatory ventilation (HFOV)	High-frequency oscillating gas flow used to facilitate gas exchange. Titrated against blood gases
Extracorporeal membrane oxygenation (ECMO)	Oxygenation and CO_2 clearance achieved using an external vascular bypass with oxygenator. Used in severe ARDS

tion may compound this problem by increasing intrathoracic pressure, which reduces venous return.

The selection of ventilator mode and settings for tidal volume, respiratory rate, positive end-expiratory pressure (PEEP) and inspiratory to expiratory ratio is dependent on the cause of the respiratory failure.

Weaning from respiratory support: The majority of patients require mechanical ventilatory support for only a few days and do not need a process of weaning. In contrast, patients who have required long-term ventilatory support for severe lung disease, e.g. ARDS, may initially be unable to sustain even a modest degree of respiratory work due to reduced lung compliance and muscle weakness; hence they require a programme of gradual weaning from ventilation.

Tracheostomy: This is usually performed electively when endotracheal intubation is likely to be prolonged (>14 days). Tracheostomies help patient comfort, aid weaning from ventilation, and allow access for tracheal toilet and intermittent respiratory support.

Anaphylaxis

Anaphylaxis is a life-threatening, systemic allergic reaction caused by IgE-mediated release of histamine and other vasoactive mediators. Clinical features are wheeze, stridor, angioedema, urticaria and a feeling of impending doom. Potential allergen triggers should be ascertained. The most common are:

• Foods (peanut, shellfish, eggs). • Latex. • Insect venom (bee and wasp). • Drugs (penicillin, anaesthetic agents).

The route of allergen exposure influences the features of the reaction; e.g. an inhaled allergen leads to wheezing. Anaphylactoid reactions result from non-IgE-mediated degranulation of mast cells by drugs (opiates, aspirin), chemicals (radiocontrast media) or other triggers (exercise, cold). The clinical presentations are indistinguishable, and in the acute situation discriminating between them is unnecessary.

Investigations

Measurement of acute and convalescent serum mast cell tryptase concentrations may be useful to confirm the diagnosis. Specific IgE tests may be preferable to skin prick tests when investigating patients with a history of anaphylaxis.

Management

Anaphylaxis is an acute medical emergency. The immediate management includes:

• Prevention of further allergen exposure (e.g. removal of bee sting). • Ensuring airway patency. • Prompt administration of adrenaline (epinephrine; 0.3–0.5 mL 1:1000 IM, repeat if needed). • Antihistamines (e.g. chlorphenamine 10 mg IM). • Corticosteroids (e.g. hydrocortisone 200 mg IV) to prevent late-phase symptoms. • Oxygen. • Restoration of BP (lay the patient flat, give IV fluids). • Nebulised β_2-agonists for wheeze.

Patients should be referred for specialist assessment. The aims are to:

• Identify the trigger factor. • Educate the patient regarding avoidance and management of subsequent episodes. • Establish whether immunotherapy is indicated.

Patients and their carers should be prescribed and taught to use self-injectable adrenaline (epinephrine) and should wear a Medic-Alert bracelet. If the trigger factor cannot be identified (~30%), recurrence is common.

Acute kidney injury

Acute kidney injury (AKI; p. 167) in the context of critical illness is usually due to pre-renal factors such as uncorrected hypovolaemia, hypotension or ischaemia causing reduced renal oxygen delivery. Acute tubular necrosis (ATN) may result from ischaemia, bacterial or chemical toxins. Nephrotoxic drugs such as NSAIDs or radiological contrast media can cause or exacerbate AKI.

Oliguria is frequently an early sign of systemic problems in critical illness and successful resuscitation is associated with restoration of good urine output, an improving acid–base balance and correction of plasma potassium, urea and creatinine. Obstruction must always be excluded early by abdominal USS; thereafter, treatment involves correcting hypotension, treating sepsis and stopping toxic drugs. If renal function does not respond, venovenous haemofiltration is the usual replacement therapy in ICU.

Gastrointestinal and hepatic disturbance

The intestinal mucosa is vulnerable in shock, and ischaemia and ulceration commonly occur. With loss of the mucosal barrier, toxins can enter the portal circulation.

Hepatic dysfunction in critical illness can take three forms:
• 'Shock liver' with necrosis, hypoglycaemia, deranged LFTs and lactic acidosis. • Hyperbilirubinaemia due to cholestasis. • Transaminitis, commonly due to drug toxicity.

Early institution of enteral nutrition is the most effective strategy for protecting the gut mucosa and providing nutrition. Total parenteral nutrition (TPN) should be started if attempts at enteral feeding have failed. Close glycaemic control (using insulin when needed) and stress ulcer prophylaxis improve outcomes.

Neurological problems in intensive care

Impaired consciousness or coma is often an early feature of severe systemic illness. Prompt assessment and management of airway, breathing and circulation are essential to prevent further brain injury, to allow diagnosis and to permit definitive treatment to be instituted. Impaired conscious level is graded according to the Glasgow Coma Scale, which is also used to monitor progress. A targeted neurological examination is very important in the unconscious patient, noting:
• Pupil size and reaction to light. • Presence or absence of neck stiffness. • Focal neurological signs. • Evidence of other organ impairment.

Management

The aim of management in acute brain injury is to optimise cerebral oxygen delivery by maintaining a normal arterial oxygen content and a cerebral perfusion pressure >60 mmHg. A rise in intracranial pressure (ICP) as a result of haematoma, contusions or ischaemic swelling is damaging both directly to the cerebral cortex and by producing downward pressure on the brain stem, and indirectly by reducing cerebral perfusion pressure. ICP can be reduced by ventilation to lower $PaCO_2$ to 4–4.5 kPa (~30–34 mmHg), by the osmotic diuretic mannitol and by craniotomy. Head-up tilt and control of epileptic seizures are also important.

Neurological monitoring must be combined with frequent clinical assessment. The motor response to pain is a particularly important prognostic sign. No response or extension of the upper limbs is associated with severe injury, and unless there is improvement within a few days, prognosis is very poor. A flexor response is encouraging and indicates that a good outcome is still possible.

Critical illness polyneuropathy is another potential complication in patients with sepsis and multiple organ failure. It can result in areflexia, gross muscle-wasting and failure to wean from the ventilator, thus prolonging the duration of intensive care.

Sepsis

The incidence of sepsis is increasing due to the ageing population, the increased frequency of invasive surgery, higher bacterial resistance and more immunosuppressed patients.

Any or all of the features of SIRS (see Box 3.3) may be present, together with an obvious focus of infection such as purulent sputum from the chest with shadowing on CXR or erythema around an IV line. However, severe sepsis may present as unexplained hypotension, and the speed of onset may simulate major pulmonary embolism or myocardial infarction.

A distinction should be made between community-acquired and hospital-acquired infections, as the likely causative microorganism may be different and this will direct the initial choice of antibiotics. The aim of management is to identify and treat the underlying cause.

Nosocomial infections are an increasing problem on critical care units; cross-infection is a major concern, particularly with regard to MRSA and multidrug-resistant Gram-negative organisms. The most important practice in preventing cross-infection is thorough hand-washing after every patient contact. Limiting the use of antibiotics helps to prevent the emergence of multidrug-resistant bacteria.

Management

Cultures should be taken from blood, urine, sputum, any vascular lines and any wounds. Prompt administration of broad-spectrum antibiotics that cover probable causative organisms (based on the site of infection, previous antibiotic therapy and local resistance patterns) is essential. The early stages of septic shock are often dominated by hypotension with relative volume depletion due to marked arteriolar and particularly venular dilatation. Sufficient IV fluid should be given to ensure that the intravascular volume is not the limiting factor in determining oxygen delivery.

Vasoactive drugs: These are often used in the ICU. The most appropriate vasoactive drug should be chosen based on a full analysis of the circulation and knowledge of the different inotropic, dilating or constricting properties of these drugs (see Box 3.5). In most cases, a vasoconstrictor such as noradrenaline (norepinephrine) is necessary to increase systemic vascular resistance and BP, while an inotrope (dobutamine) may be necessary to maintain cardiac output.

Corticosteroids: Assessment of the pituitary–adrenal axis is difficult in the critically ill but up to 30% of patients may have adrenal insufficiency. Corticosteroid replacement therapy is controversial. Recent evidence suggests that, although it is associated with earlier resolution of shock, it has no effect on survival.

Disseminated intravascular coagulation

Disseminated intravascular coagulation (DIC), also called consumptive coagulopathy, is common in critically ill patients and often heralds the onset of multiple organ failure.

It is characterised by an increase in prothrombin time, partial thromboplastin time and fibrin degradation products, and a fall in platelets and fibrinogen. It causes either widespread bleeding from vascular access points, GI tract, bronchial tree and surgical wound sites, or widespread evidence of thrombosis.

Management is supportive, with infusions of fresh frozen plasma and platelets, while the underlying cause is treated.

DISCHARGE FROM INTENSIVE CARE

Critical care discharge is a complex process and can be stressful for patients. Ideally, they should be discharged to a suitable step-down ward area during daytime working hours, and with full multidisciplinary handover. A period of physical and emotional rehabilitation is needed after critical illness, and this may be prolonged.

WITHDRAWAL OF CARE

Withdrawal of support is appropriate when it is clear that the patient has no realistic prospect of recovery or of surviving with a quality of life that he or she would value. In these situations, intensive care will only prolong the dying process and is therefore futile. Nevertheless, when active support is withdrawn, management should remain positive and be directed towards allowing the patient to die with dignity and as free from distress as possible. Patients' views are paramount and increasing use is being made of advance directives or 'living wills'. Communication with the patient, if possible, and the family is of crucial importance at this time.

OUTCOMES OF INTENSIVE CARE

Although mortality is affected by case mix, typically 20% of patients will die in the ICU and a further 30% die before leaving hospital. Long-term physical and psychological effects are common despite best treatment.

Poisoning

4

Acute poisoning accounts for ~1% of hospital admissions in the UK. In developed countries, intentional self-harm using pre-scribed or 'over-the-counter' medicines is most common, with paracetamol, antidepressants and drugs of misuse being the most frequently used. Poisoning is a major cause of death in young adults, usually before hospital admission. Accidental poisoning is also common in children and the elderly. In developing countries, self-harm with organophosphorus pesticides and herbicides is endemic, and frequently fatal.

GENERAL APPROACH TO THE POISONED PATIENT

Triage
• Assess vital signs immediately. • Identify poison(s) involved and obtain information about it/them. • Identify patients at risk of further self-harm and remove remaining hazards from them.

History
The diagnosis of poisoning is usually apparent from the history, although occasionally patients may conceal information, or exagger-ate or deliberately mislead staff. Try to establish:

• What toxin(s) have been taken and how much? • When and how were they taken? • Have alcohol or other drugs been taken too? • Can any witness corroborate the information? • What drugs have the GP prescribed? • What is the risk of suicide? • Is the patient capable of rational decisions? • Are there any other significant medical conditions?

   In envenomed patients, establish:

• When was the patient exposed to the bite/sting? • What did the causal organism look like? • How did it happen? • Were there mul-tiple bites/stings? • What first aid was given? • What are the patient's

CLINICAL EXAMINATION OF THE POISONED PATIENT

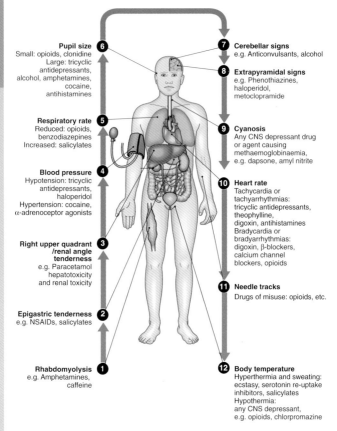

Pupil size ❻
Small: opioids, clonidine
Large: tricyclic
antidepressants,
alcohol, amphetamines,
cocaine,
antihistamines

Respiratory rate ❺
Reduced: opioids,
benzodiazepines
Increased: salicylates

Blood pressure ❹
Hypotension: tricyclic
antidepressants,
haloperidol
Hypertension: cocaine,
α-adrenoceptor agonists

Right upper quadrant
/renal angle ❸
tenderness
e.g. Paracetamol
hepatotoxicity
and renal toxicity

Epigastric tenderness ❷
e.g. NSAIDs, salicylates

Rhabdomyolysis ❶
e.g. Amphetamines,
caffeine

❼ **Cerebellar signs**
e.g. Anticonvulsants, alcohol

❽ **Extrapyramidal signs**
e.g. Phenothiazines,
haloperidol,
metoclopramide

❾ **Cyanosis**
Any CNS depressant drug
or agent causing
methaemoglobinaemia,
e.g. dapsone, amyl nitrite

❿ **Heart rate**
Tachycardia or
tachyarrhythmias:
tricyclic antidepressants,
theophylline,
digoxin, antihistamines
Bradycardia or
bradyarrhythmias:
digoxin, β-blockers,
calcium channel
blockers, opioids

⓫ **Needle tracks**
Drugs of misuse: opioids, etc.

⓬ **Body temperature**
Hyperthermia and sweating:
ecstasy, serotonin re-uptake
inhibitors, salicylates
Hypothermia:
any CNS depressant,
e.g. opioids, chlorpromazine

> **i** 4.1 Risk factors for suicide
>
> - Psychiatric illness (depression, schizophrenia)
> - Male sex
> - Living alone
> - Recent bereavement, divorce or separation
> - Suicide note written
> - Age >45
> - Unemployment
> - Chronic physical ill health
> - Drug or alcohol misuse
> - Previous attempts (violent method)

symptoms? • Do they have other medical conditions, regular treatments, previous similar episodes or known allergies?

Clinical examination (p. 34)

There may be needle marks or evidence of previous self-harm, e.g. razor marks on forearms. Pupil size, respiratory rate and heart rate may help to narrow down the potential list of toxins. The Glasgow Coma Scale (GCS; Box 16.3) is most frequently used to assess the degree of impaired consciousness. The patient's weight helps to determine whether toxicity is likely to occur, given the dose ingested. When patients are unconscious and no history is available, other causes of coma must be excluded (especially meningitis, intracerebral bleeds, hypoglycaemia, diabetic ketoacidosis, uraemia and encephalopathy). Certain classes of drug cause clusters of typical signs, e.g. cholinergic or anticholinergic, sedative or opioid effects, which can aid diagnosis.

Investigations

U&Es and creatinine should be measured in all patients, and ABGs in those with circulatory or respiratory compromise. Drug levels are a useful guide treatment for some specific toxins, e.g. paracetamol, salicylate, iron, digoxin, carboxyhaemoglobin, lithium and theophylline. Urinary drug screens have a limited clinical role.

Psychiatric assessment

All patients who have taken a deliberate drug overdose should undergo psychiatric evaluation by a trained professional before discharge, but ideally after recovering from poisoning. The purpose is to establish the short-term risk of suicide and to identify potentially treatable problems, either medical, psychiatric or social. Risk factors for suicide are shown in Box 4.1.

MANAGEMENT OF THE POISONED PATIENT

Eye or skin contamination should be treated with appropriate washing or irrigation. Patients who have recently ingested

4.2 Antidotes available for the treatment of specific poisonings

Poison	Antidote
Anticoagulants (e.g. warfarin)	Vitamin K, fresh frozen plasma
β-adrenoceptor antagonists (beta-blockers)	IV glucagon, adrenaline (epinephrine)
Calcium channel blockers	Calcium gluconate, calcium chloride, glucagon
Cardiac glycosides, e.g. digoxin	Digoxin-specific antibody fragments (F_{ab})
Cyanide	Oxygen, dicobalt edetate, nitrites, sodium thiosulphate, hydroxocobalamin
Ethylene glycol/methanol	Ethanol, fomepizole
Iron salts	Desferrioxamine
Lead	DMSA, DMPS, disodium calcium edetate
Mercury	DMPS
Opioids	Naloxone
Organophosphorus insecticides, nerve agents	Atropine, oximes (e.g.pralidoxime)
Paracetamol	N-acetylcysteine, methionine

significant overdoses need further measures to prevent absorption or increase elimination:

Activated charcoal (50 g orally) can be given, if a potentially toxic amount of poison has been ingested <1 hr before presentation. Agents that do not bind to activated charcoal include ethylene glycol, iron, lithium, mercury and methanol. Whole-bowel irrigation with polyethylene glycol can be used for toxic ingestions of iron, lithium and theophylline, or to flush out packets of illicit drugs. Urinary alkalinisation using IV sodium bicarbonate enhances elimination of salicylates, methotrexate and the herbicide 2,4-D. Haemodialysis is occasionally used for serious poisoning with salicylates, theophylline, ethylene glycol, methanol or carbamazepine. Infusions of lipid emulsion can be used to reduce tissue concentrations of lipid-soluble drugs such as tricyclic antidepressants.

Specific antidotes are only available for a small number of poisons (Box 4.2). In serious cases, meticulous supportive care, including the treatment of seizures, coma and arrythmias, with ventilatory support where required, is critical to good outcome.

POISONING BY SPECIFIC PHARMACEUTICAL AGENTS

Paracetamol

In overdose, paracetamol causes hepatic damage and occasionally renal failure. The antidote of choice is N-acetylcysteine (NAC) given IV (orally in some countries), which protects against toxicity if given <8 hrs after overdose (Fig. 4.1). A patient presenting >8 hrs after ingestion should have immediate NAC administration, which can later be stopped if the paracetamol level is below the treatment line. If a patient presents >15 hrs after ingestion, LFTs, prothrombin

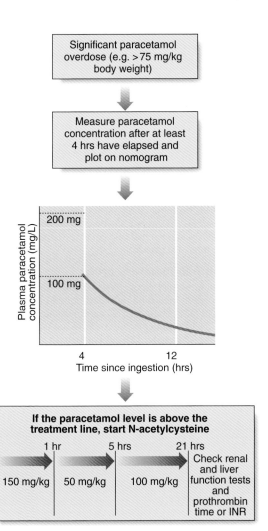

Fig. 4.1 The management of a paracetamol overdose patient.

ratio (or INR) and renal function tests should be performed, the antidote started, and a poisons information centre or liver unit contacted for advice. Liver transplantation should be considered in individuals who develop acute liver failure due to paracetamol. If multiple paracetamol ingestions have taken place over time (a staggered overdose), plasma paracetamol concentration will be uninterpretable. NAC may still be indicated, although treatment thresholds vary between countries.

Salicylates (aspirin)

Symptoms of salicylate overdose include nausea, vomiting, tinnitus and deafness. Direct stimulation of the respiratory centre produces hyperventilation. Signs of serious poisoning include vasodilation with sweating, hyperpyrexia, metabolic acidosis, pulmonary oedema, renal failure, agitation, confusion, coma and fits.

Activated charcoal is useful within 1 hr of ingestion. Plasma salicylate concentration is measured 2 hrs after ingestion in symptomatic patients, then repeated because of continued drug absorption. Concentrations >500 mg/L are serious and those >700 mg/L are life-threatening. Dehydration should be corrected by careful fluid replacement, and metabolic acidosis treated with sufficient IV sodium bicarbonate (8.4%) to normalise $[H^+]$. Urinary alkalinisation is indicated for adult patients with salicylate concentrations >500 mg/L. Haemodialysis should be considered if serum salicylate is >700 mg/L, there is resistant metabolic acidosis, or severe CNS effects (coma, convulsions) are present.

Non-steroidal anti-inflammatory drugs

Non-steroidal anti-inflammatory drug (NSAID) overdose usually causes only minor GI upset, including mild abdominal pain, vomiting and diarrhoea. Activated charcoal and symptomatic treatment is usually sufficient. Rarely, patients have convulsions; these are usually self-limiting and seldom need treatment beyond airway protection and oxygen.

Antidepressants

Tricyclic antidepressants (TCAs) in overdose: Cause anticholinergic, sodium channel-blocking and α-blocking effects. Life-threatening complications include coma, hypotension and arrhythmias, such as ventricular tachycardia/fibrillation or heart block. Activated charcoal is useful within 1 hr of ingestion. ECG monitoring is needed for at least 6 hrs. QRS or QT prolongation indicates risk of arrhythmia and should be treated with IV sodium bicarbonate (8.4%).

Selective serotonin re-uptake inhibitors in overdose: Cause nausea, tremor, insomnia and tachycardia but rarely lead to serious arrhythmia, and supportive treatment is usually sufficient.

Lithium in overdose: Causes nausea, diarrhea, polyuria, weakness, ataxia, coma and convulsions. Charcoal is ineffective and haemodialysis is used in severe cases.

Cardiovascular medications

Beta-blockers: Cause bradycardia and hypotension. Overdose is treated using IV fluids, with atropine or isoprenaline to counteract bradycardia.

Calcium channel blockers: Cause hypotension and heart block in overdose. IV fluids and calcium supplements may be effective; insulin/dextrose infusions or pacing are also used in resistant cases.

Digoxin poisoning: Usually accidental or due to renal failure. ECG monitoring is needed, as bradycardia or ventricular arrhythmias may occur. Digoxin-specific antibody fragments should be administered if serious arrhythmias occur.

Antimalarials

Chloroquine: Toxic in overdose, causing nausea, agitation, convulsions, hypotension and arrhythmias. ECG monitoring and correction of arrhythmias are essential, and diazepam infusions may be protective.

Quinine: Deaths from quinine overdose have been reported after ingestion of only 1.5 g in adults and 900 mg in children. Symptoms include visual loss, nausea, vomiting, tinnitus, deafness, headache and tremor. In large overdoses, ataxia, coma, respiratory depression, haemolysis, hypotension and arrhythmias can occur. Treatment is with activated charcoal and management of fits and arrhythmias.

Antidiabetic agents

Sulphonylureas, meglitinides and parenteral insulins can all cause hypoglycaemia in overdose, although insulin is non-toxic if ingested.

The onset and duration of hypoglycaemia vary, but can last for several days with the longer-acting agents such as isophane and lente insulins. Metformin overdose can cause lactic acidosis, particularly in elderly patients and those with renal or hepatic impairment, or if co-ingested with ethanol, when there is a significant mortality rate. Hypoglycaemia should be corrected urgently with 50 mL IV 50% dextrose, or with a sugary drink if the patient is conscious. This should be followed by an infusion of 10% or 20% dextrose titrated to the patient's blood glucose to prevent further hypoglycaemia. Blood glucose and U&Es should be checked regularly.

DRUGS OF MISUSE

Cannabis

Cannabis (grass, pot, ganja, spliff, reefer) is commonly smoked with tobacco or eaten.

In low doses, cannabis produces euphoria, perceptual alterations and conjunctival injection, followed by relaxation and drowsiness, hypertension, tachycardia, slurred speech and ataxia. High doses can produce hallucinations and psychosis. Ingestion or smoking rarely results in serious poisoning, and supportive treatment is normally sufficient.

Benzodiazepines

Taken alone, benzodiazepine overdoses are remarkably safe but benzodiazepines can enhance CNS depression when taken with other drugs, including alcohol.

Common symptoms are drowsiness, ataxia, dysarthria, nystagmus and confusion. Respiratory depression and hypotension may occur with severe poisoning, especially after IV use of short-acting agents. Activated charcoal is useful within 1 hr of ingestion. Conscious level, respiratory rate and O_2 saturation should be observed for ≥6 hrs after a substantial overdose. Flumazenil is a specific benzodiazepine antagonist that increases conscious level, but it carries the risk of convulsions and is contraindicated in those who have co-ingested TCAs, or have a history of seizures.

Cocaine

Cocaine is available as water-soluble hydrochloride crystals for nasal inhalation or as insoluble free base ('crack' cocaine) that vaporises at high temperature and produces a rapid intense effect when smoked.

Effects appear rapidly after inhalation, especially after smoking, and include euphoria, agitation and aggression. Sympathomimetic effects, including tachycardia and mydriasis, are common; and serious complications, including coronary artery spasm, myocardial infarction (even with normal coronary arteries), ventricular arrhythmias, convulsions, hypertension and stroke, may occur within 3 hrs of use. All patients should be observed with ECG monitoring for ≥4 hrs. ST elevation is common and troponin T is a useful marker of myocardial damage. Benzodiazepines and IV nitrates should be used to treat chest pain or hypertension but β-blockers should be avoided. Coronary angiography may be required and acidosis should be corrected.

Amphetamines

These include amphetamine sulphate ('speed'), methylamphetamine ('crystal meth') and 3,4-methylenedioxymethamphetamine (MDMA, ecstasy). Tolerance is common, leading regular users to seek progressively higher doses.

Toxic features appear in minutes and last 4–6 hrs, or longer after overdose. Sympathomimetic and serotonergic effects are common, and serious complications include supraventricular and ventricular arrhythmias, hyperpyrexia, rhabdomyolysis, coma, convulsions, metabolic acidosis, acute renal failure, disseminated intravascular coagulation and ARDS. A small proportion of patients who have taken ecstasy develop hyponatraemia, usually through drinking excessive amounts of water in the absence of sufficient exertion to sweat it out. Management is supportive and directed at complications.

Gamma hydroxybutyrate and gamma butyrolactone

Gamma hydroxybutyrate (GHB) and gamma butyrolactone (GBL) are sedative agents with psychedelic and body-building effects. Users drink GHB solution until they achieve the desired effects.

Toxic features include sedation, coma, hallucinations and hypotension. Nausea, diarrhoea, vertigo, tremor, myoclonus, extrapyramidal signs, fits, metabolic acidosis and hypokalaemia may also occur. The sedative effects are potentiated by other depressants, e.g. alcohol. Coma usually resolves spontaneously and abruptly within hours. Activated charcoal is useful within 1 hr of ingestion. All patients should be monitored and supported for ≥2 hrs.

D-Lysergic acid diethylamide

D-Lysergic acid diethylamide (LSD) is a synthetic hallucinogen. It is usually ingested as small squares of impregnated absorbent paper, which are often printed with a distinctive design.

Vision is affected most often, with heightened visual awareness of objects, especially colours, image distortion and hallucinations. Patients presenting to hospital usually do so because of a 'bad trip', with panic, confusion, vivid visual hallucinations or aggression, or after self-harm due to the psychosis. Patients with psychotic reactions should be observed in a quiet, dim room. Diazepam is useful if sedation is needed.

Opioids

These include heroin, morphine, methadone, codeine, oxycodone, pethidine, dihydrocodeine and dextropropoxyphene. IV use gives a rapid, intensely pleasurable experience, often accompanied by heightened sexual arousal. Physical dependence occurs within a few weeks of regular high-dose injection; as a result, the dose is escalated and the addict's life becomes increasingly centred on obtaining and taking the drug.

Opioid poisoning: Accidental overdose is common. The hallmarks of opioid poisoning are depressed respiration, hypotension, pulmonary oedema, pinpoint or small pupils, and signs of IV drug misuse (e.g. needle track marks). Death can occur by respiratory arrest or from aspiration of gastric contents. Methadone may cause QT_c prolongation and torsades de pointes.

Management of opioid poisoning: The airway should be cleared and breathing supported if necessary. High-flow oxygen should be administered. ABGs should be performed to check the adequacy of ventilation. Endotracheal intubation can often be avoided by prompt administration of the opioid antagonist naloxone. It should be used as a bolus dose (0.4–2 mg IV in adults, repeated if necessary) until the level of consciousness and respiratory rate increase and the pupils dilate. An infusion of naloxone may be needed because its half-life is much shorter than the half-lives of most opioids, but may precipitate withdrawal in chronic users.

Opioid withdrawal: Can start within 12 hrs and causes intense craving, rhinorrhoea, lacrimation, yawning, perspiration, shivering, piloerection, vomiting, diarrhoea and abdominal cramps. Examination reveals tachycardia, hypertension, mydriasis and facial flushing.

Body packers and stuffers

Body packers smuggle large quantities of illicit cocaine, heroin or amphetamines by swallowing packages wrapped in clingfilm or condoms. Body stuffers attempt to conceal illicit drugs by swallowing them (often poorly packaged) to avoid arrest. Both risk acute severe toxicity from package rupture. Packages may be visible on X-ray, CT or USS. Passage may be accelerated by whole-bowel irrigation.

ALCOHOL MISUSE AND DEPENDENCE

Alcohol consumption, associated with social, psychological and physical problems, constitutes misuse. The criteria for alcohol dependence, a more restricted term, are shown in Box 4.3. Approximately one-quarter of male patients in general hospital medical wards in the UK have a current or previous alcohol problem. Availability of alcohol and social patterns of use appear to be the most important factors. Genetic factors predispose to dependence. The majority of alcoholics do not have an associated psychiatric illness, but a few drink heavily in an attempt to relieve anxiety or depression.

Alcohol misuse may emerge during the patient's history, although patients may minimise their intake. Withdrawal symptoms in those admitted to hospital are a common presentation, as a high alcohol intake cannot be sustained in this setting.

Consequences of alcohol misuse

Acute and chronic effects of alcohol are summarised in Box 4.4. Social, psychiatric and cerebral effects are particularly damaging.

Social problems: Include absenteeism, unemployment, marital tensions, child abuse, financial difficulties and problems with the law, such as violence and traffic offences.

Psychological problems: Alcohol has acute depressant effects and chronic depression is common. Alcohol misuse is often implicated in suicide attempts. People who are socially anxious may use alcohol to relieve anxiety and develop dependence. Alcohol withdrawal increases anxiety. Alcoholic hallucinosis is a rare condition in which patients experience auditory hallucinations in clear consciousness. Symptoms of alcohol withdrawal (see Box 4.4) usually become maximal 2–3 days after the last drink, and can include seizures.

4.3 Criteria for alcohol dependence

- Narrowing of the drinking repertoire (restriction to one type of alcohol, e.g. spirits)
- Priority of drinking over other activities (salience)
- Tolerance of effects of alcohol
- Repeated withdrawal symptoms
- Relief of withdrawal symptoms by further drinking
- Subjective compulsion to drink
- Reinstatement of drinking behaviour after abstinence

4.4 Consequences of alcohol misuse

Acute intoxication

- Emotional and behavioural disturbance
- Medical problems – hypoglycaemia, aspiration of vomit, respiratory depression; accidents and injuries sustained in fights

Chronic effects

- Symptoms of withdrawal – restlessness, anxiety, panic attacks; autonomic symptoms – tachycardia, sweating, pupil dilatation, nausea, vomiting; delirium tremens – agitation, hallucinations, illusions, delusions; seizures
- Neurological – peripheral neuropathy; cerebral haemorrhage; cerebellar degeneration; dementia
- Hepatic – fatty change and cirrhosis; liver cancer
- GI – oesophagitis, gastritis; Mallory–Weiss syndrome; pancreatitis; malabsorption; oesophageal cancer; oesophageal varices
- Respiratory – pulmonary TB; pneumonia, aspiration
- Skin – spider naevi; Dupuytren's contractures; palmar erythema; telangiectasis
- Cardiac – cardiomyopathy; hypertension
- Musculoskeletal – myopathy; fractures
- Endocrine and metabolic – pseudo-Cushing's syndrome; gout; hypoglycaemia
- Reproductive – hypogonadism; infertility; fetal alcohol syndrome
- Psychiatric and cerebral – alcoholic hallucinosis; alcoholic 'blackouts'; Wernicke's encephalopathy; Korsakoff's syndrome

Delirium tremens is a form of delirium associated with severe alcohol withdrawal. It has a significant mortality and morbidity.

Effects on the brain: Acute effects include ataxia, slurred speech, aggression and amnesia after heavy drinking. Established alcoholism may cause alcoholic dementia, a global cognitive impairment resembling Alzheimer's disease but which does not progress with abstinence. Indirect effects on behaviour can result from head injury, hypoglycaemia and portosystemic encephalopathy. Wernicke–Korsakoff syndrome is a rare brain disorder caused by thiamine (vitamin B_1) deficiency that results from damage to the mamillary bodies, dorsomedial nuclei of the thalamus and adjacent grey matter. The most common cause is long-standing heavy drinking with inadequate diet. Without prompt treatment, acute Wernicke's encephalopathy (nystagmus, ophthalmoplegia, ataxia and confusion) can progress to the irreversible Korsakoff's syndrome (severe short-term memory deficits and confabulation).

Management and prognosis

Advice about the harmful effects of alcohol and safe levels of consumption is often sufficient. Altering leisure activities or changing jobs may help, if these are contributing. Psychological treatment at specialised centres is used for patients who have recurrent relapses. Support is also provided by voluntary organisations such as

Alcoholics Anonymous (AA) in the UK. Withdrawal syndromes can be prevented or treated with benzodiazepines. Large doses may be required (e.g. diazepam 20 mg 4 times daily), tailed off over 5–7 days as symptoms subside. Prevention of the Wernicke–Korsakoff complex requires immediate use of high doses of thiamine (IV Pabrinex). There is no treatment for established Korsakoff's syndrome. Acamprosate may help sustain abstinence by reducing craving. Disulfiram is used with psychological support to deter patients from relapsing. Antidepressants and antipsychotics may be needed to treat complications. Relapse is common after treatment.

CHEMICALS AND PESTICIDES

Carbon monoxide

Carbon monoxide (CO) is a colourless, odourless gas produced in faulty appliances burning organic fuels, in house fires and in vehicle exhausts. CO binds to haemoglobin (Hb) and cytochrome oxidase, reducing oxygen delivery and inhibiting cellular respiration. CO poisoning is frequently fatal, often before the patient reaches hospital.

Clinical features

Early features are misleadingly non-specific: headache, nausea, irritability, weakness and tachypnoea. Late features include lethargy, ataxia, nystagmus, drowsiness, hyperventilation, hyper-reflexia progressing to coma, convulsions, hypotension, respiratory depression and cardiovascular collapse. Myocardial infarction and arrhythmias may occur. Cerebral oedema, rhabdomyolysis and renal failure also occur.

Management

High-flow oxygen should be given as soon as possible (it reduces the half-life of COHb from 4–6 hrs to ~40 mins). The COHb concentration is of value in confirming exposure to CO, although it does not correlate well with the severity of poisoning. Pulse oximetry is misleading, as this measures both COHb and oxyhaemoglobin. ECG should be checked in all patients and ABGs in serious cases. Hyperbaric oxygen may reduce the half-life of COHb further, although the logistical difficulties of transporting sick patients to hyperbaric chambers should not be under-estimated, and improved outcome has not been proven.

Organophosphorus insecticides and nerve agents

Organophosphorus (OP) compounds are widely used as pesticides (e.g. malathion, fenthion), especially in developing countries, and also exist as highly toxic chemical warfare agents (e.g. sarin). OPs inactivate acetylcholinesterase (AChE) by phosphorylation, leading to the accumulation of acetylcholine (ACh) at cholinergic synapses.

The fatality rate following deliberate ingestion of OP pesticides in developing countries in Asia is 5–20%.

OP poisoning causes an acute cholinergic phase, which may occasionally be followed by the intermediate syndrome of OP-induced delayed polyneuropathy.

Acute cholinergic syndrome: Occurs within a few minutes of exposure. Vomiting and profuse diarrhoea typically follow oral ingestion. Bronchoconstriction, bronchorrhoea and salivation cause respiratory compromise. Miosis and muscle fasciculation occur, followed by paralysis of limb, respiratory and sometimes extraocular muscles. Coma, fits and arrhythmias can complicate severe cases. Management is as follows:

• The airways should be cleared and maintained. • Contaminated clothing should be removed, eyes irrigated, skin washed and activated charcoal given if within 1 hr of ingestion. • Early use of sufficient atropine (0.6–2 mg IV, repeated every 10–25 mins until secretions are controlled) is life-saving. • Oximes, such as pralidoxime (2 g IV over 4 mins, repeated 4–6 times daily), can reactivate phosphorylated AChE and prevent muscle weakness, convulsions or coma if given early. Cost and unavailability restrict the use of oximes in developing countries. • Intensive cardiorespiratory support is usually required for 48–72 hrs.

Intermediate syndrome: Occurs in 20% of cases 1–4 days after poisoning. Progressive muscle weakness spreads from the ocular and facial muscles to involve the limbs and ultimately causes respiratory failure. Onset is often rapid, but complete recovery is possible with adequate ventilatory care.

Organophosphate-induced delayed polyneuropathy: This rare complication occurs ~2–3 wks after acute exposure. Degeneration of long myelinated nerve fibres leads to a mixed sensory/motor polyneuropathy with paraesthesiae and progressive flaccid limb weakness, which may progress to paraplegia. Recovery is prolonged and often incomplete.

Methanol and ethylene glycol

Ethylene glycol is used in antifreeze and methanol is found in a number of solvents. Both cause ataxia, drowsiness, coma and fits. Methanol causes blindness. Ethanol and fomepizole are used as antidotes to block the formation of toxic metabolites. Dialysis speeds elimination in severe poisoning.

Drinking water contamination

In large parts of South-east Asia and South America, poisoning from contaminated drinking water is endemic. Arsenic causes chronic neuropathy with wasting; fluoride causes tooth, bone and joint disease and also occurs in the Middle East, and East and West Africa. Control of drinking water content is the key intervention.

ENVENOMING

A variety of species use venom either to acquire prey or to defend themselves. Accidental envenoming is common in the rural tropics; however, cases may occur anywhere from exotic venomous pets. Snake and scorpion bites are numerically the most important, but even bee and wasp stings can cause lethal anaphylaxis. Details of individual venoms are available at www.toxinology.com.

Clinical effects of a bite or sting vary widely, and some bites contain no venom ('dry bites').

Local effects: Vary from trivial to severe pain, swelling and necrosis. Lethal systemic effects may accompany trivial local symptoms.

General systemic effects: Include headache, nausea, shock, collapse, fits and cardiac arrest.

Specific systemic effects: Depend on the toxin present, which may be:

• Neurotoxic – flaccid paralysis or excitatory causing autonomic effects. • Cardiotoxic – usually non-specific. • Myotoxic – muscle pain, myoglobinuria, renal failure, raised CK. • Renotoxic – secondary to hypotension or myoglobin, or direct. • Coagulopathy – bruising, bleeding or thrombosis. • Necrotoxins – tissue necrosis. • Allergenic – anaphylaxis.

Management

Rapid and accurate history, examination and early intiation of treatment are vital. Multiple bites or stings are more likely to cause major envenoming.

• In the field: effective cardiopulmonary resuscitation is crucial. • Avoid harmful 'treatments', e.g. cut and suck, tourniquets. • Accurate identification of the organism. • For snake bites: immobilisation of the bitten limb to limit venom spread. • For non-necrotic snake and spider bites: pressure bandage plus immobilisation. • For fish/jellyfish stings: local heat (45°C water immersion). • ECG, O_2 saturation, blood count, U&Es, CK and coagulation screen. • In remote locations: it may be useful to check blood held in a glass container for clotting at 20 mins. • Rapid administration of the species-appropriate antivenom. • Cardiovascular, respiratory and renal support: as required. • Treatment of specific coagulopathy.

Infectious disease

Infection comprises an interaction between the human body and another organism, which may be harmless colonisation or harmful infectious disease. While it is rarely in the interests of the organism to kill the host, it is in the host's interests to kill disease-causing microorganisms, whilst preserving beneficial colonising organisms. Infection remains a major cause of disease worldwide, due to the emergence of new or resistant organisms and the cost of effective control strategies in resource-poor regions.

PRINCIPLES OF INFECTIOUS DISEASE

Infectious agents are divided into the following categories:
• Prions – misfolded proteins devoid of nucleic acids, which cause transmissible spongiform encephalopathies. • Viruses – RNA- or DNA-containing pathogens that rely on host cells for replication. • Bacteria – prokaryotes capable of independent replication but lacking a nucleus. • Eukaryotic pathogens – fungi, protozoa and helminths.

Many organisms live symbiotically in the human body as colonising normal flora, often benefiting the host (e.g. vitamins K and B_{12}, produced by gut flora). In contrast, disease results when pathogenic organisms produce virulence factors that damage host cells. Primary pathogens cause disease in healthy hosts, while opportunistic pathogens cause disease only in the immune-compromised host.

DETECTION OF INFECTION

A variety of methods are used:

Nucleic acid amplification tests (NAAT): Can not only identify viruses and bacteria but also detect strain types and toxin or resistance genes.

Culture: Largely supplanted by NAAT for viruses. Bacterial culture is still widely used for identification and antibiotic sensitivity testing, but can be slow and not all organisms grow in culture.

CLINICAL EXAMINATION OF PATIENTS WITH INFECTIOUS DISEASE

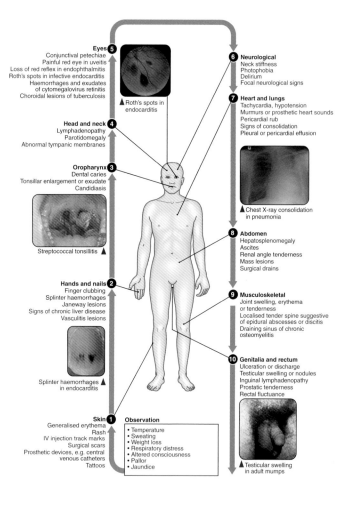

Eyes 5
Conjunctival petechiae
Painful red eye in uveitis
Loss of red reflex in endophthalmitis
Roth's spots in infective endocarditis
Haemorrhages and exudates
of cytomegalovirus retinitis
Choroidal lesions of tuberculosis

▲ Roth's spots in endocarditis

Head and neck 4
Lymphadenopathy
Parotidomegaly
Abnormal tympanic membranes

Oropharynx 3
Dental caries
Tonsillar enlargement or exudate
Candidiasis

Streptococcal tonsillitis ▲

Hands and nails 2
Finger clubbing
Splinter haemorrhages
Janeway lesions
Signs of chronic liver disease
Vasculitis lesions

Splinter haemorrhages ▲
in endocarditis

Skin 1
Generalised erythema
Rash
IV injection track marks
Surgical scars
Prosthetic devices, e.g. central
venous catheters
Tattoos

Observation
• Temperature
• Sweating
• Weight loss
• Respiratory distress
• Altered consciousness
• Pallor
• Jaundice

6 Neurological
Neck stiffness
Photophobia
Delirium
Focal neurological signs

7 Heart and lungs
Tachycardia, hypotension
Murmurs or prosthetic heart sounds
Pericardial rub
Signs of consolidation
Pleural or pericardial effusion

▲ Chest X-ray consolidation
in pneumonia

8 Abdomen
Hepatosplenomegaly
Ascites
Renal angle tenderness
Mass lesions
Surgical drains

9 Musculoskeletal
Joint swelling, erythema
or tenderness
Localised tender spine suggestive
of epidural abscesses or discitis
Draining sinus of chronic
osteomyelitis

10 Genitalia and rectum
Ulceration or discharge
Testicular swelling or nodules
Inguinal lymphadenopathy
Prostatic tenderness
Rectal fluctance

▲ Testicular swelling
in adult mumps

Specialised mass spectrometers can be used for rapid identification of organisms in blood cultures.

Immunological tests: Host antibodies can be detected using various in vitro immunological assays. A rise in titre between acute and convalescent serum samples indicates recent infection, but tests may be negative in the immunocompromised. Interferon-gamma release assays detect infection through the release of interferon from sensitised host T cells exposed to bacterial peptides.

RESERVOIRS OF INFECTION

Human reservoirs: Colonised or infected individuals may act as reservoirs, carrying organisms on the skin, throat (e.g. meningococci), nose, bowel (e.g. *Salmonella*) or blood (e.g. hepatitis B).

Animal reservoirs: Animals are a source of human infections (zoonoses), e.g. *Salmonella* from poultry, TB and brucellosis from milk. Spread may continue from cases to other humans (e.g. Q fever).

Environmental reservoirs: Environmental pathogens include *Legionella* in air conditioning or water, and enteropathogens (typhoid, cholera, *Cryptosporidia* or hepatitis A) in water. Soil may harbour spores of *Clostridia* (tetanus) or anthrax.

TRANSMISSION OF INFECTION

This occurs by several routes:
• Respiratory – inhalation. • Faecal–oral – ingestion. • Sexually transmitted – via mucous membranes. • Blood-borne – inoculation. • Via vector or fomite: an animal or object bridges the gap between host and reservoir.

Health care-acquired infection

Health care-acquired infections (HAIs) affect 6–10% of all hospital admissions and create a significant clinical and economic burden. The close proximity of hospital inpatients, the widespread use of antibiotics and the ease of transmission by health-care workers have led to the selection of multidrug-resistant organisms such as MRSA and vancomycin-resistant enterococci (VRE). Spread of these organisms, plus infections such as *Clostridium difficile* and norovirus, may lead to outbreaks of infection and necessitate ward or hospital closure.

PREVENTION OF INFECTION

HAIs have to be managed by comprehensive antibiotic policies and careful adherence to strict infection control protocols. Although environmental cleanliness and clean clothing are cosmetically important, recent evidence has confirmed the absolute importance of hand hygiene in the control of HAI. The use of alcohol hand lotion by all health-care workers between every patient contact is an effective alternative to soap and water in prevention of most HAI, but not *Clostridium difficile*.

Outbreak control

An outbreak of infection is defined as the occurrence of any disease clearly in excess of normal expectancy. Confirmation requires evidence of identical genotype in organisms isolated from cases. Cases are sought by testing and then plotted on an outbreak curve. Case-control studies may be used to establish the source. Good communication of data to health-care workers is needed to achieve control. Many countries have systems of compulsory notification of contagious conditions to public health authorities to assist outbreak control.

Immunisation

Passive immunisation means administering antibodies to a specific pathogen. This produces temporary protection after exposure but, as antibodies are obtained from blood, this may carry risks of blood-borne infection.

Active immunisation uses whole live attenuated organisms or components of organisms to prevent disease by inducing immunity. Vaccination may be applied to entire populations or to subpopulations at specific risk through travel or occupation. Usually the goal is to prevent infection, but vaccination against human papillomavirus (HPV) was introduced to prevent cervical cancer. Vaccination is successful when the number of susceptible hosts in a population becomes too low to sustain transmission (herd immunity). Naturally acquired smallpox was eradicated by vaccination in 1980. A similar programme aims to eradicate poliomyelitis.

PRESENTING PROBLEMS IN INFECTIOUS DISEASES

Fever

Fever implies an elevated core temperature of >38°C. Clinical features are used to guide appropriate investigations, which include:
• FBC and differential. • U&Es, liver function, glucose and muscle enzymes. • ESR and CRP. • Autoantibodies. • CXR and ECG. • Urinalysis and culture. • Blood culture. • Throat swab.

Additional tests are indicated by local symptoms and if the patient is immunocompromised.

Pyrexia of unknown origin

Pyrexia of unknown origin (PUO) is a common presenting problem and may be defined as a consistently elevated body temperature of >38°C persisting for >3 wks with no diagnosis after initial investigation. Many causes of PUO are listed in Box 5.1. Two or more causes of fever may coexist. Fever in old age merits special attention (Box 5.2).

5.1 Aetiology of pyrexia of unknown origin (PUO)

Infections (~30%)

- Specific locations: abscess at any site, cholecystitis/cholangitis, UTI, prostatitis, dental, sinus, bone and joint infections, endocarditis
- Specific organisms: TB (particularly extrapulmonary), brucellosis, viruses (cytomegalovirus (CMV), Epstein–Barr virus (EBV), HIV-1), fungi (*Aspergillus*, *Candida*)
- Specific patient groups: imported infections, e.g. malaria, dengue, leishmaniasis, enteric fevers, *Burkholderia pseudomallei*, nosocomial infections, HIV-related infections, e.g. *Pneumocystis jirovecii*, disseminated *Mycobacterium avium*, cytomegalovirus (CMV)

Malignancy (~20%)

- Lymphoma, myeloma and leukaemia
- Solid tumours (renal, liver, colon, stomach, pancreas)

Connective tissue disorders (~15%)

- Older patients: temporal arteritis/polymyalgia rheumatica
- Younger patients: systemic lupus erythematosus (SLE), Still's disease, polymyositis, vasculitis, Behçet's disease
- Rheumatic fever

Miscellaneous (~20%)

- Inflammatory bowel disease, alcoholic liver disease, granulomatous hepatitis, pancreatitis
- Myeloproliferative disease, haemolytic anaemia
- Sarcoidosis, atrial myxoma, thyrotoxicosis, hypothalamic lesions
- Familial Mediterranean fever, drug reactions, factitious fever

No diagnosis or resolves spontaneously (15%)

5.2 Fever in old age

- **Temperature measurement**: fever may be missed because oral temperatures are unreliable. Rectal measurement may be needed but core temperature is increasingly measured using eardrum reflectance.
- **Associated acute confusion**: common with fever, especially in those with underlying cerebrovascular disease or dementia.
- **Prominent causes of PUO**: include endocarditis, TB and intra-abdominal sepsis. Non-infective causes include polymyalgia rheumatic, temporal arteritis and tumours.
- **Common infective causes in the very frail** (e.g. nursing home residents): include pneumonia, urinary infection, soft tissue infection and gastroenteritis.

5.3 Additional investigations in PUO

- Serological tests: autoantibodies, complement, immunoglobulins, cryoglobulins
- Echocardiography
- USS of abdomen
- CT/MRI of thorax, abdomen and/or brain
- Skeletal imaging: X-rays, CT/MRI spine, isotope bone scan
- Labelled white-cell scan
- PET scan
- Biopsy: bronchoscopic, lymph node, liver, bone marrow, temporal artery, laparoscopic

Detailed history should include:

Recent travel history: Malaria, respiratory infections, viral hepatitis, typhoid and dengue are the most common causes of imported fever in the UK.

Personal and social history: Exposure to STI, illicit drug use.

Occupational or recreational history: Animal exposure, consumption of unpasteurised milk.

Investigations and management

Measure temperature and vital signs 4-hourly. Regularly review and expand history-taking. Repeat physical examination regularly for emerging signs such as cardiac murmurs, lymphadenopathy and rashes. Initial investigations are summarised above. If these are inconclusive, additional ones (Box 5.3) should be considered.

Lesions on imaging should normally be biopsied to detect pathogens by culture or nucleic acid detection.

Liver biopsy: May reveal TB, lymphoma or granulomatous disease, including sarcoidosis. It is unlikely to help unless the liver is biochemically or radiologically abnormal.

Bone marrow biopsy: Has a diagnostic yield in PUO of ~15%, the most commonly detected diseases being myelodysplasia, other haematological malignancies and TB. More rarely, brucellosis, enteric fever or visceral leishmaniasis may be detected, underlining the importance of sending samples for culture as well as microscopy.

Temporal artery biopsy: Should be considered in patients >50 yrs, even if the ESR is not significantly elevated. Since arteritis is patchy, diagnostic yield is increased if a 1.5 cm section of artery is biopsied.

Prognosis

The overall mortality of PUO is 30–40% mainly because of malignancy in older patients. If no cause is found on exhaustive investigation, the mortality is low and spontaneous recovery often occurs.

Fever in the injection drug-user

Infection is introduced by non-sterile (often shared) equipment, and is facilitated by immunodeficiency due to malnutrition or the toxic effects of drugs. Risks increase with prolonged drug use and central injection in large veins, necessitated by thrombosis of peripheral veins. Fever is usually due to soft tissue or respiratory infections.

Clinical assessment

Site: Femoral vein injections may cause DVT, of which 50% are infected; arterial injection may cause false aneurysm formation and compartment syndrome. Psoas abscess and septic arthritis also occur. *Clostridium* infection has been recorded with IM injection of heroin.

Technical details: Sharing of needles and spoons, and use of contaminated drugs or solvents increase the risk of infection (e.g. HIV-1, hepatitis B or C).

Other details: Establish what has been injected, including what solvents were used. Check recent viral test status. Beware surreptitious self-treatment with antibiotics, which may mask culture results.

Symptoms that may accompany fever: Include breathlessness, myalgia, confusion and tachycardia. It may be difficult to distinguish symptoms due to infection from those accompanying drug withdrawal.

Signs: These include:
• Rashes. • Injection site abscess. • Joint pain or swelling from injection. • DVT or compartment syndrome in the legs. • Local tenderness or referred pain from an abscess site, e.g. flexion at the hip eliciting back pain is indicative of ilio-psoas abscess. • New murmurs or evidence of cardiac decompensation: may suggest either right- or left-sided endocarditis (check nails for splinter haemorrhages), or the cardiomyopathy of generalised sepsis. The JVP may show V waves in tricuspid endocarditis. Pleural rub or effusion is seen in DVT with PE, or septic emboli from endocarditis or infected DVT. • Stupor: occurs in drug overdose or hepatic encephalopathy; agitation with drug withdrawal; headache and drowsiness in meningitis or encephalitis; local paralysis or spasms with tetanus or botulism.

Management

Management is that of the underlying condition. Flucloxacillin is useful against *Staphylococcus aureus*, although vancomycin may be needed if MRSA is present. Appropriate sedative medicines should be provided for those suffering withdrawal symptoms after a long period of dependency.

Fever in the immunocompromised host

Immunosuppression may be congenital; acquired through infection or haematological disease; or iatrogenic, induced by chemotherapy for cancer or for autoimmune diseases. These may be distinguished by history, and careful examination may reveal where infection has breached the skin or mucosal barriers. Blood and urine cultures, with imaging – including chest CT and virology of nasopharyngeal aspirates – may reveal the nature and site of infection. Patients with respiratory signs should have induced sputum or bronchoscopy for *Pneumocystis jirovecii*, bacteria and fungi.

Neutropenic fever is defined as a neutrophil count of $<0.5 \times 10^9/L$, with fever $>38.5°C$, although risk increases as the neutrophil count falls $<1.0 \times 10^9/L$. Patients with neutropenia are particularly prone to bacterial and fungal infections. Gram-positive organisms are the most common pathogens, particularly in the presence of in-dwelling catheters. Blood cultures, swabs and urine samples should be taken, potential sources removed and empirical antibiotic therapy started, with a broad-spectrum penicillin (e.g. piperacillin/tazobactam). An aminoglycoside (e.g. gentamicin) is often given too, although data suggest monotherapy is as effective. Antifungals such as caspofungin may be added if fever has not resolved in 3–5 days.

Severe skin and soft tissue infections
Necrotising fasciitis

There are two types of necrotising fasciitis:

Type 1: This is a mixed infection with Gram-negative bacteria and anaerobes, often seen following surgery or in diabetic or immuno-compromised patients.

Type 2: This is caused by group A or other streptococci. About 60% of cases are associated with streptococcal toxic shock syndrome (p. 75).

Both types produce a severe, rapidly progressive and destructive inflammation of the dermis and subcutaneous tissues, leading to intense pain, profound toxaemia and multisystem failure. The affected area is erythematous, hot and shiny. Central anaesthesia (due to cutaneous nerve damage), surrounded by exquisitely tender erythematous skin, is pathognomonic.

Treatment is with broad-spectrum antibiotics, e.g. piperacillin/tazobactam with metronidazole. Streptococcal infections respond to benzylpenicillin with clindamycin. Surgical débridement should subsequently be considered if control is not achieved.

Clostridial soft tissue infections
Gas gangrene or myonecrosis

Although *Clostridia* may colonise or contaminate wounds, no action is required unless spreading infection is present. In anaerobic cellulitis, usually due to *C. perfringens*, gas forms locally and extends along tissue planes, but bacteraemia does not occur. Prompt surgical débridement, along with penicillin or clindamycin therapy, is usually effective.

Gas gangrene is defined as acute invasion of healthy living muscle undamaged by previous trauma by *C. perfringens*. It develops following deep penetrating injury sufficient to create an anaerobic environment and allow clostridial introduction and proliferation.

Severe pain at the site of the injury progresses rapidly over 18–24 hrs. Bronze/purple discoloration develops in tense and

5.4 Causes of acute diarrhoea

Infectious

- **Toxin-mediated**: *Bacillus cereus*, *Clostridium* spp. enterotoxin, *Staph. aureus*
- **Bacterial**: *Shigella*, *Campylobacter*, *C. difficile*, *Salmonella*, enterotoxigenic *E. coli*, enteroinvasive *E. coli*, *Vibrio cholerae*
- **Viral**: rotavirus, norovirus
- **Protozoal**: *Giardia*, *Cryptosporidium*, microsporidiosis, amoebic dysentery, isosporiasis
- **Systemic**: Acute diverticulitis, sepsis, pelvic inflammatory disease, meningococcaemia, atypical pneumonia, malaria

Non-infectious

- **GI**: inflammatory bowel disease, bowel malignancy, overflow from constipation, enteral tube feeding
- **Metabolic**: diabetic ketoacidosis, thyrotoxicosis, uraemia, neuroendocrine tumours releasing 5-HT or vasoactive intestinal peptide
- **Drugs and toxins**: NSAIDs, cytotoxic agents, PPIs, antibiotics, dinoflagellates, plant toxins, heavy metals, ciguatera or scombrotoxic fish poisoning

exquisitely tender skin. Gas in tissues may cause crepitus on examination or be visible on X-ray, CT or USS. Systemic toxicity develops rapidly with high leucocytosis, multi-organ dysfunction, raised creatine kinase and disseminated intravascular haemolysis. High-dose IV penicillin, clindamycin, cephalosporins and metronidazole therapy is very effective, coupled with aggressive surgical débridement of affected tissues. Use of hyperbaric oxygen is controversial.

Acute diarrhoea and vomiting

Acute diarrhoea, sometimes with vomiting, is an extremely common presenting problem, and may result from both infectious and non-infectious causes (Box 5.4). Infectious diarrhoea is caused by transmission of viruses, bacteria or protozoa either by the faecal–oral route or via infected fomites, food or water. Psychological or physical stress may also precipitate diarrhoea. Occasionally, diarrhoea may be the presenting feature of another systemic illness, such as pneumonia.

Enterotoxic organisms, e.g. *Bacillus cereus*, *Staph. aureus* and *Vibrio cholerae*, produce vomiting and/or 'secretory' watery diarrhoea. Organisms that invade the mucosa, such as *Shigella*, *Campylobacter* and enterohaemorrhagic *E. coli* (EHEC), have longer incubation periods and may cause systemic upset and blood in the stool. Box 5.5 summarises the causes of bloody diarrhoea.

Clinical assessment

History: Should include:
• Duration and frequency of diarrhoea. • Presence of blood, abdominal pain and tenesmus. • Recent foods ingested (common associations are shown in Box 5.6). • Other family members affected.

5.5 Causes of bloody diarrhoea

Infectious

- *Campylobacter* spp., *Shigella* dysentery, non-typhoidal salmonellae, enterohaemorrhagic or enteroinvasive *E. coli*, *C. difficile*, *Vibrio parahaemolyticus*, *Entamoeba histolytica*

Non-infectious

- Diverticular disease, rectal or colonic malignancy, inflammatory bowel disease, bleeding haemorrhoids, anal fissure, ischaemic colitis, intussusception

5.6 Foods associated with infection, including gastroenteritis

- **Raw seafood**: norovirus, *Vibrio*, hepatitis A
- **Raw eggs**: *Salmonella*
- **Undercooked meat/poultry**: *Salmonella*, *Campylobacter*, EHEC, *C. perfringens*
- **Unpasteurised milk or juice**: *Salmonella*, *Campylobacter*, EHEC, *Yersinia enterocolitica*
- **Unpasteurised soft cheeses**: *Salmonella*, *Campylobacter*, enterotoxigenic *E. coli* (ETEC), *Y. enterocolitica*, *Listeria*
- **Home-made canned foods**: *Clostridium botulinum*
- **Raw hot dogs, pâté**: *Listeria*

Fever and bloody diarrhoea suggest an invasive, colitic, dysenteric process. Incubation <18 hrs suggests a toxin-mediated food poisoning; >5 days suggests protozoal or helminthic infection.

Examination:
• Assess degree of dehydration by skin turgor, pulse and BP measurement. • Measure urine output and ongoing stool losses. • Carry out regular full abdominal examination.

Investigations

• Stool microscopy (for cysts, ova and parasites), culture and *C. difficile* toxin assay. • FBC, U&Es. • Blood film for malaria if patient has been in an affected area. • Blood/urine culture and CXR: may reveal an underlying diagnosis.

Management of acute diarrhoea

Isolation: All patients with acute, potentially infective diarrhoea should be appropriately isolated to minimise person-to-person spread of infection.

Fluid replacement: Replace established losses and ongoing losses, as well as normal daily requirements. This may be done with IV fluid or with oral rehydration solution (ORS). One sachet of commercial ORS made up to 200 mL is given for each diarrhoea stool.

Antibiotics/antimicrobial therapy: Not generally used, except in severe cases (e.g. immunocompromise, comorbidity, systemic involvement). May precipitate haemolytic uraemic syndrome in EHEC infection.

Adjunctive antidiarrhoeal therapy: Anti-motility drugs are not generally recommended and may indeed prolong or worsen the course of an acute infective gastroenteritis.

Non-infectious food poisoning

Plant toxins: Those causing diarrhoea or vomiting occur in under-cooked red kidney beans, in potatoes discoloured green by light and in many fungi.

Chemical toxins: Originating in dinoflagellates and concentrated by shellfish or fish, these can cause gastrointestinal symptoms and paralysis. Scombrotoxic food poisoning results from eating contaminated tuna, mackerel or sardines.

Antimicrobial-associated diarrhoea: This is common in the elderly. Between 20 and 25% of cases are caused by *C. difficile*; if this toxin is detected, treatment with metronidazole or vancomycin is effective.

Infections acquired in the tropics
Fever in travellers recently returned from the tropics

Both tropical and non-tropical infection may present with fever after tropical travel. Frequent final diagnoses are:
• Malaria. • Typhoid fever. • Viral hepatitis. • Dengue fever.
• Travellers to West Africa may have viral haemorrhagic fevers (e.g. Marburg, Lassa or Ebola) while those in South-east Asia may have avian influenza (H5N1); all these require special isolation.

Clinical assessment

History:
• Countries and environments visited. • Travel dates. • Exposures: ill people, animals, insect bites, freshwater swimming. • Dietary history. • Sexual history. • Malaria prophylaxis – what taken and local resistance. • Any local medicines/remedies taken. • Vaccination history – if the patient was vaccinated against yellow fever and hepatitis A and B, this virtually rules out these infections. Oral and injectable typhoid vaccinations are 70–90% effective.

Examination: Careful, repeated examination is vital, paying particular attention to rashes or lesions, throat, eyes, nail beds, lymph nodes and abdomen (Fig. 5.1).

Investigations

Initial investigations in all settings should start with thick and thin blood films for malaria parasites, FBC, urinalysis and CXR if indicated. Box 5.7 gives the diagnoses that should be considered in acute fever with no localising signs, grouped according to differential WCC.

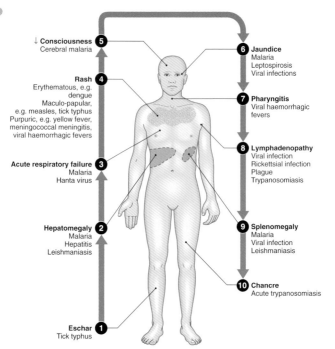

↓ Consciousness 5
Cerebral malaria

6 Jaundice
Malaria
Leptospirosis
Viral infections

Rash 4
Erythematous, e.g.
dengue
Maculo-papular,
e.g. measles, tick typhus
Purpuric, e.g. yellow fever,
meningococcal meningitis,
viral haemorrhagic fevers

7 Pharyngitis
Viral haemorrhagic
fevers

Acute respiratory failure 3
Malaria
Hanta virus

8 Lymphadenopathy
Viral infection
Rickettsial infection
Plague
Trypanosomiasis

Hepatomegaly 2
Malaria
Hepatitis
Leishmaniasis

9 Splenomegaly
Malaria
Viral infection
Leishmaniasis

10 Chancre
Acute trypanosomiasis

Eschar 1
Tick typhus

Fig. 5.1 Acute fever in/from the tropics: clinical examination.

5.7 Differential WCC: acute fever in the absence of localising signs		
WCC differential	**Potential diagnoses**	**Further investigations**
Neutrophil leucocytosis	Bacterial sepsis	Blood culture
	Leptospirosis	Culture of blood and urine, serology
	Borreliosis: tick or louse-borne relapsing fever	Blood film
	Amoebic liver abscess	USS
Normal WCC and differential	Typhoid fever	Blood, stool and culture
	Typhus	Serology
	Arboviral infection	Serology (PCR and viral culture)
Lymphocytosis	Viral fevers	Serology
	Infectious mononucleosis	Monospot test
	Rickettsial fevers	Serology

<table>
<tr><td colspan="3">i 5.8 Parasitic causes of eosinophilia</td></tr>
</table>

Infestation	Pathogen	Clinical syndrome
Strongyloidiasis	*S. stercoralis*	Larva currens
Helminth infections	Hookworm, *Ascaris*	Anaemia
	Toxocara	Visceral larva migrans
Schistosomiasis	*S. haematobium*	Katayama fever
	S. mansoni, S. japonicum	Chronic infection
Filariases	*Loa loa*	Skin nodules
	Wuchereria bancrofti	Elephantiasis
	Onchocerca volvulus	Visual disturbance
Other nematode infections	*Trichinella*	Myositis
Cestode infections	*Taenia saginatum,*	Asymptomatic, lesions
	T. solium, Echinococcus	in liver
Liver fluke infections	*Fasciola hepatica*	Hepatic symptoms
Lung fluke infections	*Paragonimus westermani*	Lung lesions

Diarrhoea acquired in the tropics

Common causes include *Salmonella*, *Campylobacter* and *Cryptosporidia* infections. Typhoid, paratyphoid, shigellosis and amoebiasis usually occur in visitors to the Indian subcontinent and sub-Saharan Africa.

Other causes to be considered are tropical sprue (p. 449), giardiasis and HIV enteropathy.

Eosinophilia acquired in the tropics

Non-parasitic causes of eosinophilia include haematological conditions (p. 548), allergic reactions and HIV-1 or human T-cell lymphotropic virus (HTLV)-1 infection. In travellers or tropical residents, however, eosinophilia is associated with parasite infections (particularly helminths). Anybody with an eosinophil count $>0.4 \times 10^9/L$ should be investigated for both parasitic (Box 5.8) and non-parasitic causes (p. 523). Eosinophilia is not a typical feature in malaria, amoebiasis, leishmaniasis, leprosy or tapeworm infections other than cysticercosis.

Clinical assessment

• Travel history, e.g. freshwater bathing in sub-Saharan Africa. • Any rashes or itching (schistosomiasis, strongyloidiasis). • Haematuria (schistosomiasis). • Subcutaneous swellings (loiasis, cutaneous larva migrans). • Febrile hepatosplenomegaly (schistosomiasis, toxocariasis). • Myositis (trichinosis, cysticercosis). • Pneumonitis (helminth infection, filariasis, strongyloidiasis). • Meningitis (strongyloidiasis).

Investigations

Direct visualisation of adult worms, larvae or ova provides the best evidence. Box 5.9 lists the initial investigations for eosinophilia.

i 5.9 **Initial investigation of eosinophilia**

Investigation	Pathogens sought
Stool microscopy	Ova, cysts and parasites
Terminal urine	Ova of *Schistosoma haematobium*
Duodenal aspirate	Filariform larvae of *Strongyloides*, liver fluke ova
Day bloods	Microfilariae of *Brugia malayi*, *Loa loa*
Night bloods	Microfilariae of *Wuchereria bancrofti*
Skin snips	*Onchocerca volvulus*
Serology	*Schistosoma*, *Filaria*, *Strongyloides*, hydatid, trichinosis, etc.

Skin conditions acquired in the tropics

The most common skin problems in the tropics are bacterial and fungal skin infections, scabies and eczema. These are described elsewhere (p. 723). In travellers, infected insect bites and cutaneous larva migrans are common. Box 5.10 summarises the types of rash commonly seen in tropical travellers/residents. Skin biopsy and culture may be required to achieve a firm diagnosis.

Infection issues in adolescence

These are shown in Box 5.11.

Infection issues in pregnancy

These are summarised in Box 5.12.

VIRAL INFECTIONS

Viruses are simple infectious agents consisting of a portion of genetic material, RNA or DNA, enclosed in a protein coat that is antigenically unique for that species. They cannot exist in a free-living state, needing to infect host cells to survive. Once inside cells, they utilise host material for protein synthesis and genetic reproduction. All viral infections must therefore originate from an infected source by either direct or vector-mediated spread.

Systemic viral infections with exanthem

Childhood exanthems are characterised by fever and widespread rash. Maternal antibodies protect for the first 6–12 mths but thereafter incidence rises. Although the incidence of exanthems has diminished as a result of vaccination programmes, incomplete uptake can increase infection in later life.

Measles

The WHO has set the objective of eradicating measles but vaccination of 95% of a population is required to prevent outbreaks. Natural illness produces lifelong immunity.

5.10 Rash in tropical travellers/residents

Maculopapular

- Dengue, HIV-1, typhoid, *Spirillum minus*, rickettsial infections, measles

Petechial or purpuric

- Viral haemorrhagic fevers, yellow fever, meningococcal sepsis, leptospirosis, rickettsial spotted fevers, malaria

Urticarial

- Schistosomiasis, toxocariasis, strongyloidiasis, fascioliasis

Vesicular

- Monkeypox, insect bites, rickettsial pox

Ulcers

- Leishmaniasis, *Mycobacterium ulcerans* (Buruli ulcer), dracunculosis, anthrax, rickettsial eschar, tropical ulcer, ecthyma

Papules

- Scabies, insect bites, prickly heat, ringworm, onchocerciasis

Nodules or plaques

- Leprosy, chromoblastomycosis, dimorphic fungi, trypanosomiasis, onchocerciasis, myiasis, tungiasis

Migratory linear rash

- Cutaneous larva migrans, *Strongyloides stercoralis*

Migratory papules/nodules

- *Loa loa*, gnathosomiasis, schistosomiasis

Thickened skin

- Mycetoma, elephantiasis

5.11 Infection issues in adolescence

Common infectious syndromes	Infectious mononucleosis, bacterial pharyngitis, whooping cough, staphylococcal skin/soft tissue infection, UTI, gastroenteritis
Life-threatening infections	Meningococcal meningitis, bacterial sepsis
STIs	HIV-1, hepatitis B, chlamydia
Travel-related infections	Diarrhoea, malaria
Infections in susceptible groups	E.g. those with cystic fibrosis, congenital immunodeficiency, acute leukaemia
Adherence to prolonged treatment	E.g. TB, antiretroviral therapy, osteomyelitis – adherence often hard to achieve in adolescence
Vaccination	HPV
Risk reduction	Education on sexual health, alcohol and recreational drug use important

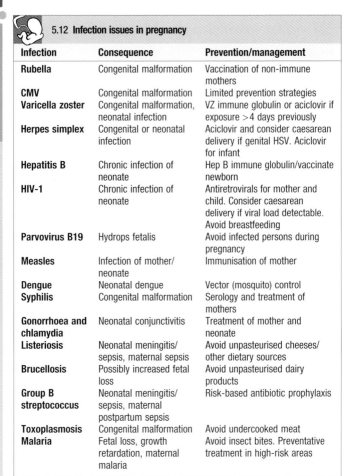

5.12 Infection issues in pregnancy

Infection	Consequence	Prevention/management
Rubella	Congenital malformation	Vaccination of non-immune mothers
CMV	Congenital malformation	Limited prevention strategies
Varicella zoster	Congenital malformation, neonatal infection	VZ immune globulin or aciclovir if exposure >4 days previously
Herpes simplex	Congenital or neonatal infection	Aciclovir and consider caesarean delivery if genital HSV. Aciclovir for infant
Hepatitis B	Chronic infection of neonate	Hep B immune globulin/vaccinate newborn
HIV-1	Chronic infection of neonate	Antiretrovirals for mother and child. Consider caesarean delivery if viral load detectable. Avoid breastfeeding
Parvovirus B19	Hydrops fetalis	Avoid infected persons during pregnancy
Measles	Infection of mother/neonate	Immunisation of mother
Dengue	Neonatal dengue	Vector (mosquito) control
Syphilis	Congenital malformation	Serology and treatment of mothers
Gonorrhoea and chlamydia	Neonatal conjunctivitis	Treatment of mother and neonate
Listeriosis	Neonatal meningitis/sepsis, maternal sepsis	Avoid unpasteurised cheeses/other dietary sources
Brucellosis	Possibly increased fetal loss	Avoid unpasteurised dairy products
Group B streptococcus	Neonatal meningitis/sepsis, maternal postpartum sepsis	Risk-based antibiotic prophylaxis
Toxoplasmosis	Congenital malformation	Avoid undercooked meat
Malaria	Fetal loss, growth retardation, maternal malaria	Avoid insect bites. Preventative treatment in high-risk areas

Clinical features

Infection is by respiratory droplets with an incubation period of 6–19 days to onset of rash. A prodromal illness 1–3 days before the rash appears heralds the most infectious stage with upper respiratory symptoms, conjunctivitis and the presence of 'Koplik's spots' (small white spots surrounded by erythema) on the internal buccal mucosa (Fig. 5.2). As natural antibody develops, the maculo-papular rash appears (Fig. 5.3), spreading from face to extremities. Lymphadenopathy and diarrhoea are common.

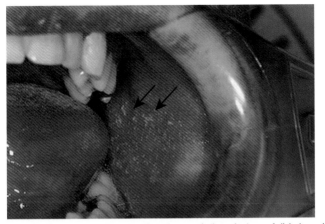

Fig. 5.2 Koplik's spots (arrows) seen on buccal mucosa in the early stages of clinical measles.

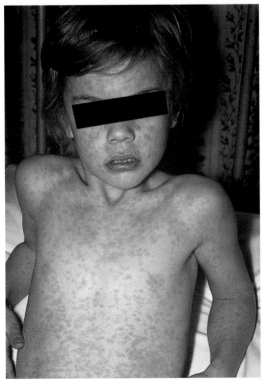

Fig. 5.3 Typical measles rash.

Complications include:

• Otitis media. • Bacterial pneumonia. • Encephalitis/convulsions. • Subacute sclerosing panencephalitis (rare, late and serious).

Management

In the immunocompetent, the disease is self-limiting; however, severity and complications are increased in the malnourished and immunosuppressed. Pregnant women should be considered for treatment with immunoglobulin. All children aged 12–15 mths should be vaccinated against measles as a combined vaccine with mumps and rubella (MMR), with a further dose at age 4 yrs. Antibiotics are only indicated for superinfection.

Rubella (German measles)

Rubella is a viral exanthem transmitted by aerosol, with infectivity from up to 10 days before to 2 wks after the onset of the rash. The incubation period is 15–20 days. Most childhood cases are subclinical, although disease can present with lymphadenopathy and a maculopapular rash that starts on the face and moves to the trunk. Complications include arthralgia, thrombocytopenia, hepatitis and rarely encephalitis.

The greatest significance of rubella is for pregnant women, as transplacental infection may result in severe congenital disease. If rubella is suspected in a pregnant woman, confirmation is provided either by rubella IgM antibodies in serum or by IgG seroconversion. In the exposed pregnant woman, the absence of rubella IgG indicates potential for infection. Children should be immunised against rubella as part of standard vaccination programmes using MMR (see above). Women of child-bearing age should be tested and vaccinated if seronegative.

Parvovirus B19

This air-borne virus causes mild or subclinical infection in normal hosts. Around 50% of children and 60–90% of adults are seropositive. In addition to the clinical manifestations summarised in Box 5.13, there may be a transient block in erythropoiesis, which is insignificant unless haemoglobinopathy or haemolysis is also present. Parvovirus B19 DNA may be detected in the serum by PCR; however, as illness is usually mild or subclinical and self-limiting, confirmatory blood tests are not always required. If infection occurs during pregnancy, the fetus should be monitored closely for signs of hydrops.

Human herpesvirus 6 and 7

These viruses are associated with a benign febrile illness of children with a maculopapular erythematous rash: 'exanthem subitum'. In the immunocompromised they cause an infectious mononucleosis-like syndrome. Around 95% of children are infected by age 2.

5.13 Clinical features of parvovirus B19 infection

Syndrome/affected age group	Clinical manifestations
Fifth disease (erythema infectiosum) Small children	Three clinical stages: a 'slapped cheek' appearance (Fig. 5.4), reticulate eruption on the body and limbs, then resolution. Often the child is quite well throughout
Gloves and socks syndrome Young adults	Fever and an acral purpuric eruption with a clear margin at the wrists and ankles. Mucosal involvement also occurs
Arthropathies Adults, occasionally children	Polyarthropathy of small joints. In children it tends to involve the larger joints in an asymmetrical distribution
Impaired erythropoiesis Adults, those with haematological disease, the immunosuppressed	Can cause a mild anaemia but in an individual with underlying haematological abnormality can precipitate an aplastic crisis
Hydrops fetalis Transplacental fetal infection	Asymptomatic or symptomatic maternal infection can cause fetal anaemia with aplastic crisis leading to non-immune hydrops fetalis and spontaneous abortion

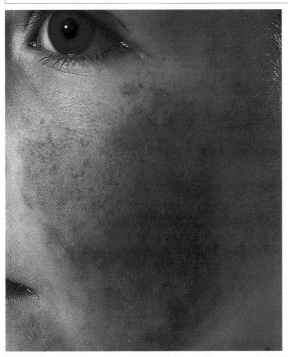

Fig. 5.4 Slapped cheek syndrome. The typical facial rash of human parvovirus B19 infection.

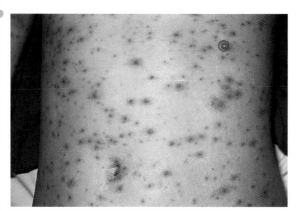

Fig. 5.5 Chickenpox.

Chickenpox

Varicella zoster virus (VZV) is a dermotropic and neurotropic virus causing primary infection, usually in childhood, which may reactivate in later life. It is spread by aerosol and direct contact and is highly infectious. Disease in children is usually better tolerated than in adults, pregnant women and the immunocompromised.

The incubation period is 11–20 days, after which a vesicular eruption begins (Fig. 5.5), often on mucosal surfaces first, followed by rapid dissemination in a centripetal fashion. New lesions occur in crops every 2–4 days, accompanied by fever. The rash progresses within 24 hrs from small pink macules to vesicles and pustules, which then crust. Infectivity lasts from 2 to 4 days before the rash appears until the last crusts separate. Diagnosis is clinical but may be confirmed by PCR of vesicular fluid.

Complications include:
• Secondary bacterial infection of rash (due to scratching). • Self-limiting cerebellar ataxia. • Congenital abnormalities if maternal disease is contracted in the first trimester. • Pneumonitis, which may be fatal.

Antiviral agents such as aciclovir and famciclovir are not required for uncomplicated childhood chickenpox. They are used when patients present within 24–48 hrs of vesicle onset, in all patients with complications, including pregnant women. Immunosuppressed patients require prolonged treatment, initially parenteral. Human VZV immunoglobulin may attenuate infection in highly susceptible contacts of chickenpox sufferers such as the immunosuppressed and pregnant women. VZV vaccine, now in use in the USA, offers effective protection.

Shingles (herpes zoster)

This is produced by reactivation of latent VZV from the dorsal root ganglion of sensory nerves and most commonly involves the

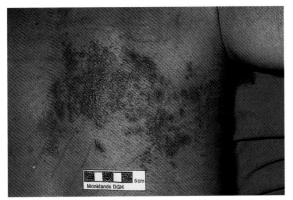

Fig. 5.6 Typical 'shingles' varicella zoster virus infection reactivating in a thoracic dermatome: 'a band of roses from Hell'.

thoracic dermatomes (Fig. 5.6) and the ophthalmic division of the trigeminal nerve.

Burning discomfort develops in the affected dermatome, followed 3–4 days later by a vesicular rash. There may be viraemia and distant 'satellite' lesions. Severe, extensive or prolonged disease suggests underlying immunosuppression, e.g. HIV. Chickenpox may be caught from shingles but not vice versa.

Complications

• Ophthalmic trigeminal involvement: may lead to corneal ulceration and requires ophthalmology review. • Ramsay Hunt syndrome: facial palsy, ipsilateral loss of taste and buccal ulceration, and a rash in the external auditory canal. • Post-herpetic neuralgia: can be difficult to treat but may respond to amitriptyline or gabapentin. • Myelitis/encephalitis: rare.

Early therapy with aciclovir helps to limit early- and late-onset pain and to prevent the development of post-herpetic neuralgia.

Dengue

The dengue flavivirus is spread by the vector mosquito *Aedes aegypti* and is endemic in South-east Asia, India, Africa and the Americas.

The incubation period following a mosquito bite is 2–7 days, with a prodrome of malaise and headache, followed by a morbilliform rash, arthralgia, pain on eye movement, headache, nausea, vomiting, lymphadenopathy and fever. The rash spreads centrifugally, spares the palms and the soles, and may desquamate on resolution. The disease is self-limiting but convalescence is slow.

Dengue haemorrhagic fever and dengue shock syndrome: These more severe manifestations occasionally complicate infection: circulatory failure, features of a capillary leak syndrome, and disseminated intravascular coagulation (DIC) with haemorrhagic complications such as petechiae, ecchymoses, epistaxis, GI bleeding and multi-organ failure. Other complications include encephalitis, hepatitis and myocarditis. Case fatality with this aggressive disease may approach 10%.

Investigations

• Detection of a 4× rise in anti-dengue IgG antibody titres.
• Amplification of dengue RNA by PCR.

Management and prevention

Management is supportive, with treatment of haemorrhage, shock and pain as required. Insecticides that control mosquito levels help to limit transmission. Aspirin should be avoided and steroids are ineffective. There is currently no licensed vaccine.

Systemic viral infections without exanthem
Mumps

Mumps is a systemic viral infection causing swelling of the parotid glands. It is endemic worldwide and peaks at 5–9 yrs of age. Vaccination has reduced childhood incidence but, if incomplete, leads to outbreaks in young adults. Infection is by respiratory droplets. Incubation lasts 15–24 days, and tender parotid swelling (bilateral in 75%) develops after a prodrome of pyrexia and headache. Diagnosis is clinical.

Complications

• Epididymo-orchitis: occurs in 25% of post-pubertal males, with testicular atrophy, although sterility is unlikely. Oophoritis is less common. • Mumps meningitis: complicates 10% of cases, with lymphocytes in CSF. • Encephalitis. • Transient hearing loss and labyrinthitis: uncommon. • Spontaneous abortion.

Management

Analgesia for symptoms is sufficient. There is no evidence that corticosteroids are of value in orchitis. Mumps vaccine, given as part of MMR vaccine, has markedly reduced incidence and, if used widely, abolishes the epidemic pattern of disease.

Influenza

This is an acute systemic viral illness predominantly affecting the respiratory system, caused by influenza A or B viruses. Seasonal changes in haemagglutinin (H) and neuraminidase (N) glycoproteins allow the organism to evade natural immunity and cause outbreaks or epidemics of varying severity.

Clinical features

Influenza is highly infectious by respiratory droplet spray from the earliest stages of infection. Incubation is 1–3 days and onset is with fever, malaise, myalgia and cough. Viral or superadded bacterial pneumonia is an important complication. Myositis, myocarditis, pericarditis and encephalitis are rare complications.

Management involves early diagnosis, scrupulous hand hygiene and infection control to limit spread by coughing and sneezing. Neuraminidase inhibitors such as oseltamivir (75 mg twice daily for 5 days) can reduce the severity of symptoms if started within 48 hrs of symptom onset.

Prevention involves seasonal vaccination of vulnerable groups, e.g. people over 65, the immunosuppressed and those with chronic illnesses.

Avian influenza is the transmission of avian influenza A from sick poultry to humans, causing severe disease. Human–human spread is rare. Swine influenza, caused by a H1N1 strain infecting humans, spread around the world from Mexico in 2009.

Infectious mononucleosis

Infectious mononucleosis (IM) is a syndrome of pharyngitis, cervical lymphadenopathy, fever and lymphocytosis, most often caused by the Epstein–Barr virus (EBV), a gamma herpesvirus. In developing countries, subclinical infection in childhood is virtually universal. In developed countries, primary infection often occurs in adolescence or later, from asymptomatic excreters. Saliva is the main means of spread, either by droplet infection or environmental contamination in childhood, or by kissing among adolescents and young adults. IM is not highly contagious, so case isolation is unnecessary.

In addition to EBV, an IM syndrome may result from infection with CMV, herpesvirus 6 or 7, HIV-1 or toxoplasmosis.

Clinical features

• Prolonged prodrome of fever, malaise and headache. • Lymphadenopathy, especially posterior cervical. • Pharyngeal inflammation or exudates. • Persisting fever and fatigue. • Splenomegaly. • Palatal petechiae. • Periorbital oedema. • Clinical or biochemical hepatitis. • A non-specific rash.

Complications

Common: Include an antibiotic-induced rash (classically amoxicillin), severe laryngeal oedema and post-viral fatigue.

Less common: Cranial nerve palsies, meningoencephalitis, haemolytic anaemia, glomerulonephritis, pericarditis, pneumonitis and haemorrhage from splenic rupture or thrombocytopenia.

Long-term: Include lymphoma in the immunosuppressed. EBV is also implicated in some forms of Hodgkin's lymphoma, Burkitt's lymphoma, and nasopharyngeal carcinoma in China and Alaska.

Investigations

• Monospot test (heterophile antibody absorption test): may initially be negative so should be repeated if clinical suspicion is high. • Atypical lymphocytes on blood film. • EBV IgM antibodies.

Management

Treatment is symptomatic, e.g. aspirin gargles to relieve a sore throat. Oral prednisolone may be required to relieve laryngeal oedema. Chronic fatigue may respond to graded exercise programmes. Contact sports should be avoided until splenomegaly has resolved to avoid splenic rupture.

Cytomegalovirus

Cytomegalovirus (CMV) circulates readily among children, in whom infection causes no symptoms. The infection is transferred by contact with an excreter, who sheds virus in saliva, urine and genital secretions. There is a second period of virus acquisition in teenagers and adults up to 35, with significant sexual and oral spread.

Most CMV infections are asymptomatic, but in adults may produce an illness resembling IM. Lymphadenopathy, pharyngitis and tonsillitis are found less often than in IM, while hepatomegaly is more common. Unusual complications include neurological involvement, autoimmune haemolytic anaemia, pericarditis, pneumonitis and arthropathy. Hepatitis, retinitis, colitis and encephalitis are among serious complications in immunosuppressed patients. CMV infection during pregnancy carries a 40% risk of fetal infection, causing rashes, hepatosplenomegaly and a 10% risk of neurological damage to the fetus.

Atypical lymphocytes are seen less commonly than in IM, and the Monospot test is negative. Detection of CMV-specific IgM antibody confirms the diagnosis and treatment is symptomatic in the immunocompetent. In immunosuppressed patients, IV ganciclovir or oral valganciclovir is useful.

Yellow fever

Yellow fever is a flavivirus infection that is a zoonosis of monkeys in the tropical rainforests of West and Central Africa and South and Central America. It is transferred to humans by infected *Aedes* or *Haemagogus* mosquitoes and is a major public health problem, causing 200 000 infections/yr, mainly in sub-Saharan Africa, with a mortality of ~15%.

The incubation period is 3–6 days, and the acute phase is usually characterised by a mild febrile illness lasting less than a week. Fever remits, then recurs in some cases after a few hours to days. In severe cases, the disease returns with rigors and high fever, severe backache, abdominal pain, nausea, vomiting, bradycardia and jaundice. This may progress to shock, DIC, hepatic and renal failure with jaundice, petechiae, mucosal haemorrhages, GI bleeding, seizures and coma.

Diagnosis is by virus isolation from blood or the identification of IgM antibodies.

Management

Treatment is supportive, with meticulous attention to fluid and electrolyte balance, urine output and BP. Blood transfusions, plasma

5.14 Common viral haemorrhagic fevers

Disease (geography)	Reservoir	Transmission	Clinical features if severe (% mortality)
Lassa fever (W Africa)	Multimammate rats	Rat urine Body fluids	Haemorrhage, encephalopathy, ARDS (responds to ribavirin) (15%)
Ebola fever (West and Central Africa)	Undefined –?bats	Body fluids Handling primates	Haemorrhage, hepatic and renal failure (25–90%)
Marburg fever (Central Africa)	Undefined	Body fluids Handling primates	Haemorrhage, diarrhoea, encephalopathy, orchitis (25–90%)
Yellow fever (Central Africa, S/ Central America)	Monkeys	Mosquitoes	Hepatic failure, renal failure, haemorrhage (~15%)
Dengue (Africa, India, S Asia, S/Central America)	Humans	*Aedes aegypti*	Haemorrhage, shock (<10%)
Crimean–Congo (Africa, Asia, E Europe)	Small vertebrates	*Ixodes* tick Body fluids	Encephalopathy, haemorrhage, hepatic/ renal failure, ARDS (30%)
Bolivian and Argentinean (S America)	Rodents (*Calomys* spp.)	Urine	Haemorrhage, shock, cerebellar signs (15–30%)
Haemorrhagic fever with renal syndrome (Hantaan fever) (N Asia, N Europe, Balkans)	Rodents	Aerosols from faeces	Renal failure, stroke, pulmonary oedema, shock (5%)

5 · INFECTIOUS DISEASE

expanders and peritoneal dialysis may be necessary. A vaccine effective for at least 10 yrs is available.

Viral haemorrhagic fevers

The viral haemorrhagic fevers are zoonoses caused by several different viruses, and occur in rural and health-care settings in defined regions, as summarised in Box 5.14. Management is supportive; ribavarin is effective in some viral haemorrhagic fevers. Transmission by infected secretions can cause major outbreaks, e.g. Ebola in West Africa in 2014. Case isolation and scrupulous infection control are essential.

Viral infections of the skin
Herpes simplex virus 1 and 2

Type 1 herpes simplex virus (HSV) typically produces mucocutaneous lesions of the head and neck, while type 2 predominantly affects the genital tract. Seroprevalence is 30–100% for HSV-1 and 20–60% for HSV-2.

Virus shed by an infected individual infects via a mucosal surface of a susceptible person. HSV infects sensory and autonomic nerve ganglia, and episodes of reactivation occur throughout life, precipitated by stress, trauma, illness or immunosuppression. Primary infection normally occurs as a vesiculating gingivostomatitis. It may also present as a keratitis (dendritic ulcer), viral paronychia, vulvovaginitis, cervicitis (often unrecognised), balanitis or rarely as encephalitis. Diagnosis is by PCR, electron microscopy or culture of vesicular fluid.

Complications

• Corneal dendritic ulcers: may produce scarring. • Encephalitis: preferentially affects the temporal lobe. • HSV infection in patients with eczema: can result in disseminated skin lesions (eczema herpeticum; Fig. 5.7). • Neonatal HSV infection: may be disseminated and potentially fatal.

Management

Treatment is with antiviral agents such as aciclovir; best results are achieved with early treatment.

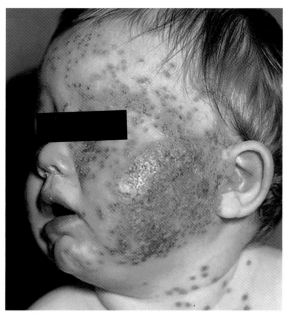

Fig. 5.7 Eczema herpeticum. Herpes simplex virus-1 infection spreads rapidly in eczematous skin.

Human herpesvirus 8

This virus, which spreads via saliva, causes Kaposi's sarcoma in both AIDS-related and endemic non-AIDS-related forms.

Enterovirus infections

Hand, foot and mouth disease: A mild febrile illness affecting children, mainly in the summer months, and caused by Coxsackie viruses or echoviruses. There is fever, lymphadenopathy, mouth ulceration and a vesicular eruption on the hands and feet.

Herpangina: Causes discrete vesicles on the palate associated with high fever, sore throat and headache.

Both of these conditions are self-limiting without treatment.

Poxvirus infections

These DNA viruses are potentially important pathogens but nowadays rarely cause significant human disease. They include smallpox, monkey pox and cow pox, as well as orf and molluscum contagiosum (p. 722).

Smallpox (variola): This severe disease, with a high mortality in the unvaccinated, was eradicated worldwide in 1980 following an international vaccination campaign. The classical form is characterised by a typical centrifugal vesicular/pustular rash, worst on the face and extremities, with no cropping (i.e. unlike chickenpox), and accompanied by fever, severe myalgia and odynophagia.

Gastrointestinal viral infections

Norovirus (Norwalk agent)

Norovirus is the most common cause of infectious gastroenteritis in the UK, causing outbreaks in closed communities such as hospital wards, cruise ships and military camps. Food handlers may also transmit norovirus. It is highly infectious by the faecal-oral route and causes prominent vomiting with diarrhoea after an incubation period of 24–48 hrs. Diagnosis is by electron microscopy or PCR of stool samples. Case isolation and scrupulous cleaning are required to control outbreaks.

Rotavirus

Rotaviruses are the major cause of diarrhoeal illness in young children worldwide and are responsible for 10–20% of deaths due to gastroenteritis in developing countries. Infection is endemic in developing countries. There are winter epidemics in developed countries, particularly in hospitals. The virus infects enterocytes, causing decreased surface absorption and loss of enzymes on the brush border. The incubation period is 48 hrs and patients present with watery diarrhoea, vomiting, fever and abdominal pain. Diagnosis is aided by commercially available enzyme immunoassay kits, which simply require fresh or refrigerated stool for effective demonstration of the pathogens. The disease is self-limiting but dehydration needs appropriate management. Effective vaccines have been developed.

Other viruses

Adenoviruses are frequently identified from stool culture and implicated as a cause of diarrhoea. Two serotypes (40 and 41) appear to be more frequently found in association with diarrhoea than the more common upper respiratory types 1–7.

PRION DISEASES

These primarily affect the nervous system and are covered on page 669.

BACTERIAL INFECTIONS

Bacterial infections of the skin, soft tissues and bones
Staphylococcal infections

Staphylococci are normal commensals of human skin and anterior nares, but they cause a variety of infections if they penetrate a break in the skin, caused either by a foreign body such as a cannula or a surgical incision, or by a primary skin condition such as eczema. Ecthyma, folliculitis, furuncles and carbuncles represent superficial skin infections with this ubiquitous organism (p. 702).

Wound and cannula-related infections caused by *Staph. aureus* are important causes of inpatient morbidity. Their incidence may be lessened by good infection control techniques. If there is evidence of spreading infection such as a surrounding cellulitis, antistaphylococcal antimicrobial therapy, e.g. flucloxacillin and benzylpenicillin, should be instituted. IV drug-users who share injecting equipment are susceptible to skin and subcutaneous tissue infections, and may also develop thrombosis in the affected limb. If staphylococcal infection reaches the blood stream (staphylococcal septicaemia), this may cause severe sepsis and needs to be treated aggressively. Growth of *Staph. aureus* in blood cultures should never be dismissed as a 'contaminant' unless all possible underlying causes have been excluded and repeat cultures are negative. Secondary spread to the heart valves, causing endocarditis, is possible in any superficial staphylococcal infection.

Meticillin-resistant Staph. aureus

Resistance to meticillin due to a penicillin-binding protein mutation has been recognised in *Staph. aureus* for over 30 yrs. Meticillin-resistant *Staph. aureus* (MRSA) is a major health-care-acquired pathogen, and the recent recognition of resistance to vancomycin/teicoplanin (glycopeptides) in either glycopeptide intermediate *Staph. aureus* (GISA) or, rarely, vancomycin-resistant (VRSA) strains threatens our ability to manage serious infections produced by such organisms. MRSA now accounts for up to 40% of staphylococcal bacteraemia in developed countries, requiring care in both control and specific therapy of these infections. Clinicians must prescribe according to sensitivity testing and take whatever appropriate infection control measures are advised locally.

Staphylococcal toxic shock syndrome

This serious and life-threatening disease is associated with infection by *Staph. aureus* that is producing toxic shock syndrome toxin 1 (TSST1). Staphylococcal toxic shock syndrome (TSS) is most commonly seen in young women in association with the use of highly absorbent tampons. The toxin acts as a 'super-antigen', triggering significant T-helper cell activation and very high peripheral polymorphonuclear leucocyte numbers.

TSS has an abrupt onset with high fever, generalised systemic upset (myalgia, headache, sore throat and vomiting), a generalised erythematous blanching rash resembling scarlet fever, and hypotension. It rapidly progresses over a matter of hours to multisystem involvement with cardiac, renal and hepatic compromise, leading to death in 10–20%. The diagnosis is clinical, supported by Gram stain of menstrual fluid demonstrating typical staphylococci. Treatment is with IV fluid resuscitation and antistaphylococcal antibiotics such as flucloxacillin or vancomycin. Recovery is accompanied at 7–10 days by desquamation (Fig. 5.8).

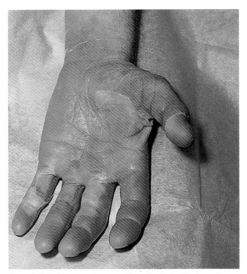

Fig. 5.8 Full-thickness desquamation after toxic shock syndrome.

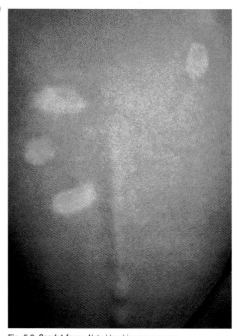

Fig. 5.9 **Scarlet fever.** Note blanching on pressure.

Streptococcal infections
Streptococcal scarlet fever

Group A and occasionally group C and G streptococci are implicated. Pharyngitis or tonsillitis may lead to scarlet fever if the organism produces pyogenic exotoxin. Common in school-age children, scarlet fever can occur in young adults in contact with young children.

A diffuse erythematous rash occurs, which blanches on pressure (Fig. 5.9), classically with circumoral pallor. The tongue, initially coated, becomes red and swollen ('strawberry tongue'). The disease lasts ~7 days; the rash disappears in 7–10 days, followed by a fine desquamation. Residual petechial lesions in the antecubital fossa may be seen. Treatment involves active therapy for the underlying infection (benzylpenicillin or orally available penicillin) plus symptomatic measures.

Streptococcal toxic shock syndrome

This is associated with severe group A, C or G streptococcal skin infections producing pyogenic exotoxin A. Initially, an influenza-like illness occurs with, in 50% of cases, signs of localised skin or soft tissue infection. A faint erythematous rash, mainly on the chest, rapidly progresses to circulatory shock then multi-organ failure.

Fluid resuscitation is essential, with parenteral antistreptococcal antibiotics, usually benzylpenicillin with clindamycin. If necrotising fasciitis is present (p. 54), urgent surgical débridement is required.

Cellulitis, erysipelas and impetigo
See pages 701 and 702.

Other streptococcal infections
These are shown in Box 5.15.

5.15 Streptococcal and related infections

Group A (*Strep. pyogenes*)

- Skin/tissue infection (erysipelas, impetigo, necrotising fasciitis)
- Puerperal sepsis
- Glomerulonephritis
- Bone and joint infection
- Streptococcal toxic shock syndrome
- Scarlet fever
- Rheumatic fever
- Tonsillitis

Group B streptococci (*Strep. agalactiae*)

- Neonatal infections, including meningitis
- Septicaemia
- Female pelvic infections
- Cellulitis

Group D enterococci (*E. faecalis*)

- Endocarditis
- Urinary tract infection

α-haemolytic *viridans* streptococci (*Strep. mitis, sanguinis, mutans, salivarius*)

- Endocarditis
- Septicaemia in immunosuppressed

α-haemolytic optochin-sensitive (*Strep. pneumoniae*)

- Pneumonia
- Meningitis
- Endocarditis
- Septicaemia
- Bacterial peritonitis
- Otitis media

Anaerobic streptococci (*Peptostreptococcus* spp.)

- Peritonitis
- Liver abscess
- Dental infections
- Pelvic inflammatory disease

N.B. All streptococci can cause septicaemia.

Treponematoses
Syphilis

This disease is described on page 125.

Endemic treponematoses

Yaws: This granulomatous disease is caused by *Treponema pertenue*, which is morphologically and serologically indistinguishable from the causative organisms of syphilis and pinta. Organisms are transmitted by bodily contact from a patient with infectious yaws through minor abrasions of the skin, producing a granulomatous primary lesion, usually on the leg or buttock. The secondary eruption usually follows a few weeks or months later. There may also be hypertrophic periosteal bone lesions, and in late yaws osteitis and gummas resembling tertiary syphilis.

Pinta and bejel: These two treponemal infections occur in poor rural populations with low standards of domestic hygiene, but are found in separate parts of the world (pinta: South and Central America; bejel: Middle East, Central Asia). They have features in common, notably that they are transmitted by contact, usually within the family and not sexually, and in the case of bejel, through common eating and drinking utensils.

For yaws, pinta and bejel, diagnosis is by microscopic detection of spirochaetes and serology; treatment involves a single IM dose of long-acting (e.g. benzathine) benzylpenicillin. Improvements in domestic hygiene greatly reduce these diseases.

Systemic bacterial infections
Brucellosis

Brucellosis is caused by an intracellular organism endemic in animals. Although six species of *Brucella* are known, only four are important to humans:

• *B. melitensis* (goats, sheep and camels). • *B. abortus* (cattle). • *B. suis* (pigs). • *B. canis* (dogs).

B. melitensis causes the most severe disease.

Infected animals may excrete brucellae in their milk for long periods and human infection is acquired by ingesting contaminated milk, cheese, yoghurt, butter and uncooked meat, or via the respiratory tract through splashes of infected secretions or excreta.

Clinical features

Acute illness is characterised by a high swinging temperature, rigors, sweating, lethargy, headache, and joint and muscle pains. Occasionally, there is delirium, abdominal pain and constipation. Physical signs are non-specific, e.g. enlarged lymph nodes or a palpable spleen that may lead to hypersplenism and thrombocytopenia. Other features are shown in Box 5.16.

Investigations

• Blood cultures: prolonged incubation may be required. *B. melitensis* is the most readily cultured species. • CSF culture in

5.16 Focal manifestations of brucellosis	
Musculoskeletal	Suppurative arthritis, synovitis, bursitis; spinal spondylitis; osteomyelitis; paravertebral or psoas abscess
CNS	Meningitis; stroke; cranial nerve palsies; myelopathy; intracranial or subarachnoid haemorrhage; radiculopathy
Ocular	Uveitis; retinal thrombophlebitis
Cardiac	Myocarditis; endocarditis
Respiratory	Pneumonitis; lung abscess; hilar adenopathy
Abdominal	Splenic abscess or calcification, hepatitis, orchitis

neurobrucellosis: positive in ~30% of cases. • Serology: a single titre of >1/320 or a fourfold rise in antibody supports the diagnosis but can take several weeks.

Management

Aminoglycosides show synergistic activity with tetracyclines when used against brucellae. Standard therapy therefore consists of 6 wks of doxycycline with IV gentamicin for the first 7 days. Rifampicin is added if there is bone involvement, and ceftriaxone if there is neurobrucellosis.

Borrelia *infections*
Lyme disease

Lyme disease (named after the town of Old Lyme in Connecticut, USA) is caused by *Borrelia burgdorferi*. The reservoir of infection is maintained in ixodid (hard) ticks that feed on a variety of large mammals, particularly deer. The organism is transmitted to humans via infected tick bites. Lyme disease is found in the USA, Europe, Russia, China, Japan and Australia.

Clinical features: There are three stages: early localised, early disseminated and late disease. Progression may be arrested at any stage.

Early localised disease: The characteristic feature is a skin reaction around the site of the tick bite, known as erythema migrans. Initially, a red macule or papule appears 2–30 days after the bite. It then enlarges peripherally with central clearing ('bull's eye macule'), and may persist for months. The rash may be accompanied by fever, headache and regional lymphadenopathy.

Early disseminated disease: Dissemination occurs via the blood stream and lymphatics. There may be a systemic reaction with malaise, arthralgia and occasionally metastatic areas of erythema migrans. Neurological involvement may follow weeks or months after infection, with lymphocytic meningitis, cranial nerve palsies (especially unilateral or bilateral facial palsy) and peripheral neuropathy. Radiculopathy, often painful, may present a year or more after initial infection. Carditis, sometimes accompanied by atrioventricular conduction defects, is common in the USA but rarer in Europe.

Late disease: Late manifestations include arthritis, polyneuritis and encephalopathy. Prolonged arthritis, particularly affecting large joints, is a well-described feature but is rare in the UK. Brain parenchymal involvement causing neuropsychiatric abnormalities may also be encountered, but again is very rare in the UK. Acrodermatitis chronica atrophicans is an uncommon late complication seen more frequently in Europe than North America. Doughy, patchy discoloration occurs on the peripheries, eventually leading to shiny atrophic skin. The lesions are easily mistaken for those of peripheral vascular disease.

Investigations: The diagnosis of Lyme borreliosis is often clinical. Anti-*Borrelia* antibody detection is frequently negative in the early stages, but 90–100% sensitive in late disease. Culture from biopsies is slow and not generally available; it has a low yield. PCR has been used to detect DNA in blood, urine and CSF.

Management: Standard therapy consists of a 14-day course of doxycycline or amoxicillin; disseminated disease will require more prolonged treatment. Some 15% of patients with early disease will develop a mild Jarisch–Herxheimer reaction during the first 24 hrs of therapy. Neuroborreliosis is treated with parenteral β-lactam antibiotics for 3–4 wks. Preventative measures (such as protective clothing and insect repellents) should be used in tick-infested areas.

Louse-borne relapsing fever

The human body louse, *Pediculus humanus*, causes itching. Borreliae (*B. recurrentis*) are liberated from the infected lice when they are crushed during scratching, which also inoculates the borreliae into the skin.

The borreliae invade most tissues of the body, including liver, spleen and meninges, causing hepatosplenomegaly, jaundice and meningism, accompanied by high fever, tachycardia and headache. Marked thrombocytopenia results in petechial rash, serosal haemorrhage and epistaxis. The acute illness lasts between 4 and 10 days. A proportion of patients may relapse.

Examination of thick and thin blood films or dark-field microscopy allows diagnosis. Treatment is with procaine penicillin followed by tetracycline. A severe Jarisch–Herxheimer reaction is seen with successful chemotherapy.

Tick-borne relapsing fever

Soft ticks (*Ornithodoros* spp.) transmit *B. duttonii* (and several other *Borrelia* species) through saliva while feeding on their host. Rodents are the reservoir in all parts of the world, except in East Africa where humans are the reservoir.

Clinical manifestations are similar to the louse-borne disease but spirochaetes are detected in fewer patients on dark-field microscopy. A 7-day course of treatment with either tetracycline or erythromycin is needed.

Leptospirosis

Leptospires are tightly coiled, thread-like organisms, ~5–7 μm in length, which are actively motile by rotating and bending. In reservoir species they persist in the convoluted tubules of the kidney without causing apparent disease, and are shed into the urine in massive numbers. Particular leptospiral serogroups are associated with characteristic animal hosts; for example, *Leptospira icterohaemorrhagica* is the classical parasite of rats, and *L. canicola* of dogs.

Leptospires can enter their human hosts through intact or injured skin or mucous membranes, e.g. following immersion in contaminated water.

Clinical features

The incubation period averages 1–2 wks. Four main clinical syndromes can be discerned:

Bacteraemic leptospirosis: A non-specific illness with high fever, weakness, muscle pain and tenderness (especially of the calf and back), intense headache and photophobia, and sometimes diarrhoea and vomiting. Conjunctival congestion is the only notable physical sign. The illness comes to an end after ~1 wk, or else merges into one of the other forms of infection.

Aseptic meningitis: Classically associated with *L. canicola*, this is very difficult to distinguish from viral meningitis. The conjunctivae may be congested but there are no other differentiating signs.

Icteric leptospirosis (Weil's disease): A dramatic, life-threatening event, accounting for <10% of symptomatic infections. It is characterised by fever, haemorrhages, jaundice and renal impairment. Conjunctival hyperaemia is a frequent feature. The patient may have a transient macular erythematous rash, but the characteristic skin changes are those of purpura, with large areas of bruising. In severe cases there may be epistaxis, haematemesis and melaena, or bleeding into the pleural, pericardial or subarachnoid spaces. Thrombocytopenia is present in 50% of cases. Jaundice is deep and the liver is enlarged, but there is usually little evidence of hepatic failure or encephalopathy. Renal failure, primarily caused by impaired renal perfusion and acute tubular necrosis, results in oliguria or anuria, with the presence of albumin, blood and casts in the urine. Myocarditis, encephalitis and aseptic meningitis are other associated features. Uveitis and iritis may appear months after apparent clinical recovery.

Pulmonary syndrome: This is particularly recognised in the Far East. It is characterised by haemoptysis, patchy lung infiltrates on CXR and respiratory failure. Total bilateral lung consolidation and ARDS develop in severe cases.

Investigations

Laboratory tests show polymorphonuclear leucocytosis, thrombocytopenia and elevated creatine phosphokinase. In jaundiced patients LFTs are mildly hepatitic in pattern, with moderately raised transaminases; the prothrombin time may be prolonged. A lumbar puncture may show moderately elevated protein level and a normal glucose content in the CSF. Definitive diagnosis requires detection of the organism, its DNA, or a rising antibody titre:

• Blood culture: most likely to be positive if taken before the 10th day of illness. • Urine culture: leptospires are present in the urine from the 2nd wk of illness. • Microscopic agglutination test (MAT): seroconversion or a fourfold rise in titre between acute and convalescent sera is confirmatory. • PCR: can detect leptospiral DNA in blood in early symptomatic disease, and is positive in urine from the 8th day and for many months afterwards.

Management and prevention

Supportive management, including the transfusion of blood and platelets, along with dialysis, is critical. Oral doxycycline or IV penicillin is effective but may not prevent renal failure. IV ceftriaxone is an effective alternative. A Jarisch–Herxheimer reaction may occur during treatment but is usually mild. Prophylactic doxycycline 200 mg weekly can prevent infection.

Plague

Plague is caused by *Yersinia pestis*, a small Gram-negative bacillus that is spread between rodents by their fleas, which may also bite humans. In the late stages of human plague, *Y. pestis* may be expectorated and spread between humans by droplets. Epidemics of plague, such as the 'Black Death', have attacked humans since ancient times, with a high fatality rate. Because it can spread by aerosol and because pneumonic plague is frequently fatal, it is also a potential bioweapon.

The incubation period is 3–6 days following access via the skin but is shorter after inhalation.

Three distinct forms are recognised.

Bubonic plague: In this, the most common form of the disease, the onset is usually sudden with a rigor, high fever, dry skin and severe headache. Soon, aching and swelling at the site of the affected lymph nodes begin. The groin is the most common site of the 'bubo' (the swollen lymph nodes and surrounding tissue). A rapid pulse, hypotension, mental confusion and splenomegaly develop rapidly.

Septicaemic plague: In this form, common in the elderly, the patient is toxic and may have GI symptoms such as nausea, vomiting, abdominal pain and diarrhoea. DIC may occur, manifested by bleeding from various orifices or puncture sites, along with ecchymoses. Hypotension, shock, renal failure and ARDS may lead to further deterioration. Meningitis, pneumonia and expectoration of blood-stained sputum may complicate the picture. There is a high mortality.

Pneumonic plague: The onset is very sudden with cough and dyspnoea. The patient soon expectorates copious blood-stained, frothy, highly infective sputum, becomes cyanosed and dies. X-rays of the lung show bilateral nodular infiltrates progressing to ARDS.

Investigations

The organism may be cultured from blood, sputum or bubo aspirates. Characteristic bipolar coccobacilli are seen in smears of these fluids after staining with Wayson's stain or by immunofluorescence. Seroconversion or a single anti-F1 antibody titre >128 confirms the diagnosis. DNA diagnosis through PCR is under evaluation. Plague is a notifiable disease.

Management

Immediate treatment is vital. Streptomycin or gentamicin is the drug of choice. Tetracycline and chloramphenicol are alternatives. Treatment may also be needed for acute circulatory failure, DIC and hypoxia. The patient should be isolated for 48 hrs, carers should wear protective clothing, and inadvertent exposure should prompt prophylactic treatment with doxycycline.

Listeriosis

Listeria monocytogenes is an environmental bacterium that can contaminate food, including cheese and undercooked meats. It outgrows other pathogens during refrigeration. It causes gastroenteritis in immunocompetent patients, but more serious invasive illness in the elderly, immunocompromised and pregnant women. In pregnancy, in addition to systemic symptoms like fever and myalgia, listeriosis causes chorioamnionitis, fetal deaths, abortions and neonatal infection. Meningitis is another common manifestation. Diagnosis is made by blood and CSF culture. The most effective treatment is a combination of IV ampicillin with an aminoglycoside. A sulfamethoxazole/trimethoprim combination can be used in those with penicillin sensitivity. Good food hygiene helps to prevent infection. Pregnant women should avoid high-risk foods (see Box 5.6 above).

Typhoid and paratyphoid (enteric) fevers

These diseases, which are transmitted by the faecal–oral route, are important causes of fever in India, sub-Saharan Africa and Latin America. Elsewhere they are relatively rare. The causative organisms are *Salmonella typhi* and *S. paratyphi* A and B.

Clinical features

Typhoid fever: The incubation period of typhoid fever is ~10–14 days, and the onset may be insidious. The temperature rises in a stepladder fashion for 4 or 5 days with malaise, increasing headache, drowsiness and aching in the limbs. Constipation may be present, although in children diarrhoea and vomiting may be prominent early in the illness. There is a relative bradycardia. At the end of the 1st wk a rash may appear on the upper abdomen and on the back as sparse, slightly raised, rose-red spots, which fade on pressure. Cough and epistaxis occur. Around the 7th–10th day the spleen becomes palpable. Constipation is then succeeded by diarrhoea and abdominal distension with tenderness. Bronchitis and delirium may develop. If untreated, by the end of the 2nd wk the patient may be profoundly ill. Following recovery, up to 5% of patients become chronic carriers of *S. typhi*.

Paratyphoid fever: The course tends to be shorter and milder than that of typhoid fever and the onset is often more abrupt, with acute enteritis. The rash may be more abundant and the intestinal complications less frequent.

Complications

Haemorrhage from, or a perforation of, the ulcerated Peyer's patches (follicles where bacilli localise) in the small intestine may occur at 2–3 wks into the illness. Additional complications include cholecystitis, myocarditis, nephritis, arthritis and meningitis. Bone and joint infection is common in children with sickle-cell disease.

Investigations

Blood culture is the most important diagnostic method in a suspected case. Blood count typically shows leucopenia. The faeces will contain the organism more frequently during the 2nd and 3rd wks.

Management

Ciprofloxacin (500 mg 4 times daily) is the drug of choice, although resistance is rising in India and the UK. Ceftriaxone or azithromycin is an alternative. Treatment should be continued for 14 days; pyrexia may persist for up to 5 days after the start of specific therapy. Improved sanitation and living conditions, and vaccination of travellers reduce the incidence of typhoid.

Tularaemia

Tularaemia is caused by a highly infectious Gram-negative bacillus, *Francisella tularensis*, and is a zoonotic disease of the northern hemisphere. Wild rabbits and domestic dogs or cats are the reservoirs; ticks and mosquitoes are the vectors.

Infection is introduced through insect bites, resulting in the most common 'ulceroglandular' variety of the disease (70–80%), characterised by skin ulceration with regional lymphadenopathy. Inhalation of the infected aerosols may result in pulmonary tularaemia, presenting as pneumonia. Rarely, the portal of entry of infection may be the conjunctiva, leading to a nodular, ulcerated conjunctivitis with regional lymphadenopathy (an 'oculoglandular' form). Demonstration of a single high titre ($\geq 1:160$) or a fourfold rise in 2–3 wks in the tularaemia tube agglutination test confirms the diagnosis. PCR is being developed for rapid, reliable diagnosis. Treatment consists of a 7–10-day course of parenteral streptomycin or gentamicin.

Melioidosis

Melioidosis is a febrile illness with pneumonia and hepatosplenomegaly; it is found in South India, East Asia and northern Australia. The CXR may resemble that in TB, and subcutaneous abscesses are also a feature. Culture of blood, sputum or pus may reveal the causative organism, *Burkholderia pseudomallei*. Treatment is with IV ceftazidime or meropenem, followed by oral doxycycline and co-trimoxazole for at least 12 wks. Abscesses should be drained.

Gastrointestinal bacterial infections
Food poisoning

Bacterial causes of acute gastroenteritis are listed in Box 5.4 above.

Staphylococcal food poisoning

Staph. aureus transmission occurs from the hands of food handlers to foodstuffs such as dairy products, including cheese, and cooked meats. Inappropriate storage permits growth and production of heat-stable enterotoxins.

Nausea and vomiting develop within 1–6 hrs. Diarrhoea may not be marked. Most cases settle rapidly but severe dehydration can occasionally be life-threatening. The mainstays of treatment are antiemetics and fluid replacement. Public health authorities should be notified if the source was a food vendor.

Bacillus cereus

Rapid onset of vomiting within hours of food consumption occurs after the ingestion of the pre-formed enterotoxins of *B. cereus*. Fried rice or sauces are frequent sources, and enterotoxin is formed during storage. Between 1 and 4 hrs after ingestion, brisk vomiting and some diarrhoea occur, with rapid resolution within 24 hrs.

If viable organisms are ingested, the toxin is produced within the gut, leading to a longer incubation period of 12–24 hrs and watery diarrhoea with abdominal cramps. The disease is self-limiting. Management simply consists of fluid replacement and public health notification.

Clostridium perfringens

Spores of *C. perfringens* are widespread in the guts of large animals and in soil. In anaerobic conditions, *C. perfringens* spores in incompletely cooked contaminated meat germinate and viable organisms multiply to give large numbers. Subsequent reheating of the food causes heat-shock sporulation of the organisms, during which they release an enterotoxin. Symptoms (diarrhoea and cramps) occur 6–12 hrs following ingestion.

'Point source' outbreaks, in which a number of cases all become symptomatic following ingestion, classically occur after school or canteen lunches where meat stews are served. Clostridial enterotoxins are potent and most people who ingest them will be symptomatic. The illness is usually self-limiting.

Campylobacter jejuni

This infection is a zoonosis carried in the gut of cattle and poultry, and is the most common cause of bacterial gastroenteritis in the UK. The most common source of the infection is meat, such as chicken, or contaminated milk products, although the organism can also survive in fresh water.

The incubation period is 2–5 days. Colicky abdominal pain ensues, along with nausea, vomiting and significant diarrhoea, frequently containing blood. Most *Campylobacter* infections affect fit young adults and are self-limiting after 5–7 days. Between 10 and 20% have prolonged symptoms and merit treatment with antibiotics such as erythromycin, as ciprofloxacin resistance is common. About 1% of cases will develop bacteraemia and possible distant foci of infection. *Campylobacter* spp. have been linked to Guillain–Barré syndrome and post-infectious reactive arthritis.

Salmonella *spp.*

These Gram-negative organisms produce two distinct clinical entities:

• The serotypes *S. typhi* and *S. paratyphi* A, B, C have a purely human reservoir and produce the septicaemic illness 'enteric fever' (see above). • Other *Salmonella* serotypes are subdivided into five distinct subgroups that produce gastroenteritis, of which *S. enteritidis* and *S. typhimurium* are the most important.

Transmission is by contaminated water or food, particularly poultry, egg products and related fast foods.

The incubation period of *Salmonella* gastroenteritis is 12–72 hrs and the predominant feature is diarrhoea, sometimes containing blood. Vomiting may be present at the outset. About 5% of cases will be bacteraemic. Reactive (post-infective) arthritis occurs in ~2% of cases. Antibiotics are not indicated unless there is bacteraemia, which is a clear indication for antibiotic therapy, as salmonellae are notorious for persistent infection and often colonise endothelial surfaces such as an atherosclerotic aorta or a major blood vessel.

Escherichia coli

E. coli is a major member of the Enterobacteriaceae and may be present without causing disease in the human gut at any given time. There are five different clinico-pathological patterns of disease, all associated with diarrhoea.

Enterotoxigenic E. coli (ETEC): These cause most cases of travellers' diarrhoea in developing countries, although other causes are possible (Box 5.17). The organisms produce either a heat-labile or a heat-stable enterotoxin, causing marked secretory diarrhoea and vomiting after 1–2 days' incubation. The illness is usually mild and self-limiting after 3–4 days. Ciprofloxacin has been used to limit the duration of symptoms but benefit is unproven.

Enteroinvasive E. coli (EIEC): This illness is very similar to *Shigella* dysentery and is caused by invasion and destruction of colonic

- Enterotoxigenic *E. coli* (ETEC)
- *Shigella* spp.
- *Campylobacter jejuni*
- *Salmonella* spp.
- *Plesiomonas shigelloides*
- Non-cholera *Vibrio* spp.
- *Aeromonas* spp.

mucosal cells. No enterotoxin is produced. Acute watery diarrhoea, abdominal cramps and some scanty blood-staining of the stool are common. The symptoms are rarely severe and are usually self-limiting.

Enteropathogenic E. coli (EPEC): These are very important in infant diarrhoea. Ability to attach to the gut mucosa is the basis of their pathogenicity. This causes destruction of microvilli and disruption of normal absorptive capacity. The symptoms vary from mild non-bloody diarrhoea to quite severe illness.

Enteroaggregative E. coli (EAEC): These strains adhere to the mucosa and produce a locally active enterotoxin. A 'stacked brick' aggregation is seen in the small bowel. They have been associated with prolonged diarrhoea in children in South America, South-east Asia and India.

Enterohaemorrhagic E. coli (EHEC): A number of distinct 'O' serotypes of *E. coli* produce two distinct enterotoxins (verocytotoxin), which are identical to toxins produced by *Shigella* ('shiga toxins 1 and 2'). *E. coli* O157:H7 is perhaps the best known of these verocytotoxigenic *E. coli* (VTEC), but others, including types O126 and O11, are also implicated. The organism has an extremely low infecting dose (10–100 organisms). The reservoir of infection is in the gut of herbivores. Contaminated milk and meat products, such as hamburgers, have long been recognised as a source of this infection. The incubation period is between 1 and 7 days. Initial watery diarrhoea becomes frankly and uniformly blood-stained in 70% of cases and is associated with severe and often constant abdominal pain. There is little systemic upset, vomiting or fever. Enterotoxins, if produced, have both a local effect on the bowel and a distant effect on particular body tissues such as glomerular apparatus, heart and brain. The potentially life-threatening haemolytic uraemic syndrome (HUS – p. 182) occurs in 10–15% of sufferers from this infection, arising 5–7 days after the onset of symptoms. It is most likely at the extremes of age, is heralded by a high peripheral leucocyte count and may be induced, particularly in children, by antibiotic therapy. HUS is treated by dialysis if necessary and may be averted by active intervention with processes such as plasma exchange.

Clostridium difficile *infection*

C. difficile is occasionally present in normal gut flora. Clinical infection usually follows up to 6 wks after antibiotic therapy, which alters gut flora. Transmission is by spores, which are resistant to alcohol hand gels, and disease results from the production of two toxins. A number of different ribotypes of the organism exist, the 027 ribotype producing particularly severe disease and significant mortality.

Infection causes diarrhoea, which may be bloody, and may be complicated by pseudomembranous colitis. Around 80% of cases are over 65 yrs of age, and many have multiple comorbidities.

C. difficile is found in the stool in 30% of cases of antibiotic-associated diarrhoea and 90% of those with pseudomembranous colitis, but also in 20% of healthy elderly patients in care. Diagnosis therefore depends on finding *C. difficile* toxin in the stool.

Precipitating antibiotics should be stopped. Treatment is with oral metronidazole for 10 days or, in severe cases, oral vancomycin. Faecal transplantation is emerging as a treatment for relapses. Prevention requires careful infection control and restriction of antibiotic prescription.

Yersinia enterocolitica

This organism, commonly found in pork, causes mild to moderate gastroenteritis and can produce significant mesenteric adenitis after an incubation period of 3–7 days. It predominantly causes disease in children but adults may also be affected. The illness resolves slowly, with 10–30% of cases complicated by persistent arthritis or Reiter's syndrome.

Cholera

Cholera, caused by *Vibrio cholerae* serotype 01, is the archetypal bacterial cause of acute watery diarrhoea. Infection spreads via the stools or vomit of symptomatic patients or those of the much larger number of subclinical cases. It survives for up to 2 wks in fresh water and 8 wks in salt water. Transmission is normally through infected drinking water, shellfish and food contaminated by flies, or on the hands of carriers.

Clinical features: Severe diarrhoea without pain or colic begins suddenly and is followed by vomiting. Following the evacuation of normal gut faecal contents, typical 'rice-water' material is passed, consisting of clear fluid with flecks of mucus, resulting in enormous loss of fluid and electrolytes. Shock and oliguria ensue, necessitating fluid and electrolyte replacement.

Investigations and management: The diagnosis should be confirmed by visualisation of the organism on stool dark-field microscopy, which shows the 'shooting star' motility of *V. cholerae*. Rectal swab or stool cultures allow identification. Cholera is notifiable under international health regulations. Replacement of fluid and

INFECTIOUS DISEASE • 5

electrolyte losses is paramount. IV Ringer's lactate is used until vomiting stops; thereafter, oral rehydration solution is ideal for this purpose. Up to 50 L may be needed in 2–5 days. Treatment with tetracycline, doxycycline or ciprofloxacin reduces the duration of excretion of *Vibrio*. Strict personal hygiene, a clean piped water supply and good food hygiene practices prevent the spread of disease.

Vibrio parahaemolyticus

This marine organism produces a disease similar to enterotoxigenic *E. coli*. It is acquired from raw seafood and is very common where ingestion of such food is widespread (e.g. Japan). After an incubation period of ~20 hrs, explosive diarrhoea, abdominal cramps and vomiting occur. Systemic symptoms of headache and fever are frequent but the illness is self-limiting, taking 4–7 days to resolve.

Bacillary dysentery (shigellosis)

Shigellae are Gram-negative rods, closely related to *E. coli*, that invade the colonic mucosa. They are often multi-resistant to antibiotics. The organism only infects humans and its spread is facilitated by its low infecting dose of ~10 organisms. Transmission by unwashed hands after defecation is by far the most common. Outbreaks occur in mental hospitals, residential schools and other closed institutions.

Disease severity varies with serotype; cases due to *Shigella sonnei* are mild, while those due to *Sh. dysenteriae* may be fulminating and cause death within 48 hrs. Symptoms include diarrhoea, which may be bloody, colicky abdominal pain and tenesmus. Arthritis or iritis may occasionally complicate bacillary dysentery (Reiter's syndrome; p. 587), and may be associated with HLA-B27.

Oral rehydration therapy is necessary to replace water and electrolytes. Antibiotic therapy with ciprofloxacin for 3 days is effective in known shigellosis and appropriate in epidemics. Hand-washing is important to prevent faecal contamination of food and milk.

Respiratory bacterial infections

Pneumonia, bronchitis and pulmonary TB are dealt with in Chapter 9.

Diphtheria

Corynebacterium diphtheriae, the causative organism, is highly contagious, and spreads by droplet infection. The average incubation period is 2–4 days. Diphtheria was eradicated from much of the developed world by mass vaccination in the mid-20th century but remains an important cause of illness in some countries, which has prompted the WHO to issue guidelines for the management of infection.

Clinical features

Acutely, the disease presents as membranous tonsillitis, nasal infection or laryngeal infection. The diagnostic feature is the 'wash-leather' elevated greyish-green membrane on the tonsils. There may be swelling of the neck ('bull-neck') and tender enlargement of the lymph nodes, or blood-stained nasal discharge. Complications occur as a result of exotoxins acting on the heart or nervous system, and include myocarditis and peripheral neuropathy. Laryngeal obstruction or paralysis may occur and is life-threatening.

Management

This should take place in a hospital for infectious diseases. Treatment should begin once appropriate swabs have been taken rather than waiting for microbiological confirmation. The three main areas of management are:
• Diphtheria antitoxin produced from hyperimmune horse serum: neutralises any toxin not fixed to tissue but can cause anaphylaxis.
• Administration of antibiotic: penicillin or amoxicillin. • Strict isolation procedures: cases must be isolated until cultures from three swabs 24 hrs apart are negative.

Prevention

Active immunisation should be given to all children. If diphtheria occurs in a closed community, contacts should be given erythromycin, which is more effective than penicillin in eradicating the organism in carriers. All contacts should also be immunised or given a booster dose of toxoid. Booster doses are required every 10 yrs to maintain immunity.

Pneumococcal infection

Streptococcus is the leading cause of pneumonia (p. 289) but also causes otitis media, meningitis and sinusitis. Asplenic individuals are at risk of fulminant pneumococcal sepsis. Penicillin and macrolide resistance is increasing, although still uncommon in the UK. Pneumococcal vaccine is helpful in those predisposed to infection, especially the elderly and those without a functioning spleen.

Anthrax

The Gram-positive *Bacillus anthracis* usually causes infection through contact with herbivores, though its spores can survive for years in soil. There are three recognised forms of infection:

Cutaneous anthrax: When hides and bones, spores are inoculated into exposed skin, producing an irritated papule on an oedematous haemorrhagic base. This develops into a black eschar.

GI anthrax: This is caused by ingestion of contaminated meat. The caecum is the seat of infection, producing nausea, vomiting, anorexia and fever, followed 2–3 days later by abdominal pain and bloody diarrhoea.

Inhalational (pulmonary) anthrax: Disease caused by inhalation of spores is very rare but is a potential form of bioterrorism. Fever, dyspnoea, cough, headache, pleural effusions and septicaemia develop 3–14 days after exposure and mortality is 50–90%.

Management
B. anthracis can be cultured from lesional skin swabs. Skin lesions are readily curable with early antibiotic therapy. Treatment is with ciprofloxacin until penicillin susceptibility is confirmed; the regimen can then be changed to benzylpenicillin IM. Aggressive fluid resuscitation and the addition of an aminoglycoside may improve the outlook. Prophylaxis with ciprofloxacin is recommended for anyone at high risk of exposure to biological warfare.

Bacterial infections with neurological involvement
Bacterial meningitis, botulism and tetanus are dealt with in Chapter 16.

Mycobacterial infections
Tuberculosis
This is described in Chapter 9.

Leprosy
Leprosy (Hansen's disease) is a chronic granulomatous disease affecting skin and nerve, and is caused by *Mycobacterium leprae*. The clinical form of the disease is determined by the degree of cell-mediated immunity (CMI) expressed by that individual towards *M. leprae*. High levels of CMI with elimination of leprosy bacilli produce tuberculoid leprosy, whereas absent CMI results in lepromatous leprosy. The medical complications of leprosy are due to nerve damage, immunological reactions and bacillary infiltration. It affects 4 million people worldwide, 70% of whom live in India, with the remainder in Brazil, Indonesia, Mozambique, Madagascar, Tanzania and Nepal.

Untreated lepromatous patients discharge bacilli from the nose. Infection occurs through the nose, followed by haematogenous spread to skin and nerve. The incubation period is 2–5 yrs for tuberculoid cases and 8–12 yrs for lepromatous cases.

Clinical features
The cardinal features are skin lesions with anaesthesia, thickened peripheral nerves and acid-fast bacilli on skin smear or biopsy. The features of the two principal types of leprosy are compared in Box 5.18.

Skin: The most common skin lesions are macules or plaques. Tuberculoid patients have a few hypopigmented lesions. In lepromatous leprosy, papules, nodules or diffuse infiltration of the skin occur. Confluent lesions on the face can lead to a 'leonine facies' (Fig. 5.10).

5.18 Clinical characteristics of the polar forms of leprosy

Clinical and tissue-specific features	Lepromatous	Tuberculoid
Skin and nerves		
No. and distribution	Wide dissemination	Few sites, asymmetrical
Skin lesions		
Margin – definition	Poor	Good
– elevation	Never	Common
Colour – dark skin	Slight hypopigmentation	Marked hypopigmentation
– light skin	Slight erythema	Coppery or red
Surface	Smooth, shiny	Dry, scaly
Central healing	None	Common
Sweat, hair	Impaired late	Impaired early
Loss of sensation	Late	Early, marked
Nerve enlargement/ damage	Late	Early, marked
Bacilli	Many	Absent
Natural history	Progressive	Self-healing
Other tissues	Upper respiratory mucosa, eye, testes, bone, muscle	None
Reactions	Immune complexes (type 2)	Cell-mediated (type 1)

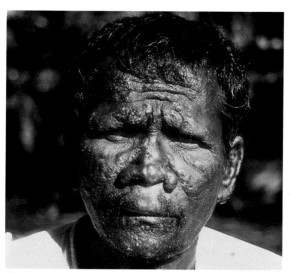

Fig. 5.10 Lepromatous leprosy. Widespread nodules and infiltration with loss of the eyebrows. This man also has early collapse of the nose.

Anaesthesia: In skin lesions, the small dermal sensory and auto-nomic nerve fibres are damaged, causing local sensory loss and loss of sweating within that area. Anaesthesia may also occur in the distribution of a large peripheral nerve, or in a 'glove and stocking' distribution.

Nerve damage: Peripheral nerve trunks are affected at 'sites of predilection', including the ulnar (elbow), median (wrist), radial (humerus, causing wrist drop), radial cutaneous (wrist), common peroneal (knee), posterior tibial and sural nerves at the ankle, facial nerve as it crosses the zygomatic arch, and great auricular in the posterior triangle of the neck. All these nerves should be examined for enlargement and tenderness, and tested for motor and sensory function. The CNS is not affected.

Eye involvement: Blindness due to leprosy is a devastating com-plication for a patient with anaesthetic hands and feet. Eyelid closure is impaired when the facial (7th) nerve is affected. Damage to the trigeminal (5th) nerve causes anaesthesia of the cornea and conjunc-tiva. The cornea is then susceptible to trauma and ulceration.

Other features: These include nasal collapse due to bony destruc-tion and hypogonadism from testicular atrophy.

Borderline cases

Borderline tuberculoid (BT): The skin lesions are more numerous than in tuberculoid leprosy, and there is more severe peripheral nerve damage. These patients are prone to type 1 reactions (see below) with consequent nerve damage.

Borderline leprosy (BB): Patients have numerous skin lesions varying in size, shape and distribution. Annular lesions are charac-teristic and nerve damage is variable.

Borderline lepromatous leprosy (BL): There are widespread small macules and nerve involvement. Patients may experience both type 1 and type 2 reactions.

Pure neural leprosy: This type occurs principally in India and accounts for 10% of cases. Asymmetrical peripheral nerve involve-ment occurs without skin lesions.

Leprosy reactions

These are events superimposed on the cardinal features described above.

Type 1 (reversal) reactions: These occur in 30% of borderline patients (BT, BB, BL) and are delayed hypersensitivity reactions. Skin lesions become erythematous; peripheral nerves become tender and painful with sudden loss of nerve function. Reversal reactions may occur spontaneously, after starting treatment or after comple-tion of multidrug therapy.

Type 2 (erythema nodosum leprosum – ENL) reactions: Partly due to immune complex deposition, these occur in BL and lepromatous patients who produce antibodies and have a high antigen load. They manifest with malaise, fever and crops of small pink nodules on the

| | 5.19 Modified WHO-recommended multidrug therapy regimens in leprosy |

Type of leprosy*	Monthly supervised treatment	Daily self-administered treatment	Duration of treatment
Paucibacillary	Rifampicin 600 mg	Dapsone 100 mg	6 mths
Multibacillary	Rifampicin 600 mg Clofazimine 300 mg	Clofazimine 50 mg Dapsone 100 mg	12 mths

In this field classification WHO recommends treatment of multibacillary patients for 12 mths only.
*WHO classification for field use when slit skin smears are not available:
• paucibacillary (1–5 skin lesions; includes old 'single-lesion' category)
• multibacillary (>5 skin lesions).

face and limbs. Iritis and episcleritis are common. Other signs are acute neuritis, lymphadenitis, orchitis, bone pain, dactylitis, arthritis and proteinuria. ENL may continue intermittently for several years.

Investigations

• Slit skin smears: dermal material is scraped on to a glass slide and acid-fast bacilli may be seen on microscopy. • Skin biopsy: histological examination may aid diagnosis. • Neither serology nor PCR testing for *M. leprae* DNA is sensitive or specific enough for diagnosis.

Management

Multidrug treatment (MDT; Box 5.19): All leprosy patients should be given MDT. Rifampicin is a potent bactericidal for *M. leprae* but resistance can arise through a single mutation so it should always be given as part of MDT. Dapsone is bacteriostatic. It commonly causes mild haemolysis but rarely anaemia. Clofazimine is a red, fat-soluble crystalline dye, weakly bactericidal for *M. leprae*. Skin discoloration (red to purple-black) and ichthyosis are troublesome side-effects, particularly on pale skins. Newer drugs such as per-floxacin, ofloxacin, clarithromycin and minocycline are now established second-line options.

Treatment of reactions: Control is most readily achieved with high-dose oral prednisolone. Thalidomide may also be used but its teratogenicity limits its use in women of child-bearing potential. Hydrocortisone eye drops may be used for ocular symptoms.

Patient education and rehabilitation: Patients should be reassured that after 3 days of chemotherapy they are not infectious and can lead a normal social life. Additional measures include:

• Scrupulous attention to skin care: required if patients are to avoid damage to their anaesthetic limb. • Appropriate footwear: should help to protect pressure points. • Ulceration: should be treated seriously, with the cause of the injury identified, and the patient advised not to weight-bear until the ulcer has healed. • Physiotherapy: can help prevent contractures and atrophy of muscles.

Prognosis

The majority of patients, especially those who have no nerve damage at the time of diagnosis, do well on MDT, with resolution of skin lesions. Borderline patients are at risk of developing type 1 reactions, which may result in devastating nerve damage.

Prevention and control

Programmes aimed at case detection and provision of MDT are now in place in many of the countries affected by leprosy. BCG vaccination has been shown to give good but variable protection against leprosy; adding killed *M. leprae* to BCG does not give enhanced protection.

Rickettsial and related intracellular bacterial infections

These are caused by Gram-negative organisms that occur in the intestines and saliva of ticks, mites, lice and fleas. Following an inoculating bite, the organisms multiply in capillary endothelial cells and cause fever, rash and organ damage. There are two main groups of rickettsial fevers: the spotted fever group and the typhus group.

Spotted fever group

Rocky Mountain spotted fever: Rickettsia rickettsii is transmitted by tick bites, largely in western and south-eastern states of the USA and also in Central and South America. The incubation period is ~7 days. The rash appears on about the 3rd or 4th day, looking at first like measles, but in a few hours the typical maculopapular eruption develops. Within 24–48 hrs the rash spreads in a centripetal fashion from wrists, forearms and ankles to the back, limbs and chest, and then to the abdomen where it is least pronounced. Larger cutaneous and subcutaneous haemorrhages may appear in severe cases. The liver and spleen become palpable. At the extremes of life the mortality is 2–12%.

Other spotted fevers: Rickettsia coronii and *R. africae* cause Mediterranean and African tick typhus. An eschar (black, necrotic sore) is associated with a maculopapular rash on trunk, limbs, palms and soles. Complications include delirium and meningism.

Typhus group

Scrub typhus fever: Caused by *Orientia tsutsugamushi*, transmitted by mites. It occurs in the Far East, Myanmar, Pakistan, Bangladesh, India, Indonesia, the South Pacific and Queensland. Initially the patient develops one or more eschars, surrounded by cellulitis with regional lymphadenopathy. The incubation period is ~9 days. Mild or subclinical cases are common. The onset of symptoms is usually sudden with headache (often retro-orbital), fever, malaise, weakness and cough. An erythematous maculopapular rash appears on about the 5th–7th day and spreads to the trunk, face and limbs, including the palms and soles, with generalised painless lymphadenopathy. The rash fades by the 14th day. The patient develops a remittent fever that falls by the 12th–18th day. In severe infection the patient is prostrate with cough, pneumonia, confusion and deafness. Cardiac failure, renal failure and haemorrhage may develop. Convalescence is often slow and tachycardia may persist for some weeks.

Epidemic (louse-borne) typhus: Caused by *Rickettsia prowazekii* and prevalent in parts of Africa, especially Ethiopia and Rwanda, and in the South American Andes and Afghanistan. Overcrowding facilitates spread, which is through scratching skin contaminated with louse faeces. The incubation period is usually 12–14 days. The onset is usually sudden, with rigors, fever, frontal headaches, pains in the back and limbs, constipation and bronchitis. The face is flushed and cyanotic, the eyes are congested and the patient becomes confused. A petechial, mottled rash appears on the 4th–6th day, first on the anterior folds of the axillae, sides of the abdomen or backs of hands, then on the trunk and forearms, sparing the neck and face. During the 2nd wk, symptoms increase, with sores on the lips and a dry, brown, shrunken and tremulous tongue. The spleen is palpable, the pulse feeble and the patient stuporous and delirious. The temperature falls rapidly at the end of the 2nd wk and the patient recovers gradually. Fatal cases usually die in the 2nd wk from toxaemia, cardiac or renal failure, or pneumonia.

Endemic (flea-borne) typhus: Flea-borne or 'endemic' typhus, caused by *Rickettsia typhi*, is endemic worldwide. Humans are infected when the faeces or contents of a crushed flea that has fed on an infected rat are introduced into the skin. The incubation period is 8–14 days. The symptoms resemble those of a mild louse-borne typhus. The rash may be scanty and transient.

Investigation of rickettsial infection

The diagnosis of rickettsial infection is essentially clinical, and may be confirmed by antibody detection or PCR in specialised laboratories. Differential diagnoses include malaria, typhoid, meningococcal septicaemia and leptospirosis.

Management of the rickettsial diseases

The different rickettsial fevers vary greatly in severity but all respond to tetracycline, doxycycline or chloramphenicol. Sedation may be required for delirium and transfusion for haemorrhage. Reservoirs of the disease, such as fleas, ticks and mites, should be controlled with insecticides.

Q fever

Q fever occurs worldwide and is caused by the rickettsia-like organism *Coxiella burnetii*, an obligate intracellular organism that can survive in the extracellular environment. Cattle, sheep and goats are important reservoirs and the organism is transmitted by inhalation of aerosolised particles. In culture, the organism undergoes antigenic shift from the infectious phase I to the non-infectious phase II form.

Clinical features

The incubation period is 3–4 wks.

The initial symptoms are non-specific with fever, headache and chills. In 20% of cases a maculopapular rash occurs. Other presentations include pneumonia and hepatitis. Chronic Q fever may present with osteomyelitis, encephalitis and endocarditis.

Investigations

Diagnosis is usually serological, and the stage of the infection can be distinguished by isotype tests and phase-specific antigens. Acute phase II IgM titres peak at 4–6 wks. In chronic infections IgG titres to phase I and II antigens may be raised.

Management

Doxycycline is the treatment of choice. Rifampicin is added in cases of Q fever endocarditis, which can require prolonged treatment, even when two antimicrobial agents are used.

Bartonellosis

This group of diseases is caused by intracellular Gram-negative rods closely related to the rickettsiae. The principal human pathogens are *Bartonella quintana* and *B. henselae*. *Bartonella* infections are associated with the following clinical conditions:

Trench fever: This is a relapsing fever with severe leg pain, which is debilitating but not fatal.

Bacteraemia and endocarditis in the homeless: The endocarditis is associated with severe damage to the heart valves.

Cat scratch disease: *B. henselae* causes this common benign lymphadenopathy in children and young adults. A vesicle or papule develops on the head, neck or arms after a cat scratch. The lesion resolves spontaneously but lymphadenopathy may persist for up to 4 mths.

Bacillary angiomatosis: This is an HIV-associated disease.

Investigations

• Blood cultures: require prolonged incubation and enriched media.
• Serological testing: haemagglutination, indirect immunofluorescence, ELISA.

Management

Bartonella spp. are susceptible to β-lactams, rifampicin, erythromycin and tetracyclines. Antibiotic use is guided by clinical need. Cat scratch disease usually resolves spontaneously but *Bartonella* endocarditis requires valve replacement and combination antibiotic therapy.

Chlamydial infections

Three organisms cause most human chlamydial infections:
• *Chlamydia trachomatis* causes trachoma (see below), lymphogranuloma venereum and sexually transmitted genital infections (p. 127).
• *C. psittaci* causes psittacosis. • *C. pneumoniae* is a cause of atypical pneumonia (p. 289).

Trachoma

Trachoma is a chronic keratoconjunctivitis caused by *C. trachomatis*, and is the most common cause of avoidable blindness. Transmission occurs in dry and dirty environments through flies, on fingers and within families. In endemic areas, the disease is most common in children.

Clinical features

The onset is usually insidious and may be asymptomatic. Early symptoms include conjunctivitis and blepharospasm, which may be difficult to distinguish from viral conjunctivitis, but hyperaemia with pale follicles on the conjunctivae are characteristic of trachoma. Lid inversion and corneal vascularisation with opacity are important complications. Infection may be latent for long periods between recrudescences, and may not be detected until vision begins to fail.

Investigations and management

Intracellular inclusions may be demonstrated in conjunctival scrapings by staining with iodine or immunofluorescence. A single dose of azithromycin (20 mg/kg) is first-choice treatment, and is more effective than tetracycline eye ointment. Deformity and scarring of the lids, and corneal opacities, ulceration and scarring require surgical treatment after control of local infection.

The WHO is promoting the SAFE strategy for trachoma control (**s**urgery, **a**ntibiotics, **f**acial cleanliness and **e**nvironmental improvement). Proper eye care of newborn and young children is essential.

PROTOZOAL INFECTIONS

Systemic protozoal infections
Malaria

Malaria is caused by *Plasmodium falciparum*, *P. vivax*, *P. ovale* and *P. malariae*, as well as the predominantly simian parasite, *P. knowlesi*. It is transmitted by the bite of female anopheline mosquitoes and occurs throughout the tropics and subtropics at altitudes below 1500 m. Recent estimates indicate 515 million clinical cases/yr, of which two-thirds occur in sub-Saharan Africa. *P. falciparum* is now resistant to chloroquine in South-east Asia and throughout Africa. Reversal of the resurgence in malaria by improved vector and disease control is a major goal of the WHO.

Due to increased travel, over 2000 cases are imported annually into Britain. Most are due to *P. falciparum*, usually from Africa, and of these 1% die because of late diagnosis. Immigrants living long term in the UK who visit family overseas are particularly at risk, because they lose their partial immunity and do not realise that they should be taking prophylaxis. A few people living near airports in Europe have acquired malaria from accidentally imported mosquitoes.

Life cycle

The female anopheline mosquito becomes infected by feeding on human blood containing malarial parasite gametocytes. Human infection starts when an infected mosquito inoculates saliva containing sporozoites into the skin during feeding; these disappear from human blood within half an hour and enter the liver. After some days merozoites leave the liver and invade red blood cells, where further multiplication takes place, producing trophozoites and then schizonts (Fig 5.11). Rupture of schizonts releases more merozoites into the blood and causes fever, the periodicity of which depends on the species of parasite (see below).

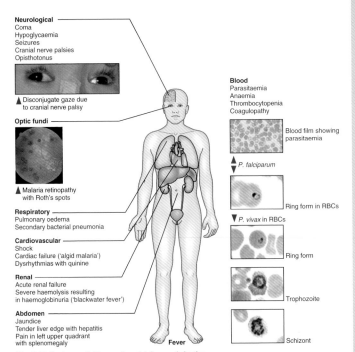

Neurological
Coma
Hypoglycaemia
Seizures
Cranial nerve palsies
Opisthotonus

▲ Disconjugate gaze due to cranial nerve palsy

Optic fundi

▲ Malaria retinopathy with Roth's spots

Respiratory
Pulmonary oedema
Secondary bacterial pneumonia

Cardiovascular
Shock
Cardiac failure ('algid malaria')
Dysrhythmias with quinine

Renal
Acute renal failure
Severe haemolysis resulting in haemoglobinuria ('blackwater fever')

Abdomen
Jaundice
Tender liver edge with hepatitis
Pain in left upper quadrant with splenomegaly

Fever

Blood
Parasitaemia
Anaemia
Thrombocytopenia
Coagulopathy

Blood film showing parasitaemia

▲▼ *P. falciparum*

Ring form in RBCs

▼ *P. vivax* in RBCs

Ring form

Trophozoite

Schizont

Fig. 5.11 Features of *Plasmodium falciparum* infection.

P. vivax and *P. ovale* may persist in liver cells as dormant forms, hypnozoites, capable of developing into merozoites months or years later. Thus the first attack of clinical malaria may occur long after the patient has left the endemic area, and the disease may relapse after treatment with drugs that kill only the erythrocytic stage of the parasite. *P. falciparum* and *P. malariae* have no persistent exo-erythrocytic phase but recrudescences of fever may result from multiplication in the red cells of parasites that have not been eliminated by treatment and immune processes.

Clinical features

The pathology in malaria is due to haemolysis of infected red cells and adherence of infected red blood cells to capillaries.

P. falciparum infection (see Fig. 5.11): This is the most dangerous of the malarias. The onset is often insidious, with malaise, headache and vomiting, and is often mistaken for influenza. Cough and mild diarrhoea are also common. Release of parasites from schizonts is asynchronous; therefore the fever has no particular pattern. Jaundice is common due to haemolysis and hepatic dysfunction. The liver and spleen enlarge and become tender, and anaemia develops rapidly. Complications of falciparum malaria are summarised in Box 5.20. Splenectomy increases the risk of severe malaria.

P. vivax and P. ovale infection: In many cases the illness starts with several days of continued fever before the development of classical bouts of fever on alternate days. Fever starts with a rigor.

5.20 Severe manifestations of *P. falciparum* malaria and their management	
Cerebral malaria	
Coma	Maintain airway, exclude other causes, ventilate if necessary
Convulsions	Diazepam or paraldehyde
Hyperpyrexia	Tepid sponging, fan, paracetamol
Hypoglycaemia	Monitor blood glucose, IV dextrose infusion
Severe anaemia (PCV <15%)	Transfusion
Acute pulmonary oedema	Nurse at 45°, venesect, limit IV fluids, diuretics, CPAP, haemofilter
Acute renal failure	Exclude other causes, dialysis (peritoneal or haemodialysis)
Bleeding/coagulopathy	Transfuse screened fresh blood, or FFP, cryoprecipitate
Metabolic acidosis	Fluids, oxygen, treat sepsis and hypoglycaemia
Shock ('algid malaria')	Suspect Gram −ve septicaemia, IV antimicrobials, fluid resuscitation
Aspiration pneumonia	IV antimicrobials, oxygen, physiotherapy
Hyperparasitaemia	Partial or full exchange transfusion, haemapheresis

From WHO. Severe falciparum malaria. In: Severe and complicated malaria. 3rd edn. Trans R Soc Trop Med Hyg 2000; 94 (suppl. 1): S1-41.

The patient feels cold and the temperature rises to ~40°C. After half an hour to an hour the hot or flush phase begins. It lasts several hours and gives way to profuse perspiration and a gradual fall in temperature. The cycle is repeated 48 hrs later. Gradually the spleen and liver enlarge and may become tender. Anaemia develops slowly. Herpes simplex is common. Relapses are frequent in the first 2 yrs after leaving the malarious area.

P. malariae infection: This is usually associated with mild symptoms and bouts of fever every 3rd day. Parasitaemia may persist for many years with the occasional recrudescence of fever, or without producing any symptoms. *P. malariae* causes glomerulonephritis and the nephrotic syndrome in children.

Investigations

Giemsa-stained thick and thin blood films should be examined. In the thick film erythrocytes are lysed, releasing all blood stages of the parasite. This facilitates the diagnosis of low-level parasitaemias. A thin film is essential to confirm the diagnosis, to identify the species of parasite and, in *P. falciparum* infections, to quantify the parasite load (by counting the percentage of infected erythrocytes).

Immunochromatographic 'dipstick' tests for *P. falciparum* antigens are now marketed and provide a useful non-microscopic means of diagnosing this infection. They should be used in parallel with blood film examination and are especially useful when the microscopist is less experienced. PCR remains largely a research tool.

Management

Mild P. falciparum malaria: P. falciparum is now resistant to chloroquine and sulfadoxine-pyrimethamine almost worldwide, so an artemisinin-based treatment is recommended. Co-artemether (artemether and lumefantrine) is given 4 tabs at 0, 8, 24, 36, 48 and 60 hrs. Alternatives are quinine (600 mg quinine salt 3 times daily for 5–7 days), followed by doxycycline or clindamycin. Doxycycline should be avoided in pregnancy and artemether in early pregnancy. WHO policy is moving towards artemisinin-based combination therapy (ACT).

Complicated P. falciparum malaria: Severe malaria (parasite count >2% in any non-immune patient) is a medical emergency. Immediate management should include IV artesunate (2.4 mg/kg IV at 0, 12 and 24 hrs, then daily for 7 days). When the patient has recovered sufficiently, oral artesunate 2 mg/kg once daily is given instead of infusions to a total cumulative dose of 17–18 mg/kg. IV quinine salt is an alternative, with ECG monitoring. Management of the complications of severe *P. falciparum* infection is summarised in Box 5.20.

Non-falciparum malaria: P. vivax, P. ovale and *P. malariae* infections should be treated with oral chloroquine (600 mg chloroquine base, followed at 6 hrs by 300 mg, then 150 mg twice daily for 2 more days). Relapses can be prevented by taking one of the antimalarial drugs in suppressive doses. Radical cure is achieved in *P. vivax* and *P. ovale* using primaquine (15 mg daily for 14 days), which destroys the hypnozoite phase in the liver. Haemolysis may develop in those who are glucose-6-phosphate dehydrogenase (G6PD)-deficient. Cyanosis due to the formation of methaemoglobin in the red cells is more common but not dangerous.

Prevention

Choice of prophylactic agent is determined by the risk of malaria in the area being visited and the degree of chloroquine resistance. A variety of agents are used, e.g. chloroquine, atovaquone plus proguanil (Malarone), doxycycline and mefloquine. Updated recommendations are summarised at www.fitfortravel.nhs.uk. Many agents require to be taken in advance of travel and continued after return. Mefloquine is useful in areas of multiple drug resistance but contraindications exist. Use of insecticide-treated bed nets, insect repellents and protective clothing are also important means of reducing infection. Vaccines against malaria are under development but not yet fully protective.

Babesiosis

This is caused by a tick-borne intra-erythrocytic protozoon parasite. Patients present with fever 1–4 wks after a tick bite. Severe illness is seen in splenectomised patients. The diagnosis is made by blood film examination. Treatment is with quinine and clindamycin.

African trypanosomiasis (sleeping sickness)

African sleeping sickness is caused by trypanosomes conveyed to humans by the bites of infected tsetse flies and is unique to sub-Saharan Africa. The disease has declined by 60% since 1990 due to improved control. *Trypanosoma brucei gambiense* has a wide distribution in West and Central Africa and accounts for 90% of cases. *T. brucei rhodesiense* is found in parts of East and Central Africa and, unlike *gambiense*, has a large reservoir in wild animals. Transmission is common at riversides and in wooded grasslands.

Clinical features

A bite by a tsetse fly is painful and commonly becomes inflamed, but if trypanosomes are introduced, the site may again become painful and swollen ~10 days later ('trypanosomal chancre') and the regional lymph nodes enlarge ('Winterbottom's sign'). Within 2–3 wks of infection the trypanosomes invade the blood stream. The early haematolymphatic stage gives way to a late encephalitic stage.

Rhodesiense infections: Acute and severe. Within days or a few weeks the patient is usually severely ill and may have developed pleural effusions and signs of myocarditis or hepatitis. There may be a petechial rash. The patient may die before there are signs of involvement of the CNS. If the illness is less acute, drowsiness, tremors and coma develop.

Gambiense infection: Slow course, with irregular bouts of fever and firm, discrete, rubbery and painless enlargement of lymph nodes. These are particularly prominent in the posterior triangle of the neck. The spleen and liver may become palpable. After some months, in the absence of treatment, the CNS is invaded. This is shown clinically by headache and changed behaviour, blunting of higher mental functions, insomnia by night and sleepiness by day, mental confusion and eventually tremors, pareses, wasting, coma and death.

Investigations

• Thick and thin blood films: stained as for the detection of malaria, will reveal trypanosomes. • Lymph node aspirate: may be more sensitive in *gambiense* infection. • Card agglutination trypanosomiasis test (CATT): simple and rapid. • Lumbar puncture: in cases of CNS involvement, CSF will reveal raised protein, WCC and IgM, and diminished glucose.

Management

Unfortunately, therapeutic options for African trypanosomiasis are limited and most of the antitrypanosomal drugs are toxic and expensive. The prognosis is good if treatment is begun early before the brain has been invaded. Treatments are summarised in Box 5.21.

American trypanosomiasis (Chagas' disease)

Chagas' disease occurs widely in South and Central America. The cause is *Trypanosoma cruzi*, transmitted to humans from the faeces of a reduviid (triatomine) bug, in which the trypanosomes develop before becoming infective to humans. Infected faeces from the bugs are rubbed in through the conjunctiva, mucosa of mouth or nose, or abrasions of the skin in humans. Blood transfusions are responsible for up to 5% of infections and congenital transmission may also occur.

Clinical features

Acute phase: The acute phase is seen in only 1–2% of infected individuals before the age of 15 yrs. Young children (1–5 yrs) are

5.21 Treatment of African trypanosomiasis		
	First-line	**Second-line**
***Gambiense* trypanosomiasis**		
Stage 1	Pentamidine	Eflornithine or melarsoprol
Stage 2	Eflornithine	Melarsoprol
***Rhodesiense* trypanosomiasis**		
Stage 1	Suramin	Melarsoprol
Stage 2	Melarsoprol	Nifurtimox with melarsoprol

most commonly affected. The entrance of *T. cruzi* through an abrasion produces a dusky-red firm swelling and regional lymphadenopathy. A conjunctival lesion, although less common, is more characteristic; the unilateral firm reddish swelling of the lids may close the eye and this constitutes 'Romaña's sign'. In a few patients an acute generalised infection soon appears, with a transient morbilliform or urticarial rash, fever, lymphadenopathy and enlargement of the spleen and liver. In a small minority of patients acute myocarditis and heart failure or neurological features, including personality changes and signs of meningoencephalitis, may be seen. The acute infection may be fatal to infants.

Chronic phase: About 50–70% of infected patients become seropositive and develop an indeterminate form when no parasitaemia is detectable. They have a normal lifespan with no symptoms but are a natural reservoir for the disease and maintain the life cycle of parasites. After a latent period of several years, 10–30% of chronic cases develop low-grade myocarditis, and damage to conducting fibres causing a cardiomyopathy. In nearly 10% of patients damage to Auerbach's plexus results in dilatation of various parts of the alimentary canal, especially the colon and oesophagus, so-called 'mega' disease. Dilatation of the bile ducts and bronchi is also a recognised sequela. Reactivation of Chagas' disease can occur in patients with HIV if the CD4 count falls <200 cells/mm^3 (p. 130).

Investigations

• Blood film: *T. cruzi* is easily detectable in the acute illness. • Xenodiagnosis: infection-free, laboratory-bred reduviid bugs are allowed to feed on the patient and the bugs' faeces are subsequently examined for parasites. • PCR: parasite DNA detection by PCR is highly sensitive in blood or in bug faeces for xenodiagnosis. • Antibody detection is also highly sensitive.

Management

Nifurtimox and benznidazole are parasiticidal drugs; either can be used in the acute and early chronic phase for 60–90 days. Adverse reactions to both drugs are frequent (30–55%). Cure rates of up to 80% may be achieved. Surgery may be required for 'mega' disease. Rates of infection may be reduced by destruction of the reduviid bugs with insecticides.

Toxoplasmosis

Toxoplasma gondii is a coccidian intracellular parasite ubiquitous in mammals. It is the most common protozoal infection in developed countries; 22% of adults in the UK are seropositive. In India and Brazil, 40–60% of pregnant women are seropositive. Congenital infection or that occurring in HIV-positive patients may cause considerable morbidity and may be fatal.

Life cycle

The sexual phase of the parasite's life cycle occurs in the small intestinal epithelium of the cat. Oöcysts shed in cat faeces are spread to intermediate hosts (pork, lamb), including humans, through contamination of soil. Once ingested by the intermediate host, the parasite transforms, in the intestinal epithelium, into rapidly dividing tachyzoites. These then infect other tissues, leading to the formation of microscopic tissue cysts containing bradyzoites, which persist for the lifetime of the host. Cats become infected or re-infected by ingesting tissue cysts in their prey.

Clinical fe atures

In most immunocompetent individuals, including children and pregnant women, the infection goes unnoticed. In ~10% of patients it causes a self-limiting illness. The peak incidence of clinical illness is in adults aged 25–35 yrs.

The most common presenting feature is painless lymphadenopathy, which may be localised or generalised. Systemic symptoms, which are 'flu-like, are infrequent. Complete resolution usually occurs within a few months, although symptoms and lymphadenopathy tend to fluctuate unpredictably and some patients do not recover completely for a year or more. Very infrequently, encephalitis, myocarditis, polymyositis, pneumonitis or hepatitis may develop. Toxoplasmosis acquired in utero by vertical spread can also cause retinochoroiditis, hydrocephalus and microcephaly.

Investigations

The Sabin–Feldman indirect fluorescent antibody test is used in immunocompetent patients. A fourfold rise in IgG or the presence of IgM indicates acute infection. The presence of high-avidity IgG excludes infection in the past 3–4 mths, which is important in pregnancy. Lymph node tissue may be used as a source of *T. gondii* DNA to be amplified by PCR, or be stained with *T. gondii* antisera to demonstrate treponemes histochemically.

Management

As the disease is usually self-limiting, treatment is reserved for rare cases of severe or progressive disease, and for infection in immunocompromised patients. *T. gondii* infection responds poorly to antimicrobial therapy but pyrimethamine, sulfadiazine and folinic acid may be used.

Leishmaniasis

Leishmaniasis is caused by unicellular flagellate intracellular protozoa belonging to the genus *Leishmania*. It comprises three broad groups of disorder:
• Visceral leishmaniasis (VL, kala-azar). • Cutaneous leishmaniasis (CL). • Mucosal leishmaniasis (ML).

Although most clinical syndromes are caused by zoonotic transmission of parasites from animals (chiefly canine and rodent reservoirs) to humans through phlebotomine sandfly vectors, humans are the only known reservoir (anthroponotic) in major VL foci in the Indian subcontinent and for transmission among injection drug users. The disease occurs in ~100 countries around the world, with an estimated annual incidence of 2 million new cases (1.5 million CL and 0.5 million VL).

Life cycle

Flagellar promastigotes (10–20 μm) are introduced by the feeding female sandfly (*Phlebotomus* in the eastern hemisphere, *Lutzomyia* and *Psychodopygus* in the western hemisphere). The promastigotes are taken up by neutrophils, which undergo apoptosis and are engulfed by macrophages in which the parasites transform into amastigotes (2–4 μm, Leishman–Donovan bodies). These multiply, ultimately causing macrophage lysis and infection of other cells. Sandflies pick up amastigotes when feeding on infected patients or animal reservoirs. In the sandfly, the parasite transforms into a flagellar promastigote, which multiplies in the gut of the vector and migrates to the proboscis to infect a new host.

Visceral leishmaniasis (kala-azar)

VL is caused by the protozoon *Leishmania donovani* complex (comprising *L. donovani*, *L. infantum* and *L. chagasi*). Rarely, a dermatotropic species (e.g. *L. tropica*) may cause visceral disease. India, Sudan, Bangladesh and Brazil account for 90% of cases of VL, while other affected regions include the Mediterranean, East Africa, China, Arabia, Israel and other South American countries. VL can present unexpectedly, e.g. after blood transfusion, in immunosuppressed patients after transplantation and in HIV infection.

Clinical features

The great majority of people infected remain asymptomatic. In the Indian subcontinent, adults and children are equally affected; elsewhere it is predominantly a childhood disease, except in adults with HIV.

Symptomatic cases feature:
• Fever: accompanied initially by rigor and chills, and decreasing over time with occasional relapses. • Splenomegaly: develops quickly in the first few weeks and may become massive. • Hepatomegaly. • Lymphadenopathy: common except in the Indian subcontinent. • Skin: a blackish discoloration of the skin ('kala azar' is Hindi for 'black skin') is a feature of advanced disease and is now rarely seen. • Haematological abnormalities: severe anaemia, thrombocytopenia and pancytopenia with retinal, GI or nasal bleeding. • Oedema and ascites: secondary to low albumin. • Secondary infection: profound immunosuppression may result in TB, dysentery,

herpes zoster and chickenpox. Skin infections, cellulitis and scabies are common.

Investigations

There is pancytopenia with granulocytopenia and monocytosis. There is polyclonal hypergammaglobulinaemia (IgG first, then IgM) and hypoalbuminaemia. Splenic smears demonstrate amastigotes (Leishman–Donovan bodies) with 98% sensitivity as a diagnostic test. PCR is performed on peripheral blood; it is sensitive especially in the immunosuppressed but only performed in specialised laboratories. Serodiagnosis by immunofluorescence is also used in developed countries. In developing countries, a highly sensitive and specific direct agglutination test of stained promastigotes and an equally efficient rapid immunochromatographic k39 strip test have been developed.

Differential diagnosis

This includes malaria, typhoid, TB, schistosomiasis and many other infectious and neoplastic conditions, some of which may coexist with VL. Fever, splenomegaly, pancytopenia and non-response to antimalarial therapy may provide clues before specific laboratory diagnosis is made.

Management

Pentavalent antimonials: Antimony (Sb) compounds, such as sodium stibogluconate and meglumine antimoniate, are the mainstay of treatment in most parts of the world; in the Indian subcontinent, however, almost two-thirds of cases are refractory to Sb. A daily dose of 20 mg/kg is given, IV or IM, for 28–30 days. Side-effects are common and include arthralgias, myalgias, raised hepatic transaminases and pancreatitis, especially in patients co-infected with HIV. Severe cardiotoxicity, manifested by concave ST segment elevation, prolongation of QT_c >0.5 msec, ventricular ectopics, ventricular dysrhythmias and sudden death, is not uncommon. The incidence of cardiotoxicity and death can be very high with improperly manufactured Sb.

Amphotericin B: Amphotericin B deoxycholate, 0.75–1 mg/kg daily for 15–20 doses, is an alternative in areas where there is Sb unresponsiveness. It has a cure rate of nearly 100%. Infusion-related side-effects, e.g. high fever with rigor, thrombophlebitis, diarrhoea and vomiting, are extremely common. Serious (occasionally fatal) adverse events, such as renal or hepatic toxicity, hypokalaemia, thrombocytopenia and myocarditis, are not uncommon. Lipid formulations of amphotericin B are less toxic. AmBisome is approved by the US FDA and is first-line therapy in Europe for VL. High daily doses of the lipid formulations are well tolerated, thus reducing hospital stay and cost. AmBisome has been made available at preferential cost in developing countries.

Other drugs: Miltefosine, paromomycin and pentamidine have also been used to treat VL. Multidrug therapy is likely to increase in order to prevent the emergence of resistance.

Response to treatment

A good response results in abatement of fever, a feeling of well-being, gradual decrease in splenic size, weight gain and recovery of blood counts. Patients should be followed regularly for a period of 6–12 mths, as a small minority may relapse. Relapse is indicated by enlargement of the spleen, return of fever, weight loss and decline in blood counts.

HIV–visceral leishmaniasis co-infection

This is declining in Europe due to antiretroviral therapy, but is increasing in Africa, South America and the Indian subcontinent.

The clinical triad of fever, splenomegaly and hepatomegaly is found in most co-infected cases, but those with a low CD4 count commonly have atypical clinical presentations. VL may present with GI involvement (stomach, duodenum or colon), ascites, pleural or pericardial effusion, or involvement of lungs, tonsil, oral mucosa or skin. Diagnostic principles remain the same as for non-HIV patients, based on the detection of amastigotes in body fluids or PCR of the blood.

Treatment of VL in a setting of HIV co-infection remains essentially the same as in immunocompetent patients, using amphotericin B or Sb, but there are some differences in outcome. There is a tendency to relapse within a year, and monthly maintenance liposomal amphotericin B may prevent this.

Post-kala-azar dermal leishmaniasis (PKDL)

After treatment and recovery from the visceral disease in India and Sudan, some patients develop dermatological manifestations. In India, dermatological changes occur in a small minority of patients (usually adults) 6 mths to ≥3 yrs after the initial infection, in contrast to Sudan where 50% of patients (usually children) develop PKDL rapidly (within 6 mths). The diagnosis is clinical, based on the characteristic appearance of macules, papules, nodules (most frequently) and plaques on the face, especially around the chin. The face often appears erythematous. Hypopigmented macules can occur and are highly variable in extent and location. There are no systemic symptoms but such patients are a human reservoir for disease. Treatment of Indian PKDL is difficult – Sb for 120 days or several courses of amphotericin B infusions are required. In Sudan, spontaneous healing occurs in about three-quarters of cases within 1 yr.

Prevention and control

Insecticides, as well as physical barriers such as mosquito nets and protective clothing, help prevent the transmission of the disease to humans. Dogs and other animals known to be infected should be destroyed. Early detection and adequate treatment of cases reduce the human reservoir of the disease.

Cutaneous and mucosal leishmaniasis
Cutaneous leishmaniasis

Cutaneous leishmaniasis (CL; oriental sore) occurs in both the Old World and the New World, causing two distinct types of leishmaniasis:

Old World CL: A mild disease found around the Mediterranean basin, throughout the Middle East and Central Asia as far as Pakistan, and in sub-Saharan West Africa and Sudan. It is caused by *Leishmania major*, *L. tropica* and *L. aethiopica*.

New World CL: A disfiguring disease, largely found in Central and South America. It is caused by the *Leishmania mexicana* complex (*L. mexicana*, *L. amazonensis* and *L. venezuelensis*) and by the *Viannia* subgenus *L. (V.) brasiliensis* complex (*L. (V.) guyanensis*, *L. (V.) panamensis*, *L. (V.) brasiliensis* and *L. (V.) peruviana*).

The incubation period is 2–3 mths (range 2 wks to 5 yrs). The characteristic lesions of CL are ulcerated papules that form at the site of a vector bite. They may be single or multiple, and may measure up to 10 cm in diameter (Fig. 5.12). There can be satellite lesions, especially in *L. major* and occasionally in *L. tropica* infections. Regional lymphadenopathy, pain, pruritus and secondary bacterial infections may occur. Lesions on the pinna of the ear are more common in New World CL. *L. mexicana* is responsible for chiclero

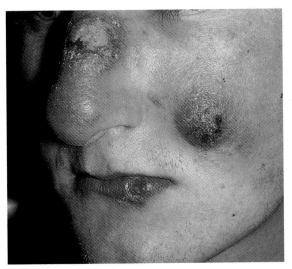

Fig. 5.12 Cutaneous leishmaniasis.

ulcers, self-healing sores seen in Mexico. If immunity is good, there is usually spontaneous healing in *L. tropica*, *L. major* and *L. mexicana* lesions. In some patients with anergy to *Leishmania*, the skin lesions of *L. aethiopica*, *L. mexicana* and *L. amazonensis* infections progress to the development of diffuse CL; this is characterised by spread of the infection from the initial ulcer, usually on the face, to involve the whole body in the form of non-ulcerative nodules. Occasionally, in *L. tropica* infections, sores that have apparently healed relapse persistently (recidivans or lupoid leishmaniasis).

Mucosal leishmaniasis

The *Viannia* subgenus (New World CL) extends from the Amazon basin to Paraguay and Costa Rica, and is responsible for deep sores and mucosal leishmaniasis (ML). Young men with chronic lesions are particularly at risk, and between 2 and 40% of infected persons develop 'espundia', metastatic lesions in the mucosa of the nose or mouth. This is characterised by thickening, erythema and later ulceration of the nasal mucosa, typically starting at the junction of the nose and upper lip. The lips, soft palate, fauces and larynx may also be invaded and destroyed. There is no spontaneous healing, and death may result from severe respiratory tract infections due to massive destruction of the pharynx.

Investigations in CL and ML

• Slit skin smear: amastigotes identified using Giemsa stain. • Culture: material obtained from sores or fine needle aspiration. • PCR: increasingly used for diagnosis and speciation, especially in ML.

Management of CL and ML

Treatment of CL should be individualised on the basis of the causative organism, severity of the lesions, availability of drugs, tolerance of the patient for toxicity, and local resistance patterns.

Small lesions may self-heal or be treated by freezing with liquid nitrogen or curettage. Topical application of paromomycin 15% plus methylbenzethonium chloride 12% is beneficial in CL. Intralesional antimony is also rapidly effective and generally well tolerated in CL. For CL with multiple lesions and for ML, parenteral Sb (20 mg/kg/day) should be used. CL requires 20 days of systemic Sb; ML is treated for 28 days. Refractory CL or ML should be treated with amphotericin B. Other effective drugs include pentamidine, fluconazole, ketoconazole and itraconazole.

Prevention of CL and ML

Personal protection against sandfly bites is important. No effective vaccine is yet available.

Gastrointestinal protozoal infections
Amoebiasis

Amoebiasis is caused by *Entamoeba histolytica*; it is common throughout the tropics and occasionally acquired in the UK. Infection can give rise to amoebic dysentery or extra-intestinal amoebiasis, e.g. amoebic liver abscess.

Clinical features

Intestinal amoebiasis or amoebic dysentery: Cysts of *E. histolytica* are ingested in water or uncooked food contaminated by human faeces. The parasite invades the mucous membrane of the large bowel, producing ulceration. The incubation period of amoebiasis ranges from 2 wks to many years, followed by a chronic course with grumbling abdominal pains (often in the right lower quadrant, mimicking appendicitis) and two or more unformed stools a day. Diarrhoea alternating with constipation is common, as is mucus, sometimes with streaks of blood. There is a dysenteric presentation, with passage of blood and mucus simulating bacillary dysentery or ulcerative colitis, especially in the elderly and those with superadded pyogenic infection.

Amoebic liver abscess: This occurs when trophozoites enter the liver via the portal vein. In the liver, usually the right lobe, they multiply and rapidly destroy the parenchyma, forming an amoebic abscess. Local symptoms of an enlarged, tender liver, cough and pain in the right shoulder are characteristic, but symptoms may remain vague and signs minimal. A high swinging fever without much systemic upset is sometimes seen. A large liver abscess may rupture through the diaphragm into the lung, from where its contents may be coughed up. Rupture into the pleural cavity, the peritoneal cavity or pericardial sac is less common but more serious.

Investigations

• Fresh stool sample: may reveal motile trophozoites on microscopy. • Sigmoidoscopy: typical flask-shaped ulcers may be seen and should be scraped for microscopy. • Antibodies: detectable by immunofluorescence in 95% of patients with hepatic amoebiasis and intestinal amoeboma but in only ~60% of dysenteric amoebiasis. • PCR: also sensitive but not widely available.

If the clinical picture suggests amoebic abscess, there may be a neutrophil leucocytosis and a raised right hemidiaphragm on CXR. Confirmation is by liver USS.

Management

Intestinal and early hepatic amoebiasis responds quickly to oral metronidazole. Diloxanide furoate should be given orally for 10 days after treatment to eliminate luminal cysts. Drainage/aspiration may be required for amoebic abscess to prevent rupture; this yields characteristic brown 'anchovy sauce' liquid. Surgical drainage is needed if rupture occurs.

Giardiasis

Infection with *Giardia lamblia* is found worldwide and is common in the tropics. It particularly affects children, tourists and immunosuppressed individuals, and is the parasite most commonly imported into the UK. The cysts remain viable in water for up to 3 mths and infection usually occurs by ingesting contaminated water.

The parasites attach to the duodenal and jejunal mucosa, causing inflammation. After an incubation period of 1–3 wks, there is diarrhoea, abdominal pain, weakness, anorexia, nausea and vomiting. On examination there may be abdominal distension and tenderness. Diagnosis is made on stool microscopy demonstrating cysts. Treatment is with a single dose of tinidazole 2 g, or metronidazole 400 mg 3 times daily for 10 days.

Cryptosporidiosis

Cryptosporidium spp. are coccidian protozoal parasites of humans and domestic animals. Infection is acquired by the faecal–oral route through contaminated water supplies. The incubation period is ~7–10 days, and is followed by watery diarrhoea and abdominal cramps. The illness is usually self-limiting, but in immunocompromised patients, especially those with HIV, it can be devastating, with persistent severe diarrhoea and substantial weight loss (p. 133).

INFECTIONS CAUSED BY HELMINTHS

Helminths (from the Greek *helmins*, meaning worm) include several classes of parasitic worm, large multicellular organisms with complex tissues and organs. Three groups of helminths parasitise humans:

Nematodes (roundworms): Intestinal (e.g. *Ancylostoma, Strongyloides, Ascaris*), tissue-dwelling (e.g. *Wuchereria bancrofti*).

Trematodes (flukes): Blood (*Schistosoma* spp.), lung (*Paragonimus* spp.), liver (e.g. *Fasciola hepatica*), intestinal (*Fasciolopsis buski*) flukes.

Cestodes (tapeworms): Intestinal (e.g. *Taenia solium, T. saginata*), tissue (e.g. *Echinococcus*).

Intestinal human nematodes
Ancylostomiasis (hookworm)

The causative organisms are *Ancylostoma duodenale* and *Necator americanus*. Ancylostomiasis is one of the main causes of anaemia in the tropics. The life cycle involves the passage of the hookworm from the soil through the skin via the blood stream to the lungs. The worms ascend the bronchi and are swallowed, the adult worm inhabiting the duodenum and jejunum. Eggs are passed in faeces, and develop through the larval stage to the filariform infective stage in the soil. Geographic distribution is as follows:

• *A. duodenale*: Far East, Mediterranean coastal regions, Africa.
• *N. americanum*: West, East and Central Africa, Central and South America, Far East.

Clinical features

• Cutaneous: allergic dermatitis of the feet at the time of infection.
• Pulmonary: paroxysmal cough, blood-stained sputum. • GI:

vomiting, epigastric pain, diarrhoea. • Systemic: symptoms of iron deficiency anaemia such as tiredness, malaise, cardiac failure.

Investigations
• Stool sample: ova on microscopy. FOB testing may be positive. • FBC: eosinophilia. • CXR: patchy consolidation.

Management
A single dose of albendazole (400 mg) is the treatment of choice. Mebendazole 100 mg twice daily for 3 days is an alternative. Oral iron supplementation is effective in patients who are anaemic.

Strongyloidiasis
Strongyloides stercoralis is a small nematode (2 mm × 0.4 mm). The life cycle involves the passage of the filariform larvae in the soil through the skin to the upper part of the small intestine, where the adult worms live. Eggs produced by the female hatch in the bowel and are passed in the larval stage in the faeces. Autoinfection may lead to a chronic form of the disease. It is found in the tropics and subtropics, especially the Far East.

Clinical features
• Cutaneous: itchy rash, urticarial papules and plaques, larva currens (linear urticarial weals on buttocks and abdomen). • GI: diarrhoea, abdominal pain, steatorrhoea, weight loss. • Disseminated infection occurs in the immunosuppressed (e.g. HIV, steroid treatment), causing pulmonary (wheeze, cough) and neurological symptoms (meningoencephalitis).

Investigations
• Stool sample: microscopy (motile larvae may be seen) and culture. • Jejunal aspirate/string test. • Blood: eosinophilia and antibodies by ELISA.

Management
• Ivermectin is first choice. • Albendazole is an alternative.

Ascaris lumbricoides (roundworm)
This pale yellow nematode is 20–35 cm long and causes up to 35% of intestinal obstruction in endemic areas of the tropics. The life cycle begins with ingestion of mature ova in contaminated food. *Ascaris* larvae hatch in the duodenum, migrate through the lungs, ascend the bronchial tree, are swallowed, and mature in the small intestine.

Clinical features
• GI: abdominal pain, severe obstructive complications (particularly at the terminal ileum), intussusception, volvulus, haemorrhagic infarction and perforation. • Hepatobiliary: blockage of the bile or pancreatic duct with worms. • Symptoms due to a generalised

hypersensitivity reaction caused by tissue migration: pneumonitis, bronchial asthma, urticaria.

Investigations

• Stool sample: adult worms visible; microscopy reveals ova. • FBC: eosinophilia. • Barium enema: may occasionally demonstrate worms.

Management

A single dose of albendazole (400 mg) is effective. Alternatives include pyrantel pamoate, ivermectin and mebendazole. Patients should be warned that they might expel numerous large worms. Intestinal obstruction is treated with nasogastric suction, piperazine and IV fluids.

Enterobius vermicularis *(threadworm)*

This helminthic infection is common throughout the world, especially in children. The life cycle begins with the ingestion of ova, which develop in the small intestine. Adult worms live in the colon. The adult female lays eggs around the anus, causing intense itching; eggs may be carried on the fingers to the mouth, causing autoinfection.

Clinical features

Intense itch in the perianal or genital area is the most common presenting symptom.

Investigations

Ova may be collected on a strip of adhesive tape applied in the morning to the perianal skin.

Management

• Single dose of mebendazole 100 mg, albendazole 400 mg or piperazine 4 g. Dosing should be repeated at 2 wks to prevent auto-reinfection. • If infection is recurrent, all family members should be treated. • General hygiene measures help to prevent spread: laundering of bedclothes, keeping nails short and clean.

Trichuris trichiura *(whipworm)*

This is common all over the world under unhygienic conditions. The life cycle begins with ingestion of ova in contaminated food. Adult worms 3–5 cm in length live in the caecum, lower ileum, appendix, colon and anal canal.

Infection is usually asymptomatic; intense infections may cause persistent diarrhoea or rectal prolapse. Diagnosis is by stool microscopy for ova. Treatment involves mebendazole or albendazole for 3 days or 5–7 days in heavy infections.

Tissue-dwelling human nematodes
Filariases

Filarial worms are tissue-dwelling nematodes. The larval stages are inoculated by biting mosquitoes or flies. The larvae develop into adult worms (2–50 cm long), which, after mating, produce millions of microfilariae (170–320 μm long) that migrate in blood or skin, causing a symptomatic immune response. Worms live 10–15 yrs and microfilariae 2–3 yrs. The life cycle is completed when the vector takes up microfilariae while feeding on humans, normally the only host.

Lymphatic filariasis

The causative organisms are *Wuchereria bancrofti* and *Brugia malayi*, which have different geographic distributions:

• *W. bancrofti*: occurs in tropical Africa, coastal areas of North Africa, Asia, Indonesia and northern Australia, the South Pacific islands, the West Indies, and North and South America. • *B. malayi*: affects Indonesia, Borneo, Malaysia, Vietnam, South China, South India and Sri Lanka.

Clinical features

Acute: Filarial lymphangitis presents with fever, pain, tenderness and erythema along the course of inflamed lymphatic vessels. Inflammation of the spermatic cord, epididymitis and orchitis is common. The whole episode lasts a few days but may recur several times a year.

Chronic: Oedema becomes persistent with regional lymphadenopathy. Progressive enlargement, coarsening, corrugation and fissuring of the skin and subcutaneous tissue develop gradually, causing irreversible 'elephantiasis'. The scrotum may reach an enormous size. Chyluria and chylous effusions are milky and opalescent.

Tropical pulmonary eosinophilia: This may develop when filariae enter pulmonary capillaries, causing a massive allergic response. Mainly seen in India, it presents with cough, wheeze and fever, and may progress to chronic interstitial lung disease.

Investigations

• FBC: massive eosinophilia (the highest of all the helminthic infections). • Indirect immunofluorescence on serum: detects filarial antibodies. • Wet blood film from a sample drawn at night: microfilariae circulate in large numbers at night. • Radiology: calcified filariae may be detected on X-ray.

Management

Diethylcarbamazine (DEC) kills microfilariae and adult worms. In the first 24–36 hrs of therapy, a severe allergic response to dying microfilariae, characterised by fever, headache, nausea, vomiting, arthralgia and prostration, may be seen, and severity is proportional to the filarial load. Antihistamines and oral steroid may be used to control the symptoms. Chronic lymphoedema should be managed with physiotherapy, tight bandaging and elevation, as well as scrupulous attention to skin care to prevent infection. Surgery is useful in selected cases. DEC can also be used for prophylaxis in endemic areas with a once-yearly dose.

Loiasis

The causative organism is the filaria *Loa loa*. The adults, 3–7 cm × 4 mm, chiefly parasitise the subcutaneous tissue of humans.

Clinical features

The infection is often symptomless. The first sign is usually a Calabar swelling, an irritating, tense, localised swelling up to a few centimetres in diameter that develops around an adult worm. The swelling is generally on a limb, and may be particularly painful if near a joint. It usually disappears after a few days but may persist for 2 or 3 wks. Other cutaneous signs include urticaria or, rarely, a visible worm wriggling under the skin (especially that of an eyelid) or across the eye under the conjunctiva.

Investigations

• Blood: direct visualisation of filariae, eosinophilia. • Immunology: antifilarial antibodies are positive in 95%. • X-rays: may demonstrate a calcified worm.

Management

DEC for 3 wks is curative but a febrile reaction to treatment is common, and may require steroids. Protective clothing and insect repellent prevent inoculation.

Onchocerciasis (river blindness)

The causative organism is *Onchocerca volvulus*; it is transmitted to humans by a bite from the *Simulium* fly. Onchocerciasis is a major cause of blindness in sub-Saharan Africa, Yemen, and parts of Central and South America. The worms live for up to 17 yrs in human tissue. Live microfilariae are poorly immunogenic, but dead ones elicit severe allergic inflammation. Death of microfilariae in the eye may cause blindness.

Clinical features

• May be symptomless in the early stages. • Itchy papular urticaria: excoriated papules, patchy hyperpigmentation, thickened, wrinkled skin. • Superficial lymphadenopathy: may become pendulous in the groin area. • Firm subcutaneous nodules (onchocercomas): result from fibrosis around adult worms. • Eyes: itch, lacrimation, conjunctivitis, progressing to sclerosing keratitis, 'snowflake' deposits on the cornea, choroidoretinitis and optic neuritis.

Investigations

• Direct microscopy of skin snip/shaving: demonstrates microfilariae. • FBC: eosinophilia. • Filarial antibodies: present in serum in 95% of cases.

Management

Ivermectin in a single dose is the treatment of choice, as it kills microfilariae with minimal toxicity. Dose is repeated 3-monthly to prevent relapses. Prevention takes the form of protective clothing, population prophylaxis with ivermectin, and insecticides to kill the *Simulium* fly.

Dracunculiasis (Guinea worm)

The Guinea worm (*Dracunculus medinensis*) is a tissue-dwelling nematode that is transmitted to humans by the ingestion of the crustacean *Cyclops*, now found only in sub-Saharan Africa. Management is by extraction of the protruding worm (which is over 1 m long), by winding it out gently over several days on a matchstick. The worm must not be broken.

Zoonotic nematodes
Trichinosis (trichinellosis)

Trichinella spiralis is a nematode that parasitises rats and pigs and is transmitted to humans by consumption of partially cooked infected pork or bear meat. Symptoms result from invasion of intestinal submucosa by ingested larvae, which develop into adult worms, and the secondary invasion of tissues, particularly striated muscle, by fresh larvae produced by these adult worms. Outbreaks have occurred in the UK, as well as in other countries where pork is eaten.

Clinical features

Infection may be asymptomatic. GI symptoms, such as nausea and diarrhoea, develop within 24–48 hrs coincident with invasion of the intestinal mucosa. Larval invasion on day 4–5 produces fever and oedema of the face, eyelids and conjunctivae. Larval invasion of muscle produces myositis. Larval migration may cause acute myocarditis and encephalitis.

Investigations

• Muscle biopsy: microscopy may demonstrate encysted larvae.
• Public health investigations: may reveal a cluster of cases who have eaten infected pork from a common source.

Management

Albendazole kills newly formed adult worms. Corticosteroids are required to counteract the effects of acute inflammation.

Cutaneous larva migrans

Larvae of the dog hookworm (*Ancylostoma caninum*) migrate 2–3-cm/day across the skin, causing intense itch and a linear serpiginous track. Treatment is with topical thiabendazole or systemic albendazole.

Trematodes (flukes)

These leaf-shaped worms are parasitic to humans and animals. Their complex life cycles may involve one or more intermediate hosts, often freshwater molluscs.

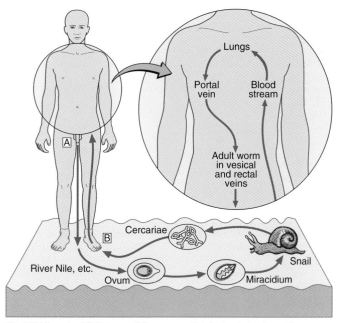

Fig. 5.13 Life cycle of *Schistosoma*. A Ova are passed into fresh water in urine and faeces.
B Cercariae in fresh water penetrate the skin of bathers, infecting a new host.

Schistosomiasis

Schistosomiasis (bilharziasis) is a major cause of morbidity in the tropics and is being spread by irrigation schemes. There are five species of the genus *Schistosoma* that commonly cause disease in humans: *S. haematobium*, *S. mansoni*, *S. japonicum*, *S. mekongi* and *S. intercalatum*. The life cycle of *Schistosoma* is illustrated in Figure 5.13. The human is the definitive host, and the freshwater snail the intermediate host.

Clinical features

These vary between species and are dependent on the stage of infection. After a symptom-free period of 3–5 wks, the acute presentation (Katayama syndrome) is with fever, urticaria, muscle aches, abdominal pain and cough. Chronic schistosomiasis is due to egg deposition. The eggs of *S. haematobium* mainly pass through the wall of the bladder, but may also involve the rectum, seminal vesicles, vagina, cervix and Fallopian tubes. Painless terminal haematuria is the most common symptom. *S. mansoni* and *S. japonicum* mainly pass through the wall of the bowel or are carried to the liver. Diarrhoea with mucus and blood is common. A summary of the symptoms of schistosomiasis as they correlate with the stage and type of infection is given in Box 5.22.

	5.22 Clinical pathology of schistosomiasis			
Stage	**Time**	***S. haematobium***	***S. mansoni* and *S. japonicum***
Cercarial penetration	Days	Papular dermatitis at site of penetration	As for *S. haematobium*
Larval migration and maturation	Weeks	Pneumonitis; myositis; hepatitis; fever; 'serum sickness'; eosinophilia; seroconversion	As for *S. haematobium*
Early egg deposition	Months	Cystitis; haematuria; ectopic granulomatous lesions: skin, CNS; immune complex glomerulonephritis	Colitis; granulomatous hepatitis; acute portal hypertension; ectopic lesions as for *S. haematobium*
Late egg deposition	Years	Fibrosis and calcification of ureters, bladder: bacterial infection, calculi, hydronephrosis, carcinoma; pulmonary granulomas and pulmonary hypertension	Colonic polyposis and strictures; periportal fibrosis; portal hypertension; pulmonary features as for *S. haematobium*

Investigations

Blood tests show eosinophilia. Serology (ELISA) aids screening but remains positive after cure.

S. haematobium: Dipstick urine testing demonstrates blood and albumin. Microscopy of a centrifuged terminal urine sample shows eggs. USS may demonstrate bladder wall thickening, hydronephrosis and bladder calcification. Cystoscopy reveals 'sandy' patches, bleeding mucosa and later distortion.

S. mansoni and S. japonicum: Stool microscopy demonstrates the characteristic egg with its lateral spine. Rectal biopsy may demonstrate schistosomes. Sigmoidoscopy may show inflammation or bleeding.

Management

Praziquantel is the drug of choice for all forms of schistosomiasis, producing parasitological cure in 80% of individuals. Side-effects are uncommon but include nausea and abdominal pain. Surgical intervention for ureteric stricture or bladder thickening may be required.

Liver flukes

Liver flukes infect at least 20 million people and remain an important public health problem in many endemic areas. They are associated with abdominal pain, hepatomegaly and relapsing cholangitis. *Clonorchis sinensis* is a major aetiological agent of bile duct cancer.

Cestodes (tapeworms)

Cestodes are ribbon-shaped worms that inhabit the intestinal tract of humans who have ingested undercooked infected beef, pork or fish. The causative organisms in each food are *Taenia saginata*, *T. solium* and *Diphyllobothrium latum*, respectively.

Some tapeworms, e.g. *T. saginata* and *D. latum*, cause only intestinal infection, while *T. solium* can cause intestinal or systemic infection (cysticercosis) and *Echinococcus granulosus* causes only systemic infection (hydatid disease).

T. solium is common in Central Europe, South Africa, South America and parts of Asia, while *T. saginata* occurs in all parts of the world. The adult worm may be several metres long. Intestinal infection is diagnosed by finding ova or segments in the stool. Praziquantel is the drug of choice, and prevention depends on efficient meat inspection and thorough cooking of meat.

Cysticercosis

Human cysticercosis is acquired either by ingesting *T. solium* ova on contaminated fingers (faecal–oral route) or by eating undercooked, contaminated pork (Fig. 5.14). The larvae are liberated from eggs in the stomach, penetrate the intestinal mucosa, and are carried to the subcutaneous tissue, skeletal muscles and brain, where they develop and form cysticerci, 0.5–1 cm cysts that contain the head of a young worm.

Clinical features

There are palpable cutaneous nodules that may calcify. Infection of the cerebral tissue may cause personality change, epilepsy, hydrocephalus or encephalitis.

Investigations

Biopsy of a cutaneous nodule may demonstrate cysticerci. CT/MRI will demonstrate cerebral cysts. X-rays of muscles may show calcified cysts. Antibody detection is available for serodiagnosis.

Management and prevention

Albendazole is the drug of choice for parenchymal neurocysticercosis. Praziquantel is another option. Prednisolone is also given for 14 days. Seizures should be controlled with appropriate anti-epileptic medicines. Good food handling and hygiene practices will reduce transmission.

Echinococcus granulosus (Taenia echinococcus) and hydatid disease

Dogs are the definitive hosts of the tiny tapeworm *E. granulosus*; ova produced by the adult worms inhabiting the dog are ingested by intermediate hosts, which include sheep, cattle, camels and humans. The embryo is liberated from the ovum in the small intestine and gains access to the blood stream and thus to the liver. The

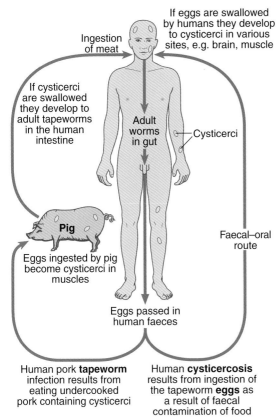

Fig. 5.14 Cysticercosis: life cycle of *Taenia solium*.

resultant cyst grows very slowly, sometimes intermittently, and may outlive the patient. It may calcify or rupture, giving rise to multiple cysts. The disease is common in the Middle East, North and East Africa, Australia and Argentina. Foci of infection persist in rural Wales and Scotland.

Clinical features

Hydatid disease is typically acquired in childhood; it causes cysts in the liver (75% of cases), lung, bone or brain. Symptoms are slow to develop and are a result of local pressure.

Investigations

USS or CT usually demonstrates the cyst. Serology is positive in 70–90%.

Management and prevention

Surgical excision is the treatment of choice, with praziquantel administered peri-operatively to kill protoscolices. Albendazole should also be used and may be effectively combined with aspiration. Good personal hygiene and animal handling practices, and regular deworming of dogs can reduce disease prevalence.

FUNGAL INFECTIONS

Superficial fungal infections of the skin are described in Chapter 17.

Subcutaneous mycoses
Chromoblastomycosis

Chromoblastomycosis is a tropical fungal disease of the cutaneous and subcutaneous tissue. The causative organism is most commonly *Fonsecaea pedrosoi*, and the disease is inoculated by trauma, particularly in those walking barefoot. Lesions may start several months after the injury in the form of a papule, which later turns into a painless, itchy, scaly nodule or plaque. Later there may be hypertrophy of the tissue, leading to a verrucous and cauliflower-like appearance.

Investigations

Biopsy shows brown, rounded sclerotic bodies. Culture confirms the aetiological agent.

Management

• Oral itraconazole or terbinafine. • Cryosurgery with liquid nitrogen.

Mycetoma

Mycetoma is a chronic suppurative infection of the deep soft tissues and bones, occurring mainly in the tropics. The limbs are most commonly affected. It is caused either by anaerobic filamentous bacteria, *Actinomycetes* (60% – actinomycetoma), or by true fungi, *Eumycetes* (40% – eumycetoma). Both groups produce characteristically coloured grains, the colour depending on the organism.

Clinical features

The causative organism is usually introduced by a thorn and the infection is most common on the foot (Madura foot). The mycetoma begins as a painless swelling at the site of implantation, which grows and spreads steadily within the soft tissues, causing further swelling and eventually penetrating bones. Nodules develop under the epidermis and these rupture, revealing sinuses through which grains (fungal colonies) are discharged. Deeper tissue invasion and involvement of bone are rapid and greater in actinomycetoma than eumycetoma. There is little pain and usually no fever or lymphaden-opathy, but there is progressive disability.

Investigations
Biopsy/aspiration of pus should be sent for microscopy, culture and determination of sensitivity.

Management
• *Eumycetes*: ketoconazole or itraconazole. • *Actinomycetes*: prolonged course of co-trimoxazole. • Surgical amputation may be required in severe cases.

Sporotrichosis
Sporotrichosis is caused by *Sporothrix schenckii*. It presents as a local-ised subcutaneous nodule at the site of inoculation (often a thorn scratch), which subsequently ulcerates with a pustular discharge (fixed cutaneous). The disease may then spread along the cutaneous lymphatic channels, forming multiple cutaneous nodules along their route, which ulcerate and discharge (lymphocutaneous). Pulmonary involvement occurs but is rare.

Investigations
Biopsy tissue should be sent for microscopy and culture.

Management
• Oral itraconazole for cutaneous and lymphocutaneous disease.
• Amphotericin B for systemic life-threatening illness.

Systemic fungal infections
Candidiasis
The species of *Candida* most commonly involved in human disease is *C. albicans*. Other species increasingly implicated are *C. tropicalis*, *C. glabrata* and *C. krusei*. Infection is most common in the immuno-suppressed, particularly neutropenic patients, as neutrophils form the body's main defence against *Candida*. The source of infection is usually endogenous, originating in flora in the patient's oropha-ryngeal and genital areas, commonly producing oropharyngeal or vaginal candidiasis or 'thrush'.

Clinical features
Systemic infection with *Candida* may be acute or chronic:

Acute disseminated candidiasis: Usually presents as candidae-mia, often in the presence of a central venous catheter. Recent abdominal surgery, antibiotics, total parenteral nutrition and IV drug misuse predispose to candidaemia. Up to 40% have ophthalmic involvement, with 'cotton wool' retinal exudates progressing to vitreous haze and threatening sight.

Chronic disseminated (hepatosplenic) candidiasis: Presents in neutropenic patients as persistent fever despite antibacterial therapy. There is abdominal pain, elevated alkaline phosphatase and multiple lesions seen in liver and spleen on imaging. This infection may last for months despite therapy.

Management

Infection detected on blood culture must be treated aggressively. In-dwelling catheters should be removed. Treatments for candidaemia include an echinocandin, amphotericin B, voriconazole and fluconazole.

Cryptococcosis

This is found worldwide and is caused by *Cryptococcus neoformans* and *Cr. gattii*. The former causes opportunistic infection, most commonly in those with HIV, while the latter causes severe disease in immunocompetent hosts. Spread is by inhalation. Disseminated cryptococcal infection mainly affects the immunocompromised. CNS manifestations include meningitis and cryptococcoma. Pulmonary cryptococcus can present as severe pneumonia in the immunocompromised, or cavitating nodules in immunocompetent patients.

Neurological disease is diagnosed by culture or recognition of spores in the CSF (India ink stain). The CSF shows a lymphocytosis and is often at high pressure (consequently, the condition may be complicated by raised intracranial pressure). Biopsy and serological detection of antigen may also be useful. Treatment is with IV antifungal agents such as amphotericin B. Recovery may be monitored by a fall in the antigen titres.

Mild pulmonary disease is treated with fluconazole or resection of nodules.

Histoplasmosis

Histoplasmosis is caused by *Histoplasma capsulatum* and is found in all parts of the USA, especially in the east central states. A variant, *H. duboisii*, is found in parts of tropical Africa. *H. capsulatum* multiplies in soil enriched by the droppings of birds and bats. Infection is by inhalation of infected dust.

Clinical features

Histoplasma infection is usually asymptomatic or self-limiting. Pulmonary symptoms may include non-productive cough, pleuritic pain and an influenza-like illness with fever. On examination, lymphadenopathy, rashes and pulmonary crackles may be found.

Investigations

• Biopsy: tissue should be sent for smear, histology and culture. • CXR: may show soft infiltrates, cavitating or calcified nodules, and hilar nodes. • Antigen or antibody detection in blood.

Management

• IV amphotericin B in severe infection. • Itraconazole for chronic infection. • Steroids may be added initially in severe pulmonary disease.

Coccidioidomycosis

This is caused by the air-borne organisms *Coccidioides immitis* and *C. posadasii*, and is found in Central and South America. It is acquired by inhalation and is asymptomatic in 60%. In others it affects the lungs, lymph nodes and skin. Meningitis is a rare but severe occurrence. Pulmonary coccidioidomycosis has two forms:

Primary coccidioidomycosis: If symptomatic, causes cough, fever, dyspnoea and rashes.

Progressive coccidioidomycosis: Marked systemic upset and lobar pneumonia; may mimic TB.

Diagnosis is by complement fixation and precipitin tests, and treatment is with antifungal azoles, or amphotericin B in severe disease.

Paracoccidioidomycosis

This is caused by *Paracoccidioides brasiliensis* and occurs in South America. Mucocutaneous lesions occur early. Involvement of lymphatic nodes and lungs is prominent and the GI tract may also be attacked. Treatment is with oral itraconazole solution.

Blastomycosis

North American blastomycosis is caused by *Blastomyces dermatitidis*. It also occurs in Africa. Systemic infection begins in the lungs and mediastinal lymph nodes and resembles pulmonary TB. Bones, skin and the genitourinary tract may also be affected. Treatment is with itraconazole or amphotericin B.

SEXUALLY TRANSMITTED BACTERIAL INFECTIONS

Syphilis

Syphilis is caused by infection, through abrasions in the skin or mucous membranes, with the spirochaete *Treponema pallidum*. In adults the infection is usually sexually acquired; however, transmission by kissing, blood transfusion and percutaneous injury has been reported. Transplacental infection of the fetus can occur.

Primary syphilis: The incubation period is usually between 14 and 28 days, with a range of 9–90 days. The primary lesion or chancre develops at the site of infection, usually in the genital area. A dull red macule develops, becomes papular and then erodes to form an indurated, painless ulcer (chancre) with associated inguinal lymphadenopathy. Without treatment, the chancre will resolve within 2–6 wks to leave a thin atrophic scar.

Secondary syphilis: This occurs 6–8 wks after the development of the chancre when treponemes disseminate to produce a multisystem disease. Constitutional features such as mild fever, malaise and headache are common. Over 75% of patients present with a maculopapular rash on the trunk and limbs that may later involve the palms and soles. Generalised non-tender lymphadenopathy is present in >50% of patients. Mucosal lesions, known as mucous patches, may affect the genitalia, mouth, pharynx or larynx and are essentially modified papules, which become eroded. Rarely, confluence produces characteristic 'snail track ulcers' in the mouth.

Tertiary syphilis: This may develop between 3 and 10 yrs after infection. The characteristic feature is a chronic granulomatous lesion called a gumma, which may be single or multiple and can affect skin, mucosa, bone, muscles or viscera. Resolution of active disease should follow treatment, though some tissue damage may be permanent.

After several years, cardiovascular syphilis, particularly aortitis with aortic incompetence, angina and aneurysm, and neurosyphilis, with meningovascular disease, tabes dorsalis or general paralysis of the insane, may develop (see p. 667).

Congenital syphilis: This is rare where antenatal serological screening is practised. Antisyphilitic treatment in pregnancy treats the fetus, if infected, as well as the mother. Treponemal infection in pregnancy may result in:

• Miscarriage or stillbirth. • A syphilitic baby (a very sick baby with hepatosplenomegaly and a bullous rash). • A baby who develops signs of congenital syphilis (condylomata lata, oral/anal/genital fissures, 'snuffles', lymphadenopathy and hepatosplenomegaly).

Adults with congenital syphilis may display the following classic features:

• Hutchinson's incisors (anterior–posterior thickening with notch on narrowed cutting edge). • Mulberry molars (imperfectly formed cusps/deficient dental enamel). • High arched palate. • Maxillary hypoplasia. • Rhagades (radiating scars around mouth, nose and anus). • Sabre tibia (from periostitis). • Bossing of frontal and parietal bones.

The treatment of choice is penicillin by injection.

Gonorrhoea

Gonorrhoea is caused by infection with *Neisseria gonorrhoeae* and may involve columnar epithelium in the lower genital tract, rectum, pharynx and eyes. Transmission is usually the result of vaginal, anal or oral sex. The incubation period is usually 2–10 days.

In men the anterior urethra is commonly infected, causing urethral discharge and dysuria, but symptoms are absent in ~10% of cases. Epididymo-orchitis may occur. In women, the urethra, paraurethral glands/ducts, Bartholin's glands/ducts or endocervical canal may be infected but 80% are asymptomatic. Acute pelvic inflammatory disease (PID, see below) is a rare complication. The rectum may also be involved, either due to contamination from a urogenital site or as a result of anal sex. Gram-negative intracellular diplococci are seen on direct smears from infected sites. Antibiotic resistance complicates treatment. The UK recommendation has changed to IM ceftriaxone 500 mg.

Chlamydial infection

Chlamydia is transmitted and presents in a similar way to gonorrhoea.

In men, urethral symptoms are usually mild and occur in <50% of cases. Epididymo-orchitis may occur. In women, the cervix and urethra are commonly involved. Infection is asymptomatic in ~80% of women but may cause vaginal discharge, dysuria, intermenstrual and/or post-coital bleeding. Lower abdominal pain, dyspareunia and intermenstrual bleeding suggest complicating PID. Examination may reveal mucopurulent cervicitis, contact bleeding from the cervix, evidence of PID or no obvious clinical signs. PID, with the risk of tubal damage and subsequent infertility or ectopic pregnancy, is an important long-term complication. Treatment options for chlamydia include a single 1-g oral dose of azithromycin, although PID requires more prolonged treatment.

SEXUALLY TRANSMITTED VIRAL INFECTIONS

Herpes simplex

Genital herpes simplex transmission is usually sexual (vaginal, anal, orogenital or oro–anal), but perinatal infection of the neonate may also occur. The manifestations of herpes simplex infection are covered on page 71.

Human papillomavirus (HPV)

Of the many subtypes of human papillomavirus (HPV), genotypes 6, 11, 16 and 18 most commonly infect the genital tract through sexual transmission.

Genotypes HPV-6 and 11 cause benign anogenital warts. Genotypes such as 16 and 18 are associated with dysplastic conditions and cancers, but not benign warts. Anogenital warts are the result of HPV-driven hyperplasia and usually develop after an incubation period of between 3 mths and 2 yrs. Local treatment with cryotherapy or podophyllotoxin may help, and condoms offer some protection. Vaccines are highly effective in preventing cervical neoplasia and are in routine use in several countries.

HUMAN IMMUNODEFICIENCY VIRUS INFECTION

The acquired immunodeficiency syndrome (AIDS) is caused by the human immunodeficiency virus (HIV-1) and was first recognised in 1981. HIV-2 causes a similar but less aggressive illness occurring mainly in West Africa. AIDS has become the second leading cause of disease worldwide and the leading cause of death in Africa (causing >20% of deaths). Immune deficiency arises from continuous HIV replication leading to virus- and immune-mediated destruction of CD4 lymphocytes.

Global epidemic and regional patterns

In 2011, the WHO estimated that there were 34.2 million people living with HIV/AIDS, 2.5 million new infections and 1.7 million deaths. Globally, new infections have declined by 20% in the past 10 yrs, although incidence is still increasing in Eastern Europe, Central Asia, the Middle East and North Africa particularly in injection drug-users. Expansion of access to combination antiretroviral therapy (ART) has resulted in improved life expectancy and a 24% decline in global AIDS-related deaths since 2005. Despite this, HIV remains important and has caused over 30 million deaths since the start of the epidemic.

HIV is transmitted:

• By sexual contact. • By exposure to blood or blood products (e.g. drug users, patients with haemophilia or occupationally in health-care workers). • Vertically from mother to child in utero, during birth or by breastfeeding.

In the Americas and Western Europe, the epidemic has until now predominantly affected men who have sex with men (MSM), whereas in Eastern Europe, Central Asia, the Middle East and Southeast Asia, IV drug use also causes many infections. In sub-Saharan Africa, the Caribbean and Oceania, most transmission is heterosexual. Worldwide, the major route of transmission is heterosexual.

A high proportion of patients with haemophilia had been infected through contaminated blood products by the time HIV antibody screening was adopted in the USA and Europe in 1985. Screening of blood products has virtually eliminated these as a mode of transmission in developed countries; however, the WHO estimates that 5–10% of blood transfusions globally are with HIV-infected blood.

The transmission risk after exposure is summarised in Box 5.23.

Virology and immunology

HIV is an enveloped RNA retrovirus of the lentivirus family. The different stages of the viral replication process offer opportunities for drug therapy (Box 5.24). A small percentage of T-helper lymphocytes enter a post-integration latent phase and represent sanctuary sites from antiretroviral drugs, which only act on replicating virus. This prevents current ART from eradicating HIV. Latently infected CD4 cells also evade CD8 cytotoxic T lymphocytes.

Diagnosis and initial testing

HIV infection is detected by testing for host antibodies; most tests are sensitive to antibodies to both HIV-1 and HIV-2. Global trends are towards more widespread testing. Counselling is essential both before testing and after the result is obtained.

Following diagnosis, the CD4 lymphocyte count should be determined. This indicates the degree of immune suppression and is used to guide treatment. Counts between 200 and 500/mm^3 have a low

5.23 Risk of HIV transmission after single exposure to an HIV-infected source	
HIV exposure	**Approximate risk**
Sexual intercourse	
Vaginal: female to male	0.05%
male to female	0.1%
Anal: insertive	0.05%
receptive	0.5%
Oral: insertive	0.005%
receptive	0.01%
Blood exposure	
Transfusion	90%
IV drug user sharing needle	0.67%
Percutaneous needle stick	0.3%
Mucous membrane splash	0.09%
Mother to child	
Vaginal delivery	15%
Breastfeeding (per month)	0.5%

5.24 Stages of viral replication and corresponding drug targets		
Stage	**Steps in replication**	**Drug targets**
1	Attachment to CD4 receptor	
2	Binding to co-receptor CCR5 or CXCR4	CCR5/CXCR4 receptor inhibitors
3	Fusion	Fusion inhibitors
4	Reverse transcription	Nucleoside and non-nucleoside reverse transcription inhibitors (NRTIs and NNRTIs)
5	Integration	Integrase inhibitors
6	Transcription	
7	Translation	
8	Cleavage of polypeptides and assembly	Protease inhibitors (PIs)
9	Viral release	

risk of major opportunistic infection; below $200/mm^3$ there is a high risk of AIDS-defining conditions. Quantitative PCR of HIV-RNA, known as viral load, is used to monitor the response to ART.

Natural history and classification of HIV
Primary infection

Primary infection is symptomatic in >50% of cases and usually occurs 2–4 wks after exposure. The major clinical manifestations resemble infectious mononucleosis:

• Fever. • Pharyngitis with lymphadenopathy. • Myalgia/arthralgia. • Headache. • Diarrhoea. • Mucosal ulceration. • Oral and genital ulceration.

The presence of a maculopapular rash or mucosal ulceration suggests HIV rather than the other causes of infectious mononucleosis. Lymphopenia with oropharyngeal candidiasis may occur. Symptomatic recovery normally takes 1–2 wks but may take up to 10 wks, and parallels the return of the CD4 count and the fall in viral load. In many patients the illness is mild and is only identified by retrospective enquiry.

Diagnosis is made by detecting HIV-RNA in the serum by PCR, as antibody tests may be negative in the early stages. The differential diagnosis includes:

• Acute Epstein–Barr virus. • Cytomegalovirus. • Streptococcal pharyngitis. • Toxoplasmosis. • Secondary syphilis.

Asymptomatic infection

This lasts for a variable period, during which the infected individual remains well with no evidence of disease, except for persistent generalised lymphadenopathy (defined as enlarged glands at ≥2 extra-inguinal sites). Viraemia peaks during this phase and high viral loads predict a more rapid rate of decline in CD4 count (Fig. 5.15). The median time from infection to development of AIDS in adults is 9 yrs.

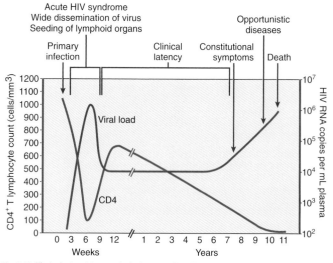

Fig. 5.15 Virological and immunological progression of HIV infection.

5.25 AIDS-defining diseases

- Oesophageal candidiasis
- Chronic cryptosporidial diarrhoea
- Chronic mucocutaneous herpes simplex
- Pulmonary or extrapulmonary TB
- Progressive multifocal leucoencephalopathy
- Recurrent non-typhi *Salmonella* septicaemia
- Invasive cervical cancer
- Kaposi's sarcoma
- HIV-associated wasting
- Primary cerebral lymphoma
- Cryptococcal meningitis
- Cytomegalovirus (CMV) retinitis or colitis
- *Pneumocystis jirovecii* pneumonia (PJP)
- Disseminated *Mycobacterium avium intracellulare* (MAI)
- Cerebral toxoplasmosis
- Extrapulmonary coccidioidomycosis
- Extrapulmonary histoplasmosis
- Non-Hodgkin's lymphoma
- HIV-associated dementia

Minor HIV-associated disorders

A wide range of disorders indicating some impairment of cellular immunity occurs in most patients before they develop AIDS. Careful examination of the mouth is important, as oral candidiasis and oral hairy leucoplakia are common and important conditions that require the initiation of ART and prophylaxis against opportunistic infections, irrespective of the CD4 count.

AIDS

AIDS is defined by the development of specified opportunistic infections, tumours and other clinical features (Box 5.25). This is accompanied by a fall in CD4 count to <200 cells/mm^3, and a change in the spectrum of associated infections (Box 5.26).

PRESENTING PROBLEMS IN HIV INFECTION

Lymphadenopathy

Lymphadenopathy in HIV can be due to malignancy (Kaposi's sarcoma or lymphoma) or infections, especially TB. Enlarging lymph nodes should undergo needle biopsy for mycobacterial culture and cytology for lymphoma.

Weight loss

The HIV wasting syndrome is an AIDS-defining condition comprising 10% weight loss and either chronic diarrhoea or chronic weakness with unexplained fever. Infections, painful oral conditions and depression should be excluded before diagnosis.

> **5.26 Correlations between CD4 count and HIV-associated diseases**
>
> **<500 cells/mm³**
>
> • TB, bacterial pneumonia, herpes zoster, oropharyngeal candidiasis, non-typhoid salmonellosis, Kaposi's sarcoma, non-Hodgkin's lymphoma, HIV-associated idiopathic thrombocytopenic purpura
>
> **<200 cells/mm³**
>
> • *Pneumocystis jirovecii* pneumonia (PJP), chronic herpes simplex ulcers, oesophageal candidiasis, *Isospora belli* diarrhoea, HIV wasting syndrome, HIV-associated dementia, peripheral neuropathy, endemic mycoses
>
> **<100 cells/mm³**
>
> • Cerebral toxoplasmosis, cryptococcal meningitis, cryptosporidiosis and microsporidiosis, primary CNS lymphoma, CMV, disseminated MAI, progressive multifocal leucoencephalopathy

Fever

Fever is a very common presentation in HIV. Non-*Salmonella* bacteraemia can present with fever without diarrhoea. PUO in HIV should be investigated with abdominal CT, which may reveal lymphadenopathy or splenic microabscesses. Bone marrow should be sampled if there are cytopenias. TB or disseminated *Mycobacterium avium* infection (MAI) are common underlying causes of fever.

Mucocutaneous disease

HIV-associated skin diseases include:

Psoriasis and drug rashes: Exacerbated by HIV.

Seborrhoeic dermatitis: Scaly patches in skin folds. Fungal infection contributes.

Herpes simplex: May affect the nasolabial and anogenital regions. Ulcers lasting >4 wks are AIDS-defining.

Herpes zoster: Usually presents with a dermatomal vesicular rash on an erythematous base. In advanced disease it may be multi-dermatomal, with a high risk of post-herpetic neuralgia.

Kaposi's sarcoma (KS; Fig. 5.16): A lympho-endothelial tumour due to sexually transmitted herpesvirus 8. Predominantly affects men and presents with red–purple papular or nodular skin lesions. May spread to lymph nodes, lungs and the GI tract. Chemotherapy is reserved for those who fail to improve on ART.

Bacillary angiomatosis: A bacterial infection caused by *Bartonella henselae*. Causes red–purple skin lesions. May become disseminated with fevers, lymphadenopathy and hepatosplenomegaly.

Oral **Candida** *infection:* Very common in HIV and nearly always caused by *C. albicans*. Treatment is with an oral azole drug.

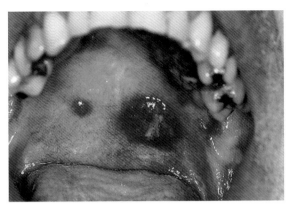

Fig. 5.16 Oral Kaposi's sarcoma. A full examination is important to detect disease that may affect the palate, gums, fauces or tongue.

Oral hairy leucoplakia: Corrugated white plaques running vertically on the side of the tongue; virtually pathognomonic of HIV. It is usually asymptomatic and is due to EBV.

Gastrointestinal disease

Oesophageal candidiasis: Causes dysphagia. Concomitant oral candidiasis is usual. Systemic fluconazole is usually curative.

Large-bowel diarrhoea: Usually caused by *Campylobacter*, *Shigella* or *Salmonella*. CMV colitis may occur in those with CD4 counts <100/mm^3.

Small-bowel diarrhoea: Presents with watery diarrhoea and wasting without fever and may be due to HIV enteropathy or have an infective cause – typically, cryptosporidiosis, microsporidiosis, isosporiasis or disseminated MAI.

Hepatobiliary disease

Because of shared risk factors, co-infection of HIV patients with hepatitis B (HBV) and/or C (HCV) is common, particularly in injection drug users and patients with haemophilia. In both HBV and HCV infection, HIV increases viraemia and also the risk of hepatic fibrosis and hepatoma. During treatment, a flare of hepatitis may be seen with immune recovery.

Hepatitis B: Treatment with anti-HBV drugs is indicated in all those with active HBV replication, hepatitis or fibrosis. The ART drugs tenofovir, lamivudine and emtricitabine are useful in this situation.

Hepatitis C: Treatment for HCV should be deferred until ART has restored the CD4 count to >350 cells/mm^3. Response to anti-HCV therapy is similar to that in HIV-negative patients, but toxicity is more common.

HIV cholangiopathy: A sclerosing cholangitis is seen in patients with severe immune suppression. Co-infection with CMV, cryptosporidiosis and microsporidiosis may be present. ERCP with cautery may be needed, and ART may also improve this condition.

Respiratory disease

Respiratory admissions in HIV patients are most frequently due to bacterial pneumonia, *Pneumocystis jirovecii* pneumonia (in high-income countries) or TB (in low-income countries).

Pneumocystis jirovecii: Clinical features include:

• Progressive dyspnoea. • Dry cough. • Fever. • Exercise-induced O_2 desaturation. • Hypoxaemia on ABGs. • Impaired carbon monoxide transfer factor. • Raised LDH (from lung damage). • Pneumothorax.

Auscultation is unremarkable and the CXR may be normal in early disease (15–20%) but classically shows perihilar ground-glass changes. Induced sputum is a sensitive diagnostic test. Co-trimoxazole is used for treatment and prophylaxis.

Pulmonary TB: TB is the most common cause of admission in countries with a high TB incidence. The clinical presentation depends on immune function. When the CD4 count is >200 cells/mm³, disease is more likely to be reactivated, upper-lobe, open cavitatory disease. As immunosuppression increases, the clinical pattern changes:

• Disease progresses more rapidly. • X-ray appearances become atypical with lymphadenopathy or effusions rather than apical cavitation. • Sputum smears are often negative in the absence of cavitation. • Many patients have disseminated disease with miliary pulmonary shadowing, pleural or lymph node disease or extrapulmonary TB. TB in HIV responds well to standard short-course therapy (p. 295).

Bacterial infections: Bacterial pneumonia (p. 289) is common in HIV.

Nervous system and eye disease

Cognitive impairment: HIV invades the nervous system early, and meningo-encephalitis may occur at seroconversion. Neuropsychiatric tests may reveal neurocognitive disorders ranging from asymptomatic impairment to dementia. Dementia is associated with cerebral atrophy on CT or MRI, but usually responds to ART. Progressive multifocal leucoencephalopathy (PMFL) is a fatal demyelinating disease caused by the JC virus; it presents with stroke-like episodes and cognitive impairment. Vision is often affected. The presence of JC-DNA in CSF is diagnostic. No specific treatment exists and the prognosis is poor. CMV encephalitis may also cause cognitive impairment, and responds poorly to treatment.

Space-occupying lesions: *Toxoplasma* infection (p. 104) is the most common cause. Cerebral toxoplasmosis is caused by reactivation of residual *Toxoplasma gondii* cysts from past infection. Imaging reveals multiple ring-enhancing space-occupying lesions with surrounding oedema. Diagnosis is by imaging supported by serology. Treatment is with sulfadiazine and pyrimethamine, although co-trimoxazole may also be effective, with improvement in 1–2 wks and shrinkage of lesions in 2–4 wks. Primary CNS lymphomas are high-grade B-cell lymphomas associated with EBV infection. Imaging typically shows a single enhancing periventricular lesion with surrounding oedema. If lumbar puncture can be safely performed, EBV-DNA can be demonstrated by PCR. Treatment is usually palliative with dexamethasone and symptom relief. The prognosis is poor. Tuberculoma is identified by lesions resembling toxoplasmosis on imaging. CSF shows features of tuberculous meningitis (p. 662).

Stroke: Atherosclerosis is enhanced by HIV and by some antiretroviral drugs. HIV can also cause vasculitis. The result is an increased incidence of stroke in patients with HIV.

Meningitis: Cryptococcus neoformans is the most common cause of meningitis in AIDS patients. It presents subacutely with a 2–3-wk history of headache, fever, vomiting and mild confusion; neck stiffness is often absent (<50%). Protein, cell counts and glucose may be normal in the CSF, although CSF cryptococcal antigen tests have sensitivity and specificity close to 100%. Treatment is 2 wks of amphotericin B followed by fluconazole. Tuberculous meningitis is also common and presents in a similar way to that in patients without HIV.

Myelopathy and radiculopathy: Myelopathy most commonly results from tuberculous spondylitis. Vacuolar myelopathy causes paraparesis in advanced HIV disease. CMV polyradiculitis causes painful legs, flaccid paraparesis, saddle anaesthesia and sphincter dysfunction. Despite ganciclovir treatment, functional recovery is poor.

Retinopathy: CMV retinitis causes painless, progressive visual loss in patients with severe immunosuppression. Haemorrhages and exudates are seen on the retina. Treatment with ganciclovir or valganciclovir may halt progression but does not restore lost vision. The eyes may also be affected by toxoplasmosis or varicella zoster infection. In addition, immune recovery with ART sometimes causes uveitis.

Rheumatological problems

HIV can cause seronegative arthritis resembling the rheumatoid type, or it can exacerbate reactive arthritis.

Diffuse infiltrative lymphocytosis syndrome is a benign lymphocytic tissue infiltration that commonly presents with bilateral parotid swelling and lymphadenopathy. Hepatitis, arthritis and polymyositis may occur. Treatment is with steroids and ART but the response is variable.

Haematological problems

Normochromic normocytic anaemia and thrombocytopenia are common in advanced HIV. Antiretroviral drugs may cause haematological disorders, e.g. zidovudine causes macrocytic anaemia and neutropenia. Immune thrombocytopenia in HIV responds to steroids or immunoglobulins, together with ART.

Renal disease

HIV-associated nephropathy is an important cause of renal failure and presents with nephrotic syndrome. Outcomes of renal transplantation on ART are good.

Cardiac disease

HIV-associated cardiomyopathy is a rapidly progressive dilated cardiomyopathy. Tuberculous pericarditis and accelerated coronary atheroma are other HIV-associated cardiac disorders.

MANAGEMENT OF HIV

Prevention of opportunistic infections

Effective ART is the best protection, but other protective measures remain important:
• Avoidance of contaminated water. • Barrier contraception. • Avoidance of animal-borne infection (cats). • Malaria vector control in endemic areas. • Co-trimoxazole prophylaxis: protects against *Pneumocystis*, toxoplasmosis and *Isospora belli*. • Vaccination against pneumococcus, seasonal influenza and hepatitis B is useful once CD4 counts are >200 cells/mm^3.

Antiretroviral therapy

The goals of ART are to:
• Reduce the viral load to an undetectable level (<50 copies/mL) for as long as possible. • Improve the CD4 count (above a level of 200 cells/mm^3 significant HIV-related events rarely occur). • Prolong life without unacceptable side-effects. • Reduce transmission.

The decision to start therapy is influenced by symptoms, CD4 count and the patient's wishes. Treatment is usually commenced when the CD4 count falls <350 cells/mm^3 or the patient is symptomatic. Earlier treatment is given if an unaffected partner is at risk. Commonly used drugs are shown in Box 5.27. The standard combination antiretroviral regimens are two NNRTIs together with an NNRTI, PI or integrase inhibitor. Subsequent ART regimen switches are guided by resistance testing.

Adherence to lifelong treatment is vital, and is enhanced by:
• Disclosure of HIV status. • Joining support groups. • Patient-nominated treatment supporters. • Management of coincident depression and substance abuse.

Treatment should be monitored by measuring viral load, which should drop tenfold in the first 4–8 wks of ART. Within 6 mths, viral load should be below the limit of detection (usually <50 copies/mL). Treatment failure is defined as a subsequent rise to >400–1000

5.27 Commonly used antiretroviral drugs	
Classes	**Drugs**
Nucleoside reverse transcriptase inhibitors (NRTIs)	Abacavir, emtricitabine, lamivudine, tenofovir, zidovudine
Non-nucleoside reverse transcriptase inhibitors (NNRTIs)	Efavirenz, nevirapine, etravirine
Protease inhibitors (PIs)	Atazanavir, darunavir, lopinavir
Integrase inhibitors	Raltegravir
Chemokine receptor inhibitor	Maraviroc

copies/mL. CD4 count rises with treatment and falls with treatment failure, and can be used for monitoring in countries where viral load is unavailable.

Pregnancy, HIV and ART

All pregnant women should be recommended for HIV screening. ART has reduced the risk of mother-to-child transmission of HIV to <1%. Caesarean section reduces the risk of transmission but makes no difference to risk in those on ART. HIV is also transmitted by breastfeeding but risk can be reduced by treating the infant with antiretrovirals.

Post-exposure prophylaxis

When risk of infection is deemed to be significant after careful risk assessment, post-exposure prophylaxis (PEP) should be given. The first dose should be given as soon as possible, preferably within 6–8 hrs; after 72 hrs PEP is ineffective. Dual NRTIs are usually recommended, with a PI or efavirenz if exposure is high-risk. HIV antibody testing should be repeated at 6, 12 and 24 wks after exposure.

Clinical biochemistry and metabolism

6

Between 60 and 70% of all critical decisions taken in regard to patients in health-care systems in developed countries involve a laboratory service or result. This chapter describes disorders whose primary manifestation is in abnormalities of biochemistry laboratory results, or whose underlying pathophysiology involves disturbance in specific biochemical pathways.

WATER AND ELECTROLYTE DISTRIBUTION

In a typical adult male, the 40 L of total body water (TBW) constitute ~60% of body weight. About 25 L is located inside cells (intracellular fluid; ICF), while the remainder is in the extracellular fluid (ECF) compartment. Plasma constitutes a small fraction (some 3 L) of the ECF while the remainder is interstitial fluid within the tissues but outside the cells.

The dominant cation in the ICF is potassium, while in the ECF it is sodium (Fig. 6.1). Phosphates and negatively charged proteins constitute the major intracellular anions, while chloride and bicarbonate dominate the ECF anions. An important difference between the plasma and interstitial ECF is that only plasma contains significant concentrations of protein.

The major force maintaining the difference in cation concentration between the ICF and ECF is the sodium–potassium pump (Na,K-activated ATPase) integral to all cell membranes. Maintenance of the cation gradients across cell membranes is essential for many cell processes, including the excitability of conducting tissues such as nerve and muscle. The difference in protein content between the plasma and the interstitial fluid compartment is maintained by the protein permeability barrier at the capillary wall. This protein concentration gradient contributes to the balance of forces across the capillary wall that favour fluid retention within the capillaries (the colloid osmotic, or oncotic, pressure of the plasma), maintaining circulating plasma volume.

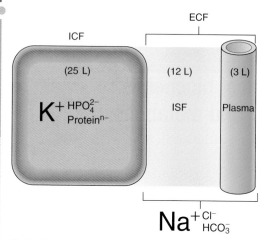

Fig. 6.1 Normal distribution of body water and electrolytes. Schematic representation of volume (L = litres) and composition (dominant ionic species only shown) of the intracellular fluid (ICF) and extracellular fluid (ECF) in a 70-kg male. Total body water (TBW) = ~60% of body weight. TBW = ICF + ECF = 40 L. The main difference in composition between the plasma and interstitial fluid (ISF) is the presence of appreciable concentrations of protein in the plasma (not shown) but not the ISF. The sodium–potassium pump maintains the cation concentration difference between the ICF and ECF. The difference in protein content between the plasma and interstitial compartments is maintained by the permeability characteristics of the capillary wall.

Investigation of water and electrolytes

Because the blood consists of both intracellular (red cell) and extra-cellular (plasma) components, it is important to avoid haemolysis of the sample, which causes contamination of the plasma by intra-cellular elements, particularly potassium. Blood should not be drawn from an arm into which an IV infusion is being given, to avoid contamination by the infused fluid.

Whole-body disturbances of fluid and electrolytes cause clinical problems, as outlined in Box 6.1.

A guide to the interpretation of disorders of urea and electrolytes is given in Box 6.2.

Since the kidney maintains body fluid composition by adjusting urine volume and composition, it is often helpful to obtain a simul-taneous sample of urine ('spot' specimen or 24-hr collection) at the time of blood analysis.

DISORDERS OF SODIUM BALANCE

When sodium balance is disturbed, as a result of imbalance between intake and excretion, any tendency for plasma sodium concentration to change is usually corrected by the osmotic mechanisms control-ling water balance (see below). As a result, disorders in sodium

6.1 Manifestations of disordered fluid and electrolytes		
Primary disturbance	**Altered physiology**	**Clinical effect**
Sodium	ECF volume	Circulatory changes
Water	ECF osmolality	Cerebral changes
Potassium	Action potential in excitable tissues	Neuromuscular and cardiac effects
Hydrogen ion	Acid–base disturbance	Altered tissue function
Magnesium	Cell membrane instability	Neuromuscular and cardiac effects
Phosphate	Cellular energetics	Widespread tissue effects

ECF = extracellular fluid.

6.2 How to interpret urea and electrolyte results	
Sodium	Largely reflects reciprocal changes in body water
Potassium	May reflect K shifts in and out of cells
	Low: usually excess loss (renal, GI)
	High: usually renal dysfunction
Chloride	Generally changes in parallel with Na
	Low in metabolic alkalosis
	High in some metabolic acidosis
Bicarbonate	Abnormal acid–base disorders – see Box 6.6
Urea	Rises with ↓glomerular filtration rate, ↓renal perfusion, ↓urine flow, catabolic states or high protein intake
Creatinine	Rises with ↓glomerular filtration rate, high muscle mass, some drugs

balance present chiefly as altered ECF volume rather than altered sodium concentration.

Sodium depletion

Aetiology includes the following factors:

• Inadequate intake. • GI sodium loss: vomiting, diarrhoea, external fistula. • Skin sodium loss: excess sweating, burns. • Renal sodium loss: diuretics, mineralocorticoid deficiency. • Internal sequestration: bowel obstruction, pancreatitis.

Clinical features

Symptoms and signs of hypovolaemia are as follows:

• Thirst. • Dizziness on standing. • Weakness. • Low JVP. • Postural hypotension. • Tachycardia. • Dry mouth. • Confusion. • Weight loss.

Supportive biochemistry includes:

• Low plasma sodium (note that plasma sodium may be in the reference range if salt and water losses proceed in parallel). • High urea. • High urine osmolality. • Low urine sodium.

Management of sodium and water depletion

This has two main components:
• Treatment of the cause where possible, to stop ongoing salt and water losses. • Replacement of salt and water deficits, and provision of ongoing maintenance requirements, by IV infusion when depletion is severe.

IV fluid therapy: A typical adult requires 2.5–3 L of water, 100–140 mmol of sodium and 70–100 mmol of potassium per day. IV normal saline distributes to the ECF; ~20% is retained in the plasma whereas IV 5% dextrose contributes <10% of the infused volume to plasma volume. The choice of fluid and rate of administration depend on the clinical circumstances and the laboratory data.

Sodium excess

In the presence of normal function of the heart and kidneys, an excessive intake of salt and water is compensated for by increased excretion and so is unlikely to lead to clinically obvious features of hypervolaemia.

Causes of sodium and water excess in clinical practice include:
• Impaired renal function: primary renal disease. • Primary hyperaldosteronism: Conn's syndrome. • Secondary hyperaldosteronism: congestive cardiac failure, cirrhotic liver disease, nephrotic syndrome.

Peripheral oedema is the most common physical sign associated with these conditions (p. 165), although it is not usually a feature of Conn's syndrome.

Management

The management of ECF volume overload involves:
• Specific treatment directed at the cause, e.g. ACE inhibitors in heart failure, corticosteroids in minimal change nephropathy. • Restriction of dietary sodium to 50–80 mmol/day. • Diuretics (loop or thiazide).

DISORDERS OF WATER BALANCE

Daily water intake can vary over a wide range, from 500 mL to several litres a day. While a certain amount of water is lost through the stool, sweat and the respiratory tract, the kidneys are chiefly responsible for adjusting water excretion to maintain a constant body water content and body fluid osmolality (reference range 280–296 mmol/kg).

Disturbances in body water metabolism, in the absence of changes in sodium balance, manifest principally as abnormalities of plasma sodium concentration, and hence of plasma osmolality. The main consequence of changes in plasma osmolality, especially when rapid, is altered cerebral function. This is because, when extracellular osmolality changes abruptly, water flows rapidly across cell membranes with resultant cell swelling (during hypo-osmolality) or shrinkage (during hyperosmolality). Cerebral cell function is very sensitive to such volume changes, particularly during cell swelling, when an increase in intracerebral pressure causes reduced cerebral perfusion.

Hyponatraemia

When hyponatraemia (plasma Na <135 mmol/L) develops gradually, it is relatively asymptomatic. More rapid changes in plasma osmolality and plasma sodium may be associated with:
• Anorexia. • Nausea. • Vomiting. • Confusion. • Lethargy. • Seizures. • Coma.

The causes of hyponatraemia are best organised according to any associated change in ECF volume status, i.e. the total body sodium. In all cases, there is retention of water relative to sodium, and it is the clinical examination rather than the electrolyte test results that gives clues to the underlying problem.

Hypovolaemic (sodium deficit with a relatively smaller water deficit): Renal Na loss (diuretics), GI Na loss (vomiting, diarrhoea).

Euvolaemic (water retention alone, i.e. 'dilutional'): Primary polydipsia, SIADH (Box 6.3).

Hypervolaemic (sodium retention with relatively greater water retention): Heart failure, cirrhosis and chronic kidney disease (without water restriction).

Investigations

Plasma and urine electrolytes and osmolality (Box 6.4) are usually the only tests required to classify the hyponatraemia.

6.3 Syndrome of inappropriate antidiuretic hormone secretion (SIADH): causes and diagnosis

Causes

- Tumours, especially small-cell lung cancer
- CNS disorders: stroke, trauma, infection, psychosis
- Pulmonary disorders: pneumonia, TB
- Drugs: anticonvulsants, psychotropics, antidepressants, cytotoxics, oral hypoglycaemics, opiates
- Idiopathic

Diagnosis

- Low plasma sodium concentration (typically <130 mmol/L)
- Low plasma osmolality (<270 mmol/kg)
- Urine osmolality not minimally low (>150 mmol/kg)
- Urine sodium concentration not minimally low (>30 mmol/L)
- Low–normal plasma urea, creatinine, uric acid
- Exclusion of other causes of hyponatraemia
- Appropriate clinical context (see above)

6.4 Urine Na and osmolality in the differential diagnosis of hyponatraemia*

Urine Na (mmol/L)	Urine osmolality (mmol/kg)	Possible diagnoses
Low (<30)	Low (<100)	Primary polydipsia, malnutrition
Low	High (>150)	Salt depletion, hypovolaemia
High (>40)	Low	Diuretic action (acute phase)
High	High	SIADH, adrenal insufficiency

*Urine analysis may give results of indeterminate significance; if so, diagnosis depends on comprehensive clinical assessment.

Management

The treatment for hyponatraemia is critically dependent on the rate of development and severity, and on the underlying cause.

If hyponatraemia has developed rapidly (over hours to days), and there are signs of cerebral oedema (patient is obtunded or convulsing), sodium levels should be rapidly restored to normal by infusion of hypertonic (3%) sodium chloride solutions.

Rapid correction of hyponatraemia that has developed slowly (over weeks to months) may lead to 'central pontine myelinolysis', which may cause permanent structural and functional cerebral changes and is generally fatal. The rate of plasma sodium correction in chronic asymptomatic hyponatraemia should not exceed 10 mmol/L/day, and an even slower rate would generally be safer.

Specific treatment should be directed at the underlying cause. For hypovolaemic patients, this will involve controlling sodium loss and giving IV saline if clinically warranted. Patients with dilutional hyponatraemia usually respond to fluid restriction in the range of 600–1000 mL/day and removal of the precipitating stimulus (e.g. a drug causing SIADH). Demeclocycline or oral urea supplements may be of use in SIADH.

Hypernatraemia

Just as hyponatraemia represents a failure of the mechanisms for diluting the urine during free access to water, so hypernatraemia (plasma Na >148 mmol/L) reflects an inadequacy of the kidney in concentrating the urine in the face of restricted water intake.

Patients with hypernatraemia generally have reduced cerebral function and cerebral dehydration. This triggers thirst and drinking, and if adequate water is obtained, is self-limiting. If adequate water is not obtained, dizziness, confusion, weakness and ultimately coma and death can result.

Similar to hyponatraemia, the causes of hypernatraemia may be classified based on the volume state of the patient:

Hypovolaemic (sodium deficit with a relatively greater water deficit): Renal Na losses (diuretics), GI Na losses (colonic diarrhoea), skin Na losses (excessive sweating).

Euvolaemic (water deficit alone): Diabetes insipidus (central or nephrogenic, p. 378).

Hypervolaemic (sodium retention with relatively less water retention): Enteral or parenteral nutrition, oral salt administration, chronic kidney disease (during water restriction).

Management

Treatment of hypernatraemia depends on both the rate of development and the underlying cause.

If there is reason to think that the condition has developed quickly, correction with appropriate volumes of IV hypotonic fluid may be attempted relatively rapidly.

In older, institutionalised patients, however, it is more likely that the disorder has developed slowly and extreme caution should be exercised in lowering the plasma sodium, to avoid the risk of cerebral oedema.

DISORDERS OF POTASSIUM BALANCE

Potassium is the major intracellular cation (see Fig. 6.1), and the steep concentration gradient for potassium across the cell membrane of excitable cells plays an important part in generating the resting membrane potential and allowing the propagation of the action potential, which is crucial to normal functioning of nerve, muscle and cardiac tissues.

Hypokalaemia

Hypokalaemia is asymptomatic if mild (3–3.3 mmol/L). Larger reductions cause:

• Muscular weakness. • Tiredness. • Cardiac effects: ventricular ectopics or more serious arrhythmias, potentiation of the adverse effects of digoxin. The ECG shows typical T wave changes (Fig. 6.2). • Functional bowel obstruction due to paralytic ileus. • Long-standing hypokalaemia causes damage to renal tubules (hypokalaemic nephropathy) and interference with the tubular response to ADH (acquired nephrogenic diabetes insipidus), causing polyuria and polydipsia.

Causes of hypokalaemia include:

Redistribution into cells: Alkalosis, insulin excess, β_2-agonists.
Reduced potassium intake: Dietary, IV therapy.
Excessive losses: These may be renal or GI.
Renal losses may be caused by the following factors:

• With hypertension: primary/secondary hyperaldosteronism, Cushing's syndrome, corticosteroids, ectopic ACTH. • With normal to low BP: diuretics, renal tubular acidosis, post-obstructive diuresis, recovery after acute tubular necrosis, inherited tubular disorders.

GI losses may be caused by:

• Vomiting. • Diarrhoea. • Bowel obstruction. • Laxative abuse.

HYPOKALAEMIA

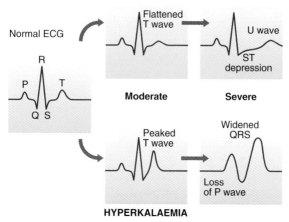

Fig. 6.2 The ECG in hypokalaemia and hyperkalaemia.

Investigations

Measurement of plasma electrolytes, bicarbonate, urine potassium and sometimes calcium and magnesium is usually sufficient to establish the diagnosis.

Plasma renin activity and aldosterone levels identify patients with primary hyperaldosteronism (p. 366) and other mineralocorticoid excess when renin is suppressed; in other causes of hypokalaemia, renin is elevated.

Occasionally, the cause of hypokalaemia is obscure, especially when the history is incomplete or unreliable, and the urine potassium is indeterminate. Many such cases are associated with metabolic alkalosis, and in this setting the measurement of urine chloride concentration can provide a helpful guide to diagnosis.

• A low urine chloride (<30 mmol/L) is characteristic of vomiting (spontaneous or self-induced). • A chloride >40 mmol/L suggests diuretic therapy (acute phase) or a tubular disorder.

Management

If the problem is redistribution of potassium into cells, reversal of the underlying cause (e.g. correction of alkalosis) may restore plasma potassium without supplements.

In most cases, potassium replacement (oral or IV) will be required. The rate of administration depends on the severity of hypokalaemia and the presence of cardiac or neuromuscular complications, but should generally not exceed 10 mmol of potassium/hr. If higher rates are needed, the concentration of potassium infused may be increased to 40 mmol/L if a peripheral vein is used, but higher concentrations must be infused into a large 'central' vein with continuous cardiac monitoring.

Hyperkalaemia

Hyperkalaemia typically presents with progressive muscular weakness, but sometimes there are no symptoms until cardiac arrest occurs (caused by the marked slowing of action potential conduction in the presence of potassium levels >7 mmol/L).

Typical ECG changes are shown in Figure 6.2. Peaking of the T wave is an early ECG sign, but widening of the QRS complex presages a dangerous cardiac arrhythmia.

Causes of hyperkalaemia include:

Redistribution out of cells: Acidosis, insulin deficiency, β-blockers, severe hyperglycaemia.

Increased intake: Exogenous (diet, IV therapy); endogenous (haemolysis, rhabdomyolysis).

Renal potassium retention: Renal failure (acute and chronic); tubular secretory failure – drugs (NSAIDs, ACE inhibitors, spironolactone), tubulo-interstitial disease, Addison's disease.

Spurious result: in vitro haemolysis.

Investigations

Plasma electrolyte, creatinine and bicarbonate results, together with consideration of the clinical scenario, will usually provide the explanation for hyperkalaemia. Addison's disease should be excluded, unless there is an obvious alternative diagnosis, as described on page 364.

Management

Treatment of hyperkalaemia depends on the severity and rate of development. In the absence of neuromuscular symptoms or ECG changes, reduction of potassium intake and correction of underlying abnormalities may be sufficient. In acute and/or severe hyperkalaemia, more urgent measures must be taken (Box 6.5).

6.5 Treatment of hyperkalaemia

Mechanism	Therapy
Stabilise cell membrane potential[1]	IV calcium gluconate (10 mL of 10% solution)
Shift K into cells	Inhaled β$_2$-agonist, e.g. salbutamol
	IV glucose (50 mL of 50% solution) and insulin (5 U Actrapid)
	IV sodium bicarbonate[2] (100 mL of 8.4% solution)
Remove K from body	IV furosemide and normal saline[3]
	Ion exchange resin (e.g. Resonium) orally or rectally
	Dialysis

[1]If ECG changes suggestive of hyperkalaemia (K typically >7 mmol/L).
[2]If acidosis present.
[3]If adequate residual renal function.

DISORDERS OF ACID–BASE BALANCE

Patients with disturbances of acid–base balance may present clinically either with the effects of tissue malfunction due to disturbed pH (such as altered cardiac and CNS function), or with secondary changes in respiration as a response to the underlying metabolic change (e.g. Kussmaul respiration during metabolic acidosis). The clinical picture is often dominated by the cause of the acid–base change, such as uncontrolled diabetes or primary lung disease. Frequently, the acid–base disturbance only becomes evident when the venous plasma bicarbonate concentration is noted to be abnormal, or when a full ABG analysis shows abnormalities in the pH, PCO_2 or bicarbonate.

The common abnormalities in blood gas parameters in acid–base disturbances are shown in Box 6.6. Interpretation of blood gas results is made easier by blood gas diagrams (e.g. Fig. 6.3), which indicate whether any acidosis or alkalosis is due to acute or chronic respiratory derangements of $PaCO_2$ or to metabolic causes.

In metabolic disturbances, respiratory compensation is almost immediate; i.e. the compensatory change in PCO_2 is achieved soon after the onset of the metabolic disturbance. In respiratory disorders, on the other hand, a small initial change in bicarbonate occurs as a result of chemical buffering of CO_2, largely within red blood cells, but further compensatory changes in bicarbonate occur via long-term adjustments in acid secretory capacity by the kidney, requiring days to weeks. When clinically obtained acid–base parameters do not accord with the predicted compensation shown, a mixed acid–base disturbance should be suspected.

Metabolic acidosis

Metabolic acidosis occurs when an acid other than carbonic acid (due to CO_2 retention) accumulates in the body, resulting in a fall in the plasma bicarbonate. The pH fall that would otherwise occur is blunted by hyperventilation, resulting in a reduced PCO_2. If the kidneys are intact (i.e. not the cause of the initial disturbance), renal excretion of acid increases gradually over days to weeks, raising the

---

i | 6.6 Principal patterns of acid–base disturbance

Disturbance	H[+]	Primary change	Compensatory response
Metabolic acidosis	>40[1]	$HCO_3^- <24$ mmol/L	$PCO_2 <5.33$ kPa[2]
Metabolic alkalosis	<40[1]	$HCO_3^- >24$ mmol/L	$PCO_2 >5.33$ kPa[2,3]
Respiratory acidosis	>40[1]	$PCO_2 >5.33$ kPa[2]	$HCO_3^- >24$ mmol/L
Respiratory alkalosis	<40[1]	$PCO_2 <5.33$ kPa[2]	$HCO_3^- <24$ mmol/L

[1]H[+] of 40 nmol/L = pH of 7.40.
[2]PCO_2 of 5.33 kPa = 40 mmHg.
[3]PCO_2 does not rise above 7.33 kPa (55 mmHg) because hypoxia intervenes to drive ventilation.

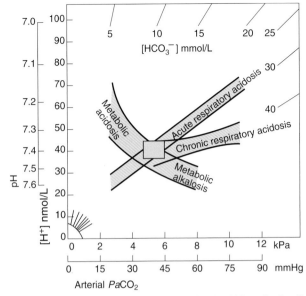

Fig. 6.3 Changes in blood [H⁺], PaCO₂ and plasma [HCO₃⁻] in acid–base disorders. The shaded rectangle indicates the limits of normal. The bands represent 95% confidence limits of single disturbances in human blood in vivo. The diagonal lines (top and right) indicate bicarbonate levels. For any measured value of $[H^+]$, the corresponding value of $PaCO_2$ indicates whether the acidosis or alkalosis is primarily respiratory or metabolic in origin.

plasma bicarbonate and hence the pH towards normal in the new steady state.

Causes of metabolic acidosis are classified according to the anion gap, which is the difference between the main measured cations $[Na^+ + K^+]$ and the main measured cations $[Cl^- + HCO_3^-]$. This is normally 12–16 mmol/L but increases when an acid accumulates accompanied by a corresponding anion.

Metabolic acidosis with normal anion gap: GI base loss (loss of HCO_3^- in diarrhoea, small bowel fistula, urinary diversion procedure). Renal tubular acidosis (urinary loss of HCO_3^- in proximal RTA, impaired tubular acid secretion in distal RTA). Therapeutic infusion or poisoning with HCl or NH_4Cl.

Metabolic acidosis with increased anion gap: Diabetic ketoacidosis (accumulation of ketones with hyperglycaemia). Lactic acidosis (shock or liver disease). Renal failure. Poisoning (aspirin, methanol, ethylene glycol).

Management

Identify and correct the underlying cause. As metabolic acidosis is frequently associated with sodium and water depletion, resuscitation with appropriate IV fluids will often be needed. Use of IV bicarbonate in this setting is controversial.

Metabolic alkalosis

Metabolic alkalosis is characterised by an increase in the plasma bicarbonate concentration and the plasma pH (see Box 6.6). There is a compensatory rise in PCO_2 due to hypoventilation but this is limited by the respiratory response to hypoxia.

Clinically, apart from manifestations of the underlying cause, there may be few symptoms or signs related to alkalosis itself. When the rise in systemic pH is abrupt, plasma ionised calcium falls and signs of increased neuromuscular irritability, such as tetany, may develop (p. 356).

The causes are best classified by the accompanying disturbance of ECF volume:

Hypovolaemic metabolic alkalosis (most common pattern): Sustained vomiting – acid-rich fluid is lost from the body, hypokalaemia stimulates renal H^+ excretion. Diuretics (not potassium-sparing diuretics) increase acid loss into the urine.

Normovolaemic (or hypervolaemic) metabolic alkalosis: Occurs when both bicarbonate retention and volume expansion are found together:

• Corticosteroid excess (Conn's syndrome, Cushing's syndrome, corticosteroid therapy). • Overuse of antacids.

Management

Metabolic alkalosis associated with hypovolaemia is treated with IV fluids, specifically isotonic sodium chloride. Replacement of potassium helps correct the hypokalaemia and its consequences in the kidney.

In metabolic alkalosis associated with normal or increased volume, treatment should focus on correcting the underlying cause.

Respiratory acidosis

Respiratory acidosis occurs when there is accumulation of CO_2 due to type II respiratory failure (p. 275). This results in a rise in the PCO_2, with a compensatory increase in plasma bicarbonate concentration, particularly when the disorder is of long duration and the kidney has fully developed its capacity for increased acid excretion.

The aetiology, clinical features and management of respiratory acidosis are covered in Chapter 9.

Respiratory alkalosis

Respiratory alkalosis develops when there is a period of hyperventilation resulting in a reduction of PCO_2 and increase in plasma pH. If the condition is sustained, renal compensation occurs, such that tubular acid secretion is reduced and the plasma bicarbonate falls.

This acid–base disturbance is frequently of short duration, as in anxiety states or over-vigorous assisted ventilation. It can be prolonged in the context of pregnancy, pulmonary embolism, chronic liver disease, and ingestion of certain drugs that stimulate the brainstem respiratory centre (e.g. salicylates).

Clinical features of hyperventilation are described on page 266; the characteristic perioral and digital tingling is due to a reduction in ionised calcium caused by increased binding of calcium to albumin in the alkalotic ECF. In severe cases, Trousseau's sign and Chvostek's sign may be positive, and tetany or seizures may develop (p. 357).

Mixed acid–base disorders

In patients with complex illnesses, it is not uncommon for more than one independent disturbance of acid–base metabolism to be present at the same time. In these situations, the arterial pH will represent the net effect of all primary and compensatory changes. Indeed, the pH may be normal, but the presence of underlying acid–base disturbances can be gauged from concomitant abnormalities in the PCO_2 and bicarbonate concentration (see Fig. 6.3).

DISORDERS OF DIVALENT ION METABOLISM

Disorders of calcium metabolism are covered in Chapter 10.

Magnesium is mainly an intracellular cation, functionally important for many enzymes, including the Na/K ATPase. It can also regulate potassium and calcium channels.

Free plasma magnesium (~70% of the total) is filtered at the glomerulus, with the majority of this reabsorbed in the loop of Henle and tubules. Reabsorption is enhanced by parathyroid hormone (PTH).

Hypomagnesaemia

Aetiology involves:

• Inadequate intake: starvation, parenteral nutrition. • Excessive losses: GI (vomiting, diarrhoea, fistulae), renal (diuretics, alcohol, acute tubular necrosis). • Complex formation: acute pancreatitis.

Clinical features

The clinical features of hypomagnesaemia and hypocalcaemia are similar: tetany, arrhythmias, especially torsades de pointes (p. 223), and seizures. Hypomagnesaemia is associated with hypocalcaemia because magnesium is required for normal PTH secretion in response to a fall in serum calcium; also, hypomagnesaemia induces resistance to PTH in bone. Hypomagnesaemia is also associated with hyponatraemia and hypokalaemia, and these may mediate some of the clinical manifestations.

Management

Treat the underlying cause. Oral magnesium is poorly absorbed and may cause diarrhoea. If disease is symptomatic, correct with IV magnesium. If due to diuretic use, adjunctive use of a potassium-sparing diuretic will also reduce renal magnesium losses.

Hypermagnesaemia

Hypermagnesaemia is much less common than hypomagnesaemia. It may be due to:
• Acute or chronic renal failure. • Adrenocortical insufficiency.
• Increased intake (antacids, laxatives, parenteral therapy).

Clinical features
• Bradycardia. • Hypotension. • Reduced consciousness. • Respiratory depression.

Management
• Restrict magnesium intake. • Optimise renal function. • Promote renal magnesium excretion with IV hydration and a loop diuretic. • Use calcium gluconate to reverse overt cardiac effects. • Consider dialysis, ultimately.

DISORDERS OF PHOSPHATE METABOLISM

Inorganic phosphate is involved in energy metabolism, intracellular signalling and bone/mineral balance. It is freely filtered at the glomerulus, with ~65% reabsorbed in the proximal tubule and a further 10–20% reabsorbed in the distal tubules. Proximal reabsorption is reduced by PTH.

Hypophosphataemia

Aetiology involves:
• Redistribution into cells: refeeding after starvation, respiratory alkalosis. • Inadequate intake or absorption: malabsorption, diarrhoea. • Increased renal excretion: hyperparathyroidism, volume expansion.

Clinical features
• Impaired function and survival of all blood cell lines. • Muscle weakness, respiratory failure, congestive cardiac failure, ileus. • Decreased consciousness, coma. • Osteomalacia.

Management
• Oral phosphate supplements. • IV sodium or potassium phosphate salts: may be used in critical situations but there is a risk of hypocalcaemia and metastatic calcification.

Hyperphosphataemia

Aetiology involves:
• Reduced renal excretion: acute and chronic renal failure, hypoparathyroidism. • Redistribution from cells: tumour lysis syndrome. • All of the above will be aggravated when the patient is taking phosphate-containing preparations.

Clinical features
These relate to hypocalcaemia and metastatic calcification, especially in chronic renal failure and tertiary hyperparathyroidism, where a high calcium phosphate product occurs.

Management

• Volume expansion with normal saline: this promotes renal phosphate excretion if renal function is normal. • Dietary phosphate restriction and phosphate binders in chronic renal failure.

DISORDERS OF AMINO ACID METABOLISM

These usually present in the neonatal period and involve lifelong treatment regimens.

Phenylketonuria

This autosomal recessive condition causes deficiency of phenylalanine hydroxylase. Affected infants accumulate phenylalanine, causing mental retardation, which can be prevented by neonatal screening and dietary phenylalanine restriction.

Homocystinuria

An autosomal recessive deficiency of cystathionine β-synthase results in increased urinary homocystine and methionine. Clinical manifestations involve:

• Eyes (displacement of the lens). • CNS (mental retardation, seizures, psychiatric disturbances). • Skeleton (Marfan-like, with osteoporosis). • Vascular system (thrombosis). • Skin (hypopigmentation).

Treatment involves a methionine-restricted, cystine-supplemented diet and large doses of pyridoxine.

DISORDERS OF CARBOHYDRATE METABOLISM

Diabetes is described in Chapter 11.

Galactosaemia

Galactosaemia is caused by an autosomal recessive mutation in the galactose-1-phosphate uridylyltransferase (*GALT*) gene. The neonate is unable to metabolise galactose, leading to vomiting or diarrhoea after milk ingestion. Treatment involves lifelong avoidance of galactose- and lactose-containing foods.

DISORDERS OF LIPID METABOLISM

Abnormalities of lipid metabolism most commonly come to light following routine blood testing. A comprehensive lipid profile should include plasma cholesterol, triglyceride and HDL cholesterol obtained after a 12-hr fast. LDL cholesterol may be calculated based on these.

Lipid measurements are usually performed for the following reasons:

• Screening for primary or secondary prevention of cardiovascular disease. • Investigation of patients with clinical features of lipid

> ### 6.7 Causes of secondary hyperlipidaemia
>
> **Secondary hypercholesterolaemia**
>
> - Hypothyroidism*
> - Pregnancy*
> - Cholestatic liver disease*
> - Drugs (diuretics, ciclosporin, corticosteroids, androgens, antiretrovirals)*
> - Nephrotic syndrome
> - Anorexia nervosa
> - Hyperparathyroidism
>
> **Secondary hypertriglyceridaemia**
>
> - Diabetes mellitus (type 2)
> - Chronic renal disease
> - Abdominal obesity
> - Excess alcohol
> - Hepatocellular disease
> - Drugs (β-blockers, retinoids, corticosteroids, antiretrovirals)
>
> *Common causes.

disorders. • Testing of relatives of patients with one of the single-gene defects causing dyslipidaemia.

Following the exclusion of secondary causes (Box 6.7), primary lipid abnormalities may be diagnosed.

Predominant hypercholesterolaemia

This is usually polygenic but may be dominant or recessive. Familial hypercholesterolaemia is usually autosomal dominant and carries a high risk of cardiovascular disease.

Clinical features include:

• Xanthelasma. • Corneal arcus. • Tendon xanthomas.

Predominant hypertriglyceridaemia

If this is primary, it is most commonly polygenic, but many cases are secondary to alcohol, diabetes or insulin resistance syndrome (p. 384).

Clinical features in severe elevation include:

• Lipaemia retinalis. • Lipaemic blood and plasma. • Eruptive xanthomas (typically on trunk and buttocks). • Acute pancreatitis. • Hepatosplenomegaly.

Mixed hyperlipidaemia

This is usually polygenic with no pathognomonic features.

Management of dyslipidaemia

Risk and benefit should be assessed individually using prediction charts.

Non-pharmacological management

Patients with lipid abnormalities should receive medical advice and, if necessary, dietary counselling to:

• Reduce intake of saturated and trans-unsaturated fat to <7–10% of total energy. • Reduce cholesterol intake to < 250 mg/day. • Replace sources of saturated fat and cholesterol with alternative foods such as lean meat, low-fat dairy products, polyunsaturated spreads and low glycaemic index carbohydrates. • Reduce energy-dense foods, such as fats and soft drinks, whilst increasing activity and exercise to maintain or lose weight. • Increase consumption of cardioprotective and nutrient-dense foods, such as vegetables, unrefined carbohydrates, fish, nuts, pulses, legumes, fruit, etc. • Adjust alcohol consumption, reducing intake if excessive or if associated with hypertension, hypertriglyceridaemia or central obesity. • Achieve additional benefits with supplementary intake of foods containing lipid-lowering nutrients, such as n-3 fatty acids, dietary fibre and plant sterols.

Response to diet is usually apparent within 3–4 wks but dietary adjustment may need to be introduced gradually. Hyperlipidaemia in general, and hypertriglyceridaemia in particular, can be very responsive to these measures. Explanation, encouragement and other measures should be undertaken to reinforce patient compliance. Even minor weight loss can substantially reduce cardiovascular risk, especially in centrally obese patients.

All other modifiable cardiovascular risk factors should be assessed and treated. Where possible, intercurrent drug treatments that adversely affect the lipid profile should be replaced.

Pharmacological management

Drugs used to lower cholesterol fall into the following categories:
• Statins (HMG-CoA reductase inhibitors). • Cholesterol absorption inhibitors. • Bile acid sequestering resins. • Nicotinic acid.

High triglyceride levels are treated with fibrates and fish oils. These are discussed further in Chapter 18.

OTHER BIOCHEMICAL DISORDERS

Amyloidosis

Amyloidosis is characterised by the extracellular deposition of insoluble proteins. These deposits consist of amyloid protein fibrils linked to glycosaminoglycans and proteoglycans, and serum amyloid P (SAP). The diagnosis should be considered in unexplained nephrotic syndrome, cardiomyopathy and peripheral neuropathy. Amyloid diseases are classified by aetiology and type of protein deposited:

Reactive (AA) amyloidosis: Increased production of serum amyloid A due to chronic infection (e.g. TB, bronchiectasis) or inflammation (e.g. rheumatoid arthritis). Around 90% of patients have proteinuria.

Light chain (AL) amyloidosis: Increased production of monoclonal light chains due to monoclonal gammopathies (myeloma, plasmacytoma). Clinical features include restrictive cardiomyopathy, neuropathy and macroglossia (pathognomonic). The condition has a poor prognosis.

Dialysis-associated (Aβ2M) amyloidosis: Accumulation of β_2-microglobulin due to dialysis. It occurs 5–10 yrs after starting dialysis, and presents with carpal tunnel syndrome, arthropathy and pathological fractures due to amyloid bone cysts.

Investigations

Biopsy of an affected organ, rectum or subcutaneous fat, when stained with Congo red dye, shows the pathognomonic apple-green birefringence of amyloid deposits under polarised light. Quantitative scintigraphy with radiolabelled SAP determines distribution of amyloid deposits.

Management

The aims of treatment are to support affected organs and, in acquired amyloidosis, to prevent further amyloid deposition through treatment of the primary cause. Liver transplantation may provide definitive treatment in selected patients with hereditary amyloidosis.

DISORDERS OF COMPLEX LIPID METABOLISM

These include the lysosomal storage disorders that have diverse clinical manifestations, typically including mental retardation. Some are now treatable using human enzyme replacement therapy, whilst others can be prevented through genetic screening.

DISORDERS OF HAEM METABOLISM: THE PORPHYRIAS

These are rare disorders due to inherited enzyme deficiencies of the haem biosynthetic pathway. They are divided into hepatic or erythropoietic, depending on the major site of excess porphyrin production. Inheritance is dominant with low penetrance, and environmental factors influence expression.

Clinical features

Two patterns are recognised:

Photosensitive skin manifestations: Pain, erythema, bullae, erosions, hirsutism and hyperpigmentation are characteristic of the most common porphyria, porphyria cutanea tarda (PCT).

Acute neurological syndrome: Presents with acute abdominal pain and autonomic dysfunction (tachycardia, hypertension and constipation), and is characteristic of acute intermittent porphyria (AIP).

Attacks are often provoked by drugs such as anticonvulsants, sulfonamides, oestrogen and progesterone (oral contraceptive pill), or by alcohol and even fasting. In some cases, no precipitant can be identified.

Investigations

Measure porphyrins, their precursors and metabolites in blood, urine and faeces. It is now possible to measure some of the affected enzymes. Identification of the underlying gene mutations has made family testing possible for some variants.

Management

With neurovisceral attacks, patients should avoid any known precipitants of acute porphyria. IV glucose can terminate acute attacks through a reduction in δ-aminolevulinic acid (ALA) synthetase activity. For photosensitive manifestations, the primary goal is to avoid sun exposure and skin trauma. Barrier sun creams containing zinc or titanium oxide are the most effective products.

Kidney and urinary tract disease

Renal medicine ranges from the management of common conditions (e.g. urinary tract infection (UTI)) to the use of complex technology to replace renal function (e.g. dialysis and transplantation). This chapter describes the common disorders of the kidneys and urinary tract, and also gives an overview of the highly specialised field of renal replacement therapy.

MEASUREMENT OF RENAL FUNCTION

The key measurement of renal function, glomerular filtration rate (GFR), is normally assessed using the serum level of endogenously produced creatinine, using a formula that allows for gender and age, e.g.:

$$\text{eGFR} = 186 \times (\text{creatinine } \mu mol/L/88.4)^{-1.154} \times (\text{age in yrs})^{-0.203} \times (0.742 \text{ if female}) \times (1.21 \text{ if black})$$

(To convert creatinine in mg/dL to μmol/L, multiply by 88.4.)

Degrees of chronic kidney disease (CKD) are defined according to GFR (see Box 7.8 below).

PRESENTING PROBLEMS IN RENAL AND URINARY TRACT DISEASE

Dysuria

Dysuria refers to painful micturition, often with suprapubic pain, frequency and a feeling of incomplete emptying. The cause is usually UTI (p. 192), but sexually transmitted diseases and bladder stone may also present with dysuria.

Loin pain

Dull ache in the loin is often musculoskeletal in origin but may be caused by renal stone, renal tumour, acute pyelonephritis or obstruction of the renal pelvis. Acute loin pain radiating to the groin ('renal

CLINICAL EXAMINATION OF THE KIDNEY AND URINARY TRACT

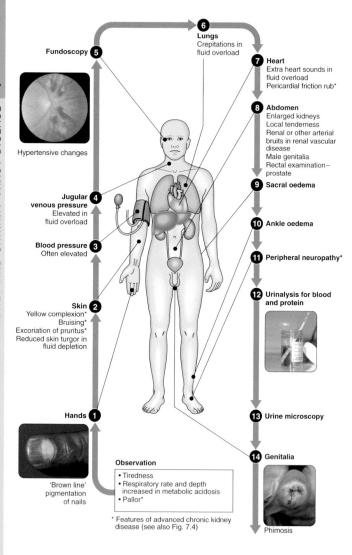

6 Lungs
Crepitations in fluid overload

5 Fundoscopy

Hypertensive changes

7 Heart
Extra heart sounds in fluid overload
Pericardial friction rub*

8 Abdomen
Enlarged kidneys
Local tenderness
Renal or other arterial bruits in renal vascular disease
Male genitalia
Rectal examination– prostate

9 Sacral oedema

4 Jugular venous pressure
Elevated in fluid overload

3 Blood pressure
Often elevated

10 Ankle oedema

11 Peripheral neuropathy*

2 Skin
Yellow complexion*
Bruising*
Excoriation of pruritus*
Reduced skin turgor in fluid depletion

12 Urinalysis for blood and protein

13 Urine microscopy

1 Hands

'Brown line' pigmentation of nails

14 Genitalia

Phimosis

Observation
- Tiredness
- Respiratory rate and depth increased in metabolic acidosis
- Pallor*

* Features of advanced chronic kidney disease (see also Fig. 7.4)

> **i** **7.1 Causes of polyuria**
>
> - Excess fluid intake
> - Hyperglycaemia
> - Cranial diabetes insipidus
> - Nephrogenic diabetes insipidus:
>   Lithium, diuretics
>   Interstitial nephritis
>   Hypokalaemia, hypercalcaemia

colic'), together with haematuria, is typical of ureteric obstruction most commonly due to calculi (p. 189).

Oliguria/anuria

Daily urine volumes <300 mL are termed oliguria. Anuria is the (almost) total absence of urine (<50 mL/day). A low measured urine volume is an important finding and is a consequence of reduced production, obstruction to urine flow or both. Patients should be assessed for signs of dehydration or hypotension, and for signs of urinary obstruction (enlarged bladder). Catheterisation relieves distal obstruction and allows monitoring of urine flow rate. USS reveals the site of obstruction.

Polyuria

Causes of an inappropriately high urine volume (>3 L/day) are shown in Box 7.1. In the assessment of polyuria accurate documentation of intake is essential.

Nocturia

Waking up at night to void urine may be a consequence of polyuria but may also result from fluid intake or diuretic use in the late evening. Nocturia also occurs in CKD, and in prostatic enlargement where it is associated with poor stream, hesitancy, incomplete bladder emptying, terminal dribbling and urinary frequency.

Frequency

Frequency describes micturition more often than a patient's expectations. It may be a consequence of polyuria, when urine volume is normal or high, but is also found in patients with dysuria or prostatic disease when urine volumes are low.

Urinary incontinence

Urinary incontinence is defined as any involuntary leakage of urine. Urinary tract pathology causing incontinence is described below. It may also occur with a normal urinary tract, e.g. in association with dementia or poor mobility, or transiently during an acute illness or hospitalisation, especially in older people. Diuretics, alcohol and caffeine may worsen incontinence.

Incontinence syndromes

Stress incontinence: Leakage occurs because passive bladder pressure exceeds the urethral pressure, due to either poor pelvic floor support or a weak urethral sphincter, most often both. This is very common in women, especially following childbirth. It is rare in men, in whom it usually follows prostate surgery. It presents with incontinence during coughing, sneezing or exertion. In women, perineal inspection may reveal leakage of urine with coughs.

Urge incontinence: Leakage usually occurs when detrusor over-activity produces an increased bladder pressure that overcomes the urethral sphincter. Urgency with or without incontinence may also be driven by a hypersensitive bladder resulting from UTI or bladder stone. Detrusor over-activity may be neurogenic (in spina bifida or multiple sclerosis) or idiopathic. The incidence of urge incontinence increases with age, and is also seen in men with lower urinary tract obstruction; it most often remits after the obstruction is relieved.

Continual incontinence: This is suggestive of a vesicovaginal or ureterovaginal fistula, often complicating previous surgery or radiotherapy.

Overflow incontinence: This occurs when the bladder becomes chronically over-distended. It is most common in men with benign prostatic hyperplasia or bladder neck obstruction, but may occur in either sex as a result of detrusor muscle failure (atonic bladder). This may be idiopathic but more commonly results from pelvic nerve damage from surgery (e.g. hysterectomy or rectal excision), trauma or infection, or from compression of the cauda equina from disc prolapse, trauma or tumour.

Post-micturition dribble: This is very common in men, even in the relatively young. It is due to a small amount of urine becoming trapped in the U-bend of the bulbar urethra, which leaks out when the patient moves. It is more pronounced if associated with a urethral diverticulum or urethral stricture. It may occur in females with a urethral diverticulum and may mimic stress incontinence.

Clinical assessment and investigations

A voiding diary is used to record the pattern of micturition, including the measured volume voided, frequency of voiding, precipitating factors and associated features, e.g. urgency. Cognitive function and mobility are assessed. Neurological assessment reveals disorders such as MS that may affect the nervous supply of the bladder. Perineal sensation and anal sphincter tone should be examined since the same sacral nerve roots also supply the bladder and urethral sphincter. The lumbar spine should be inspected for features of spina bifida occulta. Rectal examination is needed to assess the prostate in men and to exclude faecal impaction. Urinalysis and culture should be performed in all patients. An assessment of post-micturition volume should be made, either by post-micturition USS or catheterisation. Urine flow rates and full urodynamic assessment may also be helpful in selected cases.

Erectile dysfunction

This is most commonly caused by psychological, vascular or neuropathic factors. With the exception of diabetes mellitus, endocrine causes are uncommon and are characterised by simultaneous loss of libido. If the patient has erections on wakening in the morning, vascular and neuropathic causes are much less likely and a psychological cause should be suspected.

Haematuria

This indicates bleeding anywhere within the urinary tract, and may be visible (macroscopic) or only detectable on urinalysis (microscopic). Macroscopic haematuria is more likely to be caused by tumours, severe infections and renal infarction. Causes of dipstick-positive haematuria are shown in Box 7.2. Investigations and management of haematuria are outlined in Figure 7.1.

Proteinuria and nephrotic syndrome

Moderate amounts of low molecular weight protein do pass through the glomerular basement membrane (GBM). These are normally reabsorbed by tubular cells so that <150 mg/day appears in urine. Quantification and interpretation of proteinuria are covered in Box 7.3.

7.2 Interpretation of dipstick-positive haematuria

Dipstick test positive	Urine microscopy	Suggested cause
Haematuria	White blood cells	Infection
	Abnormal epithelial cells	Tumour
	Red cell casts, dysmorphic RBC	Glomerular bleeding
Haemoglobinuria	No red cells	Intravascular haemolysis
Myoglobinuria	No red cells	Rhabdomyolysis

7.3 Quantification and interpretation of proteinuria

ACR	PCR	Dipstick results	Significance
<3.5 female		–	Normal
<2.5 male			
~3.5–15		–	Microalbuminuria
~15–50	~15–50	+ to ++	Dipstick positive; equivalent to 24-hr protein <0.5 g
50–200	>250	++ to +++	Glomerular disease more likely
>200	>300	+++ to ++++	Nephrotic; always glomerular disease, equivalent to 24-hr protein excretion >3 g

ACR = urinary albumin (mg/L)/urine creatinine (mmol/L); PCR = urine protein (mg/L)/urine creatinine (mmol/L)

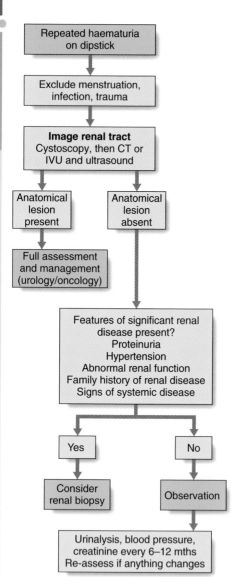

Fig. 7.1 Investigation and management of haematuria.

Clinical assessment

Proteinuria is usually asymptomatic and detected on urinalysis. It can occur transiently after exercise, during fever, in heart failure and with UTI. 'Orthostatic proteinuria', with positive daytime samples and negative morning samples, is usually benign.

Heavy proteinuria, which indicates underlying glomerular damage, can cause the nephrotic syndrome, which presents with oedema extending from the lower limbs to the abdomen, or to the face if severe. Stimulation of the renin–angiotensin system leads to avid renal sodium retention. Hypercholesterolaemia and hypercoagulability are other features. Infection is common due to urinary loss of immunoglobulins. Management includes treating the underlying renal disease, plus supportive therapy with diuretics, low-sodium diet, statins, prophylactic anticoagulation and vaccination against infection.

Microalbuminuria is a clear sign of glomerular abnormality and can identify very early glomerular disease, e.g. in diabetic nephropathy (p. 408). Persistent microalbuminuria has also been associated with an increased risk of atherosclerosis and cardiovascular mortality.

Investigation of proteinuria is summarised in Figure 7.2.

Oedema

Causes of oedema are shown in Box 7.4.

Investigations

The cause of oedema is usually apparent from the history and examination of the cardiovascular system and abdomen, combined with measurement of urinary protein and the serum albumin level. Where ascites or pleural effusion in isolation is causing diagnostic difficulty, aspiration of fluid with measurement of protein and glucose, and microscopy for cells, will usually clarify the diagnosis (p. 273).

Management

Mild fluid retention will respond to a diuretic such as a thiazide or low-dose furosemide or bumetanide. Restrict sodium (and sometimes fluid) in resistant cases. In nephrotic syndrome, renal failure

7.4 Causes of oedema	
Increased extracellular fluid	Heart failure, renal failure, liver disease
High local venous pressure	DVT, pregnancy, pelvic tumour
Low plasma oncotic pressure	Nephrotic syndrome, liver failure, malabsorption
Increased capillary permeability	Infection, sepsis, calcium channel blockers
Lymphatic obstruction	Infection (filariasis), malignancy, radiation injury

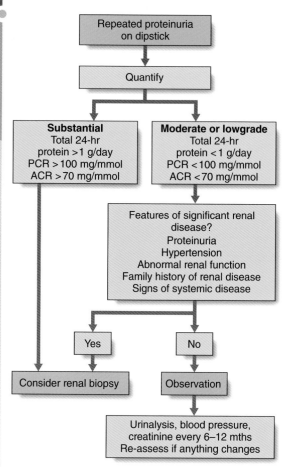

Fig. 7.2 Investigation of proteinuria. (ACR = albumin : creatinine ratio; PCR = protein : creatinine ratio)

and severe cardiac failure, very large doses of diuretics, sometimes in combination, may be required. Specific causes (e.g. venous thrombosis) should be treated.

Hypertension

Hypertension is a very common feature of renal parenchymal and vascular disease, and is an early feature of glomerular disorders. As GFR declines, hypertension becomes increasingly common, regardless of the renal diagnosis. Control of hypertension is very important in patients with renal impairment because of its close relationship

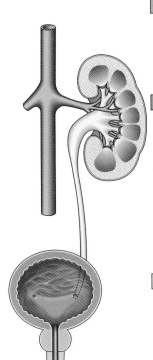

PRE-RENAL

Impaired perfusion:
• Cardiac failure
• Sepsis
• Blood loss
• Dehydration
• Vascular occlusion

RENAL

Glomerulonephritis
Small-vessel vasculitis
Acute tubular necrosis
• Drugs
• Toxins
• Prolonged hypotension
Interstitial nephritis
• Drugs
• Toxins
• Inflammatory disease
• Infection

POST-RENAL

Urinary calculi
Retroperitoneal fibrosis
Benign prostatic
enlargement
Prostate cancer
Cervical cancer
Urethral stricture/valves
Meatal stenosis/phimosis

Fig. 7.3 Causes of acute kidney injury.

with further decline of renal function (p. 175) and with the adverse cardiovascular risk in renal disease.

ACUTE KIDNEY INJURY

Acute kidney injury (AKI) refers to a sudden and often reversible loss of renal function, which develops over a period of days or weeks. There are many possible causes (Fig. 7.3) and AKI is frequently multifactorial.

Clinical features

Patients are usually oliguric (urine volume <500 mL daily). Anuria (no urine) is rare and usually indicates acute urinary tract obstruction or vascular occlusion. In ~20% of cases, the urine volume is normal or increased, but with a low GFR and a reduction of tubular reabsorption (non-oliguric AKI). Excretion is inadequate despite good urine output, and the plasma urea and creatinine increase.

Clinical features of advancing uraemia include anorexia, nausea and vomiting followed by drowsiness, apathy, confusion, muscle-twitching, hiccoughs, fits and coma. Respiratory rate may be increased due to acidosis, pulmonary oedema or respiratory infection. Anaemia is common, and is caused by blood loss, haemolysis or decreased erythropoiesis. Bleeding occurs because of disordered platelet function and disturbances of the coagulation cascade. Severe infections may complicate AKI because immune mechanisms are depressed.

Pre-renal AKI: Patients with pre-renal AKI are typically hypotensive and tachycardic, with signs of hypovolaemia including postural hypotension (>20/10 mmHg fall from lying to standing). Patients with sepsis may have peripheral vasodilatation and yet have relative under-filling of the arterial tree and renal vasoconstriction leading to AKI with acute tubular necrosis (ATN). Although the cause of renal hypoperfusion may be obvious, concealed blood loss may occur following trauma (e.g. pelvic fractures) or into a pregnant uterus. Also, large volumes of intravascular fluid may be lost after injuries and burns, and in severe inflammatory skin diseases or sepsis. Finally, pre-renal AKI may occur without hypotension in those taking NSAIDs or ACE inhibitors. Hyperkalaemia is common. Dilutional hyponatraemia occurs if the patient has continued to drink freely despite oliguria or has received inappropriate IV dextrose. Metabolic acidosis develops unless prevented by loss of hydrogen ions through vomiting or aspiration of gastric contents. Hypocalcaemia, due to reduced renal production of 1,25-dihydroxycholecalciferol, is common.

Renal and post-renal AKI: Factors that can differentiate the causes of renal and post-renal AKI are summarised in Box 7.5. Patients should be examined clinically and by USS for bladder enlargement and hydronephrosis.

Investigations

Box 7.6 indicates appropriate initial investigations in AKI. Investigations related to specific causes are covered in Box 7.7.

Management

Establish and correct the underlying cause: If hypovolaemia is present, restore blood volume as rapidly as possible (with blood or balanced salt solutions such as Hartmann's). CVP monitoring may help to guide the rate of administration of fluid, as over-filling can cause pulmonary oedema and worsen outcomes. Critically ill patients may require inotropic drugs to restore an effective BP (p. 25), but recent trials do not support the use of low-dose dopamine in severely ill patients at risk of AKI. Nephrotoxic drugs should be withdrawn. Obstruction to urine flow should be relieved either with a catheter or by nephrostomy for ureteric obstruction.

Correct metabolic derangements: Hyperkalaemia >6.5 mmol/L should be treated immediately to prevent arrhythmias. Correct

7.5 Acute kidney injury in a haemodynamically stable, non-septic patient

Urinary tract obstruction

- Suggested by a history of loin pain, haematuria, renal colic or difficulty in micturition but often clinically silent
- Can usually be excluded by renal USS – essential in any patient with unexplained AKI
- Prompt relief of obstruction restores renal function

Drugs

- Poisoning, e.g. paraquat, paracetamol, snake bite, herbal medicines
- Therapeutic agents – direct toxicity (aminoglycosides, amphotericin) or haemodynamic effects (NSAIDs, ACE inhibitors); phosphate crystallisation from IV or bowel administration

Rapidly progressive glomerulonephritis (RPGN) (p. 185)

- Typically, significant haematuria and/or proteinuria
- Causes include systemic vasculitis, systemic lupus erythematosus (SLE) and Goodpasture's (anti-GBM) disease)
- Useful blood tests include: ANCA, ANA, anti-GBM antibodies, complement, immunoglobulins
- Renal biopsy shows aggressive glomerular inflammation, usually with crescent formation

Acute interstitial nephritis (p. 186)

- Usually caused by an adverse drug reaction
- Characterised by small amounts of blood and protein in urine, often with leucocyturia
- Kidneys are normal size
- Requires cessation of drug and often prednisolone treatment

metabolic acidosis. Restoration of blood volume will correct acidosis by restoring kidney function. Severe acidosis may be treated with sodium bicarbonate (e.g. 50 mL of 8.4%) if volume status allows.

Nutrition: Parenteral or enteral tube feeding may be needed in hypercatabolic patients. Feed should include sufficient energy and adequate protein, although high protein intake should be avoided.

Infection control: Patients with AKI are at risk of intercurrent infection, and prompt diagnosis and treatment are essential.

Immunosuppression: Patients with glomerulonephritis may require immunosuppressive drugs, plasma infusion and plasma exchange.

Renal replacement therapy: If uraemia and hyperkalaemia fail to respond to the above measures, a period of renal replacement therapy may be required. The two main options for AKI are haemo-dialysis or high-volume haemofiltration. Both carry risks, including haemodynamic instability and infected catheters, so careful assessment of individual cases is required. Peritoneal dialysis can be used if haemodialysis is unavailable.

7.6 Investigation of patients with established AKI

Urea and creatinine	Compare to previous results
Electrolytes	If potassium >6.5 mmol/L, treat urgently
Calcium and phosphate	Low Ca, high PO_4 suggest CKD. Ca low in rhabdomyolysis; check CK. Hypercalcaemia in myeloma
Albumin	Low in nephritic syndrome and sepsis
FBC	Anaemia in CKD. Fragmented RBC with raised LDH in thrombotic microangiopathy. Low platelets and abnormal clotting in DIC
CRP	High in sepsis and inflammatory disease. ESR misleading in AKI
Urinalysis	Marked haematuria suggests glomerulonephritis, tumour or bleeding disorder. Heavy proteinuria suggests glomerular disease
Urine microscopy	Casts or dysmorphic RBCs suggest glomerulonephritis
	Leucocytes suggest infection or interstitial nephritis
	Crystals in drug-induced or uric acid nephropathy
Renal USS	Reveals hydronephrosis/obstruction. Small kidneys suggest CKD. Asymmetric kidneys in congenital or vascular disease
Cultures	Blood, urine, sputum, wound as appropriate
CXR	May reveal pulmonary oedema, pericardial effusion, fibrotic change in systemic inflammatory diseases, pulmonary haemorrhage
Serology	HIV and hepatitis status in case dialysis needed
ECG	If patient >40, electrolyte abnormalities or cardiac risk factors

Recovery from AKI: A gradual return of urine output and a steady improvement in biochemistry accompany recovery. Some patients, primarily those with ATN or those in whom chronic urinary obstruction has been relieved, develop a 'diuretic phase'. Sufficient fluid to replace the urine output should be given. After a few days, urine volume falls to normal as the concentrating mechanisms recover. During the diuretic phase, supplements of sodium, chloride, potassium and phosphate may be necessary to compensate for increased urinary losses.

CHRONIC KIDNEY DISEASE

Chronic kidney disease (CKD) refers to an irreversible deterioration in renal function that classically develops over a period of years (Box 7.8). Initially, it is manifest only as a biochemical abnormality. Eventually, loss of the excretory, metabolic and endocrine functions of the kidney leads to the development of the clinical symptoms and signs of renal failure, which are referred to as uraemia. When death

7.7 Clinical features and investigation of specific causes of AKI

Diagnosis	Features	Consider
Vascular occlusion	Absent pulses, anuria	Doppler USS or arteriography
Malignant hypertension	High BP, haemolysis	Examine fundi, prior BP records
Scleroderma	Sclerodactyly, ↑BP	Extractable nuclear antigen (ENA) autoantibodies
Systemic inflammatory disease	Rashes, glomerulonephritis, multi-organ involvement	Complement, ANCA, ANF, anti-GBM, cryoglobulins, tissue biopsy
Glomerular disease	Heavy proteinuria ± haematuria	Screen for systemic inflammatory disease, urgent renal biopsy
Interstitial nephritis	Recent drug use, urine WBC	Eosinophils (blood and urine), renal biopsy
Myeloma	Bone pain, hypercalcaemia, oliguria	Protein electrophoresis, skeletal survey, immunoglobulins, urinary light chains
Infections	Leptospirosis, syphilis, post-streptococcal glomerulonephritis	ASO titre, serology for specific infections

7.8 Stages of chronic kidney disease

Stage	Definition	Description	Clinical presentation
1	Kidney damage* with normal or high GFR >90	Mild CKD	Asymptomatic
2	Kidney damage and GFR 60–89		Asymptomatic
3A	GFR 45–59	Moderate CKD	Usually asymptomatic
3B	GFR 30–44		Anaemia in some. Most are non-progressive
4	GFR 15–29	Severe CKD	Symptoms usually with GFR <20. Electrolyte problems
5	GFR <15 or on dialysis	Kidney failure	Significant symptoms and complications. Dialysis usually at GFR <10

*Kidney damage means pathological abnormalities or markers of damage, including abnormalities in blood or urine tests or imaging studies. Two GFR measurements 3 mths apart are required to assign a stage. All GFR values are mL/min/1.73m^2.

7.9 Causes of chronic kidney disease	
Diabetes mellitus	20–40%
Interstitial diseases	20–30%
Glomerular diseases	10–20%
Hypertension	5–20%
Systemic inflammatory diseases	5–10%
Renovascular disease	5%
Congenital and inherited	5%
Unknown	5–20%

is likely without renal replacement therapy, the condition is called end-stage renal disease (ESRD).

CKD may be caused by any condition that destroys the normal structure and function of the kidney. Common causes are shown in Box 7.9.

Clinical features

Patients may remain asymptomatic until GFR falls <30 mL/min (stage 4 or 5; see Box 7.8). Thereafter, due to the widespread effects of renal failure, symptoms and signs may develop that are related to almost every body system (Fig. 7.4).

General symptoms: In ESRD (stage 5; see Box 7.8) patients appear ill and anaemic. Nocturia is common, due to diminished concentrating ability, together with tiredness and breathlessness. There may be unusually deep respiration related to metabolic acidosis (Kussmaul's respiration), anorexia and nausea. Later, hiccoughs, pruritus, vomiting, muscular twitching, fits, drowsiness and coma ensue.

Immune dysfunction: Cellular and humoral immunity are impaired in CKD, leading to infections – the second most common cause of death in dialysis patients, after cardiovascular disease. These range from infected access devices to pneumonias.

Haematological: CKD leads to a bleeding tendency through impaired platelet function, and this risk is increased if anticoagulants are used. Anaemia is common and, in part, related to the relative deficiency of erythropoietin; it usually correlates with the severity of renal failure and contributes to many of the non-specific symptoms of CKD.

Fluid and electrolyte abnormalities: Disproportionate fluid retention in milder renal failure, sometimes leading to episodic pulmonary oedema, is particularly associated with renal artery stenosis. Conversely, some patients with tubulointerstitial disease develop salt-wasting disease and need sodium supplements. Declining renal function is associated with metabolic acidosis (p. 148). This is often asymptomatic but may also contribute to reduced renal function and increased tissue catabolism.

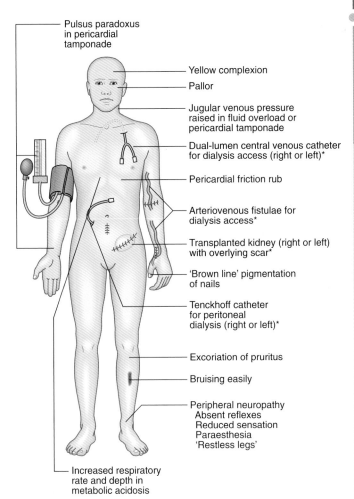

Fig. 7.4 Physical signs in chronic kidney disease. (*Features of renal replacement therapy)

In the figure, the following labels appear:

- Pulsus paradoxus in pericardial tamponade
- Yellow complexion
- Pallor
- Jugular venous pressure raised in fluid overload or pericardial tamponade
- Dual-lumen central venous catheter for dialysis access (right or left)*
- Pericardial friction rub
- Arteriovenous fistulae for dialysis access*
- Transplanted kidney (right or left) with overlying scar*
- 'Brown line' pigmentation of nails
- Tenckhoff catheter for peritoneal dialysis (right or left)*
- Excoriation of pruritus
- Bruising easily
- Peripheral neuropathy
  Absent reflexes
  Reduced sensation
  Paraesthesia
  'Restless legs'
- Increased respiratory rate and depth in metabolic acidosis

Endocrine function: Hyperprolactinaemia may produce loss of libido. Insulin half-life is prolonged, and insulin resistance occurs in CKD, complicating the treatment of diabetes.

Myopathy and neuropathy: Generalised myopathy is due to a combination of poor nutrition, hyperparathyroidism, vitamin D deficiency and electrolyte disorders. Muscle cramps are common. The 'restless leg syndrome', in which the patient's legs are jumpy during the night, may be troublesome. Sensory/motor/autonomic

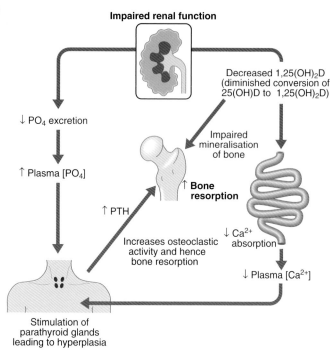

Impaired renal function

↓ PO₄ excretion

↑ Plasma [PO₄]

Decreased 1,25(OH)₂D (diminished conversion of 25(OH)D to 1,25(OH)₂D)

Impaired mineralisation of bone

↑ **Bone resorption**

↑ PTH

Increases osteoclastic activity and hence bone resorption

↓ Ca²⁺ absorption

↓ Plasma [Ca²⁺]

Stimulation of parathyroid glands leading to hyperplasia

Fig. 7.5 Pathogenesis of renal osteodystrophy. The net result of decreased 1,25(OH)₂ cholecalciferol levels and increased parathyroid hormone (PTH) levels in the presence of high [PO₄] is bone that exhibits increased osteoclastic activity and increased osteoid as a consequence of decreased mineralisation.

neuropathy appears late in the course of CKD but may improve or resolve on dialysis.

Cardiovascular disease: The risk of cardiovascular disease is substantially increased in CKD stage 3 or worse. Left ventricular hypertrophy due to hypertension increases the risk of sudden death with arrhythmia. Vascular calcification, associated with increased phosphate levels, may be sufficient to cause limb ischaemia. Pericarditis is common in untreated or inadequately treated end-stage renal disease (ESRD) and can cause pericardial tamponade and, later, constrictive pericarditis.

Metabolic bone disease: Disturbances of calcium and phosphate metabolism occur in CKD, leading to metabolic bone diseases such as osteomalacia, hyperparathyroid bone disease (osteitis fibrosa) and osteoporosis (Fig. 7.5).

Investigations

Initial screening tests in CKD are similar to those for established AKI (see Box 7.6). The aims are to:

• Identify the underlying cause. • Address reversible factors that are making renal function worse, e.g. hypertension, urinary tract obstruction or infection, and nephrotoxic medications. • Screen for complications such as osteodystrophy or anaemia. • Screen for cardiovascular risk factors.

Management

This is aimed at preventing further renal damage, managing and limiting metabolic and cardiovascular complications, and preparing for renal replacement therapy if required.

Antihypertensive therapy: Lowering BP slows the rate of decline of renal function in CKD, with associated reductions in the risk of heart failure, stroke and peripheral vascular disease. No threshold for this effect has been identified and any reduction appears beneficial. Suggested target BP is 130/80 mmHg for uncomplicated CKD and 125/75 mmHg for CKD with proteinuria >1 g/day. Achieving these limits often requires multiple drugs together with good adherence to treatment.

Reduction of proteinuria: The degree of proteinuria is clearly related to the rate of progression of renal disease, and reducing proteinuria slows progression. ACE inhibitors and angiotensin II receptor blockers (ARBs) reduce proteinuria and retard progression of CKD, as well as reducing cardiovascular events and all-cause mortality. They may produce an initial reduction in GFR but can be continued, provided the reduction is not >20% or progressive.

Dietary and lifestyle modifications: Evidence that restricting dietary protein is beneficial in humans is not clear-cut. Patients with stage 4 or 5 CKD should be advised to avoid excessive protein, but to take sufficient calories and to avoid excessive dietary potassium and phosphate. Severe protein restriction is not recommended. Smoking cessation slows disease progression and reduces cardiovascular risk. Exercise and weight loss may also be beneficial.

Lipid-lowering therapy: Hypercholesterolaemia is almost universal in patients with significant proteinuria, and increased triglycerides are common in CKD. Control of dyslipidaemia with statins may slow disease progression.

Treatment of anaemia: Recombinant human erythropoietin is effective in correcting the anaemia of CKD. The target haemoglobin is between 100 and 120 g/L. Complications of treatment include hypertension and thrombosis. Erythropoietin is less effective in the presence of iron deficiency, active inflammation or malignancy. These factors should be sought and, if possible, corrected before treatment.

Maintenance of fluid and electrolyte balance: Patients with fluid retention should have dietary sodium intake limited to 100 mmol/day, but in addition loop diuretics are often needed to treat fluid overload. Hyperkalaemia may require restriction of intake to <70 mmol/day and the withdrawal of potassium-sparing diuretics, ACE inhibitors and ARBs. Potassium-binding resins, such as calcium resonium, are useful for short-term use only. Correction of acidosis using sodium bicarbonate supplements to keep plasma bicarbonate >22 mmol/L may be beneficial. If the corresponding sodium load causes oedema, calcium carbonate may be used as an alternative.

Renal bone disease: Hypocalcaemia is corrected by giving 1α-hydroxylated synthetic analogues of vitamin D, adjusting the dose to avoid hypercalcaemia, and to reduce parathyroid hormone (PTH) levels to between 2 and 9 times normal. This will usually prevent or control osteomalacia. Hyperphosphataemia is controlled by dietary restriction of high-phosphate foods (milk, cheese, eggs) and the use of phosphate-binding drugs with food. These agents form insoluble complexes with dietary phosphate and prevent its absorption (e.g. calcium carbonate). Secondary hyperparathyroidism is usually controlled by these measures but, in severe bone disease with autonomous parathyroid function, parathyroidectomy may become necessary.

RENAL REPLACEMENT THERAPY

Renal replacement therapy (RRT) may be required temporarily for AKI or permanently for CKD. In the UK the median age of starting dialysis is 65, and 24% of patients have CKD due to diabetic nephropathy. Following initiation of dialysis in the UK, survival is 84% at 1 yr and 50% at 5 yrs. The aim of RRT is to replace the excretory functions of the kidney, and to maintain normal water and electrolyte balance. Options include haemodialysis, haemofiltration, peritoneal dialysis and transplantation (Fig. 7.6). The major side-effects of dialysis relate to haemodynamic disturbance caused by fluid removal or the extracorporeal circulation of blood, and reactions between blood and components of the dialysis system (bioincompatibility) (see Box 7.10 below).

Preparation for renal replacement therapy

When patients are known to have progressive CKD and are under regular clinic review, preparation for RRT should begin at least 12 mths before the predicted start date. This involves psychological and social support, assessment of home circumstances and discussion about choice of treatment. The principal decisions required are

7.10 Problems with haemodialysis

- Hypotension during dialysis
- Cardiac arrhythmias
- Haemorrhage
- Air embolism
- Dialyser hypersensitivity
- Emergencies between treatments (pulmonary oedema, sepsis)

Haemodialysis

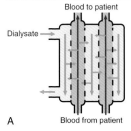

Haemofiltration

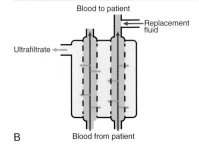

Peritoneal dialysis

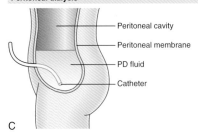

Transplantation

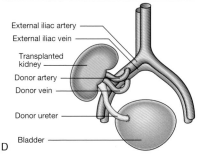

Fig. 7.6 Options for renal replacement therapy. A In haemodialysis, there is diffusion of solutes from blood to dialysate across a semi-permeable membrane down a concentration gradient. **B** In haemofiltration, both water and solutes are filtered across a semi-permeable membrane by a pressure gradient. Replacement fluid is added to the filtered blood before it is returned to the patient. **C** In peritoneal dialysis, fluid is introduced into the abdominal cavity using a catheter. Solutes diffuse from blood across the peritoneal membrane into the fluid down a concentration gradient. **D** In transplantation, the blood supply of the transplanted kidney is anastomosed to the internal iliac vessels and the ureter to the bladder. The transplanted kidney replaces all the functions of the failed kidneys.

the choice between haemodialysis and peritoneal dialysis, and referral for renal transplantation.

The average estimated GFR at the time of initiating RRT in the UK is 8 mL/min/1.73 m^2. The aim is to start RRT when symptoms of CKD have appeared but before serious complications develop.

Conservative treatment

In older patients with stage 5 CKD and multiple comorbidities, conservative, symptomatic treatment is viewed increasingly as a positive choice. Survival may be similar and patients are spared hospitalisation and invasive procedures. Patients are offered full medical, psychological and social support to optimise and sustain existing renal function for as long as possible, and appropriate palliative care in the terminal phases of disease. Many patients enjoy a good quality of life for several years. It is also appropriate to discontinue dialysis, with the consent of the patient, and to offer conservative therapy and palliative care when quality of life on dialysis is inadequate.

Haemodialysis

Haemodialysis (see Fig. 7.6A) is the most common form of RRT used for ESRD and is also used in AKI. Vascular access must be gained using either a central venous catheter or an arteriovenous shunt. The composition of the dialysate can be varied to achieve the desired solute flows and the pressure varied to remove water from the circulation if required. Anticoagulation with heparin during dialysis is standard practice. Haemodialysis for CKD may be performed at home or hospital and typically takes 3–5 hrs 3 times weekly. Complications are shown in Box 7.10.

Haemofiltration

Haemofiltration (see Fig. 7.6B) is principally used for AKI. It may be either intermittent or continuous and also allows control of intravascular volume by adjustment of the rate of fluid replacement.

Peritoneal dialysis

Peritoneal dialysis (see Fig. 7.6C) is used principally for CKD, and is useful in children and in adults with residual renal function. In continuous ambulatory peritoneal dialysis (CAPD), 2 L of sterile isotonic dialysis fluid are introduced and left in the abdomen for 4–6 hrs. Automated peritoneal dialysis is similar but fluid exchanges are performed by a pump overnight, reducing the daily treatment burden. Complications are summarised in Box 7.11.

Renal transplantation

Renal transplantation (see Fig. 7.6D) offers the best chance of long-term survival in patients with ESRD. It can restore normal kidney function and correct all the metabolic abnormalities of CKD. All patients should be considered for transplantation unless there are active contraindications (Box 7.12).

7.11 Problems with continuous ambulatory peritoneal dialysis

- CAPD peritonitis
- Catheter exit site infection
- Ultrafiltration failure
- Peritoneal membrane failure
- Sclerosing peritonitis

7.12 Contraindications to renal transplantation

Absolute

- Active malignancy – a period of at least 2 yrs of complete remission is recommended for most tumours prior to transplantation
- Active vasculitis or anti-GBM disease, with positive serology – at least 1 yr of remission is recommended prior to transplantation
- Severe heart disease
- Severe occlusive aorto-iliac vascular disease

Relative

- Age – while practice varies, transplants are not routinely offered to very young children (<1 yr) or older people (>75 yrs)
- High risk of disease recurrence in the transplant kidney
- Disease of the lower urinary tract – in patients with impaired bladder function, an ileal conduit may be considered
- Significant comorbidity

Kidney grafts may be taken from a cadaver or from a living donor. The matching of a donor to a specific recipient is strongly influenced by immunological factors, since graft rejection is the major cause of failure of the transplant. ABO (blood group) compatibility between donor and recipient is essential, and the degree of matching for major histocompatibility (MHC) antigens – particularly HLA–DR – influences the incidence of rejection. Tests should be performed for antibodies against HLA antigens, and antibodies that can bind to donor lymphocytes; both predict early rejection. Some ABO- and HLA-incompatible transplants are now possible with pre-transplant plasma exchange or immunosuppression, but the preparation required restricts this to live donor transplants.

Perioperative problems include:

Fluid balance: Careful matching of input to output is required.

Primary graft non-function: Causes include hypovolaemia, ATN or other pre-existing renal damage, hyperacute rejection, vascular occlusion and urinary tract obstruction.

Sepsis: Related to immunosuppression.

Once the graft begins to function, normal or near-normal biochemistry is usually achieved within a few days.

Management after transplantation

All transplant patients require regular lifelong clinic follow-up to monitor renal function and immunosuppression. Common immuno-suppressive regimens combine prednisolone with ciclosporin or tacrolimus together with azathioprine or mycophenolate mofetil. Treatment is associated with an increased incidence of infection, particularly opportunistic infections such as cytomegalovirus and *Pneumocystis jirovecii*. There is also an increased risk of malignancy, especially of the skin. Approximately 50% of white patients develop skin malignancy by 15 yrs post-transplant. Lymphomas are rare but may occur early and are often related to infection with herpes viruses, especially Epstein–Barr virus.

In the UK, the prognosis for transplants from cadaver donors is 96% patient and 93% graft survival at 1 yr, and 88% patient and 84% graft survival at 5 yrs. Even better results follow living donor trans-plantation (91% graft survival at 5 yrs). Living donor operations are becoming more common in the UK and can even be performed successfully with genetically unrelated donors.

RENAL VASCULAR DISEASES

Diseases that affect renal blood vessels may cause renal ischaemia, leading to acute or chronic renal failure or secondary hypertension. The rising prevalence of atherosclerosis and diabetes in ageing populations has made renovascular disease an important cause of ESRD.

Renal artery stenosis

Atherosclerosis is the most common cause of renal artery stenosis, especially in older patients with widespread arterial disease. In patients <50 yrs, fibromuscular dysplasia is a more likely cause of renal artery stenosis. This is an uncommon congenital disorder of unknown cause; it affects the media ('medial fibroplasia'), which narrows the artery but rarely leads to total occlusion. It most commonly presents with hypertension in patients aged 15–30 yrs, and in women more frequently than men.

Clinical features

Hypertension: This is driven by activation of the renin–angiotensin system in response to renal ischaemia. In atherosclerotic renal artery disease, there is usually evidence of arterial disease elsewhere, particularly in the legs. Factors that predict renovascular disease are shown in Box 7.13.

Deterioration of renal function on ACE inhibitors: When renal perfusion pressure drops, the renin–angiotensin–aldosterone system is activated and angiotensin-mediated glomerular efferent arteriolar vasoconstriction maintains glomerular filtration pressure. ACE inhibitors or ARBs block this physiological response. A drop in GFR (or >25% rise in creatinine) on ACE inhibitors raises the possibility of renal artery stenosis.

7.13 Renal artery stenosis

Renal artery stenosis is more likely if:
- Hypertension is severe, *or* of recent onset, *or* difficult to control
- Kidneys are asymmetrical in size
- Flash pulmonary oedema occurs repeatedly
- There is peripheral vascular disease of lower limbs
- Renal function has deteriorated on ACE inhibitors

Flash pulmonary oedema: Repeated episodes of acute pulmonary oedema associated with severe hypertension, without other obvious cause (e.g. myocardial infarction) in patients with normal or mildly impaired renal and cardiac function, can indicate renal artery stenosis.

Renal impairment: This may be the presenting feature in bilateral renal artery stenosis.

Investigations

Imaging of the renal arteries with CT or MRI angiography should confirm the diagnosis. USS may reveal asymmetry of kidney size. Biochemistry may show impaired renal function and elevated plasma renin, sometimes with hypokalaemia due to hyperaldosteronism.

Management

First-line management is with antihypertensives supplemented by statins and low-dose aspirin in those with atherosclerotic disease. Interventions to correct vessel narrowing should be considered in all patients <40, those with hypertension that is hard to control medically, those with deteriorating renal function and those with episodes of 'flash' pulmonary oedema. Angioplasty with stenting is of proven value in fibromuscular dysplasia, but results are less certain in atherosclerotic disease. Risks include renal infarction and failure to improve due to distal small-vessel disease.

Acute renal infarction

Sudden occlusion of the renal arteries usually presents as acute loin pain with haematuria on urine dipstick or microscopy, but pain is occasionally absent. Severe hypertension is common but not universal, presumably because some perfusion is required for renin release. LDH and CRP are commonly raised. Infarction may be caused by local atherosclerosis or by thromboemboli from a distant source, which may cause occlusion in branch arteries with multiple parenchymal infarcts, visible on CT scanning. Bilateral infarction or infarction of a single functioning kidney results in AKI with anuria. Patients with bilateral occlusion usually have widespread vascular disease and may show evidence of aortic occlusion, with absent femoral pulses and reduced leg perfusion.

7.14 Microvascular disorders associated with acute renal damage

- Thrombotic microangiopathy (haemolytic uraemic syndrome and thrombotic thrombocytopenic purpura)
    Associated with verotoxin-producing *E. coli*
    Other (familial, drugs, cancer)
- DIC
- Malignant hypertension
- Small-vessel vasculitis
- Systemic sclerosis (scleroderma)
- Atheroemboli ('cholesterol' emboli)

Management is largely supportive, and includes anticoagulation for an identified source of thromboemboli. It is sometimes possible to restore renal blood flow and function by stenting an acutely blocked main renal artery.

Diseases of small intrarenal vessels

A number of conditions are associated with acute damage and occlusion of small blood vessels (arterioles and capillaries) in the kidney (Box 7.14). They may be associated with similar changes elsewhere in the body. A common feature of these syndromes is microangiopathic haemolytic anaemia, in which fragmented red cells can be seen on a blood film as a consequence of damage during passage through the abnormal vessels.

GLOMERULAR DISEASES

Glomerular diseases may cause acute and chronic renal failure, and may follow a number of insults: immunological injury, inherited abnormality (e.g. Alport's syndrome), metabolic stress (e.g. diabetes mellitus), deposition of extraneous materials (e.g. amyloid), or other direct glomerular injury. The response of the glomerulus to injury varies according to the nature of the insult (Fig. 7.7). At one extreme, specific podocyte injury, or structural alteration of the glomerulus affecting podocyte function (e.g. by scarring or deposition of excess matrix or other material), causes proteinuria and nephrotic syndrome (p. 163). At the other end of the spectrum, inflammation leads to cell damage and proliferation, breaks form in the GBM and blood leaks into urine. In its extreme form, with acute sodium retention and hypertension, such disease is labelled nephritic syndrome.

Disease of the glomeruli may be immunological (glomerulonephritis), genetic or secondary to other disease, e.g. diabetes.

Glomerulonephritis

Glomerulonephritis means 'inflammation of glomeruli', although inflammation is not apparent in all varieties. Most types of glomerulonephritis are immunologically mediated and several respond to

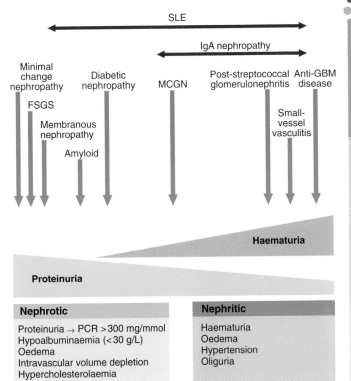

Fig. 7.7 Spectrum of glomerular diseases. (FSGS = focal and segmental glomerulosclerosis; GBM = glomerular basement membrane; IgA = immunoglobulin A; MCGN = mesangiocapillary glomerulonephritis; SLE = systemic lupus erythematosus); PCR = protein (mg/L)/creatinine (mmol/L) ratio

immunosuppressive drugs. Classifications of glomerulonephritis are largely histopathological. The clinically important types are described below.

Minimal change nephropathy

Minimal change disease occurs at all ages but accounts for nephrotic syndrome (PCR >300 mg/mmol, hypoalbuminaemia (<30 g/L), oedema and fluid retention) in most children and about one-quarter of adults. It is caused by reversible dysfunction of podocytes. It typically remits with high-dose corticosteroid therapy (1 mg/kg prednisolone for 6 wks). Some patients who respond incompletely or relapse frequently need maintenance corticosteroids, cytotoxic therapy or other agents. Minimal change disease does not progress to CKD but can present with problems related to the nephrotic syndrome and complications of treatment.

Focal segmental glomerulosclerosis

Focal segmental glomerulosclerosis (FSGS) can occur at any age. Specific causes include HIV, podocyte toxins and massive obesity, but in most cases the cause is unknown (primary FSGS). Primary FSGS presents with massive proteinuria and nephrotic syndrome. Histology shows sclerosis affecting segments of the glomeruli, with positive immunofluorescence staining for C3 and IgM. Since disease is focal, abnormal glomeruli may be missed on small renal biopsies. Some patients present with the histology of FSGS but less proteinuria. This may reflect healing of previous focal glomerular injury, such as haemolytic uraemic syndrome, cholesterol embolism or vasculitis. Such secondary FSGS has a different course and treatments.

Primary FSGS can respond to high-dose corticosteroid therapy (0.5–2.0 mg/kg/day) but most patients show little or no response. Immunosuppressant drugs have also been used to uncertain effect. Progression to CKD is common in patients who do not respond to steroids and the disease frequently recurs after renal transplantation, sometimes immediately.

Membranous nephropathy

This is the most common cause of nephrotic syndrome in adults. Some cases are associated with known causes (malignancy, hepatitis B virus) but most are idiopathic. Of this group, approximately one-third remit spontaneously, one-third remain in a nephrotic state, and one-third show progressive loss of renal function. Short-term immunosuppressive treatment may improve both the nephrotic syndrome and the long-term prognosis. However, because of the toxicity of these regimens, most nephrologists reserve such treatment for those with severe nephrotic syndrome or deteriorating renal function.

IgA nephropathy and Henoch–Schönlein purpura

IgA nephropathy is the most common glomerulonephritis and a common cause of ESRD. Presentation is with haematuria (almost universal), proteinuria (usual) and hypertension (very common). There may be severe proteinuria and nephrotic syndrome, or in some cases progressive loss of renal function. Some individuals develop acute exacerbations, often with gross haematuria, a few days after minor respiratory infections. These episodes usually subside spontaneously.

In children and occasionally in adults a systemic vasculitis occurring in response to similar infections is called Henoch–Schönlein purpura. A characteristic petechial rash (cutaneous vasculitis, typically affecting buttocks and lower legs) and abdominal pain (GI vasculitis) usually dominate the clinical picture, with mild glomerulonephritis indicated by haematuria. The glomerulonephritis is usually more prominent in older children or adults. Renal biopsy shows mesangial IgA deposition and appearances indistinguishable from acute IgA nephropathy.

Management of IgA nephropathy is largely directed towards control of BP and proteinuria reduction in an attempt to prevent or retard progressive renal disease.

Mesangiocapillary glomerulonephritis

Mesangiocapillary glomerulonephritis (MCGN) is characterised by increased mesangial cellularity, glomerular capillary thickening and subendothelial deposition of immune complexes and/or complement. It presents with proteinuria and haematuria. There are two main subtypes:

• The first features deposition of immunoglobulins within the glomeruli and is associated with chronic infections, autoimmune diseases and monoclonal gammopathy. • The second features glomerular deposition of complement and is associated with inherited or acquired abnormalities in the complement pathway.

Management of MCGN with immunoglobulin deposits consists of treatment of the underlying disease and the use of immunosuppressive drugs. There is no specific treatment for MCGN with deposition of complement in the glomeruli.

Glomerulonephritis associated with infection

Bacterial infections, usually subacute (typically subacute bacterial endocarditis), may cause a variety of histological patterns of glomerulonephritis, but usually with extensive immunoglobulin deposition and evidence of complement consumption. In the developed world, hospital-acquired infections are now a common cause of these syndromes. Worldwide, glomerulonephritis associated with malaria, HIV, hepatitis B, hepatitis C, schistosomiasis, leishmaniasis and other chronic infections is very common. The usual histological patterns are membranous and mesangiocapillary lesions, although FSGS may complicate HIV infection.

Post-streptococcal glomerulonephritis: This is most common following infection with certain strains of streptococcus (post-streptococcal nephritis), but can occur after other infections. It is much more common in children than adults but is now rare in the developed world. The latency is usually ~10 days after a throat infection or longer after skin infection, suggesting an immune mechanism rather than direct infection. An acute nephritis of varying severity occurs. Sodium retention, hypertension and oedema are particularly pronounced. There is also a reduction of GFR, proteinuria, haematuria and reduced urine volume. Characteristically, this gives the urine a red or smoky appearance. There are low serum concentrations of C3 and C4 and evidence of streptococcal infection. Renal function begins to improve spontaneously within 10–14 days, and management by fluid and sodium restriction and use of diuretic and hypotensive agents is usually followed by full recovery.

Rapidly progressive glomerulonephritis

This inflammatory nephritis causes rapid loss of renal function over days to weeks. Renal biopsy shows crescentic lesions often associated with necrotising lesions within the glomerulus. It is typically seen in Goodpasture's disease, where there are specific anti-GBM antibodies, and in small-vessel vasculitides (p. 198), but can also be seen in SLE (p. 198) and occasionally IgA and other nephropathies. Management normally includes corticosteroids and immunosuppressants.

Inherited glomerular diseases

Alport's syndrome is an uncommon X-linked condition in which abnormal collagen deposition results in haematuria, progressive renal failure and sensorineural deafness. ACE inhibitors slow but do not prevent loss of function, and many require RRT.

TUBULO-INTERSTITIAL DISEASES

These diseases affect renal tubules and the surrounding interstitium. The clinical presentation is with tubular dysfunction and electrolyte abnormalities, moderate proteinuria and varying degrees of renal impairment.

Acute interstitial nephritis

Acute interstitial nephritis (AIN) may be caused by allergic reactions (e.g. penicillins, NSAIDs), autoimmune nephritis, infections (e.g. pyelonephritis, TB) or toxins (e.g. mushrooms or myeloma light chains). Clinical presentation is with non-oliguric renal impairment or an eosinophilic reaction with fever and rash.

Investigations

Urinalysis shows leucocytes and eosinophils in 70% of patients. Renal biopsies show intense inflammation surrounding tubules and blood vessels and invading tubules, with occasional eosinophils (especially in drug-induced disease). Only ~30% of patients with drug-induced AIN have a generalised drug hypersensitivity reaction (e.g. fever, rash, eosinophilia).

Management

Remove/treat the cause. Steroids may accelerate recovery and prevent long-term scarring. Short-term dialysis is sometimes required.

Chronic interstitial nephritis

Known causes of chronic interstitial nephritis (CIN) are shown in Box 7.15; however, it is often diagnosed late and has no apparent aetiology.

Clinical features, investigations and management

Most patients present in adult life with moderate CKD (stage 3), hypertension and small kidneys. Due to tubular dysfunction, electrolyte abnormalities (e.g. hyperkalaemia, acidosis) may be severe. Urinalysis is non-specific.

- Acute interstitial nephritis
- Glomerulonephritis
- Immune/inflammatory (sarcoid, Sjögren's, systemic lupus erythematosus)
- Toxic (mushrooms, Balkan nephropathy, lead)
- Drugs (ciclosporin, tacrolimus, tenofovir, lithium, analgesics)
- Infection (severe pyelonephritis)
- Congenital/developmental (reflux, sickle cell nephropathy)
- Metabolic and systemic diseases (hypokalaemia, hyperoxaluria)

Management is supportive, with correction of electrolyte abnormalities and RRT if required.

Reflux nephropathy (chronic pyelonephritis)

This chronic interstitial nephritis is associated with vesico-ureteric reflux (VUR) in early life, and with the appearance of scars in the kidney.

Clinical features

Usually the renal scarring and renal/ureteric dilatation are asymptomatic. Presentation may be at any age, with hypertension, proteinuria or features of CKD. Frequency, dysuria and lumbar back pain may be present; however, there may be no history of UTIs. There is an increased prevalence of urinary calculi.

Investigations

• USS: will exclude significant obstruction but is not helpful in identifying renal scarring. • Longitudinal CT/MRI: may be useful to assess progression. • Radionuclide scans: sensitive but seldom required, as surgery for VUR is uncommon. • Urinalysis shows leucocytes and proteinuria (usually <1 g/24 hrs).

Management and prognosis

Treat infection. If recurrent, use prophylactic therapy. Nephrectomy is indicated if infection recurs in an abnormal kidney with minimal function. Hypertension is occasionally cured by the removal of a diseased kidney when disease is unilateral. Otherwise, surgery is rarely indicated as most childhood reflux disappears spontaneously. Children and adults with small or unilateral renal scars have a good prognosis, provided renal growth is normal. Deteriorating renal function, hypertension and proteinuria predict a poor prognosis in more severe bilateral disease. If the serum creatinine is normal and hypertension and proteinuria are absent, long-term prognosis is good.

Sickle-cell nephropathy

The longer survival of patients with sickle-cell disease (p. 541) means that a larger proportion live to develop chronic complications of microvascular occlusion.

KIDNEY AND URINARY TRACT DISEASE • 7

Clinical features

Damage to medullary vasa recta is most common. There is early loss of urine concentrating ability with polyuria. Distal renal tubular acidosis with hyperkalaemia is typical. Papillary necrosis is common. A minority of patients develop ESRD.

CYSTIC KIDNEY DISEASES

Polycystic kidney disease

Adult polycystic disease (PKD) is a common condition (prevalence ~1:1000) that is inherited as an autosomal dominant trait. Small cysts lined by tubular epithelium develop from infancy or childhood and enlarge slowly and irregularly. Surrounding normal kidney tissue is progressively attenuated. Renal failure is associated with grossly enlarged kidneys. PKD is not a pre-malignant condition. Mutations in *PKD1* account for 85% of cases and *PKD2* for ~15%. ESRD occurs in ~50% of patients with *PKD1* with a mean age of onset of 52 yrs, but in a minority of patients with *PKD2* with a mean age of onset of 69 yrs. Between 5 and 10% of patients on RRT have adult PKD.

Clinical features
See Box 7.16.

Investigations and screening
• These are based on family history, clinical examination and USS. USS demonstrates cysts in ~95% of affected patients over 20 yrs but may not detect smaller cysts in younger patients. • Genetic diagnosis is possible but not routinely used. • Screening for intracranial aneurysms is not generally indicated but can be done using MRI in those with a family history of subarachnoid haemorrhage.

7.16 Adult polycystic kidney disease: common clinical features

- Asymptomatic until later life
- Vague discomfort in loin or abdomen due to increasing mass of renal tissue
- One or both kidneys palpable, with nodular surface
- Acute loin pain or renal colic due to haemorrhage into a cyst
- Hypertension gradually develops over age 20 yrs
- Haematuria (with little or no proteinuria)
- Urinary tract or cyst infections
- Gradual-onset renal failure
- Associated features:
    - Hepatic cysts (30%)
    - Berry aneurysms of the cerebral vasculature
    - Mitral and aortic regurgitation (common but rarely severe)
    - Colonic diverticula
    - Abdominal wall hernias

Management

Good BP control is important because of cardiovascular morbidity and mortality, but there is no evidence that this retards the development of renal failure in PKD. There is some evidence that the vasopressin V2 receptor antagonist tolvaptan may slow cyst formation but this is not yet established treatment. Patients with PKD are usually good candidates for dialysis and transplantation. Sometimes kidneys are so large that one or both have to be removed to make space for a renal transplant.

Other cystic diseases

Medullary sponge kidney: Characterised by cysts confined to papillary collecting ducts, this disease is not inherited and its cause is unknown. Patients usually present as adults with renal stones. These are often recurrent, but the prognosis is generally good. The diagnosis is made by USS or intravenous urography (IVU). Contrast medium is seen to fill dilated or cystic tubules, which are sometimes calcified.

Acquired cystic disease: Patients with a very long history of renal failure (and usually on long-term dialysis) often develop multiple renal cysts in their shrunken kidneys: acquired cystic kidney disease. Kidneys are enlarged but not to the size seen in PKD. Acquired cystic disease is associated with increased erythropoietin production and an increased risk of renal cell carcinoma.

RENAL STONE DISEASE

Renal stones vary in frequency around the world, probably as a consequence of dietary and environmental factors, but genetic factors may also contribute. In Europe, 80% of renal stones contain crystals of calcium salts, ~15% contain magnesium ammonium phosphate, and small numbers of pure cystine or uric acid stones are found. In developing countries, bladder stones are common, particularly in children. In developed countries, the incidence of childhood bladder stones is low; renal stones in adults are more common. Several risk factors for renal stone formation are known (Box 7.17); however, in developed countries, most calculi occur in healthy young men with no clear predisposing cause.

Clinical features

Most renal stones are asymptomatic. Ureteric obstruction by stone causes:
• Renal colic: sudden pain in the loin, which radiates to the groin, testis or labium, in the first lumbar dermatome. Intensity steadily increases to reach a peak in a few minutes; the patient may groan in agony. • Pallor, sweating, restlessness and often vomiting. • Frequency, dysuria and haematuria. • Intense pain that usually subsides within 2 hrs but may continue for hours or days. It is usually constant during attacks, although slight fluctuations in severity may

7.17 Predisposing factors for kidney stones

- Low urine volumes: high ambient temperatures, low fluid intake
- Diet: high protein intake, high sodium, low calcium
- High urinary sodium/oxalate/urate/citrate excretion
- Hypercalcaemia of any cause (p. 355)
- Ileal disease or resection (leads to increased oxalate absorption and urinary excretion)
- Renal tubular acidosis type I (distal, p. 191)
- Familial hypercalciuria
- Medullary sponge kidney
- Cystinuria

7.18 Investigations for renal stones

Sample	Test	First stone	Recurrent stone
Stone	Chemical composition – most valuable test if stone can be recovered		✓
Blood	Calcium	✓	✓
	Phosphate	✓	✓
	Uric acid	✓	✓
	U&Es	✓	✓
	Bicarbonate	✓	✓
	Parathyroid hormone (PTH) – only if serum calcium or urine calcium excretion high		(✓)
Urine	Dipstick test for protein, blood, glucose	✓	✓
	Amino acids		✓
24-hr urine	Urea		✓
	Creatinine clearance		✓
	Sodium		✓
	Calcium		✓
	Oxalate		✓
	Uric acid		✓

occur. A dull loin ache may follow. • Similar colic that may occur with ureteric obstruction by clot or tumour.

Investigations

• Urinalysis: shows red cells. • AXR: ~90% of stones are radio-opaque. • CT of the kidneys, ureters and bladder (CTKUB) or IVU: CTKUB is superior, as it can show non-opaque stones. IVU may show delayed excretion of contrast from the kidney and a dilated ureter down to the stone. • USS may show stones and dilatation of the renal pelvis above an obstruction, and saves the patient radiation exposure.

Patients with a first renal stone should have a minimum set of investigations (Box 7.18); more detailed investigation is reserved for those with recurrent or multiple stones, or complicated or unexpected presentations. Since most stones pass spontaneously, urine should be sieved for a few days after an episode of colic to collect the calculus for analysis.

Management

• Powerful analgesia, e.g. morphine (10–20 mg), pethidine (100 mg) IM or diclofenac (100 mg) by suppository. • Antiemetics are often required.

Around 90% of stones <4 mm in diameter pass spontaneously, but only 10% of stones of >6 mm pass and these may require active intervention. Immediate action is required if there is anuria or infection in the stagnant urine proximal to the stone (pyonephrosis). Most stones can be fragmented by extracorporeal shock wave lithotripsy, in which shock waves generated outside the body are focused on the stone, breaking it into small pieces that can pass easily down the ureter.

Ureteroscopy may be required if lithotripsy is unsuccessful or unavailable, but open or percutaneous laparoscopic removal is now rarely needed except for large bladder stones. Measures to prevent recurrent stone formation depend on the results of investigations (see Box 7.18) and include dietary modifications, adequate fluid intake and diuretics.

ISOLATED DEFECTS OF TUBULAR FUNCTION

An increasing number of disorders (e.g. renal glycosuria and cystinuria) are now known to be due to specific defects of transporter molecules in renal tubular cells.

The term 'Fanconi syndrome' is used to describe generalised proximal tubular dysfunction. It is not related to Fanconi anaemia. Notable abnormalities include low blood phosphate and uric acid, the finding of glucose and amino acids in urine, and proximal renal tubular acidosis. Renal tubular acidosis describes the common endpoint of a variety of diseases affecting distal (classical or type 1) or proximal (type 2) renal tubular function. They cause metabolic acidosis with a normal anion gap (p. 149).

DISEASES OF THE COLLECTING SYSTEM AND URETERS

Congenital abnormalities

These include single kidneys, duplex kidneys with two ureters and obstruction at the pelvi-ureteric junction. The latter causes hydronephrosis in children and can be treated by laparoscopic pyeloplasty.

Retroperitoneal fibrosis

Fibrosis of retroperitoneal connective tissue may compress and obstruct the ureters.

Causes include idiopathic (most commonly), drugs, radiation, aortic aneurysm or malignancy. Presentation is with symptoms of ureteric obstruction. Investigations show high ESR/CRP; IVU/CT shows obstruction and medial deviation of ureters. Immediate treatment is usually by ureteric stenting. The idiopathic type responds to steroids; surgical ureterolysis is necessary if there is no response.

INFECTIONS OF THE URINARY TRACT

Urinary tract infection (UTI) is the most common bacterial infection managed in general medical practice and accounts for 1–3% of consultations. Prevalence in women is 3% at age 20, rising by 1% per decade thereafter. The term covers a range of conditions of varying severity from simple urethritis and cystitis to acute pyelonephritis with septicaemia.

Clinical features

Typical features of cystitis and urethritis include:
• Abrupt onset of frequency of micturition. • Scalding pain in the urethra during micturition (dysuria). • Suprapubic pain during and after voiding. • Intense desire to pass more urine after micturition, due to spasm of the inflamed bladder wall (urgency). • Cloudy urine with an unpleasant odour. • Microscopic or visible haematuria.

Systemic symptoms are usually slight or absent. However, infection in the lower urinary tract can spread; prominent systemic symptoms with fever, rigors and loin pain suggest acute pyelonephritis and may be an indication for hospitalisation.

The differential diagnosis includes urethritis due to an STI (p. 126) or Reiter's syndrome.

Investigations

An approach to investigation is shown in Box 7.19. Typical organisms causing UTI in the community include:

7.19 Investigation of patients with UTI

All patients

- Urinalysis looking for blood/protein/nitrite/glucose
- Urine microscopy and culture (MSU or urine obtained by suprapubic aspiration)
- Blood tests: U&Es, FBC

Other investigations

- Blood culture: if evidence of sepsis
- Pelvic examination: women with recurrent UTI
- Rectal examination: men (to examine prostate)
- Renal USS/CT/IVU: women who have acute pyelonephritis, recurrent UTI despite antibiotics, or UTI in pregnancy
- Cystoscopy: patients with haematuria or suspected bladder lesion

- *Escherichia coli* derived from the GI tract (~75% of infections).
- *Proteus.* • *Pseudomonas* spp. • Streptococci. • *Staphylococcus epidermidis.*

In hospital, *E. coli* still predominates, but *Klebsiella* and streptococci are more common. Certain strains of *E. coli* have a particular propensity to invade the urinary tract.

Investigation for UTI should be used selectively, most commonly in children, men and those with recurrent infections.

Management

Antibiotics are recommended in all cases of proven UTI. If urine culture has been performed, treatment may be started while awaiting the result. Treatment for 3 days is the norm and is less likely to induce alterations in bowel flora than more prolonged therapy. Trimethoprim is the usual choice for initial treatment; however, 10–40% of organisms causing UTI are resistant, the lower rates being seen in community-based practice. Nitrofurantoin, ciprofloxacin and cefalexin are also generally effective. High fluid intake and urinary alkalinising agents are often recommended but are not evidence-based.

Persistent or recurrent UTI

Treatment failure with persistence of organisms on repeat culture suggests an underlying cause such as:
- Incomplete bladder emptying (prostatic disease, neurological problems). • Foreign body (catheter, stone). • Failure of host defences (diabetes, post-menopausal atrophic urethritis).

Re-infection with a different organism, or with the same organism after an interval, may also occur. In women, recurrent infections are common and further investigation is only justified if infections are severe or frequent (>2/yr).

If the cause cannot be removed, suppressive antibiotic therapy can be used to prevent recurrence and reduce the risk of septicaemia and renal damage. Regular urine culture and a regimen of two or three antibiotics in sequence, rotating every 6 mths, are used to reduce the emergence of resistant organisms. Other simple measures to prevent recurrence include:
- Fluid intake >2 L/day. • Regular complete bladder emptying.
- Good personal hygiene. • Emptying of bladder before and after sexual intercourse. • Cranberry juice.

Asymptomatic bacteriuria

This is defined as $>10^5$/mL organisms in the urine of apparently healthy asymptomatic patients. There is no evidence that this condition causes renal scarring in adults who are not pregnant and have a normal urinary tract, and in general, treatment is not indicated. Up to 30% of patients will develop symptomatic infection within 1 yr.

Acute pyelonephritis

Acute renal infection (pyelonephritis) occurs in a minority of patients with lower UTI by ascending infection from the bladder. Rarely, bacteraemia leads to complications, including renal or perinephric abscesses, and papillary necrosis.

Clinical features

• Acute onset of pain in one or both loins, which may radiate to the iliac fossae and suprapubic area. • Lumbar tenderness and guarding. • Dysuria due to associated cystitis in 30%. • Fever with rigors, vomiting and hypotension. • Neutrophils, organisms, red cells and tubular epithelial cells in urine.

The differential diagnosis of acute pyelonephritis includes acute appendicitis, diverticulitis, cholecystitis and salpingitis. In perinephric abscess, there is marked pain and tenderness, and often bulging of the loin on the affected side. Patients are extremely ill, with fever, leucocytosis and positive blood cultures. Urinary symptoms are absent, and urine contains neither pus cells nor organisms.

Investigations and management

Bacteria and neutrophils in the urine with typical clinical features confirm the diagnosis. Renal tract USS or CT excludes a perinephric collection and obstruction as a predisposing factor. Adequate fluid intake must be ensured, if necessary IV. Antibiotics (first-line co-amoxiclav and ciprofloxacin) are given for 7–14 days. Severe cases require initial IV therapy, with a cephalosporin, quinolone or gentamicin. Urine should be cultured during and after treatment.

Tuberculosis of the kidney and urinary tract

TB of the kidney and urinary tract results from haematogenous spread of infection from elsewhere in the body.

Clinical features

• Bladder symptoms, haematuria, malaise, fever, night sweats, loin pain. • CKD as a result of urinary tract obstruction or destruction of renal tissue. • Renal calcification and ureteric strictures are typical.

Investigations and management

Urine reveals neutrophils but is negative on routine culture. Early morning urine cultures should be sent to identify tubercle bacilli. Perform cystoscopy if there is bladder involvement. Radiology of urinary tract and CXR are mandatory. Anti-TB chemotherapy (p. 295) is effective. Surgical relief of obstruction and nephrectomy are sometimes necessary for severe infection.

BENIGN PROSTATIC ENLARGEMENT (BPE)

From 40 yrs of age the prostate increases in volume by 2.4 cm^3/yr on average. Approximately 50% of men over 80 yrs will have lower urinary tract symptoms associated with BPE. Benign prostatic hyperplasia is the accompanying histological abnormality.

Clinical features

There is hesitancy, urinary frequency and urgency, poor urine flow and a sensation of incomplete voiding. Presentation may be with acute urinary retention, often precipitated by alcohol, constipation or prostatic infection. The painful distended bladder requires emergency catheter drainage. Chronic urinary retention involves a painless distended bladder that may lead to dilatation of the ureters and kidneys, with eventual renal failure. These patients may develop acute-on-chronic retention.

Investigations

• Symptom scoring systems: allow baseline values to be established and further deterioration/improvement to be assessed. • Urine flow meter readings. • Prostate volume assessment (PR and transrectal USS). • Urodynamic studies. • Renal function and renal USS.

Management

Medical treatment (α-adrenoceptor blockers, e.g. tamsulosin; 5α-reductase inhibitors, e.g. finasteride alone or in combination) may relieve obstruction. Transurethral resection of prostate (TURP) or enucleation by holmium laser is effective; open prostatectomy is rarely needed unless the prostate is very large.

TUMOURS OF THE KIDNEY AND URINARY TRACT

Renal adenocarcinoma

This is by far the most common malignant tumour of the kidney in adults, with a prevalence of 16 cases per 100 000 population. It is twice as common in males as in females. The peak incidence is between 65 and 75 yrs of age, and it is uncommon before 40. Spread may be local, lymphatic or blood-borne.

Clinical features

• 50% are asymptomatic and discovered incidentally • If symptomatic: haematuria (60%), loin pain (40%), abdominal mass (25%), pyrexia of unknown origin (PUO). • Systemic effects include fever, raised ESR and coagulopathy. • Tumour may secrete ectopic hormones, e.g. erythropoietin (EPO), PTH, renin. The effects of these disappear when the tumour is removed.

Investigations

• USS: allows differentiation between solid tumour and simple renal cysts. • CT abdomen/chest: for staging. • USS- or CT-guided biopsy: avoids nephrectomy for benign disease.

Management and prognosis

Radical nephrectomy should be performed whenever possible (even in the presence of metastases, which may regress after surgery).

Partial nephrectomy is appropriate if the tumour is <4 cm in diameter. Renal adenocarcinoma is resistant to radiotherapy and most chemotherapy, but some benefit has been seen in recent years with tyrosine kinase inhibitors and mTOR inhibitors. If the tumour is confined to the kidney, 5-yr survival is 75%. This falls to only 5% when there are distant metastases.

Urothelial tumours

These usually have a transitional cell origin and can affect the renal pelvis, ureter, bladder or urethra. They are three times more common in men than women and rare under the age of 40; they most commonly occur in the bladder. The appearance of a transitional cell tumour ranges from a delicate papillary structure, which usually indicates good prognosis, to a solid ulcerating mass, which usually signifies aggressive disease.

Clinical features and investigations

Some 80% of patients have painless, visible haematuria (see p. 164 for investigation of haematuria). Obstructive symptoms may occur. Examination is generally unhelpful. Cystoscopy is mandatory for suspected bladder cancer CT urogram or IVU demonstrates lesions in the upper urinary tract. CT chest/abdomen/pelvis allows invasive tumour staging.

Management and prognosis

Superficial tumours are treated by transurethral surgery and/or intravesical chemotherapy; cystectomy is rarely required. Regular cystoscopy is needed to detect recurrence. Carcinoma in situ responds well to intravesical BCG treatment. Invasive bladder tumours are generally treated with radical cystectomy and urinary diversion. Overall, 5-yr survival for patients with muscle-invasive bladder cancer is 50–70%.

Prostate cancer

Prostatic cancer is common in northern Europe and the USA but rare in China and Japan. In the UK the prevalence is 105 per 100000 population. It rarely occurs before the age of 50 yrs and has a mean age at presentation of 70 yrs.

Almost all prostate cancers are adenocarcinomas. Metastatic spread to pelvic lymph nodes occurs early and metastases to bone, mainly the lumbar spine and pelvis, are common.

Clinical features

Patients are either asymptomatic or there are urinary symptoms indistinguishable from BPE. Symptoms and signs due to metastases are much less common and include back pain, weight loss, anaemia and obstruction of the ureters. Prostate may feel nodular and hard on digital rectal examination with loss of the central sulcus (although up to 45% of tumours are impalpable).

Investigations

• Prostate specific antigen (PSA): a good tumour marker – 40% of patients with a serum PSA >4.0 ng/mL will have prostate cancer on biopsy. Screening programmes remain unproven, however, as the pickup rate is low. • Transrectal USS-guided needle biopsy: to confirm diagnosis. • USS of urinary tract and U&Es. • If diagnosis is confirmed: pelvic MRI and isotope bone scans are useful for staging, although high levels of serum PSA (>100 ng/mL) almost always indicate distant bone metastases. • PSA: most useful for monitoring response to treatment and disease progression.

Management and prognosis

Tumour confined to the prostate is potentially curable by either radical prostatectomy, radical radiotherapy or brachytherapy (implantation of radioactive particles), and these options should be considered in all patients with life expectancy >10 yrs. A small focus of tumour found incidentally at TURP does not significantly alter life expectancy and only requires follow-up.

Approximately half of men with prostate cancer will have metastatic disease at the time of diagnosis. Prostatic cancer is sensitive to hormonal influences; androgen depletion, either by orchidectomy or more commonly by androgen-suppressing drugs, leads to a high initial response rate in locally advanced or metastatic prostate cancer; however, the disease progresses after a year or two. A small proportion of patients fail to respond to endocrine treatment. Radiotherapy is useful for localised bone pain.

The 10-yr survival of patients with focal prostate carcinoma is 95%, but if metastases are present this falls to 10%.

Testicular tumours

These uncommon tumours occur mainly in men between 20 and 40 yrs of age; 85% are either seminomas or teratomas. Seminomas are relatively lowgrade but may metastasise to the lungs. Teratomas may contain differentiated bone, cartilage or other tissue. Testicular tumours may secrete α-fetoprotein (AFP) or β-human chorionic gonadotrophin (β-hCG).

Presentation is with a testicular lump. CT of chest, abdomen and pelvis is required for staging. Treatment is by orchidectomy with radiotherapy and/or chemotherapy for metastases.

RENAL INVOLVEMENT IN SYSTEMIC DISORDERS

Diabetes mellitus

Patients with diabetes show a steady advance from microalbuminuria to dipstick-positive proteinuria, the development of hypertension and progression to renal failure. Few require renal biopsy for diagnosis, but atypical features should raise suspicion of an alternative condition.

Management with ACE inhibitors and other hypotensive agents to slow progression has been dramatically effective. In some patients, proteinuria may be eradicated and progression completely halted, even if renal function is abnormal.

Malignant diseases

These may affect renal function in several ways:
- Direct involvement by tumour (renal, urothelial, cervical).
- Immune-mediated damage (glomerulonephritis). • Metabolic derangements (hypercalcaemia, hyperuricaemia). • Tumour products (e.g. light chains in myeloma).

Systemic vasculitis
Small-vessel vasculitis

This causes a focal inflammatory glomerulonephritis, often with crescentic changes. It may be a kidney-limited disorder with rapidly deteriorating renal function, or associated with a systemic illness with acute phase response, weight loss and arthralgia; in some patients it causes pulmonary haemorrhage, which can be life-threatening.

The most important cause is antineutrophil cytoplasmic antibody (ANCA)-positive vasculitis (p. 598), of which two subtypes occur. Microscopic polyangiitis presents with glomerulonephritis and pulmonary haemorrhage, and polyangiitis with granulomatosis (formerly Wegener's granulomatosis) presents with glomerulonephritis with granulomas of the lung and upper airway. Antibodies are non-specific, so biopsy is often required.

Treatment of small-vessel vasculitis is with steroids, immunosuppressive drugs and biological agents such as rituximab. Plasma exchange offers additional benefit in patients with progressive renal damage who are not responding to drugs.

Medium- to large-vessel vasculitis (e.g. polyarteritis nodosa)

This only causes renal disease when arterial involvement leads to hypertension, renal infarction or haematuria.

Systemic lupus erythematosus

Subclinical renal involvement, with low-level haematuria and proteinuria but minimally impaired or normal renal function, is common in systemic lupus erythematosus (SLE). Usually this is due to glomerular disease, although interstitial nephritis may also occur in overlap syndromes (e.g. mixed connective tissue disease, Sjögren's syndrome). SLE can produce almost any histological pattern of glomerular disease and an accordingly wide range of clinical features, ranging from florid rapidly progressive glomerulonephritis to nephrotic syndrome. High-dose steroids and cyclophosphamide reduce the risk of ESRD in lupus nephritis.

DRUGS AND THE KIDNEY

The kidney is susceptible to damage due to concentration of drugs and metabolites during excretion. Specific examples are shown in Box 7.20.

7.20 Drug-induced renal dysfunction: examples and mechanisms

Drug or toxin	Comments
Haemodynamic	
NSAIDs	↓ renal blood flow by inhibition of prostaglandin synthesis
ACE inhibitors	↓ efferent glomerular arteriolar tone. Toxic in renal artery stenosis/other renal hypoperfusion
Radiographic contrast media	May cause intense vasoconstriction, among other toxic effects
Acute tubular necrosis	
Aminoglycosides, amphotericin	Direct tubular toxicity but haemodynamic factors probably contribute
Paracetamol	± serious hepatotoxicity
Radiographic contrast media	May precipitate in tubules. Furosemide is a co-factor
Loss of tubular/collecting duct function	
Lithium, cisplatin	Loss of concentrating ability. Occurs at lower
Aminoglycosides, amphotericin	exposures than cause acute tubular necrosis
Glomerulonephritis (immune-mediated)	
Penicillamine, gold	Membranous nephropathy
Penicillamine	Crescentic or focal necrotising glomerulonephritis in association with ANCA +ve small-vessel vasculitis
NSAIDs	Minimal change nephropathy
Interstitial nephritis (immune-mediated)	
NSAIDs, penicillins, PPIs	Acute interstitial nephritis
Interstitial nephritis (toxicity)	
Lithium	Acute toxicity
Ciclosporin, tacrolimus	The major problem with these drugs
Tubular obstruction (crystal formation)	
Aciclovir	Drug crystallises in tubules
Chemotherapy	Uric acid crystals form as a consequence of tumour lysis
Nephrocalcinosis	
Bowel-cleansing agents	Ca, PO_4 precipitation – mild but sometimes irreversible damage
Retroperitoneal fibrosis	
Methysergide, practolol	No longer used in UK. Idiopathic form is more common

Cardiovascular disease

8

Cardiovascular disease is the leading cause of adult death in the Western world, with most deaths arising from ischaemic heart disease. Although the incidence of ischaemic heart disease is declining in many developed countries, it continues to rise in Eastern Europe and Asia. Valvular heart disease is also common, but while rheumatic fever still predominates in the Indian sub-continent and Africa, calcific aortic valve disease is now the most common problem in developed nations. Prompt recognition of the development of heart disease is limited by two factors. Firstly, patients often remain asymptomatic despite the presence of advanced disease and, secondly, the diversity of symptoms attributable to heart disease is limited and so different conditions frequently present similarly.

PRESENTING PROBLEMS IN CARDIOVASCULAR DISEASE

A close relationship between symptoms and exercise is a hallmark of cardiovascular disease. The New York Heart Association (NYHA) functional classification is often used to grade disability (Box 8.1).

Chest pain

Chest pain may arise from cardiac disease, from disease of the lungs, musculoskeletal system or GI system, or from anxiety.

Characteristics of cardiac pain

Site: Typically located in the centre of the chest.

Radiation: To the neck, jaw, and upper or lower arms. Occasionally, cardiac pain may be experienced only at the sites of radiation or in the back. Pain over the left anterior chest, radiating laterally, is unlikely to be cardiac ischaemia.

Character: Typically described as dull, constricting, choking, heavy, squeezing, crushing, burning or aching but not sharp, stabbing, pricking or knife-like. Patients typically use characteristic hand

CLINICAL EXAMINATION OF THE CARDIOVASCULAR SYSTEM

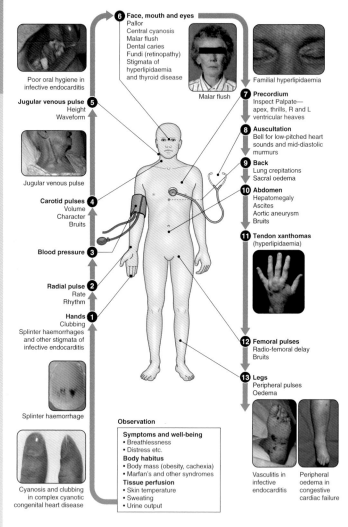

6 Face, mouth and eyes
Pallor
Central cyanosis
Malar flush
Dental caries
Fundi (retinopathy)
Stigmata of
hyperlipidaemia
and thyroid disease

Poor oral hygiene in
infective endocarditis

Malar flush

Familial hyperlipidaemia

Jugular venous pulse 5
Height
Waveform

Jugular venous pulse

Carotid pulses 4
Volume
Character
Bruits

Blood pressure 3

Radial pulse 2
Rate
Rhythm

Hands 1
Clubbing
Splinter haemorrhages
and other stigmata of
infective endocarditis

Splinter haemorrhage

Cyanosis and clubbing
in complex cyanotic
congenital heart disease

7 Precordium
Inspect Palpate—
apex, thrills, R and L
ventricular heaves

8 Auscultation
Bell for low-pitched heart
sounds and mid-diastolic
murmurs

9 Back
Lung crepitations
Sacral oedema

10 Abdomen
Hepatomegaly
Ascites
Aortic aneurysm
Bruits

11 Tendon xanthomas
(hyperlipidaemia)

12 Femoral pulses
Radio-femoral delay
Bruits

13 Legs
Peripheral pulses
Oedema

Observation

Symptoms and well-being
• Breathlessness
• Distress etc.
Body habitus
• Body mass (obesity, cachexia)
• Marfan's and other syndromes
Tissue perfusion
• Skin temperature
• Sweating
• Urine output

Vasculitis in
infective
endocarditis

Peripheral
oedema in
congestive
cardiac failure

8.1 New York Heart Association (NYHA) functional classification

Class I	No limitation during ordinary activity
Class II	Slight limitation during ordinary activity
Class III	Marked limitation of normal activities without symptoms at rest
Class IV	Unable to undertake physical activity without symptoms; symptoms may be present at rest

gestures (e.g. open hand or clenched fist). Some may describe discomfort or breathlessness rather than pain.

Provocation: Anginal pain occurs during exertion and is relieved by rest in less than 5 minutes. It may also be precipitated by emotion, a large meal or a cold wind. In crescendo or unstable angina, pain may occur on minimal exertion or at rest. Lying down may also provoke pain (decubitus angina).

Onset: The pain of myocardial infarction (MI) typically takes several minutes to develop; similarly, angina builds up gradually in proportion to exertion. Pain that occurs after, rather than during, exertion is usually musculoskeletal or psychological. The pain of aortic dissection, massive pulmonary embolism (PE) or pneumothorax usually starts suddenly.

Associated features: The pain of MI, massive PE or aortic dissection is often accompanied by sweating, nausea and vomiting. Breathlessness, due to pulmonary congestion from ischaemic left ventricular dysfunction, is often a prominent, and occasionally the dominant, feature of MI or angina (angina equivalent).

Differential diagnosis of chest pain

Psychological aspects of chest pain: Atypical chest pain is common in patients with anxiety, in whom it usually lacks a predictable relationship with exercise. Anxiety may also amplify the effects of organic disease or lead to exercise avoidance and secondary deconditioning.

Myocarditis and pericarditis: Pain is characteristically felt retrosternally, to the left of the sternum, or in the left or right shoulder. It varies in intensity with movement and with phase of respiration. It is usually described as 'sharp' and may 'catch' the patient during inspiration or coughing; there is occasionally a history of a prodromal viral illness.

Mitral valve prolapse: Causes sharp left-sided chest pain.

Aortic dissection: The pain is severe, sharp and tearing, often felt in or penetrates through to the back, and is typically abrupt in onset.

Oesophageal pain: Can mimic angina very closely, is sometimes precipitated by exercise and may be relieved by nitrates. However, it is usually possible to elicit a history relating chest pain to supine posture or to eating, drinking or oesophageal reflux. May radiate to the interscapular region and dysphagia may be present.

Bronchospasm: May be described by patients as exertional chest tightness, which can be difficult to distinguish from myocardial ischaemia. Persistent tightness after exercise, associated wheeze, cough and symptoms of atopy suggest the diagnosis.

Musculoskeletal chest pain: Common, with a very variable presentation. The pain may vary with posture or occur with specific movements (bending, stretching, turning). It is sometimes accompanied by local tenderness over a rib or costal cartilage. Causes include minor soft tissue injuries, arthritis, costochondritis and Coxsackie viral infection.

Massive pulmonary embolism: May produce severe central chest pain with breathlessness and autonomic disturbance, and can mimic MI. Sudden onset is typical. ECG may show right heart strain, and echocardiography right heart dilatation. CXR is frequently normal.

Initial evaluation of suspected cardiac pain

Stable angina: History indicates a reproducible and predictable relationship to exertion. Examination is often normal but may reveal signs of hyperlipidaemia, arterial disease, or exacerbating conditions such as anaemia. A murmur may reveal underlying aortic valve disease or hypertrophic cardiomyopathy. Investigations should include:

• FBC. • Lipids. • TFTs. • Blood glucose. • Resting and exercise ECGs.

Acute coronary syndromes: Prolonged, severe chest pain may be due to unstable angina (which comprises recent-onset limiting angina, rapidly worsening or crescendo angina, and angina at rest) or acute MI; these are known collectively as the acute coronary syndromes. Although there may be a history of antecedent chronic stable angina, an episode of chest pain at rest is often the first presentation of coronary disease. Examination may reveal comorbidity such as peripheral or cerebrovascular disease, autonomic disturbance (pallor or sweating) and complications (arrhythmia, hypotension or heart failure). A 12-lead ECG may show features of ischaemia (ST elevation or depression) and helps guide initial treatment. An ECG obtained during the episode of pain is particularly useful. Plasma troponin concentrations should be measured and, if these are normal, the test should be repeated 6–12 hrs after the onset of symptoms. If these tests are negative, an exercise test or CT coronary angiogram can help to diagnose underlying coronary disease.

Breathlessness (dyspnoea)

The differential diagnosis of dyspnoea is wide and includes many respiratory disorders (p. 265,). However, both acute and chronic dyspnoea may have a cardiac aetiology.

Acute left heart failure: May be triggered by an MI in a previously healthy heart or the onset of an arrhythmia such as atrial fibrillation (AF) in a patient with mitral stenosis. Increased left atrial pressure raises pulmonary capillary pressure, causing pulmonary oedema. Clinical features include:

• Agitation and sweating. • Frothy pink sputum. • Extensive crepitations: may be heard in the chest. • Signs of right heart failure (e.g. elevated JVP, peripheral oedema): may be present. • History of chronic heart failure or MI: often present. • CXR: shows perihilar haze or more extensive interstitial shadowing. • Underlying causes: may be revealed by ECG (e.g. MI, arrhythmia) and echocardiography (e.g. acute valvular regurgitation).

Chronic heart failure: Causes chronic exertional dyspnoea, initially on hills, and later during simple daily tasks like washing. Lying down increases venous return to the heart and provokes breathlessness (orthopnoea). Patients may wake up during the night profoundly breathless (paroxysmal nocturnal dyspnoea).

Some patients with heart failure develop a cyclical pattern of breathing with alternating apnoea and hyperventilation (Cheyne–Stokes respiration) due to prolonged circulation time and disordered respiratory control.

Breathlessness may also be the dominant or sole feature of myocardial ischaemia ('angina equivalent'). Patients sometimes describe chest tightness as 'breathlessness' but ischaemia may also cause dyspnoea by inducing transient left ventricular (LV) dysfunction. Associated chest tightness, close correlation of symptoms with exercise, and objective evidence of myocardial ischaemia from stress testing may all help to establish the diagnosis.

Acute circulatory failure (cardiogenic shock)

Shock indicates critical impairment of tissue perfusion. Causes of cardiogenic shock include:

• Myocardial infarction. • Massive PE. • Pericardial tamponade. • Mitral valve endocarditis. • Acute arrhythmia (e.g. ventricular tachycardia complicating myocarditis or MI).

Specific conditions are covered below, and the treatment of shock on page 23.

Heart failure

Heart failure describes the state that develops when the heart cannot maintain an adequate cardiac output or can do so only at the expense of elevated filling pressures. The prevalence rises from ~1% in the age group 50–59 yrs to between 5 and 10% of those aged 80–89 yrs. Overall, the prognosis is poor; ~50% of patients with severe heart failure due to LV dysfunction die within 2 yrs, many from ventricular arrhythmias or MI.

Almost all forms of heart disease can lead to heart failure (Box 8.2). Cardiac output is a function of the preload, the afterload and myocardial contractility (Fig. 8.1). When cardiac output falls, stimulation of the renin–angiotensin–aldosterone system leads to vasoconstriction, sodium and water retention, and activation of the sympathetic nervous system. These effects are mediated by release

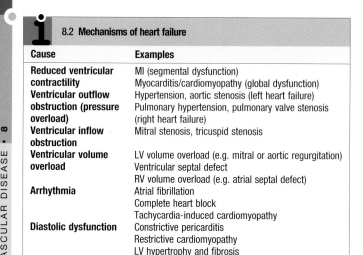

i 8.2 Mechanisms of heart failure

Cause	Examples
Reduced ventricular contractility	MI (segmental dysfunction)
	Myocarditis/cardiomyopathy (global dysfunction)
Ventricular outflow obstruction (pressure overload)	Hypertension, aortic stenosis (left heart failure)
	Pulmonary hypertension, pulmonary valve stenosis (right heart failure)
Ventricular inflow obstruction	Mitral stenosis, tricuspid stenosis
Ventricular volume overload	LV volume overload (e.g. mitral or aortic regurgitation)
	Ventricular septal defect
	RV volume overload (e.g. atrial septal defect)
Arrhythmia	Atrial fibrillation
	Complete heart block
	Tachycardia-induced cardiomyopathy
Diastolic dysfunction	Constrictive pericarditis
	Restrictive cardiomyopathy
	LV hypertrophy and fibrosis
	Cardiac tamponade

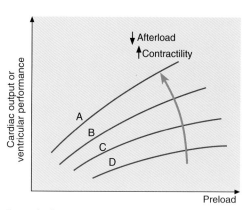

Fig. 8.1 Starling's Law. Normal (A), mild (B), moderate (C) and severe (D) heart failure. Ventricular performance is related to the degree of myocardial stretching. An increase in preload (end-diastolic volume, end-diastolic pressure, filling pressure or atrial pressure) will therefore enhance function; however, overstretching causes marked deterioration. In heart failure the curve moves to the right and becomes flatter. An increase in myocardial contractility or a reduction in afterload will shift the curve upwards and to the left.

of angiotensin II, aldosterone, endothelin-1 and antidiuretic hormone (ADH). Sympathetic activation may initially maintain cardiac output through increased myocardial contractility, heart rate and venous return. However, prolonged stimulation leads to cardiac myocyte apoptosis, hypertrophy and focal myocardial necrosis ($\downarrow$contractility), with peripheral vasoconstriction ($\uparrow$afterload). These changes produce a further fall in cardiac output, which leads to even greater neurohormonal activation, thus establishing a vicious circle. The onset of pulmonary and/or peripheral oedema is due to high atrial pressures compounded by salt and water retention.

Types of heart failure

Left-sided heart failure: This causes a reduction in LV output and/or an increase in the left atrial or pulmonary venous pressure. An acute increase in left atrial pressure may cause pulmonary oedema; a more gradual increase leads to reflex pulmonary vasoconstriction and pulmonary hypertension.

Right-sided heart failure (e.g. chronic lung disease, multiple pulmonary emboli): This causes a reduction in right ventricular (RV) output for any given right atrial pressure.

Biventricular heart failure: This may develop because disease affects both ventricles (e.g. dilated cardiomyopathy), or because left heart failure leads to chronic elevation of left atrial pressure, pulmonary hypertension and right heart failure. Heart failure may develop suddenly (acute heart failure) or gradually (chronic heart failure).

Diastolic dysfunction: In addition to the causes of systolic dysfunction above, heart failure may occur due to a stiff non-compliant ventricle causing poor filling (diastolic dysfunction). LV hypertrophy is the most common cause.

High output failure: This may occur with large arteriovenous shunts or thyrotoxicosis, due to an excessively high cardiac output.

'Compensated heart failure': This term describes a patient with impaired cardiac function in whom adaptive changes have prevented the development of overt heart failure.

Clinical features
Acute left heart failure

This usually presents with sudden-onset dyspnoea at rest with acute respiratory distress, orthopnoea and prostration. A precipitant (e.g. acute MI) may be apparent from the history. The patient appears agitated, pale and clammy. The peripheries are cool to the touch, the pulse is rapid and the JVP is usually elevated. The apex is not displaced, as there has been no time for ventricular dilatation. Auscultation may reveal a triple 'gallop' rhythm and crepitations are heard at the lung bases. Acute-on-chronic heart failure will have additional features of long-standing heart failure (see below).

Potential precipitants (e.g. arrhythmia, changes in medication, inter-current infective illness) should be identified.

Chronic heart failure

This commonly follows a relapsing and remitting course, with periods of stability interrupted by episodes of decompensation. A low cardiac output causes fatigue, listlessness and a poor effort tolerance; the peripheries are cold and BP is low. Pulmonary oedema due to left heart failure may present with breathlessness, orthopnoea, paroxysmal nocturnal dyspnoea and inspiratory crepitations over the lung bases. Right heart failure produces a high JVP, with hepatic congestion and dependent peripheral oedema. In ambulant patients the oedema affects the ankles, whereas in bed-bound patients it collects around the thighs and sacrum.

In advanced heart failure a number of non-specific complications may occur. Marked weight loss (cardiac cachexia) is caused by a combination of anorexia and impaired absorption due to GI congestion. Renal failure arises from poor renal perfusion due to a low cardiac output and may be exacerbated by diuretic therapy, ACE inhibitors and angiotensin receptor blockers. Hypokalaemia is caused by diuretics. Hyperkalaemia may occur due to the effects of drug treatment (particularly the combination of ACE inhibitors and spironolactone) and renal dysfunction. Hyponatraemia is caused by diuretic therapy or inappropriate water retention due to high ADH secretion and is a poor prognostic sign. Atrial and ventricular arrhythmias are very common and may be related to electrolyte changes (e.g. hypokalaemia, hypomagnesaemia), underlying structural heart disease, and the pro-arrhythmic effects of sympathetic activation. Sudden death occurs in up to 50% of patients, often due to ventricular arrhythmias.

Investigations

• ECG: may give clues to the aetiology of heart failure (e.g. LV hypertrophy, evidence of previous MI). • CXR: may reveal cardiomegaly and shows characteristic changes in pulmonary oedema (Fig. 8.2), including distension of upper lobe pulmonary veins, Kerley B lines (horizontal lines in the costophrenic angles indicating interstitial oedema), hazy hilar opacification (alveolar oedema) and pleural effusions. • U&Es, LFTs, TFTs and FBC: may help to identify some of the associated features listed above, as well as exacerbating factors such as anaemia. • Brain natriuretic peptide (BNP): elevated in heart failure and can be used as a screening test in breathless patients and those with oedema. • Echocardiography: should be considered in all patients with heart failure to determine the aetiology (e.g. valvular disease, regional wall motion defect in MI) and assess the severity of LV impairment.

Management of acute pulmonary oedema

This is summarised in Box 8.3.

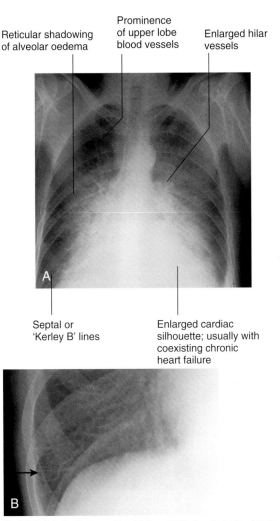

Reticular shadowing of alveolar oedema

Prominence of upper lobe blood vessels

Enlarged hilar vessels

A

Septal or 'Kerley B' lines

Enlarged cardiac silhouette; usually with coexisting chronic heart failure

B

Fig. 8.2 Radiological features of heart failure. A CXR of a patient with pulmonary oedema. **B** Enlargement of lung base showing septal or 'Kerley B' lines (arrow).

8.3 Management of acute pulmonary oedema

- Sit the patient up in order to reduce pulmonary congestion
- High-concentration oxygen (e.g. 60%)
- Continuous positive airway pressure (CPAP) 5–10 mmHg by mask
- Continuous monitoring of cardiac rhythm, BP and oxygen saturation
- Nitrates (e.g. IV glyceryl trinitrate 10–200 µg/min or buccal glyceryl trinitrate 2–5 mg) titrated upwards every 10 mins, until clinical improvement or systolic BP falls <110 mmHg
- A loop diuretic, e.g. furosemide 50–100 mg IV

Consider

- IV opiates – with caution; can cause respiratory depression

If above measures are ineffective, consider

- Inotropic agents (particularly in hypotensive patients)
- Insertion of an intra-aortic balloon pump (for cardiogenic pulmonary oedema and shock)

Management of chronic heart failure

General measures

These include:

• Effective education about the condition. • Maintenance of nutritional status. • Smoking cessation. • Avoidance of excessive salt or alcohol intake. • Regular moderate exercise. • Vaccinations for influenza and pneumococcus.

Treatment of the underlying cause (e.g. coronary artery disease (CAD), valvular disease, hypertension) is important to prevent progression.

Drug therapy

Drugs that reduce preload are indicated if there is pulmonary or systemic venous congestion. Drugs that increase contractility are useful if cardiac output is low.

Diuretics: Reduce plasma volume, thereby reducing preload and improving pulmonary and systemic venous congestion. In some patients with severe chronic heart failure, IV loop diuretics or combination therapy with a loop and thiazide diuretic may be required. Aldosterone receptor antagonists such as spironolactone are potassium-sparing diuretics that improve long-term outcome in patients with severe heart failure and those with heart failure following MI.

ACE inhibitors: Interrupt the vicious circle of neurohormonal activation in chronic heart failure, preventing salt and water retention, peripheral arterial and venous vasoconstriction, and sympathetic nervous system activation. They improve effort tolerance and mortality in moderate to severe heart failure and following MI. They may cause hypotension in hypovolaemic and elderly patients, and should therefore be started cautiously.

Angiotensin receptor blockers (ARBs): Produce haemodynamic and mortality benefits similar to those of ACE inhibitors, and are a useful alternative for patients intolerant of ACE inhibitors.

Vasodilators: May be useful in the treatment of chronic heart failure when ACE inhibitors or ARBs are contraindicated. Venodilators (e.g. nitrates) and arterial dilators (e.g. hydralazine) may be used, but may cause hypotension.

β-blockers: Help to counteract the adverse effects of enhanced sympathetic stimulation in chronic heart failure and reduce the risk of arrhythmias and sudden death. They must be introduced gradually to avoid precipitating acute-on-chronic failure, but when used appropriately have been shown to increase ejection fraction, improve symptoms and reduce mortality.

Ivabradine: Acts on the sinoatrial (SA) node to reduce heart rate. It reduces mortality and admissions in moderate to severe LV dysfunction, and is useful if β-blockers are not tolerated or not effective.

Digoxin: Can be used for rate control in heart failure with AF. It may reduce episodes of hospitalisation in patients with severe heart failure but has no effect on long-term survival.

Amiodarone: Useful for controlling arrhythmias in patients with poor LV function, as it has little negative inotropic effect.

Non-drug therapies

Cardiac resynchronisation therapy (p. 229): Restores the normal contraction pattern of the left ventricle, which may be dysynchronous in patients with impaired LV function and left bundle branch block.

Implantable cardiac defibrillators (p. 229): Reduce the risk of sudden death in selected patients with chronic heart failure, particularly those with a history of ventricular arrhythmia.

Coronary revascularisation: Bypass grafting or percutaneous coronary intervention may improve function in areas of 'hibernating' myocardium with inadequate blood supply, and can be used to treat carefully selected patients with heart failure and coronary artery disease.

Cardiac transplantation: An established and successful form of treatment for patients with intractable heart failure. Coronary artery disease and dilated cardiomyopathy are the most common indications. The use of transplantation is limited by the availability of donor hearts and so is generally reserved for young patients with severe symptoms. Serious complications include rejection, infection (due to immunosuppressive therapy) and accelerated atherosclerosis.

Ventricular assist devices: Have been employed as a bridge to cardiac transplantation, and more recently as potential long-term therapy. They assist cardiac output by using a roller, centrifugal or pulsatile pump. There is currently a high rate of complication (e.g. haemorrhage, systemic embolism, infection).

CARDIOVASCULAR DISEASE • 8

Syncope and presyncope

'Syncope' means sudden loss of consciousness due to reduced cerebral perfusion. 'Presyncope' means episodes of lightheadedness in which the patient feels they may black out. Both cause significant incapacity, particularly in the elderly. There are three principal mechanisms:

• Cardiac syncope due to mechanical dysfunction or arrhythmia. • Neurocardiogenic syncope, in which abnormal autonomic reflexes cause bradycardia and/or hypotension. • Postural hypotension, in which impaired peripheral vasoconstriction causes syncope on standing.

Other causes of blackouts include epilepsy, cerebrovascular disease and hypoglycaemia.

An accurate history from the patient and a witness is invaluable. In cardiac syncope, onset is usually sudden and recovery rapid. Patients with neurocardiogenic syncope often feel nauseated and experience malaise for several minutes before and after the episode. If standing up triggers syncope, postural hypotension is likely. Patients with seizures may exhibit abnormal movements, usually take many minutes to recover and are confused on recovery.

Cardiac syncope

Arrhythmias: May cause lightheadedness or blackouts, the latter indicating profound bradycardia or malignant ventricular tachyarrhythmias. Ambulatory ECG recordings may establish the diagnosis, as recording the ECG during symptoms is crucial to diagnosis. Patient-activated ECG recorders are useful for patients with recurrent dizziness but clearly unhelpful in sudden collapse. Where necessary, an implantable 'loop recorder' can be placed beneath the skin of the upper chest under local anaesthesia. This device continuously records an ECG, storing arrhythmic events in its digital memory for subsequent analysis.

Structural heart disease: Severe aortic stenosis, hypertrophic obstructive cardiomyopathy and severe coronary artery disease can cause lightheadedness or syncope on exertion. Profound hypotension occurs when cardiac output fails to rise normally as peripheral vascular resistance falls during exercise. Syncope may also result from an arrhythmia in these conditions.

Neurocardiogenic syncope

This can be triggered by particular situations (e.g. cough syncope or micturition syncope) but is more commonly triggered by reduced venous return due to prolonged standing, excessive heat or a large meal. Initial sympathetic activation causes vigorous contraction of the relatively underfilled ventricles. This stimulates ventricular mechanoreceptors, causing parasympathetic activation and sympathetic withdrawal, and leading in turn to bradycardia, vasodilatation or both. The diagnosis may be clear from the history, but can be confirmed using head-up tilt testing (the patient lies on a table tilted to an angle of 70° for up to 45 mins with monitoring of ECG and BP). In severe cases, drug treatment (e.g. fludrocortisone or disopyramide) may be helpful.

Hypersensitive carotid sinus syndrome may cause lightheadedness or syncope through inappropriate bradycardia and vasodilatation. Monitoring of the ECG and BP during carotid sinus massage can establish the diagnosis but should not be performed in patients with suspected carotid vascular disease (risk of embolic stroke).

Postural hypotension

May result from hypovolaemia (e.g. excessive diuretic therapy), sympathetic degeneration (e.g. diabetes mellitus, ageing) and drug therapy (e.g. vasodilators, antidepressants). Withdrawal of unnecessary medication, graduated elastic stockings and, in some cases, treatment with fludrocortisone may be helpful.

Palpitation

The term 'palpitation' may be used to describe a variety of sensations, including an erratic, fast, slow or forceful heart beat. A detailed description is essential (Box 8.4) and patients should be asked to tap out the heart beat on the table.

• Recurrent but short-lived bouts of an irregular heart beat, such as dropped or missed beats, are usually due to atrial or ventricular extrasystoles. • Attacks of a pounding, forceful, fast heart beat are a common manifestation of anxiety but may also occur in anaemia, pregnancy and thyrotoxicosis. • Discrete bouts of a very rapid (>120/min) heart beat suggest a paroxysmal arrhythmia. • AF typically presents with a completely irregular tachycardia.

An ECG recording during an attack of palpitation (ambulatory monitoring or patient-activated recorder) may be necessary to establish a definitive diagnosis. Most cases are due to an awareness of the normal heart beat, sinus tachycardia or benign extrasystoles triggered by stress, intercurrent illness, caffeine or alcohol. In such cases, careful explanation and reassurance will often suffice but a low-dose

---

8.4 How to evaluate palpitation

• Is the palpitation continuous or intermittent?
• Is the heart beat regular or irregular?
• What is the approximate heart rate?
• Do symptoms occur in discrete attacks?
• Is the onset abrupt? How do attacks terminate?
• Are there any associated symptoms, e.g. chest pain, lightheadedness, polyuria (a feature of supraventricular tachycardia, p. 220)?
• Are there any precipitating factors, e.g. exercise, alcohol?
• Is there a history of structural heart disease, e.g. coronary artery disease, valvular heart disease?

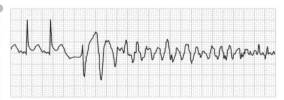

Fig. 8.3 Ventricular fibrillation. A bizarre chaotic rhythm, initiated in this case by two ectopic beats in rapid succession.

β-blocker may be helpful in patients with distressing symptoms. Arrhythmia management is described on pages 217–226.

Cardiac arrest

Cardiac arrest describes the sudden, complete loss of cardiac output. The patient is unconscious and pulseless. Death is inevitable without prompt effective treatment.

Ventricular fibrillation and pulseless ventricular tachycardia

These rhythms frequently arise in patients with MI or a history of previous MI.

• Ventricular fibrillation (VF): provokes rapid, uncoordinated movement of the ventricles, which produces no pulse. The ECG (Fig. 8.3) shows rapid, bizarre, irregular ventricular complexes.
• Ventricular tachycardia (VT): can cause cardiac arrest by preventing effective mechanical contraction and relaxation, and may degenerate into VF.

Defibrillation restores cardiac output in >80% of patients if delivered immediately.

Asystole

Asystole occurs when there is no electrical activity within the ventricles due to failure of the conducting tissue or massive ventricular damage. A precordial thump, external cardiac massage or IV atropine or adrenaline (epinephrine) may restore a rhythm, and pacing may be required.

Pulseless electrical activity (PEA)

Pulseless electrical activity (PEA) refers to the absence of cardiac output despite the presence of organised electrical activity. It may arise from treatable causes (e.g. cardiac tamponade, hypovolaemia or tension pneumothorax) but is more often due to a catastrophic event such as cardiac rupture or massive PE, so prognosis is poor.

Management of cardiac arrest

The management of cardiac arrest is shown in Figure 8.4.

Basic life support (BLS) encompasses manœuvres that attempt to maintain a low level of circulation pending more definitive treatment with advanced life support (ALS). ALS aims to restore cardiac

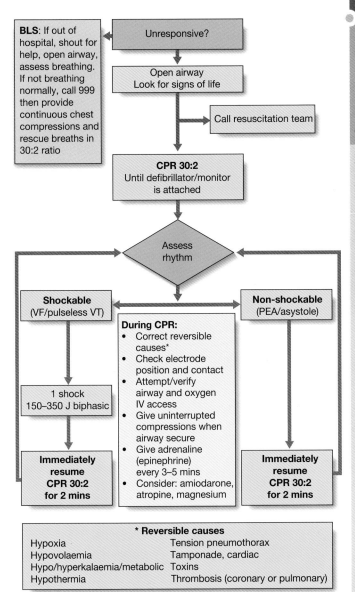

BLS: If out of hospital, shout for help, open airway, assess breathing. If not breathing normally, call 999 then provide continuous chest compressions and rescue breaths in 30:2 ratio

Unresponsive?

Open airway
Look for signs of life

Call resuscitation team

CPR 30:2
Until defibrillator/monitor is attached

Assess rhythm

Shockable
(VF/pulseless VT)

Non-shockable
(PEA/asystole)

During CPR:
- Correct reversible causes*
- Check electrode position and contact
- Attempt/verify airway and oxygen IV access
- Give uninterrupted compressions when airway secure
- Give adrenaline (epinephrine) every 3–5 mins
- Consider: amiodarone, atropine, magnesium

1 shock
150–350 J biphasic

Immediately resume CPR 30:2 for 2 mins

Immediately resume CPR 30:2 for 2 mins

* Reversible causes

Hypoxia	Tension pneumothorax
Hypovolaemia	Tamponade, cardiac
Hypo/hyperkalaemia/metabolic	Toxins
Hypothermia	Thrombosis (coronary or pulmonary)

Fig. 8.4 Algorithm for basic and adult advanced life support. For further information see www.resus.org.uk. (BLS = basic life support; CPR = cardiopulmonary resuscitation; PEA = pulseless electrical activity; VF = ventricular fibrillation; VT = pulseless ventricular tachycardia).

output by defibrillation or correction of other reversible causes of cardiac arrest. In the absence of an identifiable, treatable cause (e.g. ischaemia, aortic stenosis), survivors of VT or VF arrest should be considered for anti-arrhythmic therapy or an implantable cardiac defibrillator (p. 229). Patients who survive cardiac arrest in the context of acute MI require no specific additional treatment.

Abnormal heart sounds and murmurs

The first clinical manifestation of heart disease may be the incidental discovery of an abnormal sound on auscultation. Clinical evaluation (Box 8.5) is helpful but an echocardiogram is often necessary to confirm the nature of an abnormal heart sound or murmur. Some added sounds are physiological but may also occur in pathological conditions; for example, a third sound is common in young people and in pregnancy but is also a feature of heart failure. Similarly, an ejection systolic murmur may occur in hyperdynamic states (e.g. anaemia, pregnancy) but also in aortic stenosis. Benign murmurs do not occur in diastole, and systolic murmurs that radiate or are associated with a thrill are almost always pathological. Individual murmurs are dealt with below (pp. 248–255).

8.5 How to assess heart murmurs

When does it occur?

- Time the murmur using heart sounds, carotid pulse and apex beat. Is it systolic or diastolic?
- Does the murmur extend throughout systole or diastole, or is it confined to a shorter part of the cardiac cycle?

How loud is it? (intensity)

- Grade 1 Very soft (only audible in ideal conditions)
- Grade 2 Soft
- Grade 3 Moderate
- Grade 4 Loud with associated thrill
- Grade 5 Very loud
- Grade 6 Heard without stethoscope

N.B. Diastolic murmurs are sometimes graded 1–4.

Where is it heard best? (location)

- Listen over the apex and base of the heart, including the aortic and pulmonary areas

Where does it radiate?

- Evaluate radiation to the neck, axilla or back

What does it sound like? (pitch and quality)

- Pitch is determined by flow (high pitch indicates high-velocity flow)
- Is the intensity constant or variable?

Arrhythmias can cause palpitation, dizziness, syncope, chest pain or breathlessness, and trigger heart failure or even sudden death. They are generally classified as either tachycardias (heart rate >100/min) or bradycardias (heart rate <60/min).

• 'Supraventricular' (sinus, atrial or junctional) arrhythmias: usually produce narrow QRS complexes because the ventricles are depolarised via normal pathways. • Ventricular arrhythmias: give rise to broad QRS complexes because the ventricles are activated in an abnormal sequence.

Sinoatrial nodal rhythms

Sinus arrhythmia: Refers to a physiological increase of the sinus rate during inspiration and a slowing during expiration. It is mediated by the parasympathetic nervous system and may be pronounced in children.

Sinus bradycardia: May occur in healthy people at rest, especially athletes. Pathological causes include MI, raised intracranial pressure, hypothermia, hypothyroidism, cholestatic jaundice and drug therapy (e.g. β-blockers, verapamil, digoxin). Asymptomatic sinus bradycardia requires no treatment; symptomatic patients may require IV atropine or a pacemaker.

Sinus tachycardia: Usually due to an increase in sympathetic activity with exercise or emotion. Pathological causes include anaemia, fever, thyrotoxicosis, phaeochromocytoma, cardiac failure, shock and drug therapy (e.g. inhaled β-agonists).

Sinoatrial disease (sick sinus syndrome)

Sinoatrial disease results from degeneration of the sinus node and is common in the elderly. It may present with palpitation, dizzy spells or syncope, due to intermittent tachycardia, bradycardia, or pauses with no atrial or ventricular activity (sinus arrest or sinoatrial block). A permanent pacemaker may benefit patients with symptomatic bradycardias but is not indicated in asymptomatic patients.

Tachyarrhythmias

There are two main mechanisms of tachycardia:

Increased automaticity: The tachycardia is produced by repeated spontaneous depolarisation of an ectopic focus, often in response to catecholamines.

Re-entry: This occurs when there are two alternative pathways with different conducting properties (e.g. an area of normal tissue and an area of ischaemic tissue). In sinus rhythm, each impulse passes down both pathways before entering a common distal pathway. However, owing to different refractory periods, a premature impulse may travel selectively down one pathway, then retrogradely up the alternative pathway, establishing a closed loop or re-entry circuit and thus initiating a tachycardia.

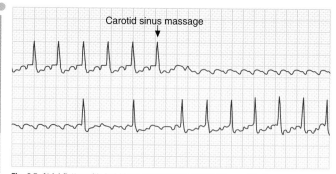

Fig. 8.5 Atrial flutter with 2:1 block: flutter waves revealed by carotid sinus massage.

Atrial tachyarrhythmias

Atrial ectopic beats (extrasystoles): Usually cause no symptoms but can give the sensation of a missed beat or abnormally strong beat. The ECG shows a premature but otherwise normal QRS complex; the preceding P wave has a different morphology because the atria activate from an abnormal site. Treatment is rarely necessary.

Atrial tachycardia: Produces a narrow-complex tachycardia with abnormal P-wave morphology caused by increased atrial automaticity, sinoatrial disease or digoxin toxicity. It may respond to β-blockers, which reduce automaticity, or class I or III antiarrhythmic drugs (p. 750). Catheter ablation may be useful for recurrent tachycardias.

Atrial flutter: Results from a large re-entry circuit within the right atrium. The atrial rate is ~300/min, but associated 2:1, 3:1 or 4:1 atrioventricular (AV) block usually produces a ventricular heart rate of 150, 100 or 75/min. The ECG shows saw-toothed flutter waves. With regular 2:1 AV block these may be buried in the QRS complexes and T waves but can be revealed by transiently increasing the degree of AV block through carotid sinus massage (Fig. 8.5) or IV adenosine. Digoxin, β-blockers or verapamil can limit the ventricular rate but electrical or chemical cardioversion using amiodarone or flecainide is often preferable. Beta-blockers or amiodarone may be used to prevent recurrent episodes of atrial flutter, but catheter ablation is now the treatment of choice for patients with persistent and troublesome symptoms.

Atrial fibrillation

Atrial fibrillation (AF) is the most common sustained cardiac arrhythmia, its prevalence rising with age. The atria beat rapidly but in an uncoordinated and ineffective manner. The ventricles are activated irregularly at a rate determined by conduction through the AV node, giving rise to an 'irregularly irregular' pulse. The ECG

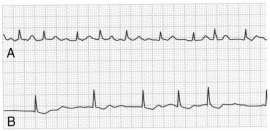

Fig. 8.6 Two examples of atrial fibrillation. The QRS complexes are irregular and there are no P waves. **A** There is usually a fast ventricular rate, often between 120 and 160/min, at the onset of AF. **B** In chronic AF the ventricular rate may be much slower due to the effects of medication and AV nodal fatigue.

8.6 Common causes of atrial fibrillation

- Coronary artery disease (including acute MI)
- Valvular heart disease, especially rheumatic mitral valve disease
- Hypertension
- Sinoatrial disease
- Hyperthyroidism
- Alcohol
- Cardiomyopathy
- Congenital heart disease
- Chest infection
- Pulmonary embolism
- Pericardial disease
- Idiopathic (lone AF)

(Fig. 8.6) shows normal but irregularly spaced QRS complexes with absent P waves.

AF can be classified as:

• Paroxysmal (intermittent, self-terminating episodes). • Persistent (prolonged episodes that can be terminated by electrical or chemical cardioversion). • Permanent.

Initially, classification may be difficult, but paroxysmal AF often becomes permanent with progression of the underlying disease. Common disease associations are shown in Box 8.6; however, many patients have 'lone atrial fibrillation', where no underlying cause is identified.

AF is often asymptomatic but can cause palpitation, breathlessness and fatigue. It may provoke myocardial ischaemia in patients with underlying coronary disease or precipitate cardiac failure in those with poor ventricular function or valve disease. The risk of stroke and systemic embolism is increased.

Management

Paroxysmal AF: All patients should have an ECG, echocardiogram and TFTs. When AF complicates an acute illness (e.g. chest infection), treatment of the primary disorder usually restores sinus rhythm. Occasional attacks of paroxysmal AF do not necessarily need treatment. For repeated symptomatic episodes, β-blockers can be used to reduce the ectopics that initiate AF and are the usual first-line therapy, especially in patients with associated ischaemic heart disease, hypertension or cardiac failure. Flecainide, along with β-blockers, prevents episodes but should be avoided in coronary disease or LV dysfunction. Amiodarone is also effective but side-effects restrict use. Digoxin and verapamil limit rate in AF but do not prevent episodes. Catheter ablation is useful in drug-resistant cases.

Persistent and permanent AF: Rhythm control – within 48 hrs of AF onset, heparinisation and cardioversion with drugs (flecainide or amiodarone) or synchronised DC shock can be attempted. Beyond 48 hrs, the ventricular rate should be controlled and cardioversion deferred until anticoagulation with warfarin (INR >2) has been established for more than 4 wks. Anticoagulation should be maintained for at least 3 mths following successful cardioversion. Unfortunately, relapse is common, particularly if AF has been present for >3 mths. After further cardioversion, amiodarone may help reduce recurrence, as may catheter ablation; however, results are less good than in paroxysmal AF. *Rate control* – β-blockers and rate-limiting calcium antagonists (e.g. verapamil) are more effective than digoxin at controlling heart rate during exercise. In resistant cases, AF can be treated by inducing complete heart block with catheter ablation after first implanting a permanent pacemaker.

Prevention of thromboembolism: Left atrial dilatation and loss of contraction cause stasis of blood and may lead to atrial thrombus formation, predisposing patients to stroke and systemic embolism. Warfarin (target INR 2.0–3.0) reduces the risk of stroke by two-thirds (with an annual risk of bleeding of 1–1.5%), while aspirin reduces it by only one-fifth. Risk stratification scores (Box 8.7) can be used to select which patients will benefit from warfarin. Risk is only loosely related to frequency and duration of episodes in intermittent AF, so guidelines do not distinguish between paroxysmal, persistent and permanent AF.

Direct thrombin inhibitors such as dabigatran have the advantage over warfarin in that they do not require blood monitoring; however, they cannot be rapidly reversed. Comorbid conditions (e.g. frequent falls) and drug interactions must be considered before anticoagulation is recommended.

'Supraventricular' tachycardias
AV nodal re-entry tachycardia

AV nodal re-entry tachycardia (AVNRT) is due to re-entry in the right atrium and AV node, and tends to occur in hearts that are

8.7 CHA₂DS₂-VASc stroke risk score for non-valvular atrial fibrillation

	Parameter	Score
C	Congestive heart failure	1 point
H	Hypertension history	1 point
A$_2$	Age $\geq$75 yrs	2 points
D	Diabetes mellitus	1 point
S$_2$	Previous stroke or transient ischaemic attack (TIA)	2 points
V	Vascular disease	1 point
A	Age 65–74 yrs	1 point
S$_c$	Sex category female	1 point
	Maximum total score	9 points

Annual stroke risk

0 points = 0% (no prophylaxis required)

1 point = 1.3% (oral anticoagulant recommended)

2+ points = >2.2% (oral anticoagulant recommended)

European Society of Cardiology Clinical Practice Guidelines: Atrial Fibrillation (Management of) 2010 and Focused Update (2012). Eur Heart J 2012; 33:2719–2747.

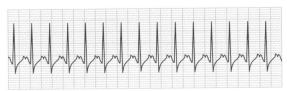

Fig. 8.7 **Supraventricular tachycardia.** The rate is 180/min and the QRS complexes are normal.

otherwise normal. It produces episodes of regular tachycardia with a rate of 140–220/min that last from a few seconds to many hours.

The patient is usually aware of a fast regular heart beat and may feel faint or breathless. Polyuria may occur. The ECG (Fig. 8.7) usually shows a regular tachycardia with normal QRS complexes but occasionally there may be rate-dependent bundle branch block. Attacks may be terminated by carotid sinus pressure or Valsalva manœuvre, but if not, IV adenosine or verapamil will restore sinus rhythm in most cases. When there is severe haemodynamic compromise, the tachycardia should be terminated by DC cardioversion (p. 226). If attacks are frequent or disabling, catheter ablation (p. 228) is the most effective therapy and is preferable to long-term drug treatment with β-blockers or verapamil.

Wolff–Parkinson–White syndrome and atrioventricular re-entrant tachycardia

An abnormal band of rapidly conducting tissue ('accessory pathway') connects the atria and ventricles. In around half of cases, premature activation of ventricular tissue via the pathway produces a short PR interval and a 'slurring' of the QRS complex, called a delta

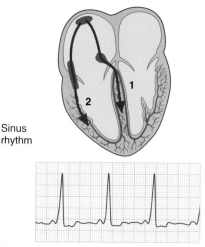

Sinus
rhythm

Fig. 8.8 Wolff–Parkinson–White syndrome. A strip of accessory conducting tissue allows electricity to bypass the AV node and spread from atria to ventricles without delay. When ventricular activation occurs through the AV node (1), the ECG is normal; however, when it occurs through the accessory pathway (2), a very short PR interval and a broad QRS complex are seen. In sinus rhythm, ventricular activation occurs by both paths, causing the characteristic short PR and slurring of the upstroke of the QRS complex (delta wave). The proportion of activation occurring via the accessory pathway may vary; therefore, at times, the ECG can look normal.

wave (Fig. 8.8). As the AV node and bypass tract have different conduction speeds and refractory periods, a re-entry circuit can develop, causing tachycardia; when associated with symptoms, the condition is known as Wolff–Parkinson–White syndrome.

The ECG appearance of atrioventricular re-entrant tachycardia (AVRT) may be indistinguishable from that of AVNRT. Carotid sinus pressure, Valsalva manœuvre or IV adenosine can terminate the tachycardia. If AF occurs, it may produce a dangerously rapid ventricular rate (since the accessory pathway lacks the rate-limiting properties of the AV node) and should be treated as an emergency, usually with DC cardioversion. Catheter ablation (p. 228) of the accessory pathway is now first-line therapy and is nearly always curative. Prophylactic treatment with flecainide or propafenone can be used but long-term drug therapy cannot be justified, as ablation is safer and more effective. Digoxin and verapamil shorten the refractory period of the accessory pathway and must be avoided.

Ventricular tachyarrhythmias
Ventricular ectopic beats (extrasystoles, premature beats)

Ventricular ectopic beats (VEBs) produce a low stroke volume and premature broad, bizarre abnormal QRS complexes on ECG.

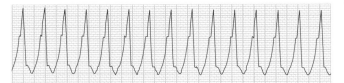

Fig. 8.9 Ventricular tachycardia: rhythm strip. Typical broad, bizarre QRS complexes with a rate of 160/min.

Patients are usually asymptomatic but may complain of an irregular heart beat, missed beats or abnormally strong beats. VEBs are frequently found in healthy people and treatment (β-blockers) is only necessary in highly symptomatic cases. Frequent VEBs in patients with heart failure or those who have survived the acute phase of MI are associated with an adverse prognosis. Treatment should be directed at the underlying cause.

Ventricular tachycardia

Ventricular tachycardia (VT) usually occurs in patients with coronary heart disease or cardiomyopathies and may cause haemodynamic compromise or degenerate into VF (p. 214). The ECG shows tachycardia with broad, abnormal QRS complexes and a rate >120/min (Fig. 8.9). VT is by far the most common cause of a broad-complex tachycardia but may be difficult to distinguish from supraventricular tachycardia with bundle branch block or Wolff–Parkinson–White syndrome. When there is doubt, it is safer to manage the problem as VT.

Emergency DC cardioversion is required if systolic BP is <90 mmHg, but if VT is well tolerated then IV amiodarone may be tried. Hypokalaemia, hypomagnesaemia, acidosis and hypoxaemia must be corrected. Beta-blockers and/or amiodarone may be effective for subsequent prophylaxis. Long-term treatment with class I anti-arrhythmic drugs is dangerous in patients with ischaemic heart disease. An implantable cardiac defibrillator may be indicated in patients with refractory VT or those at high risk of arrhythmic death (e.g. poor LV function, associated haemodynamic compromise). VT occasionally occurs in patients with otherwise healthy hearts; in such cases prognosis is good and catheter ablation can be curative.

Torsades de pointes

This form of VT complicates prolonged ventricular repolarisation, which may be congenital or secondary to drugs (e.g. class Ia, Ic and III anti-arrhythmics, macrolide antibiotics, tricyclic antidepressants, phenothiazines) or electrolyte disturbance ($\downarrow Ca^{2+}$, $\downarrow Mg^{2+}$, $\downarrow K^+$). The ECG shows rapid irregular complexes that oscillate from an upright to an inverted position, seeming to twist around the baseline. It is typically non-sustained but may degenerate into VF. The ECG in sinus rhythm shows a prolonged QT interval (>0.43 sec in men, >0.45 sec in women when corrected to a heart rate of 60).

IV magnesium should be given in all cases. Atrial pacing or IV isoprenaline shortens the QT interval by increasing heart rate. Otherwise, treatment is directed at the underlying cause. Patients with congenital long QT syndrome often require an implantable cardiac defibrillator.

Atrioventricular block

AV conduction is influenced by autonomic activity. Block may only be apparent when atrial tachycardias stress the conducting tissue.

First-degree AV block

AV conduction is delayed, producing a prolonged PR interval (>0.20 sec). It rarely causes symptoms.

Second-degree AV block

In second-degree AV block some atrial impulses fail to conduct to the ventricles, resulting in dropped beats.

Mobitz type I block ('Wenckebach's phenomenon'): There is progressive lengthening of the PR intervals, culminating in a dropped beat. The cycle then repeats itself. It is sometimes observed at rest or during sleep in athletic young adults with high vagal tone.

Mobitz type II block: The PR interval of conducted impulses remains constant but some P waves are not conducted. It is usually caused by disease of the His–Purkinje system and carries a risk of asystole. In 2:1 AV block (Fig. 8.10) alternate P waves are conducted, so it is impossible to distinguish between Mobitz type I and type II block.

Third-degree (complete) AV block

AV conduction fails completely, the atria and ventricles beat independently (AV dissociation, Fig. 8.11), and ventricular activity is maintained by an escape rhythm arising in the AV node or bundle of His (narrow QRS complexes) or the distal Purkinje tissues (broad QRS complexes). Distal escape rhythms are completely regular but slower and less reliable. Cannon waves may be visible in the neck, and the intensity of the first heart sound varies due to the loss of AV synchrony.

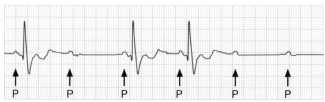

Fig. 8.10 Second-degree atrioventricular block (Mobitz type II). The PR interval of conducted beats is normal but some P waves are not conducted. The constant PR interval distinguishes this from Wenckebach's phenomenon.

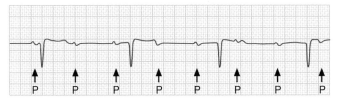

Fig. 8.11 Complete (third-degree) atrioventricular block. There is complete dissociation of atrial and ventricular complexes. The atrial rate is 80/min and the ventricular rate is 38/min.

Stokes–Adams attacks

Episodes of ventricular asystole may complicate complete heart block, Mobitz type II second-degree AV block and sinoatrial disease, resulting in recurrent syncope ('Stokes–Adams' attacks). Episodes are characterised by a sudden loss of consciousness, typically without warning, which may result in a fall. Convulsions (due to cerebral ischaemia) can occur if asystole is prolonged. There is pallor and a death-like appearance during the attack, but when the heart starts beating again there may be a characteristic flush. In contrast to epilepsy, recovery is rapid.

Management

AV block complicating acute MI: Acute inferior MI is often complicated by transient AV block because the right coronary artery supplies the AV junction. There is usually a reliable escape rhythm, and if the patient remains well, no treatment is required. Symptomatic second-degree or complete heart block may respond to IV atropine or, if this fails, a temporary pacemaker. In most cases the AV block will resolve within 7–10 days. Second-degree or complete heart block complicating acute anterior MI is usually a sign of extensive ventricular damage involving both bundle branches and carries a poor prognosis. Asystole may ensue and a temporary pacemaker should be inserted as soon as possible. If the patient presents with asystole, IV atropine (3 mg) or IV isoprenaline (2 mg in 500 mL 5% dextrose, infused at 10–60 mL/hr) may help to maintain the circulation until a temporary pacing electrode can be inserted.

Chronic AV block: Patients with symptomatic bradyarrhythmias associated with AV block should receive a permanent pacemaker. Asymptomatic first-degree or Mobitz type I second-degree AV block does not require treatment, but a permanent pacemaker is usually indicated in patients with asymptomatic Mobitz type II second-degree or complete heart block on prognostic grounds.

Bundle branch block

Interruption of the right or left branch of the bundle of His delays activation of the corresponding ventricle, broadens the QRS complex (≥0.12 sec) and produces characteristic alterations in QRS morphology (Figs 8.12 and 8.13). Right bundle branch block (RBBB) can be a

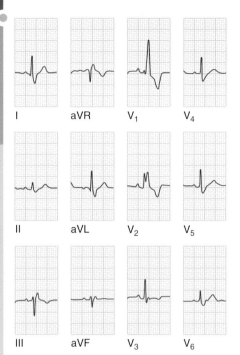

Fig. 8.12 Right bundle branch block. Note the wide QRS complexes with 'M'-shaped configuration in leads V_1 and V_2 and a wide S wave in lead I.

normal variant but left bundle branch block (LBBB) usually signifies important underlying heart disease (Box 8.8).

ANTI-ARRHYTHMIC DRUGS

These are covered on page 750.

THERAPEUTIC PROCEDURES

External defibrillation and cardioversion

The heart can be depolarised by passing an electrical current through it from an external source. This will interrupt any arrhythmia and produce a brief period of asystole, usually followed by the resumption of normal sinus rhythm. For elective cardioversion under general anaesthetic, a low-amplitude shock is synchronised to immediately after the R wave; shocks during the T wave are dangerous, as they may provoke VF. Patients with long-standing atrial arrhythmias are at risk of systemic embolism before and after cardioversion, so should be anticoagulated for at least 4 wks either side of the procedure. Defibrillation for cardiac arrest uses successive

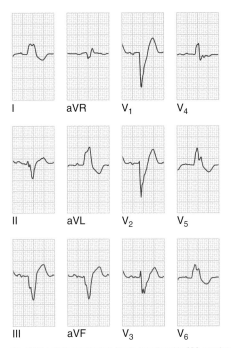

I	aVR	V₁	V₄
II	aVL	V₂	V₅
III	aVF	V₃	V₆

Fig. 8.13 Left bundle branch block. Note the wide QRS complexes with the loss of the Q wave or septal vector in lead I and 'M'-shaped QRS complexes in V_5 and V_6.

8.8 Common causes of bundle branch block

Right

- Normal variant
- RV hypertrophy or strain, e.g. PE
- Congenital heart disease, e.g. atrial septal defect
- Coronary artery disease

Left

- Coronary artery disease
- Aortic valve disease
- Hypertension
- Cardiomyopathy

unsynchronised shocks of 150 then 200 joules until sinus rhythm is restored.

Catheter ablation

Catheter ablation therapy is the treatment of choice for many patients with supraventricular tachycardia or atrial flutter, and is useful for some patients with AF or ventricular arrhythmias. A series of catheter electrodes are inserted into the heart via the venous system and used to record the activation sequence of the heart in sinus rhythm, during tachycardia and after pacing manœuvres. Once the arrhythmia focus or circuit is identified, a catheter is placed into this critical zone and the culprit tissue is selectively ablated using radio-frequency current or cryoablation. Serious complications are rare (<1%) but include inadvertent complete heart block requiring pace-maker implantation, and cardiac tamponade. Successful ablation spares the patient long-term drug treatment.

Temporary and permanent pacemakers

Temporary pacemakers

Transvenous pacing: Delivered by positioning a pacing electrode at the apex of the right ventricle via the internal jugular, subclavian or femoral vein using fluoroscopic imaging. The electrode is then connected to an external pulse generator, which can be adjusted to alter the energy output or pacing rate. Temporary pacing may be indicated in the management of transient heart block or of other causes of transient bradycardia (e.g. drug overdose), or as a prelude to permanent pacing. Complications include:

• Pneumothorax. • Brachial plexus or subclavian artery injury. • Infection (usually *Staphylococcus aureus*). • Pericarditis.

Transcutaneous pacing: Administered by delivering an electrical stimulus sufficient to induce cardiac contraction through two adhesive gel pad electrodes placed externally over the apex and upper right sternal edge. It is easy and quick to set up, but causes significant discomfort.

Permanent pacemakers

Permanent pacemakers utilise the same principles but the pulse generator is implanted under the skin. Electrodes can be placed in the right ventricular apex, the right atrial appendage or both (dual-chamber). Atrial pacing may be appropriate for patients with sinoatrial disease without AV block. In dual-chamber pacing the atrial electrode can be used to detect spontaneous atrial activity and trigger ventricular pacing, thereby preserving AV synchrony and allowing the ventricular rate to increase together with the atrial rate during exercise, leading to improved exercise tolerance. A code is used to signify the pacing mode (Box 8.9). Most dual-chamber pacemakers are programmed to a mode termed DDD. Rate-responsive pacemakers trigger a rise in heart rate in response to movement or increased respiratory rate and are used in patients unable to mount

8.9 International generic pacemaker code

Chamber paced	Chamber sensed	Response to sensing
0 = none	0 = none	0 = none
A = atrium	A = atrium	T = triggered
V = ventricle	V = ventricle	I = inhibited
D = both	D = both	D = both

8.10 Key indications for implantable cardiac defibrillator therapy

Primary prevention

- After MI, if LV ejection fraction <30%
- Mild to moderate symptomatic heart failure, on optimal drug therapy, with LV ejection fraction <35%

Secondary prevention

- Survivors of VF or VT cardiac arrest not due to transient or reversible cause
- VT with haemodynamic compromise or significant LV impairment (LV ejection fraction <35%)

* CARDIOVASCULAR DISEASE • 8

an increase in heart rate during exercise. Complications of permanent pacing include:

Early:

- Pneumothorax. • Cardiac tamponade. • Lead displacement.
- Infection.

Late:

- Infection. • Erosion of the generator or lead. • Lead fracture due to mechanical fatigue.

Implantable cardiac defibrillators

Implantable cardiac defibrillators (ICDs) sense rhythm and deliver current through leads implanted in the heart via the subclavian or cephalic vein. They automatically sense and terminate life-threatening ventricular arrhythmias. These devices have all of the functions of a pacemaker (to deal with bradycardias) but in addition can treat ventricular tachyarrhythmias using overdrive pacing, synchronised cardioversion, or defibrillation. ICD implantation is subject to similar complications as pacemaker implantation (see above). Indications for ICDs are shown in Box 8.10.

Cardiac resynchronisation therapy

Cardiac resynchronisation therapy (CRT) is a treatment for selected patients with heart failure and LBBB. This conduction defect is associated with uncoordinated LV contraction, which may exacerbate heart failure. CRT systems have an additional lead that is placed via the coronary sinus into one of the veins on the epicardial surface of the LV. Simultaneous septal and LV epicardial pacing resynchronises LV contraction, improving exercise tolerance in selected patients.

CORONARY ARTERY DISEASE

Coronary artery disease (CAD) is the leading cause of premature death in the developed world and is estimated to become, by 2020, the major cause of death worldwide. In the UK 1 in 3 men and 1 in 4 women die from CAD. Disease of the coronary arteries is almost always due to atherosclerosis and its complications, particularly thrombosis. Atherosclerosis is a progressive inflammatory disorder of the arterial wall, characterised by focal lipid-rich deposits of atheroma that remain clinically silent until they become large enough to impair arterial perfusion or until disruption of the lesion results in thrombotic occlusion or embolisation of the affected vessel. The pathogenesis of atherosclerosis is complex but several risk factors have been identified:

Age and sex: Age is the most powerful independent risk factor for atherosclerosis. Pre-menopausal women have lower rates of disease than men but thereafter risk is similar. Hormone replacement therapy has no role in prevention of atherosclerosis, however.

Family history: A 'positive' family history is present when clinical problems occur in first-degree relatives aged <50 yrs (male) or <55 yrs (female). Increased risk reflects a combination of shared genetic and environmental (e.g. smoking, exercise, diet) factors.

Hypertension: The incidence of atherosclerosis increases as BP (systolic and diastolic) rises. Antihypertensive therapy reduces cardiovascular mortality and stroke.

Hypercholesterolaemia: Risk rises with plasma cholesterol concentration. Lowering low-density lipoprotein (LDL) and total cholesterol reduces the risk of cardiovascular events (death, MI, stroke).

Diabetes mellitus: This is a potent risk factor for all forms of atherosclerosis and is often associated with diffuse disease. Insulin resistance (normal glucose homeostasis with high levels of insulin) is also a risk factor for CAD.

Lifestyle factors: There is a strong, dose-linked relationship between cigarette smoking and CAD. Alcohol is associated with reduced rates of coronary disease, but alcohol excess is associated with hypertension and cerebrovascular disease. Physical inactivity and obesity are independent risk factors for atherosclerosis; regular exercise appears to have a protective effect. Diets deficient in fresh fruit, vegetables and polyunsaturated fatty acids are associated with an increased risk of vascular disease.

Stable angina

Angina pectoris is the symptom complex occurring when an imbalance between myocardial oxygen supply and demand causes transient myocardial ischaemia. Coronary atheroma is by far the most common cause of angina; however, the symptom may also be a manifestation of other forms of heart disease, such as aortic valve disease, hypertrophic cardiomyopathy or coronary vasopasm (Prinzmetal's angina). Occasionally, the coronary arteries are involved in other disorders, such as polyarteritis and other connective tissue disease.

Clinical features

The history is by far the most important factor in making the diagnosis of stable angina (p. 201). Stable angina is characterised by central chest pain, discomfort or breathlessness that is precipitated by exertion or other forms of stress, and is promptly relieved by rest. Physical examination is frequently negative but may reveal evidence of:

• Aortic stenosis (an occasional cause of angina). • CAD risk factors (e.g. hypertension, diabetes; examine for retinopathy). • LV dysfunction (e.g. cardiomegaly). • Other arterial disease (e.g. carotid bruits, peripheral vascular disease). • Conditions that exacerbate angina (e.g. anaemia, thyrotoxicosis).

Investigations

Resting ECG: This may show evidence of previous MI but is often normal, even in patients with severe coronary artery disease. The most convincing ECG evidence of myocardial ischaemia is obtained by demonstrating reversible ST segment depression or elevation, with or without T-wave inversion, during symptoms.

Exercise ECG: The patient's ECG and BP are monitored during exercise using a standard treadmill or bicycle ergometer protocol. Planar or down-sloping ST segment depression of ≥1 mm is indicative of ischaemia; up-sloping ST depression is less specific. Exercise testing is also a useful means of assessing the severity of coronary disease and identifying high-risk individuals. However, false negatives and positives do occur and the predictive accuracy of exercise testing is lower in women than men.

Myocardial perfusion scanning: This is particularly helpful in patients who are unable to exercise or who have an equivocal or uninterpretable exercise test. Scintiscans of the myocardium are obtained at rest and during stress (exercise or pharmacological, e.g. dobutamine) after IV administration of a radioactive isotope that is taken up by viable perfused myocardium. A perfusion defect present during stress but not at rest indicates reversible myocardial ischaemia; a persistent defect suggests previous MI.

Stress echocardiography: This alternative to myocardial perfusion scanning has similar predictive accuracy (superior to exercise ECG). Ischaemic segments of myocardium exhibit reversible defects in contractility (on echocardiography) during exercise or pharmacological stress; areas of infarction do not contract at rest or during stress. The technique is particularly useful for identifying areas of viable 'hibernating' myocardium in patients with heart failure and CAD being considered for revascularisation (p. 211).

Coronary arteriography: Provides detailed anatomical information about the extent and nature of CAD. It may be indicated when non-invasive tests have failed to elucidate the cause of atypical chest pain but is usually performed with a view to revascularisation.

Management

• Identification and control of risk factors. • Symptom control. • Identification of high-risk patients for treatment to improve life expectancy.

Symptoms alone are a poor guide to the extent of coronary artery disease. Stress testing is therefore advisable in all potential candidates for revascularisation.

Identification and control of risk factors: The most important lifestyle modification is smoking cessation but other steps include regular exercise and aiming for ideal body weight. All patients with CAD should receive statin therapy, irrespective of serum cholesterol concentration. BP should be treated to a target of ≤140/85 mmHg, although ACE inhibitors (unless contraindicated) are of benefit in all patients with vascular disease. Aspirin reduces the risk of adverse events such as MI and should be prescribed indefinitely for all patients with CAD; clopidogrel is an equally effective alternative in patients intolerant of aspirin.

Relief of symptoms: Patients should be advised to avoid vigorous exertion after a heavy meal or in cold weather. Sublingual glyceryl trinitrate (GTN) in spray or tablet form will usually relieve an attack of angina in 2–3 mins. Patients should be encouraged to use GTN prophylactically before engaging in exercise that is liable to provoke symptoms.

Anti-anginal drugs: Five groups of drugs are used to prevent the symptoms of angina:

• Nitrates. • β-blockers. • Calcium antagonists. • Potassium channel activators (nicorandil). • If channel antagonists (ivabradine).

These drugs are discussed in detail on page 749. There is little convincing evidence that one group is more effective than another, although it is conventional to start with low-dose aspirin, a statin, sublingual GTN and a β-blocker, then add a calcium channel antagonist or a long-acting nitrate later, if necessary. The goal is control of angina with minimum side-effects and the simplest possible drug regimen. Revascularisation should be considered if symptoms persist despite the use of two drugs.

Percutaneous coronary intervention (PCI): This is performed by passing a fine guidewire across a coronary stenosis under radiographic control and using it to position a balloon, which is then inflated to dilate the stenosis. A coronary stent is a piece of coated metallic 'scaffolding' that can be deployed on a balloon and used to maximise and maintain dilatation of a stenosed vessel. PCI is an effective symptomatic treatment but has not been shown to improve survival in patients with stable angina. It is mainly used in single or two-vessel disease; coronary artery bypass graft (CABG) surgery is usually the preferred option in patients with three-vessel or left main disease. The main acute complication is vessel occlusion by thrombus or dissection, which may lead to myocardial damage (2–5%) requiring stenting or emergency CABG. The overall mortality risk is <0.5%. The main long-term complication is restenosis. The routine use of stents in appropriate vessels reduces both acute complications and the incidence of restenosis. Drug-eluting stents can reduce this risk even further at the cost of a small risk of late stent thrombosis. In combination with aspirin and heparin, adjunctive therapy with potent platelet inhibitors, such as clopidogrel or glycoprotein IIb/IIIa receptor antagonists, improves the outcome of PCI, with lower short- and long-term rates of death and MI.

Coronary artery bypass grafting (CABG): The internal mammary arteries, radial arteries or reversed segments of saphenous vein can be used to bypass coronary artery stenoses, usually under cardiopulmonary bypass. The operative mortality is ~1.5%, but higher in elderly patients and those with poor LV function or significant comorbidity (e.g. renal failure). There is a 1–5% risk of perioperative stroke. Approximately 90% of patients are free of angina 1 yr after surgery, but <60% of patients are asymptomatic ≥5 yrs after CABG. Arterial grafts have much better long-term patency rates than vein grafts. Treatment with aspirin or clopidogrel improves graft patency, while intensive lipid-lowering therapy slows progression of disease in the native coronary arteries and grafts. Persistent smokers are twice as likely to die in the 10 yrs following surgery compared with those who give up at surgery. CABG improves survival in patients with left main coronary stenosis and those with symptomatic three-vessel coronary disease; the benefit is greatest in those with impaired LV function or positive stress testing prior to surgery.

Acute coronary syndrome

This term encompasses unstable angina and myocardial infarction (MI). Unstable angina refers to new-onset or rapidly worsening (crescendo) angina, and angina on minimal exertion or at rest without myocardial damage. In MI there are symptoms at rest and myocardial necrosis occurs, leading to partial thickness, non-ST elevation MI (NSTEMI) or full-thickness, ST elevation MI (STEMI).

Acute coronary syndrome may present de novo or against a background of chronic stable angina. The underlying pathophysiology is usually a fissured atheromatous plaque with adherent thrombus formation.

Clinical features

• Pain: like that of angina but more severe and prolonged. • Breathlessness. • Vomiting: due to vagal stimulation, particularly in inferior MI. • Syncope or sudden death due to arrhythmia. • MI may occasionally be painless, especially in diabetic or elderly patients.

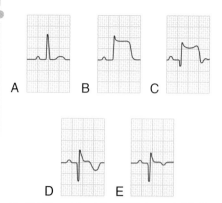

Fig. 8.14 The serial evolution of ECG changes in full-thickness myocardial infarction. **A** Normal ECG complex. **B** (Minutes) Acute ST elevation. **C** (Hours) Progressive loss of the R wave, developing Q wave, resolution of the ST elevation and terminal T-wave inversion. **D** (Days) Deep Q wave and T-wave inversion. **E** (Weeks or months) Old or established infarct pattern; the Q wave tends to persist but the T-wave changes become less marked.

Investigations

The ECG is the most important investigation in the assessment of acute chest pain and guides initial therapy. It shows a characteristic series of changes in MI (Fig. 8.14):

The earliest change is usually ST elevation followed by diminution in the size of the R wave, and development of a Q wave (indicating full-thickness infarction). Subsequently, the T wave becomes inverted and this change persists after the ST segment has returned to normal. ECG changes are best seen in the leads that 'face' the infarcted area. With anteroseptal infarction, abnormalities are found in one or more leads from V_1 to V_4. Anterolateral infarction produces changes from V_4 to V_6, in aVL and lead I. Inferior infarction is best shown in leads II, III and aVF. Infarction of the posterior wall of the left ventricle does not cause ST elevation or Q waves in the standard leads, but can be diagnosed by the presence of reciprocal changes (ST depression and a tall R wave in leads V_1–V_4). Occasionally, new-onset LBBB is the only ECG change.

Patients with ST elevation or new LBBB block require immediate reperfusion therapy. In patients with unstable angina or NSTEMI, the ECG may show ST/T-wave changes, including ST depression, transient ST elevation and T-wave inversion. These conditions carry a high risk of progression to STEMI or death.

Plasma biochemical markers (Fig. 8.15): The plasma concentration of enzymes and proteins normally concentrated within cardiac cells is increased in MI. The most useful markers are creatine kinase (CK) and CK-MB (a cardiospecific isoform) and the cardiac troponins T and I. CK starts to rise at 4–6 hrs, peaks at ~12 hrs and falls to normal within 48–72 hrs. Troponins T and I are released within 4–6 hrs and remain elevated for up to 2 wks.

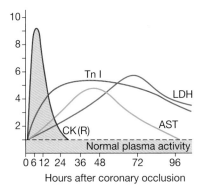

Fig. 8.15 Changes in plasma cardiac biomarker concentrations after myocardial infarction. Creatine kinase (CK) and troponin I (Tn I) are the first to rise, followed by aspartate aminotransferase (AST) and then lactate (hydroxybutyrate) dehydrogenase (LDH). In patients treated with reperfusion therapy, a rapid rise in plasma creatine kinase (curve CK (R)) occurs, due to a washout effect.

8.11 RISK stratification in acute coronary syndrome: GRACE score

Clinical feature	Points range		
Heart failure score (Killip class)	No failure: 0	to	Cardiogenic shock: 59
Systolic BP (mmHg)	≥200: 0	to	≤80: 58
Heart rate	≤50: 0	to	≥200: 46
Age (yrs)	≤30: 0	to	≥90: 100
Serum creatinine (μmol/L)	0–34: 1	to	≥353: 28
Cardiac arrest at admission	39		
ST-segment deviation	28		
Elevated cardiac enzyme levels	14		

The first five factors score points according to defined ranges (see SIGN Guideline 93; Feb 2007; pp 42 (annex 1) and 47 (annex 4): http://www.sign.ac.uk/guidelines/fulltext/93/).
Sum of points predicts in-hospital death:
0.2% for points ≤60, rising to 52% for points total >240

Echocardiography: This is useful for assessing LV and RV function and for detecting important complications, such as mural thrombus, cardiac rupture, ventricular septal defect, mitral regurgitation and pericardial effusion.

Risk stratification

Risk stratification using defined scores (e.g. the GRACE score; Box 8.11) guides the use of more complex pharmacological and interventional treatment. Additional markers of an adverse prognosis include:

• Recurrent ischaemia. • Extensive ECG changes. • Elevated troponin.
• Arrhythmias. • Haemodynamic complications (e.g. hypotension) during ischaemic episodes.

Immediate management: the first 12 hrs

Urgent hospital admission is required, as appropriate medical therapy reduces the risk of death and recurrent ischaemia by at least 60%. Initial therapy is summarised in Figure 8.16.

Analgesia is essential to relieve distress, and also to lower adrenergic drive and susceptibility to arrhythmias. IV opiates with an appropriate antiemetic (e.g. metoclopramide) should be titrated until the patient is comfortable.

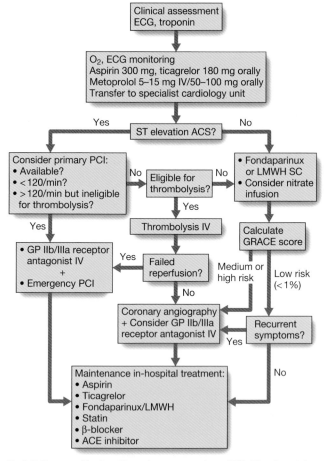

Fig. 8.16 Summary of treatment for acute coronary syndrome (ACS). (GP = glycoprotein; LMWH = low molecular weight heparin)

Antithrombotic therapy

Antiplatelet therapy with oral aspirin (300 mg initially, then 75 mg daily) improves survival (25% reduction in mortality). In combination with aspirin, the early (within 12 hrs) use of clopidogrel (600 mg, then 150 mg daily for a week, then 75 mg daily) confers a further reduction in mortality; however, in acute coronary syndrome, ticagrelor (180 mg, then 90 mg twice daily) is more effective.

Anticoagulation reduces thromboembolic complications and reinfarction. The pentasaccharide fondaparinux (2.5 mg SC daily) has the best safety and efficacy profile, but unfractionated or low molecular weight heparin is a useful alternative. Anticoagulation should be continued for 8 days or until hospital discharge.

Anti-anginal therapy

Sublingual GTN is valuable first aid in unstable angina, and IV nitrates are useful for the treatment of LV failure and the relief of recurrent or persistent ischaemic pain. IV β-blockers relieve pain, reduce arrhythmias and improve short-term mortality in patients who present within 12 hrs of the onset of symptoms, but should be avoided if there is heart failure, hypotension or bradycardia.

Reperfusion therapy in non-ST elevation MI

Immediate reperfusion therapy has no demonstrable benefit and thrombolytic therapy may be dangerous in these patients. Selected medium- and high-risk patients benefit from in-hospital coronary angiography and revascularisation but this does not need to be within 12 hrs.

Reperfusion therapy in ST elevation acute coronary syndrome

Immediate reperfusion preserves function and improves survival in these patients.

Primary percutaneous coronary intervention (PCI): The treatment of choice for STEMI. Outcomes are best when it is used in combination with glycoprotein IIb/IIIa receptor antagonists and intracoronary stent implantation. Compared to thrombolytic therapy, it is associated with a greater reduction in the risk of death, recurrent MI or stroke. The use of primary PCI has been limited by availability of this highly specialised emergency service. Thus, IV thrombolytic therapy remains first-line treatment in many hospitals, especially in rural or remote areas. When primary PCI cannot be achieved within 2 hrs, thrombolytic therapy should be administered.

Thrombolysis: Helps to restore coronary patency, preserves LV function and reduces the mortality of MI by 25–50%. Successful thrombolysis leads to reperfusion with relief of pain and resolution of acute ST elevation. It is indicated only in patients presenting within 12 hrs of the onset of symptoms and with ECG changes of LBBB or ST segment elevation of >1 mm in the limb leads or 2 mm in the chest leads. The benefit is greatest when treatment is given within the first few hours. Alteplase (human tissue plasminogen activator (tPA) 15 mg bolus, then 0.75 mg/kg up to 50 mg over 30 mins, then 0.5 mg/kg, up to 35 mg over 60 mins) is associated with better survival rates than other agents such as streptokinase, but carries a slightly higher risk of intracerebral bleeding. Newer-generation analogues of tPA, such as tenecteplase and reteplase, have equivalent efficacy to alteplase but have a longer plasma half-life and can be given by bolus administration. The major hazard of thrombolytic therapy is bleeding, particularly cerebral haemorrhage. Relative contraindications to thrombolytic therapy are summarised in Box 8.12.

Complications of acute coronary syndrome
Arrhythmias

Nearly all patients with acute MI have some form of arrhythmia; pain relief, rest and the correction of hypokalaemia are important preventative measures. VF occurs in ~5–10% of patients who reach hospital. Prompt defibrillation usually restores sinus rhythm. Early VF (within the first 48 hrs) does not adversely alter long-term prognosis, provided patients are promptly resuscitated. AV block complicating inferior infarction is usually temporary and often resolves following reperfusion. AV block complicating anterior infarction carries a risk of asystole and a prophylactic temporary pacemaker should be inserted. Other common peri-infarct arrhythmias include sinus tachycardia, sinus bradycardia, AF, VT and idioventricular rhythm; management of these is covered on page 239.

Ischaemia

Patients with recurrent angina following acute coronary syndrome are at high risk and should be considered for coronary angiography and urgent revascularisation. Angiography is also indicated in all those who have had successful thrombolysis, to treat residual stenosis.

Acute circulatory failure

Acute circulatory failure usually reflects extensive myocardial damage and indicates a bad prognosis. The assessment and management of heart failure is covered on page 210.

Pericarditis

This is particularly common on the second and third days following infarction. A distinct new pain develops, which is often positional or exacerbated by inspiration. Opiate analgesics are preferred over non-steroidal and steroidal anti-inflammatory drugs, as the latter may increase the risk of aneurysm formation and myocardial rupture. Dressler's syndrome is an autoimmune disorder that occurs weeks to months after the infarct and is characterised by persistent fever, pericarditis and pleurisy. Severe symptoms may require treatment with an NSAID or corticosteroids.

Mechanical complications

Papillary muscle rupture: May cause acute pulmonary oedema and shock with a pansystolic murmur due to the sudden onset of severe mitral regurgitation. Emergency mitral valve replacement may be necessary.

Rupture of the interventricular septum: Usually presents with sudden haemodynamic deterioration accompanied by a new loud pansystolic murmur. It may be difficult to distinguish from acute mitral regurgitation but tends to cause right heart failure rather than pulmonary oedema. Doppler echocardiography will confirm the diagnosis. Without prompt surgery, the condition is usually fatal.

Rupture of the ventricle: Leads to cardiac tamponade and is usually fatal.

Other recognised peri-infarct complications

These include:

• Systemic embolism from a cardiac thrombus. • Development of a ventricular aneurysm.

Late management
Risk stratification and further investigation

Scores (e.g. GRACE score) predict early mortality and are used to select patients for intensive therapy. Prognosis of survivors of acute coronary syndrome is related to:

Myocardial damage: Damage is assessed by echocardiography early in the recovery phase.

Ischaemia: Patients with early ischemia need urgent coronary angiography and revascularisation. Others should undergo an exercise tolerance test ~4 wks after the infarct; coronary angiography is required for those with a strongly positive test.

Ventricular arrhythmias: During convalescence from acute coronary syndrome these may indicate poor ventricular function and risk of sudden death. Although empirical anti-arrhythmic treatment is of no value, selected patients may benefit from specific anti-arrhythmic therapy (e.g. ICDs).

Lifestyle and risk factor modification

Smoking: Giving up smoking is much the most effective thing a patient can do after acute coronary syndrome, as cessation halves mortality at 5 yrs. Cessation success rates are improved by supportive advice and pharmacological therapy.

Hyperlipidaemia: Lowering serum cholesterol with statins following acute coronary syndrome reduces the risk of death, reinfarction, stroke and the need for revascularisation. Lipids should be measured within 24 hrs of presentation because cholesterol often falls in the 3 mths following infarction. Irrespective of serum cholesterol, all patients should receive statins after acute coronary syndrome, but those with LDL cholesterol concentrations >3.2 mmol/L (~120 mg/dL) benefit from more intensive therapy, such as atorvastatin 80 mg daily.

Other risk factors: Maintaining an ideal weight, eating a Mediterranean-style diet, taking regular exercise, and controlling hypertension and diabetes mellitus all improve the long-term outlook.

Mobilisation and rehabilitation

When there are no complications, the patient can return home in 5 days and gradually increase activity, with the aim of returning to work in 4–6 wks. The majority of patients may resume driving after 4–6 wks. Emotional problems, such as anxiety and depression, are common, and must be recognised and dealt with accordingly. Formal rehabilitation programmes, based on graded exercise protocols with individual and group counselling, are often very successful.

Secondary prevention and drug therapy

Low-dose aspirin therapy reduces the risk of further infarction and other vascular events by ~25% and should be continued indefinitely. Clopidogrel should be given in addition to aspirin for at least 3 mths and is a suitable alternative in aspirin-intolerant patients. Long-term β-blocker therapy reduces mortality by ~25% in survivors of acute MI and should be prescribed unless there are specific contraindications (p. 745). ACE inhibitors can prevent the onset of heart failure, improve survival and reduce hospitalisation, and should be considered in all patients with acute coronary syndrome. Patients with acute MI complicated by heart failure and LV dysfunction, and either pulmonary oedema or diabetes, further benefit from additional mineralocorticoid receptor antagonism (e.g. eplerenone 25–50 mg daily). ICDs reduce the incidence of sudden cardiac death in patients with severe LV impairment (ejection fraction ≤30%) post-MI.

Prognosis

Of those who survive an acute attack, >80% live for a further year, ~75% for 5 yrs and 50% for 10 yrs. Early death is usually due to an arrhythmia but, later on, the outcome is determined by the extent of myocardial damage. Unfavourable features include poor LV function, AV block and persistent ventricular arrhythmias. The prognosis is worse for anterior than for inferior infarcts.

Peripheral arterial disease

Almost all peripheral arterial disease (PAD) is due to atherosclerosis and it shares the same risk factors as CAD. Around 20% of UK adults aged 55–75 yrs have PAD, but only one-quarter have symptoms. PAD affects the leg eight times more often than the arm. The presence and severity of lower limb ischaemia can be determined by clinical examination (Box 8.13) and measurement of the ankle:brachial pressure index, the ratio between systolic ankle and brachial BPs (ABPI, normal >1.0). Chronic lower limb ischaemia presents as two distinct clinical entities: intermittent claudication (IC; ABPI 0.5–0.9) and critical limb ischaemia (CLI; ABPI <0.5).

Intermittent claudication

IC refers to ischaemic pain of the leg muscles precipitated by walking and relieved by rest. It is usually felt in the calf muscles (superficial femoral artery disease) but may occur in the thigh or buttock (iliac artery disease). Typically, the pain comes on after a reasonably constant 'claudication distance' and rapidly resolves on stopping.

All patients with PAD should receive 'best medical therapy' (BMT), which comprises standard secondary prevention measures for atherosclerosis (smoking cessation, regular exercise, low-dose aspirin, reduction of cholesterol, diagnosis and treatment of hypertension and diabetes) and optimisation of exacerbating conditions (e.g. heart failure, anaemia). Peripheral vasodilators such as cilostazol can improve walking distance. Intervention (angioplasty, stenting, endarterectomy or bypass) is usually only considered after 6 mths of BMT, and then only in patients whose disability is severe or threatens their livelihood. Provided patients comply with BMT, only 1–2%/yr will require amputation and/or revascularisation, but the annual mortality rate exceeds 5%, reflecting a high incidence of MI and stroke.

8.13 Features of chronic lower limb ischaemia

- Pulses – diminished or absent
- Bruits – denote turbulent flow but bear no relationship to the severity of the underlying disease
- Reduced skin temperature
- Pallor on elevation and rubor on dependency (Buerger's sign)
- Superficial veins that fill sluggishly and empty ('gutter') upon minimal elevation
- Muscle-wasting
- Skin and nails – dry, thin and brittle
- Loss of hair

Critical limb ischaemia

CLI is defined as rest (night) pain, requiring opiate analgesia, and/or tissue loss (ulceration or gangrene), present for >2 wks, in the presence of an ankle BP <50 mmHg. Whereas IC is usually due to single-segment plaque, CLI is always due to multi-level disease. Patients are at risk of losing their limb (or life) in a matter of weeks or months without surgical bypass or endovascular revascularisation, but treatment is difficult because they are often elderly with significant multisystem comorbidity and have severe multi-level disease.

Imaging is performed using duplex ultrasonography. More detailed non-invasive imaging can be provided by contrast MRI or CT. Intra-arterial digital subtraction angiography is indicated for patients suitable for endovascular revascularisation.

Diabetic vascular disease

Diabetes is present in 30–40% of those with severe limb ischaemia. It does not cause obstructive capillary microangiopathy; revascularisation is therefore effective when used together with control of infection and protection from pressure.

Buerger's disease

This inflammatory obliterative arterial disease usually affects male smokers aged 20–30 yrs, causing claudication and finger pain, with absent wrist and ankle pulses. Smoking cessation is essential, and sympathectomy and prostaglandin infusions may help.

Acute limb ischaemia

Acute limb ischaemia (ALI) is most frequently caused by acute thrombotic occlusion of a pre-existing arterial stenosis or thromboembolism (often secondary to AF). All suspected acutely ischaemic limbs (Box 8.14) must be discussed immediately with a vascular surgeon. If there are no contraindications, an IV bolus of heparin (3000–5000 U) should be given to limit thrombus propagation and protect the collateral circulation. Distinguishing thrombosis from embolism is frequently difficult. Evidence of chronic lower limb

✚	8.14 Symptoms and signs of acute limb ischaemia	
Symptoms/signs	**Comment**	
Pain **P**allor **P**ulselessness	May be absent in complete acute ischaemia, and can be present in chronic ischaemia	
Perishing cold	Unreliable, as the ischaemic limb takes on the ambient temperature	
Paraesthesia **P**aralysis	Important features of impending irreversible ischaemia	

ischaemia (e.g. previous IC symptoms, bruits, diminished contralateral pulses) favours thrombosis, while the absence of such features and the presence of AF favour embolism.

ALI due to thrombosis can often be treated medically with IV heparin (target APTT 2.0–3.0), antiplatelet agents, high-dose statins, IV fluids and oxygen. ALI due to embolus (no collateral circulation) normally results in extensive tissue necrosis within 6 hrs unless the limb is revascularised. Irreversible ischaemia mandates early amputation or palliative therapy.

Diseases of the aorta
Abdominal aortic aneurysms

An aortic aneurysm is an abnormal dilatation of the aortic wall. The most important risk factors are male gender, family history, hypertension and smoking. Median age at presentation is 65 yrs for elective and 75 yrs for emergency cases.

Many abdominal aortic aneurysms (AAAs) are asymptomatic and found incidentally or on screening, but they may cause central abdominal pain or lower limb embolic complications. USS establishes the diagnosis and is used to monitor asymptomatic AAAs; elective repair is considered if the diameter exceeds 5.5 cm. All symptomatic AAAs should be considered for repair, not least because pain often predates rupture. Distal embolisation is a strong indication for repair. Rupture of an AAA produces severe abdominal pain with hypovolaemic shock and is rapidly fatal. Operative mortality for ruptured AAA is ~50% but survivors have a good prognosis. Endovascular repair using a stent-graft introduced through the femoral artery is used increasingly to replace open surgery.

Thoracic aortic aneurysm

This may produce chest pain, aortic regurgitation, stridor, hoarseness or superior vena cava syndrome. If it erodes into adjacent structures, massive heamorrhage occurs. In Marfan's syndrome, an autosomal dominant connective tissue disorder caused by mutation in the fibrillin gene, weakening of the aortic media leads to aortic root dilatation that may be complicated by aortic regurgitation and aortic dissection (see below). CXR, echocardiography, MRI or CT may detect aortic dilatation at an early stage and can be used to monitor the disease. Treatment with β-blockers reduces the rate of aortic dilatation and the risk of rupture.

Aortic dissection

A breach in the intima of the aortic wall allows arterial blood to enter the media, which is then split into two layers, creating a 'false lumen' alongside the existing or 'true lumen'. Aortic dissection is classified into type A and type B, involving or sparing the ascending aorta, respectively. Aortic atherosclerosis and hypertension are common aetiological factors but other predisposing conditions include thoracic aortic aneurysm, aortic coarctation, previous aortic surgery, Marfan's syndrome, trauma and pregnancy.

The patient typically presents with sudden-onset, severe, 'tearing' chest pain, often associated with collapse. In type A dissection, the aortic valve may be damaged, causing acute regurgitation. Occlusion of aortic branches may cause stroke, MI or paraplegia, as well as asymmetry of the brachial, carotid or femoral pulses. The CXR may show broadening of the upper mediastinum and distortion of the aortic 'knuckle', but these findings are absent in 10% of cases. Transthoracic echocardiography can only image the first 3–4 cm of the ascending aorta but transoesophageal echocardiography, CT and MRI are all very useful. Early mortality of acute dissection is 1–5%/hr. Initial management comprises pain control and IV labetalol (target systolic BP <120 mmHg). Endoluminal repair with fenestration of the intimal flap or insertion of a stent-graft may be effective.

HYPERTENSION

High BP represents a quantitative rather than a qualitative deviation from the norm and any definition of hypertension is therefore arbitrary. The British Hypertension Society defines hypertension as a BP >140/90 mmHg. However, the incidence of cardiovascular disease (particularly stroke and CAD) is closely related to average BP at all ages, even when readings are within the 'reference range'.

In >95% of cases, no specific underlying cause of hypertension can be found and such patients are said to have essential hypertension. Important predisposing factors for essential hypertension include:

• Ethnicity (higher incidence in African Americans and Japanese). • Genetic factors. • High salt intake. • Alcohol excess. • Obesity. • Lack of exercise. • Impaired intrauterine growth.

In ~5% of cases, hypertension results from a specific underlying disorder (secondary hypertension). Causes include:

• Renal disease (renal vascular disease, glomerulonephritis, polycystic kidney disease; see Ch. 7). • Endocrine disorders (phaeochromocytoma, Cushing's syndrome, Conn's syndrome, acromegaly, thyrotoxicosis, congenital adrenal hyperplasia; see Ch. 10). • Pregnancy. • Drugs (corticosteroids, oestrogen-containing oral contraceptive pill, anabolic steroids). • Coarctation of the aorta.

Approach to newly diagnosed hypertension

Hypertension occasionally causes headache but most patients remain asymptomatic. Accordingly, the diagnosis is usually made at routine examination or when a complication arises. The history may reveal a family history, lifestyle factors (exercise, salt intake, smoking, alcohol intake) and potential drug causes. There may be symptoms suggesting a secondary cause such as phaeochromocytoma

Grade 1	Arteriolar thickening, tortuosity and increased reflectiveness ('silver wiring')
Grade 2	Grade 1 plus constriction of veins at arterial crossings ('arteriovenous nipping')
Grade 3	Grade 2 plus evidence of retinal ischaemia (flame-shaped or blot haemorrhages and 'cotton wool' exudates)
Grade 4	Grade 3 plus papilloedema

(paroxysmal headache, palpitation and sweating) or complications such as CAD (e.g. angina).

Examination may reveal radio-femoral delay (coarctation of the aorta), enlarged kidneys (polycystic kidney disease), abdominal bruits (renal artery stenosis) or features of endocrine disease. More commonly, there may be signs attributable to the complications of hypertension, such as LV hypertrophy (apical heave, fourth heart sound) or retinopathy (Box 8.15).

Target organ damage

Blood vessels: Smooth muscle hypertrophy and fibrosis are seen in larger arteries. Atheroma may lead to coronary and/or cerebrovascular disease, particularly if other risk factors are present. Structural changes in the vasculature aggravate hypertension by increasing peripheral vascular resistance and reducing renal blood flow. Hypertension is also implicated in the pathogenesis of aortic aneurysm and aortic dissection.

CNS: Stroke, due to either cerebral haemorrhage or infarction, and transient ischaemic attacks (TIAs) are common complications. Subarachnoid haemorrhage is also associated with hypertension. Hypertensive encephalopathy is a rare condition characterised by high BP, neurological symptoms (e.g. speech and visual disturbance, disorientation, fits) and evidence of haemorrhage in and around the basal ganglia on CT scan. The neurological deficit is usually reversible with adequate control of hypertension.

Retina: The optic fundi reveal a gradation of changes linked to the severity of hypertension (see Box 8.15). Hypertension is also associated with central retinal vein thrombosis.

Heart: The excess cardiac mortality and morbidity associated with hypertension are largely due to a higher incidence of CAD. High BP also places a pressure load on the heart and may lead to LV hypertrophy or, if severe, LV failure, even in the absence of coronary disease. ECG or echocardiographic evidence of LV hypertrophy is highly predictive of cardiovascular complications and therefore particularly useful in risk assessment.

Kidneys: Long-standing hypertension may cause proteinuria and progressive renal failure (p. 170) by damaging the renal vasculature.

'Malignant' or 'accelerated' phase hypertension

This rare condition is characterised by accelerated microvascular damage and intravascular thrombosis. The diagnosis is based on evidence of high BP and rapidly progressive end organ damage, such as retinopathy (grade 3 or 4), renal dysfunction (especially proteinuria) and/or hypertensive encephalopathy.

Investigations

Antihypertensive therapy is commonly lifelong treatment, so it is vital that the BP readings on which the treatment decision is based are as accurate as possible. Sphygmomanometry, particularly when performed by a doctor, can cause an unrepresentative surge in BP ('white coat' hypertension). A series of automated ambulatory BP measurements, obtained over 24 hrs or longer, provides a better profile than a limited number of clinic readings. These may be particularly helpful in patients with unusually labile BP, those with refractory hypertension, those who may be experiencing symptomatic hypotension, and those in whom white coat hypertension is suspected.

Routine investigations in all hypertensive patients should include urinalysis for blood, protein and glucose, U&Es, blood glucose, serum lipids and 12-lead ECG. Additional investigations are appropriate in selected patients to identify target organ damage (e.g. echocardiography) or potential causes of secondary hypertension (e.g. renal USS, urinary catecholamines).

Management

The sole objective of antihypertensive therapy is to reduce the incidence of adverse cardiovascular events. The relative benefit of BP reduction (~30% reduction in risk of stroke and 20% reduction in risk of CAD) is similar in all patient groups, so the absolute benefit of treatment is greatest in those at highest risk (e.g. diabetic patients). Decisions on treatment should therefore be guided by an overall assessment of cardiovascular risk. The British Hypertension Society management guidelines are summarised in Figure 8.17.

The following lifestyle measures can not only lower BP but also reduce cardiovascular risk:

• Correcting obesity. • Reducing alcohol intake. • Restricting salt intake. • Taking regular physical exercise. • Increasing consumption of fruit and vegetables.

The major classes of hypertensive drug are:

• Thiazide diuretics. • ACE inhibitors. • Angiotensin receptor blockers. • Calcium channel antagonists. • β-blockers. • α-blockers.

A detailed description of these agents is provided in Chapter 18. Combination therapy is often required to achieve adequate control,

Fig. 8.17 (opposite) Management of hypertension: British Hypertension Society guidelines. Consider specialist referral for stage 1 hypertension in those aged <40 yrs. (ABPM = ambulatory blood pressure monitoring; HBPM = home blood pressure monitoring)

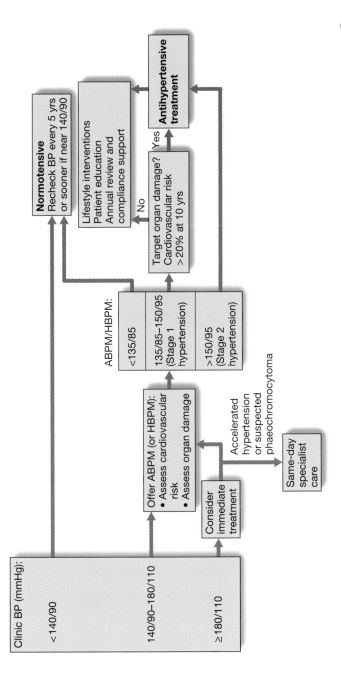

Clinic BP (mmHg):

< 140/90

140/90–180/110

≥ 180/110

Offer ABPM (or HBPM):
• Assess cardiovascular risk
• Assess organ damage

Consider immediate treatment

Accelerated hypertension or suspected phaeochromocytoma

Same-day specialist care

ABPM/HBPM:

< 135/85

135/85–150/95 (Stage 1 hypertension)

> 150/95 (Stage 2 hypertension)

Target organ damage? Cardiovascular risk > 20% at 10 yrs

No

Yes

Lifestyle interventions
Patient education
Annual review and compliance support

Normotensive
Recheck BP every 5 yrs or sooner if near 140/90

Antihypertensive treatment

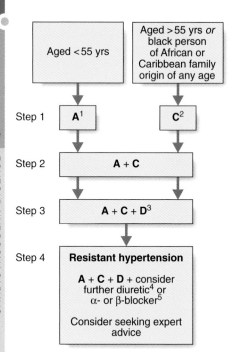

Fig. 8.18 Antihypertensive drug combinations. [1]A = ACE inhibitor or angiotensin II receptor blocker (ARB). [2]C = calcium channel blocker (CCB); consider thiazide if CCB not tolerated or in heart failure. [3]D = thiazide. [4]Low-dose spironolactone or higher-dose thiazide. [5]Consider an α- or β-blocker if further diuretics not tolerated, contraindicated or ineffective.

and a recommended treatment algorithm is shown in Figure 8.18. However, comorbid conditions may have an important influence on initial drug selection (e.g. a β-blocker might be the most appropriate treatment for a patient with angina but should be avoided in asthma).

In accelerated phase hypertension, rapid lowering of BP may compromise tissue perfusion, leading to cerebral damage or to coronary or renal insufficiency. A controlled reduction, to a level of ~150/90 mmHg, over a period of 24–48 hrs, is ideal. In most patients it is possible to bring BP under control with oral agents. Where necessary, IV labetalol, GTN and sodium nitroprusside are all effective remedies but require careful supervision, preferably in a high-dependency unit.

DISEASES OF THE HEART VALVES

A diseased valve may be narrowed (stenosed) or it may fail to close adequately, and thus permit regurgitation of blood. Doppler echocardiography is the best technique for assessing patients with valvular heart disease but often detects minor, unimportant abnormalities, e.g. trivial mitral regurgitation. Some valve disease may progress with time, so regular review is needed to detect deterioration before complications such as heart failure ensue. Patients with valvular heart disease are susceptible to bacterial endocarditis, which can be prevented by good dental hygiene. Routine antibiotic prophylaxis at times of bacteraemia is no longer recommended.

Acute rheumatic fever

Acute rheumatic fever (ARF) usually affects children or young adults. It has become very rare in Western Europe and North America but remains endemic in parts of Asia, Africa and South America. It is triggered by an immune-mediated delayed response to infection with specific strains of group A streptococci that have antigens that cross-react with cardiac myosin and sarcolemmal membrane protein. Antibodies produced against the streptococcal antigens mediate inflammation in the endocardium, myocardium and pericardium, as well as the joints and skin.

Clinical features

ARF typically follows 2–3 wks after an episode of streptococcal pharyngitis and presents with fever, anorexia, lethargy and joint pains. The diagnosis is based on the revised Jones criteria (Box 8.16).

8.16 Jones criteria for the diagnosis of rheumatic fever

Major manifestations

- Carditis
- Polyarthritis
- Chorea
- Erythema marginatum
- Subcutaneous nodules

Minor manifestations

- Fever
- Arthralgia
- Previous rheumatic fever
- Raised ESR or CRP
- Leucocytosis
- First-degree AV block

Notes

- Diagnosis depends on two or more major manifestations, or one major and two or more minor manifestations PLUS supporting evidence of preceding streptococcal infection: recent scarlet fever, raised antistreptolysin O (ASO) or other streptococcal antibody titre, positive throat culture
- Evidence of recent streptococcal infection is particularly important if there is only one major manifestation

Carditis may involve the endocardium, myocardium and pericardium to varying degrees, and manifests as breathlessness (heart failure or pericardial effusion), palpitations or chest pain (pericarditis). Other features include tachycardia, cardiac enlargement, new murmurs (especially mitral regurgitation), or a soft mid-diastolic murmur due to mitral valvulitis (Carey Coombs murmur). Acute, painful, asymmetric and migratory arthritis of the large joints (knees, ankles, elbows, wrists) is the most common major manifestation. Erythema marginatum appears as red macules, which fade in the centre but remain red at the edges; they occur mainly on the trunk and proximal extremities but not the face. Subcutaneous nodules are small, firm, painless and best felt over extensor surfaces of bone or tendons. They usually appear >3 wks after the onset of other manifestations. Sydenham's chorea (St Vitus dance) is a late (>3 mths) neurological manifestation characterised by emotional lability and purposeless involuntary choreiform movements of the hands, feet or face; spontaneous recovery usually occurs within a few months.

Investigations

Evidence of preceding streptococcal infection is required (Box 8.17). Raised WCC, ESR and CRP indicate systemic inflammation and are useful for monitoring progress of the disease. ECG (AV block, pericarditis) and echocardiography (cardiac dilatation, valve abnormalities) may reveal evidence of carditis.

Management

Penicillin is given to eliminate any residual streptococcal infection. Bed rest lessens joint pain and reduces cardiac workload. Cardiac failure should be treated as necessary. High-dose aspirin (60–100 mg/kg up to 8 g per day) usually relieves the symptoms of arthritis and a response within 24 hrs helps to confirm the diagnosis. Prednisolone 1–2 mg/kg produces more rapid symptomatic relief and is indicated

---

8.17 Investigations in acute rheumatic fever

Evidence of a systemic illness (non-specific)

- Leucocytosis, raised ESR, raised CRP

Evidence of preceding streptococcal infection (specific)

- Throat swab culture: group A β-haemolytic streptococci (also from family members and contacts)
- ASO titres: rising titres, or levels of >200 U (adults) or >300 U (children)

Evidence of carditis

- CXR: cardiomegaly; pulmonary congestion
- ECG: first- and rarely second-degree heart block; features of pericarditis; T-wave inversion; reduction in QRS voltages
- Echocardiography: cardiac dilatation; valve abnormalities

for carditis or severe arthritis, until the ESR returns to normal. Patients are susceptible to further attacks of rheumatic fever if subsequent streptococcal infection occurs, and long-term prophylaxis with penicillin should be given, usually until the age of 21.

Chronic rheumatic heart disease

This is characterised by progressive valve fibrosis and develops in at least half of those affected by rheumatic fever with carditis. Some episodes of rheumatic fever may pass unrecognised and it is only possible to elicit a positive history in about half of patients. The mitral valve is affected in >90% of cases, with the aortic valve the next most frequently involved.

Mitral stenosis

Mitral stenosis is almost always rheumatic in origin. The valve orifice is slowly diminished by progressive fibrosis, leaflet calcification and fusion of the cusps and subvalvular apparatus. Restricted blood flow from left atrium to ventricle causes a rise in left atrial pressure, leading to pulmonary venous congestion and breathlessness, while low cardiac output may cause fatigue. Patients usually remain asymptomatic until the mitral valve area is <2 cm^2 (normal =5 cm^2). AF occurs frequently due to progressive left atrial dilatation, and the onset of AF often causes rapid decompensation with pulmonary oedema because ventricular filling depends on left atrial contraction and adequate diastolic filling time. More gradual rises in left atrial pressure cause pulmonary hypertension, RV hypertrophy and dilatation, tricuspid regurgitation and right heart failure.

Clinical features

Effort-related dyspnoea is usually the dominant symptom and produces a gradual reduction in exercise tolerance over many years, culminating in dyspnoea at rest. Acute pulmonary oedema or pulmonary hypertension may cause haemoptysis. On examination, the patient is usually in AF and a malar flush may be apparent. All patients with mitral stenosis, and particularly those with AF, are at risk from left atrial thrombosis and systemic thromboembolism. The apex beat is characteristically tapping in nature. On auscultation there may be a loud first heart sound, an opening snap and a low-pitched mid-diastolic murmur. An elevated JVP, RV heave, loud pulmonary component of the second heart sound and features of tricuspid regurgitation all signify the presence of pulmonary hypertension.

Investigations

• ECG: may show bifid P waves (P mitrale) due to left atrial hypertrophy, or AF. • CXR: may show an enlarged left atrium and features of pulmonary congestion. • Doppler echocardiography: provides the definitive evaluation of mitral stenosis, allowing estimation of valve area, pressure gradient across the valve and pulmonary artery pressure.

8.18 Causes of mitral regurgitation

- Mitral valve prolapse
- Dilatation of the LV and mitral valve ring (e.g. coronary artery disease, cardiomyopathy)
- Damage to valve cusps and chordae (e.g. rheumatic heart disease, endocarditis)
- Ischaemia or infarction of papillary muscle
- MI

Management

Medical management consists of diuretics for pulmonary congestion, with anticoagulants and rate-limiting agents in the presence of AF. For persistent symptoms or pulmonary hypertension, balloon valvuloplasty is the treatment of choice, although valvotomy is an alternative. Valve replacement is indicated for severe reflux or rigid, calcified valves.

Mitral regurgitation

Causes of mitral regurgitation are shown in Box 8.18. Chronic mitral regurgitation causes gradual dilatation of the left atrium with little increase in pressure; progressive LV dilatation occurs due to chronic volume overload. Acute mitral regurgitation causes a rapid rise in left atrial pressure, resulting in pulmonary oedema.

Mitral valve prolapse: A common cause of mild mitral regurgitation, it arises from congenital anomalies or degenerative myxomatous changes and is sometimes a feature of connective tissue disorders such as Marfan's syndrome. In mild mitral prolapse, the valve remains competent but bulges back into the atrium during systole, causing a mid-systolic click but no murmur. In the presence of a regurgitant valve, the click is followed by a late systolic murmur. The condition is associated with a variety of benign arrhythmias and atypical chest pain but the overall long-term prognosis is good. If regurgitation becomes severe, mitral valve repair can be used to treat most forms of mitral valve prolapse and is preferred to mitral valve replacement.

Clinical features

Chronic mitral regurgitation typically causes progressive exertional dyspnoea and fatigue, while sudden-onset mitral regurgitation usually presents with acute pulmonary oedema. The regurgitant jet causes an apical systolic murmur that radiates to the axilla. The first heart sound is quiet and there may be a third heart sound. The apex beat feels hyperdynamic and is usually displaced to the left, indicating LV dilatation. Signs of AF, pulmonary venous congestion and pulmonary hypertension may be present.

Investigations

• CXR: may show left atrial or ventricular enlargement or features of pulmonary venous congestion (pulmonary oedema if acute).
• Echocardiography: reveals chamber dimensions, LV function, the severity of regurgitation, and structural abnormalities of the valve.
• Cardiac catheterisation: allows assessment by ventriculography and the detection of pulmonary hypertension or coexisting coronary disease.

Management

Medical treatment includes diuretics and afterload reduction with vasodilators (e.g. ACE inhibitors). AF requires digoxin and anticoagulation. Regular review is important to detect worsening symptoms, progressive cardiac enlargement and LV impairment, as these are all indications for surgical intervention (mitral valve replacement or repair). Acute severe mitral regurgitation necessitates emergency valve replacement or repair.

Aortic stenosis

The three common causes of aortic stenosis are:
• Rheumatic fever (usually associated with mitral valve disease).
• Calcification of a congenitally bicuspid valve. • In the elderly, senile degenerative aortic stenosis.

Cardiac output is initially maintained but the left ventricle becomes increasingly hypertrophied. Eventually it can no longer overcome the outflow tract obstruction and heart failure supervenes. Patients with aortic stenosis typically remain asymptomatic for many years but deteriorate rapidly when symptoms develop.

Clinical features

Mild to moderate aortic stenosis is usually asymptomatic but may be detected incidentally on routine examination. The three cardinal symptoms are angina, syncope and breathlessness.

• Angina: arises because of the increased oxygen demands of the hypertrophied LV working against the high-pressure outflow tract obstruction (or coexisting CAD). • Syncope: usually occurs on exertion when cardiac output fails to rise to meet demand because of severe outflow obstruction, causing a fall in BP. • Exertional breathlessness: suggests cardiac decompensation as a consequence of chronic excessive pressure overload.

The characteristic clinical signs are:
• Harsh ejection systolic murmur radiating to the neck (often with a thrill). • Soft second heart sound.• Slow-rising carotid pulse.
• Narrow pulse pressure. • Heaving but undisplaced apex beat.

Investigations

• The ECG: usually shows features of LV hypertrophy, often with down-sloping ST segments and T inversion ('strain pattern'), but can be normal despite severe stenosis. • Doppler echocardiography:

demonstrates restricted opening and any structural abnormalities, and permits calculation of the systolic pressure gradient. • Cardiac catheterisation: is usually necessary to assess the coronary arteries before aortic valve replacement.

Management

Patients with asymptomatic aortic stenosis have a good prognosis with conservative management but should be kept under review, as the development of symptoms is an indication for prompt aortic valve replacement. Old age is not a contraindication to valve replacement and results are very good, even for those in their eighties. Balloon valvuloplasty is useful in congenital stenosis but not in calcific stenosis.

Aortic regurgitation

This condition may be due to disease of the aortic valve cusps (e.g. rheumatic fever, infective endocarditis) or dilatation of the aortic root (e.g. ankylosing spondylitis, Marfan's syndrome, aortic dissection). The LV dilates and hypertrophies to compensate for the regurgitation, producing a large increase in stroke volume. As disease progresses, LV diastolic pressure rises and breathlessness develops.

Clinical features

In mild to moderate aortic regurgitation, patients are frequently asymptomatic but may experience an awareness of the heart beat due to the increased stroke volume. Exertional dyspnoea is the dominant symptom in more severe disease. The pulse is typically of large volume and collapsing in nature, the pulse pressure is wide and the apex beat is heaving and displaced. The characteristic soft early diastolic murmur is usually best heard to the left of the sternum with the patient leaning forward, with the breath held in expiration. A systolic murmur due to the increased stroke volume is common. In acute severe regurgitation (e.g. perforation of aortic cusp in endocarditis) there may be no time for compensatory LV hypertrophy and dilatation to develop and the features of heart failure may predominate.

Investigations

• CXR: may show dilatation of the heart and possibly of the ascending aorta. • ECG: typically shows evidence of LV hypertrophy. • Echocardiography: confirms the diagnosis and may show a dilated, hyperdynamic left ventricle. • Cardiac catheterisation and aortography: can also be helpful in assessing the severity of regurgitation, aortic dilatation and the presence of coexisting coronary artery disease.

Management

Underlying conditions, such as endocarditis and syphilis, should be treated. Replacement of the aortic valve (and aortic root, if dilated) is indicated in symptomatic regurgitation. Asymptomatic patients should also be followed up annually to detect the development of symptoms or increasing ventricular size on echocardiography; if the end-systolic dimension increases to ≥55 mm, then aortic valve replacement should be undertaken. Systolic BP should be controlled with vasodilating drugs such as nifedipine or ACE inhibitors.

Tricuspid valve disease

Tricuspid stenosis: Uncommon, usually rheumatic in origin and almost always associated with mitral and aortic valve disease. It may cause signs and symptoms of right heart failure.

Tricuspid regurgitation: Common and most frequently 'functional' as a result of RV dilatation. It may also be caused by endocarditis (especially in IV drug-users), rheumatic fever or carcinoid syndrome. Symptoms result from reduced forward flow (tiredness) and venous congestion (oedema, hepatic enlargement). The most prominent sign is a large systolic wave in the JVP. Other features include a pansystolic murmur at the left sternal edge and pulsatile hepatomegaly. Tricuspid regurgitation due to RV dilatation often improves when the cause of RV overload is corrected, e.g. diuretic and vasodilator therapy in congestive cardiac failure.

Pulmonary valve disease

Pulmonary stenosis: Can occur in the carcinoid syndrome but is usually congenital, when it may be isolated or associated with other abnormalities, such as Fallot's tetralogy (p. 259). On examination there is an ejection systolic murmur, loudest to the left of the upper sternum and radiating towards the left shoulder. Mild to moderate pulmonary stenosis is non-progressive, does not require treatment and carries a low risk of infective endocarditis. Severe pulmonary stenosis is treated by percutaneous balloon valvuloplasty or, if this is not available, surgical valvotomy.

Pulmonary regurgitation: Rarely an isolated phenomenon and usually associated with pulmonary artery dilatation due to pulmonary hypertension.

Infective endocarditis

Infective endocarditis is due to microbial infection of a heart valve (native or prosthetic), the lining of a cardiac chamber or blood vessel, or a congenital anomaly (e.g. ventricular septal defect (VSD)). It typically occurs at sites of pre-existing endocardial damage, although infection with particularly virulent organisms (e.g. *Staph. aureus*) can cause endocarditis in a previously normal heart. Areas of endocardial damage caused by a high-pressure jet of blood (e.g. VSD, mitral regurgitation, aortic regurgitation) are particularly vulnerable. When the infection is established, vegetations, composed of organisms, fibrin and platelets, grow and may break away as emboli. Adjacent tissues are destroyed, abscesses may form and valve regurgitation may develop through cusp perforation, distortion or rupture of chordae. Extracardiac manifestations, such as vasculitis and skin lesions, are due to emboli or immune complex deposition.

Microbiology

• The *viridans* group of streptococci (from the upper respiratory tract or gums) and enterococci (from the gut or urinary tract) may enter the blood stream and are common causes of subacute endocarditis, while *Staph. aureus* is increasingly responsible for acute endocarditis, especially in IV drug-users. • *Staph. epidermidis*, a normal skin commensal, is the most common organism in post-operative endocarditis after cardiac surgery. • Other offending organisms include the Gram-negative HACEK group (*Haemophilus* spp., *Actinobacillus actinomycetemcomitans*, *Cardiobacterium hominis*, *Eikenella* spp. and *Kingella kingae*). • *Coxiella burnetii* (Q fever) and *Brucella* cause occasional cases in patients exposed to farm animals. • Yeasts and fungi may be responsible in immunocompromised patients.

Clinical features

Subacute endocarditis: Should be suspected when a patient with congenital or valvular heart disease develops a persistent fever, unusual tiredness, night sweats, weight loss or new signs of valve dysfunction. Other features include embolic stroke, petechial rash, splinter haemorrhages and splenomegaly. Osler's nodes (painful swellings at the fingertips) are rare and finger clubbing is a late sign.

Acute endocarditis: Usually presents as a severe febrile illness with prominent and changing heart murmurs and petechiae. Clinical stigmata of chronic endocarditis are usually absent but embolic events (e.g. cerebral) are common, and cardiac or renal failure may develop rapidly.

Post-operative endocarditis: Should be considered in any patient who develops an unexplained fever after heart valve surgery. The pattern may resemble subacute or acute endocarditis, depending on the virulence of the organism. Morbidity and mortality are high and redo surgery is often required.

Investigations

• Diagnosis: based on the modified Duke criteria (Box 8.19). • Blood culture: the crucial investigation because it may identify the infection and guide antibiotic therapy; 3–6 sets should be taken, using scrupulous aseptic technique, prior to commencing therapy. • Echocardiography: allows detection of vegetations and abscess formation, as well as assessment of valve damage. Transoesophageal echo has a higher sensitivity than transthoracic echo for detecting vegetations (90% vs 65%) and is particularly valuable for investigating patients with prosthetic heart valves. Failure to detect vegetations does not exclude the diagnosis. • A normochromic, normocytic anaemia and elevated WCC, ESR and CRP: common. CRP is superior to ESR for monitoring progress. • Microscopic haematuria: usually present. • ECG: may show the development of AV block

8.19 Diagnosis of infective endocarditis (modified Duke criteria)

Major criteria

- Positive blood culture: typical organism from two cultures; persistent positive blood cultures taken >12 hrs apart; three or more positive cultures taken over >1 hr
- Endocardial involvement: positive echocardiographic findings of vegetations; new valvular regurgitation

Minor criteria

- Predisposing valvular or cardiac abnormality
- IV drug misuse
- Pyrexia ≥38°C
- Embolic phenomenon
- Vasculitic phenomenon
- Blood cultures suggestive – organism grown but not achieving major criteria
- Suggestive echocardiographic findings

Definite endocarditis: two major, or one major and three minor, or five minor
Possible endocarditis: one major and one minor, or three minor

(due to abscess formation). • CXR: may show evidence of cardiac failure.

Management

Any source of infection (e.g. dental abscess) should be removed as soon as possible. Empirical antibiotic therapy is with flucloxacillin and gentamicin if the presentation is acute, or with benzylpenicillin and gentamicin if it is subacute or indolent. Subsequent antibiotic treatment is guided by culture results and is usually continued for at least 4 wks. Indications for surgery (débridement of infected material, valve replacement) include heart failure, abscess formation, failure of antibiotic therapy and large vegetations on left-sided heart valves (high risk of systemic emboli).

Prevention

Patients with valvular or congenital heart disease should be made aware of the risk of endocarditis and of the importance of maintaining good dental health. Former advice for routine antibiotic prophylaxis to cover invasive or dental procedures is not supported by evidence and prophylaxis is no longer recommended.

CONGENITAL HEART DISEASE

Persistent ductus arteriosus

During fetal life, before the lungs begin to function, most of the blood from the pulmonary artery passes through the ductus arteriosus into the aorta. Normally, the ductus closes soon after birth but sometimes it fails to do so. Since the pressure in the aorta is higher than that in the pulmonary artery, there will be a continuous left to right shunt.

Usually there is no disability in infancy but cardiac failure may eventually ensue, dyspnoea being the first symptom. A continuous 'machinery' murmur is heard, maximal in the second left intercostal space below the clavicle. Closure of the patent ductus is usually performed by catheterisation using an implantable occlusive device in early childhood.

Coarctation of the aorta

This condition is associated with other abnormalities, including bicuspid aortic valve and 'berry' aneurysms of the cerebral circulation. It is an important cause to consider in younger patients with hypertension.

• BP: raised in the upper body but normal or low in the legs. • Femoral pulses: weak, and delayed in comparison with the radial pulse. • Systolic murmur: usually heard posteriorly, over the coarctation. • CXR: may show changes in the contour of the aorta and notching of the under-surfaces of the ribs from collateral vessel development. • MRI: ideal for demonstrating the lesion. • Surgical correction: advisable in all but the mildest cases. If this is done sufficiently early in childhood, persistent hypertension can be avoided but patients repaired in late childhood or adult life often remain hypertensive. • Recurrence of stenosis: may be managed by balloon dilatation, which can also be used as the primary treatment in some cases.

Atrial septal defect

This common congenital defect results in shunting of blood from left to right atrium, and then to the RV and pulmonary arteries. As a result, there is gradual enlargement of the right side of the heart and of the pulmonary arteries.

The condition is frequently asymptomatic but may cause cardiac failure or arrhythmias, e.g. AF. Characteristic physical signs include wide fixed splitting of the second heart sound and a systolic flow murmur over the pulmonary valve. The CXR typically shows enlargement of the heart and the pulmonary artery, as well as pulmonary plethora. The ECG usually shows incomplete RBBB. The defect is often first detected when a CXR or ECG is carried out for incidental reasons. Echocardiography can directly demonstrate the defect and may show RV dilatation or hypertrophy. Atrial septal defects in which pulmonary flow is increased by 50% above systemic flow should be closed either surgically or by catheter implantation of a closure device.

Ventricular septal defect

This is the most common congenital cardiac defect; it may be isolated or form part of complex congenital heart disease.

Flow from the high-pressure LV to the low-pressure RV produces a pansystolic murmur, usually best heard at the left sternal edge but radiating all over the precordium. Ventricular septal defect may present as cardiac failure in infants, as a murmur with only minor haemodynamic disturbance in older children or adults, or rarely as Eisenmenger's syndrome (see below). The CXR shows pulmonary plethora and the ECG demonstrates bilateral ventricular hypertrophy. Small ventricular septal defects require no specific treatment. Eisenmenger's syndrome is avoided by monitoring for signs of rising pulmonary resistance (serial ECG and echocardiography) and carrying out surgical repair when appropriate. Long-term prognosis is very good, except in the case of Eisenmenger's syndrome.

Eisenmenger's syndrome

Persistently raised pulmonary flow (e.g. with left to right shunting) leads to increased pulmonary resistance and pulmonary hypertension. In severe pulmonary hypertension, a left to right shunt may reverse, resulting in right to left shunting and marked cyanosis (Eisenmenger's syndrome). Patients with Eisenmenger's syndrome are at particular risk from changes in afterload that exacerbate right to left shunting, e.g. vasodilatation, anaesthesia, pregnancy.

Tetralogy of Fallot

This is the most common cause of cyanotic disease in childhood and comprises:
• Ventricular septal defect. • Right ventricular outflow obstruction (usually subvalvular). • Aorta overriding the septum. • Right ventricular hypertrophy.

The subvalvular obstruction may increase suddenly after feeding or crying, causing apnoea and unconsciousness ('Fallot's spells'). In older children, Fallot's spells are uncommon but cyanosis increases as rising RV pressure causes increasing right to left shunting across the ventricular septal defect, together with stunted growth, clubbing and polycythaemia. A loud ejection systolic murmur is heard in the pulmonary area. Cyanosis may be absent in the newborn or in patients with only mild RV outflow obstruction. Investigation is by ECG (RV hypertrophy), CXR (a 'boot-shaped' heart) and echocardiography, which is diagnostic. Definitive management is by surgical relief of the outflow obstruction and closure of the ventricular septal defect, and the prognosis is good following surgery in childhood.

Adult congenital heart disease

Many patients who would not previously have survived childhood now do so following corrective surgery; in Western countries, there are now more adults than children with congenital heart disease. These patients may develop problems in adult life. For example, following correction of coarctation of the aorta, adults may develop hypertension. Adults with repaired ventricular defects may develop ventricular arrhythmias secondary to post-operative ventricular scarring, and may require an implantable defibrillator. All such patients require careful follow-up from the teenage years through adult life in specialist clinics.

DISEASES OF THE MYOCARDIUM

Acute myocarditis

This is an acute inflammatory condition of the myocardium, caused by infection, autoimmune disease (e.g. lupus) or toxins (e.g. cocaine). Viral infection is the most common cause, particularly Coxsackie and influenza viruses A and B. Other causes include Lyme disease (p. 79), Chagas' disease (p. 103) and acute rheumatic fever.

Four presentations occur:

Fulminant myocarditis: Follows a viral illness, causing severe heart failure or cardiogenic shock.

Acute myocarditis: Presents more gradually with heart failure; it can lead to dilated cardiomyopathy.

Chronic active myocarditis: Rare, with chronic myocardial inflammation.

Chronic persistent myocarditis: Can cause chest pain and arrhythmia, sometimes without ventricular dysfunction.

Troponins and CK are elevated in proportion to the extent of damage. Echocardiography may reveal LV dysfunction, which is sometimes regional (focal myocarditis).

In most patients, the disease is self-limiting and the immediate prognosis is good; however, death may occur due to ventricular arrhythmia or rapidly progressive heart failure. Some forms of myocarditis (e.g. Chagas' disease) may lead to chronic low-grade myocarditis or dilated cardiomyopathy. Treatment for cardiac failure or arrhythmias may be required and intense physical exertion should be avoided.

Dilated cardiomyopathy

This condition is characterised by dilatation and impaired contraction of the left (and sometimes the right) ventricle. The differential diagnosis includes coronary artery disease, which must be excluded first. Other causes include:

• Alcohol. • Inherited mutations of cytoskeletal proteins. • X-linked muscular dystrophies. • Autoimmune reactions to viral myocarditis.

Most patients present with heart failure. Arrhythmia, thromboembolism and sudden death are common and may occur at any stage. Echocardiography and MRI are useful in establishing the diagnosis. Treatment is aimed at controlling the resulting heart failure and preventing arrhythmias. The prognosis is variable and cardiac transplantation may be required.

Hypertrophic cardiomyopathy

This is the most common form of cardiomyopathy and is characterised by elaborate LV hypertrophy with malalignment of the myocardial fibres. The hypertrophy may be generalised or confined largely to the interventricular septum. Heart failure develops because the stiff non-compliant ventricles impede diastolic filling.

8.20 Risk factors for sudden death in hypertrophic cardiomyopathy

- A history of previous cardiac arrest or sustained VT
- Recurrent syncope
- An adverse genotype and/or family history
- Exercise-induced hypotension
- Non-sustained VT on ambulatory ECG
- Marked increase in LV wall thickness

Septal hypertrophy may also cause dynamic LV outflow tract obstruction (hypertrophic obstructive cardiomyopathy). The condition is a genetic disorder with autosomal dominant transmission, a high degree of penetrance and variable expression.

Effort-related symptoms (angina and breathlessness), arrhythmia and sudden death (mainly from ventricular arrhythmias) are the dominant clinical problems. Signs are similar to those of aortic stenosis, except that in hypertrophic cardiomyopathy the character of the arterial pulse is jerky. The ECG is usually abnormal and may show features of LV hypertrophy or deep T-wave inversion. Echocardiography is usually diagnostic. Beta-blockers and rate-limiting calcium antagonists can help to relieve symptoms and sometimes prevent syncopal attacks but no pharmacological treatment is definitely known to improve prognosis. Outflow tract obstruction can be improved by partial surgical resection or by iatrogenic infarction of the basal septum using a catheter-delivered alcohol solution. An ICD should be considered in patients with clinical risk factors for sudden death (Box 8.20).

Restrictive cardiomyopathy

In this rare condition, ventricular filling is impaired because the ventricles are 'stiff'. This leads to high atrial pressures with atrial hypertrophy, dilatation and later AF. Amyloidosis is the most common cause in the UK.

Diagnosis can be very difficult and requires complex Doppler echocardiography, CT or MRI, and endomyocardial biopsy. Treatment is symptomatic but the prognosis is poor and transplantation may be indicated.

Other specific diseases affecting the myocardium are summarised in Box 8.21.

DISEASES OF THE PERICARDIUM

Acute pericarditis

Pericardial inflammation may be due to infection (viral, bacterial, TB), immunological reaction (e.g. post-MI, connective tissue disorder), trauma, uraemia or neoplasm. Pericarditis and myocarditis often coexist, and all forms of pericarditis may produce a pericardial effusion (see below).

8.21 Specific diseases of heart muscle

Infections

- Viral, e.g. Coxsackie A and B, influenza, HIV
- Bacterial, e.g. diphtheria, *Borrelia burgdorferi*
- Protozoal, e.g. trypanosomiasis

Endocrine and metabolic disorders

- e.g. Diabetes, hypo- and hyperthyroidism, acromegaly, carcinoid syndrome, phaeochromocytoma, inherited storage diseases

Connective tissue diseases

- e.g. Systemic sclerosis, systemic lupus erythematosus, polyarteritis nodosa

Infiltrative disorders

- e.g. Haemochromatosis, haemosiderosis, sarcoidosis, amyloidosis

Toxins

- e.g. Doxorubicin, alcohol, cocaine, irradiation

Neuromuscular disorders

- e.g. Dystrophia myotonica, Friedreich's ataxia, X-linked muscular dystrophies

Clinical features

The characteristic pain of pericarditis is retrosternal, radiates to the shoulders and neck, and is aggravated by deep breathing and movement. A low-grade fever is common. A pericardial friction rub is a high-pitched, superficial scratching or crunching noise produced by movement of the inflamed pericardium, and is diagnostic of pericarditis.

Investigations

The ECG shows ST elevation with upward concavity over the affected area, which may be widespread. PR interval depression is a very sensitive indicator of acute pericarditis.

Management

The pain is usually relieved by aspirin but a more potent anti-inflammatory agent, such as indometacin, may be required. Corticosteroids may suppress symptoms but there is no evidence that they accelerate cure. Tuberculous pericarditis causes effusion, is diagnosed on periocardiocentesis and responds to antituberculous therapy and corticosteroids.

Pericardial effusion

This refers to accumulation of fluid within the pericardial sac. Cardiac tamponade describes acute heart failure due to compression of the heart by a large or rapidly developing effusion.

Typical physical findings include hypotension, tachycardia, a markedly raised JVP that rises paradoxically with inspiration

(Kussmaul's sign), pulsus paradoxus (dramatic fall in BP during inspiration) and muffled heart sounds. The QRS voltages on the ECG are often reduced in the presence of a large effusion. CXR may show an increase in the size of the cardiac shadow, which may have a globular appearance if the effusion is large. Echocardiography confirms the diagnosis and helps identify the optimum site for aspiration of fluid. The patient usually responds promptly to percutaneous pericardiocentesis or surgical drainage; the latter is safer in cardiac rupture and aortic dissection.

Chronic constrictive pericarditis

Constrictive pericarditis is due to progressive thickening, fibrosis and calcification of the pericardium. In effect, the heart is encased in a solid shell and cannot fill properly. It often follows tuberculous pericarditis but can also complicate haemopericardium, viral pericarditis, rheumatoid arthritis and purulent pericarditis.

Clinical features

The symptoms and signs of systemic venous congestion are the hallmarks of constrictive pericarditis; AF is common and there is often dramatic ascites and hepatomegaly. Breathlessness is not prominent because the lungs are seldom congested. The condition should be suspected in any patient with unexplained right heart failure and a small heart. CXR (pericardial calcification) and echocardiography often help to establish the diagnosis, though it may be difficult to distinguish from restrictive cardiomyopathy.

Management

Surgical resection of the diseased pericardium can lead to a dramatic improvement but carries a high morbidity and produces disappointing results in up to 50% of patients.

Respiratory disease

Respiratory diseases are responsible for much morbidity and avoidable mortality, with tuberculosis (TB), pandemic influenza and pneumonia the most important in world health terms. Increasing prevalence of allergy, asthma and chronic obstructive pulmonary disease (COPD), together with a rise in worldwide smoking rates, contributes to a high burden of chronic disease. Despite improved detection and treatment, the outlook for lung cancer remains poor.

PRESENTING PROBLEMS IN RESPIRATORY DISEASE

Cough

Cough is the most common respiratory symptom and the underlying cause is often clear from other clinical features, particularly in more serious disease. Common causes of acute or transient cough are:

• Viral lower respiratory tract infection. • Post-nasal drip (rhinitis/sinusitis). • Foreign body aspiration. • Laryngitis or pharyngitis. • Pneumonia. • Congestive heart failure. • Pulmonary embolism.

Chronic cough presents more of a challenge, especially if physical examination, CXR and lung function are normal. In this context, consider:

• Post-nasal drip. • Cough-variant asthma. • Gastro-oesophageal reflux with aspiration. • Drug-induced cough (ACE inhibitors). • *Bordetella pertussis* infection.

While most patients with bronchogenic carcinoma have an abnormal CXR on presentation, fibreoptic bronchoscopy or thoracic CT is advisable for an unexplained cough of recent onset in adults (especially smokers), as this may reveal a small endobronchial tumour, unexpected foreign body, or early interstitial lung disease.

Breathlessness (dyspnoea)

Breathlessness or dyspnoea can be defined as the feeling of an uncomfortable need to breathe. It is unusual among sensations in

CLINICAL EXAMINATION OF THE RESPIRATORY SYSTEM

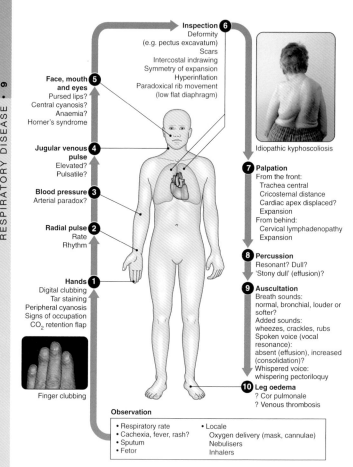

Inspection 6
Deformity
(e.g. pectus excavatum)
Scars
Intercostal indrawing
Symmetry of expansion
Hyperinflation
Paradoxical rib movement
(low flat diaphragm)

Idiopathic kyphoscoliosis

Face, mouth and eyes 5
Pursed lips?
Central cyanosis?
Anaemia?
Horner's syndrome

Jugular venous pulse 4
Elevated?
Pulsatile?

Blood pressure 3
Arterial paradox?

Radial pulse 2
Rate
Rhythm

Hands 1
Digital clubbing
Tar staining
Peripheral cyanosis
Signs of occupation
CO_2 retention flap

Finger clubbing

Palpation 7
From the front:
Trachea central
Cricosternal distance
Cardiac apex displaced?
Expansion
From behind:
Cervical lymphadenopathy
Expansion

Percussion 8
Resonant? Dull?
'Stony dull' (effusion)?

Auscultation 9
Breath sounds:
normal, bronchial, louder or softer?
Added sounds:
wheezes, crackles, rubs
Spoken voice (vocal resonance):
absent (effusion), increased (consolidation)?
Whispered voice:
whispering pectoriloquy

Leg oedema 10
? Cor pulmonale
? Venous thrombosis

Observation
- Respiratory rate
- Cachexia, fever, rash?
- Sputum
- Fetor
- Locale
  Oxygen delivery (mask, cannulae)
  Nebulisers
  Inhalers

having no defined receptors, no localised representation in the brain, and multiple causes both in health (e.g. exercise) and in diseases of the lungs, heart or muscles.

Chronic exertional breathlessness

The cause of breathlessness is often apparent from a careful clinical history. Key questions include:

How is your breathing at rest and overnight?

In COPD, there is a fixed, structural limit to maximum ventilation, and progressive hyperinflation during exercise. Breathlessness occurs with mobilisation, and patients usually experience minimal symptoms at rest and overnight. In contrast, patients with significant asthma are often woken overnight by breathlessness with chest tightness and wheeze.

Orthopnoea, however, is common in COPD, as well as in heart disease, because airflow obstruction is made worse by cranial displacement of the diaphragm by the abdominal contents when recumbent, so patients often sleep propped up. Orthopnoea is therefore not a useful symptom for distinguishing respiratory and cardiac dyspnoea.

How much can you do on a good day?

The approximate distance the patient can walk on the level should be documented, along with capacity to climb inclines or stairs. Variability within and between days is characteristic of asthma; in mild asthma, the patient may have days with no symptoms. Gradual, progressive exercise limitation over years, with consistent disability over days, is typical of COPD. When asthma is suspected, the degree of variability should be documented by peak flow monitoring.

Relentless progressive breathlessness, present also at rest, often with a dry cough, suggests interstitial disease. Impaired left ventricular function can also cause chronic exertional breathlessness, cough and wheeze. A history of angina, hypertension or myocardial infarction (MI) suggests a cardiac cause. This may be confirmed by a displaced apex beat, a raised JVP and cardiac murmurs (although these signs can occur in severe cor pulmonale). The CXR may show cardiomegaly, and an ECG and echocardiogram may reveal left ventricular disease. Measurement of ABGs may help, as, in the absence of an intracardiac shunt or pulmonary oedema, the PaO_2 in cardiac disease is normal and the $PaCO_2$ is low or normal.

Did you have breathing problems in childhood or at school?

When present, a history of childhood wheeze increases the likelihood of asthma, although this history may be absent in late-onset asthma. A history of atopic allergy also increases the likelihood of asthma.

Do you have other symptoms with your breathlessness?

Digital or perioral paraesthesiae and a feeling that 'I cannot get a deep enough breath in' are typical of psychogenic hyperventilation, but this cannot be diagnosed until other potential causes are excluded. Additional symptoms include lightheadedness, central chest discomfort or even carpopedal spasm due to respiratory alkalosis. These alarming symptoms may provoke further anxiety, exacerbating hyperventilation. Psychogenic breathlessness rarely disturbs sleep, frequently occurs at rest, may be provoked by stress and may even be relieved by exercise. ABGs show normal PO_2, low PCO_2 and alkalosis.

Pleuritic chest pain in a patient with chronic breathlessness, particularly if it occurs in more than one site over time, suggests pulmonary thromboembolism. This may occasionally present as chronic breathlessness with no other specific features, and should always be considered before diagnosing psychogenic hyperventilation.

Morning headache is an important symptom in patients with breathlessness, as it may indicate carbon dioxide retention and respiratory failure. This occurs particularly in patients with musculoskeletal disease impairing ventilation (e.g. kyphoscoliosis or muscular dystrophy).

Acute severe dyspnoea

This is one of the most common and dramatic medical emergencies.

It is important to ascertain the rate of onset and severity of the breathlessness, and whether associated cardiovascular symptoms (chest pain, palpitations, sweating and nausea) or respiratory symptoms (cough, wheeze, haemoptysis and stridor) are present. A previous history of repeated episodes of left ventricular failure, asthma or exacerbations of COPD is valuable. In children, the possibility of inhalation of a foreign body or acute epiglottitis should always be considered.

Common causes of acute breathlessness and their clinical features are listed in Box 9.1.

Investigations and management

ABGs, CXR and ECG will confirm the clinical diagnosis. Oxygen should be given pending results. Urgent endotracheal intubation may become necessary if the conscious level declines or severe respiratory acidosis is present.

Chest pain

Pleural or chest wall involvement by lung disease gives rise to peripheral chest pain, which is exacerbated by deep breathing or coughing ('pleuritic' pain). Central chest pain suggests heart disease but can occur with oesophageal disease, mediastinal tumours or massive pulmonary embolism. Tracheitis produces raw upper retrosternal pain that is worse on coughing. Musculoskeletal chest wall pain is usually exacerbated by movement and associated with local tenderness.

9.1 Differential diagnosis of acute severe dyspnoea

Condition	History	Signs	CXR	ABG	ECG
Pulmonary oedema	Chest pain, orthopnoea, palpitations, cardiac history*	Central cyanosis, ↑JVP, sweating, cool extremities, basal crackles*	Cardiomegaly, oedema/pleural effusions*	↓PaO_2, ↓$PaCO_2$	Sinus tachycardia, ischaemia*, arrhythmia
Massive pulmonary embolus	Risk factors (see Box 9.15), chest pain, pleurisy, syncope*, dizziness*	Central cyanosis, ↑JVP*, absence of signs in the lung* (tachycardia, hypotension)	Often normal. Prominent hilar vessels, oligaemic lung fields*	↓PaO_2, ↓$PaCO_2$	Sinus tachycardia, RBBB, $S_1Q_3T_3$ pattern, inverted T (V_1–V_4)
Acute severe asthma	History of asthma, wheeze*	Tachycardia, pulsus paradoxus, cyanosis (late), JVP→*, ↓peak flow, wheeze*	Hyperinflation only (unless complicated by pneumothorax)*	↓PaO_2, ↓$PaCO_2$ (↑$PaCO_2$ in extremis)	Sinus tachycardia (bradycardia in extremis)
Acute exacerbation of COPD	Previous episodes*. If in type II respiratory failure, possible drowsiness	Cyanosis, hyperinflation*, signs of CO_2 retention (flapping tremor, bounding pulses)*	Hyperinflation*, bullae, complicating pneumothorax	↓ or ↓↓ PaO_2; In type II failure: ↑$PaCO_2$±↑H⁺; ↑HCO_3^-	Nil, or signs of right ventricular strain
Pneumonia	Prodromal illness*, fever*, rigors*, pleurisy*	Fever, confusion, pleural rub*, consolidation*, cyanosis (if severe)	Pneumonic consolidation*	↓PaO_2, ↓$PaCO_2$ (↑$PaCO_2$ in extremis)	Tachycardia
Metabolic acidosis	Diabetes/renal disease, aspirin or ethylene glycol overdose	Fetor (ketones), hyperventilation without heart or lung signs*, dehydration*, air hunger	Normal	PaO_2 normal, ↓$PaCO_2$, ↑H⁺	Normal
Psychogenic	Previous episodes, digital or perioral paraesthesiae	No cyanosis, no heart or lung signs; carpopedal spasm*	Normal	PaO_2 normal*, ↓$PaCO_2$, ↓H⁺*	Normal

*Denotes a valuable discriminatory feature. (RBBB = right bundle branch block)

269

Haemoptysis

Coughing up blood, irrespective of the amount, is an alarming symptom and nearly always brings the patient to the doctor.

A clear history should be taken to establish that it is true haemoptysis and not haematemesis, gum bleeding or nosebleed. Haemoptysis must always be assumed to have a serious cause until proven otherwise. A history of repeated small haemoptyses, or blood-streaking of sputum, is highly suggestive of bronchial carcinoma. Fever, night sweats and weight loss suggest TB. Pneumococcal pneumonia is often the cause of 'rusty'-coloured sputum but can cause frank haemoptysis, as can all the pneumonic infections that lead to suppuration or abscess formation. Bronchiectasis and intra-cavitary mycetoma can cause catastrophic bronchial haemorrhage, and in these patients there may be a history of previous TB or pneumonia in early life. Pulmonary thromboembolism is a common cause of haemoptysis and should always be considered. Many episodes of haemoptysis are unexplained, even after full investigation, and are likely to be caused by simple bronchial infection.

Investigations and management

In severe acute haemoptysis, the patient should be nursed upright (or on the side of the bleeding, if this is known); oxygen should be given and the patient should be haemodynamically resuscitated. In the vast majority of cases, however, haemoptysis itself is not life-threatening and it is possible to follow a logical sequence of investigations that include: CXR, FBC, clotting screen, bronchoscopy and CT pulmonary angiography (CTPA).

The incidental pulmonary nodule

The incidental finding of a pulmonary nodule is common, particularly with the widespread use of thoracic CT scanning, and the differential diagnosis is broad (Box 9.2). Whilst most are benign, it is important to identify potentially treatable malignancies.

A lesion may be confidently described as benign if it appears unchanged over 2 yrs. If previous images showing this are available, no further investigation may be necessary. Otherwise, the likelihood of malignancy is assessed by considering the patient's age, smoking history and history of prior malignancy, and the appearance of the nodule in terms of its size, margin, density and location. Further investigation is required in most cases.

Pulmonary nodules are invariably beyond the vision of the bronchoscope and, unless infection is revealed, bronchoscopy is usually unrewarding as the yield from blind washings is low. Tissue is most commonly obtained using percutaneous needle biopsy under CT guidance. This is complicated by pneumothorax in ~20% of cases, and although only 3% require intercostal drainage, CT biopsy should only be attempted in those with good respiratory reserve.

PET scanning provides useful information about nodules of at least 1 cm in diameter, in which the presence of high metabolic

> **9.2 The solitary pulmonary nodule**
>
> **Common causes**
>
> - Bronchial carcinoma
> - Single metastasis
> - Localised pneumonia
> - Lung abscess
> - Tuberculoma
> - Pulmonary infarct
>
> **Uncommon causes**
>
> - Benign tumours
> - Lymphoma
> - Arteriovenous malformation
> - Hydatid cyst
> - Pulmonary haematoma
> - Bronchogenic cyst
> - Rheumatoid nodule
> - Pulmonary sequestration
> - Granulomatosis with polyangiitis
> - Aspergilloma ('halo' sign)

activity is strongly suggestive of malignancy, while an inactive 'cold' nodule is consistent with benign disease. False-positive results may occur with some infectious or inflammatory nodules, and false-negative results with neuro-endocrine tumours and bronchiolo-alveolar cell carcinomas.

Where biopsy is contraindicated or the lesion is too small to be confidently assessed by PET, interval CT scanning may be considered, but must be repeated at intervals for up to 2 yrs to exclude malignancy. The radiation exposure inherent in this approach, and the fact that further benign nodules are often detected, need to be considered. If the nodule is highly likely to be malignant and the patient is fit, the best option may be to proceed to resection.

Pleural effusion

The accumulation of fluid within the pleural space is termed pleural effusion. Accumulations of frank pus (empyema) or blood (haemothorax) represent separate conditions. Pleural fluid accumulates due either to increased hydrostatic pressure or decreased osmotic pressure ('transudative effusion', as seen in cardiac, liver or renal failure), or to increased microvascular permeability caused by disease of the pleural surface itself, or injury in the adjacent lung ('exudative effusion'). Some causes of pleural effusion are shown in Box 9.3.

Symptoms and signs of pleurisy often precede the development of an effusion, especially in patients with underlying pneumonia, pulmonary infarction or connective tissue disease. However, the onset may be insidious. Breathlessness is often the only symptom

9.3 Causes of pleural effusion

Common

- Pneumonia ('para-pneumonic effusion')
- TB
- Pulmonary infarction
- Malignant disease
- Cardiac failure
- Subdiaphragmatic disease (subphrenic abscess, pancreatitis)

Uncommon

- Hypoproteinaemia (nephrotic syndrome, liver failure)
- Connective tissue diseases (systemic lupus erythematosus, rheumatoid arthritis)
- Post-MI syndrome
- Acute rheumatic fever
- Meigs'syndrome (ovarian tumour + pleural effusion)
- Myxoedema
- Uraemia
- Asbestos-related benign pleural effusion

related to the effusion and its severity depends on the size and rate of accumulation.

Investigations

Radiology: The classical appearance of pleural fluid on CXR is that of a curved shadow at the lung base, blunting the costophrenic angle and ascending towards the axilla. Fluid appears to track up the lateral chest wall. In fact, fluid surrounds the whole lung at this level, but casts a radiological shadow only where the X-ray beam passes tangentially through the fluid against the lateral chest wall. Around 200 mL of fluid is required to be detectable on a PA CXR, but smaller effusions can be identified by USS or CT. Previous scarring or adhesions in the pleural space can cause localised effusions. USS is more accurate than plain CXR for determining the volume of pleural fluid and may reveal floating debris, indicating an exudate. The presence of loculation suggests an evolving empyema or resolving haemothorax. CT displays pleural abnormalities more readily than either plain radiography or USS, and may distinguish benign from malignant pleural disease.

Pleural aspiration and biopsy: In some conditions (e.g. left ventricular failure) it should not be necessary to sample fluid unless atypical features are present. In most other circumstances, diagnostic aspiration is indicated. Pleural aspiration reveals the colour and texture of fluid and on appearance alone may immediately suggest an empyema or chylothorax. The presence of blood is consistent with pulmonary infarction or malignancy, but may represent a traumatic tap. Biochemical analysis allows classification into transudate

> **9.4 Light's criteria for distinguishing pleural transudate from exudate**
>
> Pleural fluid is an exudate if one or more of the following criteria are met:
> - Pleural fluid protein : serum protein ratio > 0.5
> - Pleural fluid LDH : serum LDH ratio > 0.6
> - Pleural fluid LDH > two-thirds of the upper limit of normal serum LDH

and exudate (Box 9.4) and Gram stain and culture may reveal infection. The predominant cell type provides useful information, and cytological examination is essential. A low pH suggests infection but may also be seen in rheumatoid arthritis, ruptured oesophagus or advanced malignancy. USS- or CT-guided pleural biopsy provides tissue for pathological and microbiological analysis. If results are inconclusive, video-assisted thoracoscopy allows the operator to visualise the pleura and guide the biopsy directly.

Management

Therapeutic aspiration may be required to palliate breathlessness, but removing >1.5 L in one episode is inadvisable, as this can cause re-expansion pulmonary oedema. An effusion should never be drained to dryness before establishing a diagnosis, as further biopsy may be precluded until further fluid accumulates. Treatment of the underlying cause – e.g. heart failure, pneumonia, pulmonary embolism or subphrenic abscess – will often be followed by resolution of the effusion. The management of pleural effusion in association with pneumonia, TB and malignancy is dealt with later in this chapter.

Empyema

Empyema means pus in the pleural space. The pus may be as thin as serous fluid or so thick that it is impossible to aspirate, even through a wide-bore needle. Microscopically, neutrophils are present in large numbers. The causative organism may or may not be isolated from the pus. An empyema may involve the whole pleural space or only part of it ('loculated' or 'encysted' empyema) and is usually unilateral. Empyema is always secondary to infection in a neighbouring structure, usually the lung (bacterial pneumonias and TB). Over 40% of patients with community-acquired pneumonia develop an associated pleural effusion ('para-pneumonic' effusion) and ~15% of these become secondarily infected, often where there is a delay in diagnosis or treatment.

Clinical features

• Persistence or recurrence of pyrexia in pulmonary infections, despite the administration of a suitable antibiotic. • Rigors, sweating, malaise and weight loss. • Pleural pain, breathlessness, cough, sputum (copious amounts if empyema ruptures into a bronchus – bronchopleural fistula). • Clinical signs of a pleural effusion.

Investigations

• Blood tests: reveal a polymorphonuclear leucocytosis and high CRP. • CXR: demonstrates a pleural effusion, which often appears loculated ('D-shaped opacity'). When air is present in addition to pus (pyopneumothorax), a horizontal 'fluid level' marks the air/liquid interface. • USS shows the position of the fluid, the extent of pleural thickening and whether fluid is in a single collection or multiloculated by fibrin and debris. • CT: can be useful in assessing the underlying lung parenchyma and patency of the major bronchi. • USS-guided aspiration of pus: confirms the presence of an empyema; the pus is frequently sterile when antibiotics have already been given.

The distinction between tuberculous and non-tuberculous disease can be difficult and often requires pleural histology and culture.

Management

When the patient is acutely ill and the pus is thin, a large intercostal tube should be inserted for drainage of the pleural space. If the initial aspirate reveals turbid fluid or frank pus, or if loculations are seen on USS, the tube should be put on suction (-5 to -10 cmH$_2$O) and flushed regularly with 20 mL normal saline. An antibiotic directed against the organism causing the empyema should be given for 2–4 wks. Intrapleural fibrinolytic therapy is of no benefit. If the pleural fluid is difficult to drain, which can happen when the pus is thick or loculated, surgery is required to clear the empyema cavity. Surgical 'decortication' of the lung may be required if thickening of the visceral pleura is preventing re-expansion of the lung.

Tuberculous empyema: Anti-TB chemotherapy must be started immediately and the pus in the pleural space drained until it ceases to re-accumulate. In many patients, no other treatment is necessary but surgery is occasionally required to ablate a residual empyema space.

Respiratory failure

The term respiratory failure is used when pulmonary gas exchange fails to maintain normal arterial oxygen and carbon dioxide levels. Its classification into type I and type II relates to the absence or presence of hypercapnia (raised PaCO$_2$). The main causes are shown in Box 9.5.

Acute respiratory failure
Management

Prompt diagnosis and management of the underlying cause is crucial. In type I respiratory failure, high concentrations of oxygen (40–60% by mask) will usually relieve hypoxia but occasionally mechanical ventilation may be needed.

Acute type II respiratory failure is an emergency. It is useful to distinguish between patients with high ventilatory drive who

9.5 Respiratory failure: underlying causes and blood gas abnormalities

	Type I		Type II	
	Hypoxia (PaO_2 <8.0 kPa (60 mmHg))		Hypoxia (PaO_2 <8.0 kPa (60 mmHg))	
	Normal or low $PaCO_2$ (<6.6 kPa (50 mmHg))		Raised $PaCO_2$ (>6.6 kPa (50 mmHg))	
	Acute	**Chronic**	**Acute**	**Chronic**
H^+	→ or ↑	→	←	→ or ↑
Bicarbonate	→	→	→	↑
Causes	Acute asthma	Emphysema	Acute severe asthma	COPD
	Pulmonary oedema	Lung fibrosis	Acute exacerbation of COPD	Sleep apnoea
	Pneumonia	Lymphangitis carcinomatosa	Upper airway obstruction	Kyphoscoliosis
	Lobar collapse	Right-to-left shunts	Acute neuropathies/paralysis	Myopathies/muscular dystrophy
	Pneumothorax		Narcotic drugs	Ankylosing spondylitis
	Pulmonary embolus		Primary alveolar hypoventilation	
	ARDS		Flail chest injury	

cannot move sufficient air, and those with reduced or inadequate respiratory effort. In the former, particularly if inspiratory stridor is present, acute upper airway obstruction (e.g. foreign body inhalation or laryngeal obstruction) must be considered, as the Heimlich manœuvre, immediate intubation or tracheostomy may be life-saving.

More commonly, the problem is severe COPD or asthma, or acute respiratory distress syndrome (ARDS; p. 25). High-concentration (e.g. 60%) oxygen should be administered with monitoring of ABGs. Patients with asthma or COPD should be treated with nebulised salbutamol 2.5 mg with oxygen, repeated until bronchospasm is relieved. Failure to respond to initial treatment, declining conscious level and worsening respiratory acidosis (H^+ >50 nmol/L (pH <7.3), $PaCO_2$ >6.6 kPa (50 mmHg)) on blood gases are all indications that supported ventilation is required (p. 26).

Patients with acute type II respiratory failure with reduced drive or conscious level may be suffering from sedative poisoning, CO_2 narcosis or a primary failure of neurological drive (e.g. following intracerebral haemorrhage or head injury). History from a witness may be invaluable, and reversal of sedatives using antagonists occasionally helps, but should not delay intubation and supported mechanical ventilation in appropriate cases.

Chronic and 'acute on chronic' type II respiratory failure

In severe COPD or neuromuscular disease, $PaCO_2$ may be persistently raised, but renal retention of bicarbonate corrects arterial pH to normal. This 'compensated' pattern may be disturbed by further acute illness, such as an exacerbation of COPD, causing 'acute on chronic' respiratory failure, with acidaemia and respiratory distress followed by drowsiness and coma. These patients have lost their chemosensitivity to elevated $PaCO_2$, and depend on hypoxia for respiratory drive; they therefore develop respiratory depression if given high concentrations of oxygen.

The aims of treatment in acute on chronic type II respiratory failure are to achieve a safe PaO_2 (>7.0 kPa (52 mmHg)) without increasing $PaCO_2$ and acidosis.

Patients who are conscious and have adequate respiratory drive may benefit from non-invasive ventilation (NIV), which has been shown to reduce the need for intubation and shorten hospital stay. Those who are drowsy and have low respiratory drive require an urgent decision regarding intubation and ventilation. Important factors to consider include patient and family wishes, presence of a potentially remediable precipitating condition, prior functional capacity and quality of life.

Respiratory stimulant drugs, such as doxapram, have been superseded by intubation and mechanical ventilation in patients with CO_2 narcosis.

Home ventilation for chronic respiratory failure

Some patients with chronic respiratory failure due to spinal deformity, neuromuscular disease or advanced lung disease, e.g. cystic fibrosis, benefit from home NIV. In these conditions, morning headache (due to elevated $PaCO_2$) and fatigue may occur but the diagnosis may also be revealed by sleep studies or morning blood gas analysis. Overnight home-based NIV is often sufficient to restore the daytime PCO_2 to normal, and to relieve fatigue and headache. In advanced disease, daytime NIV may also be required.

Lung transplantation

This is an established treatment for carefully selected patients with advanced lung disease unresponsive to medical treatment. Single-lung transplantation may be used for selected patients with advanced emphysema or lung fibrosis. It is contraindicated in patients with chronic bilateral pulmonary infection, such as cystic fibrosis, because immunosuppression makes the transplanted lung vulnerable to cross-infection; for these conditions, bilateral lung transplantation is the standard procedure. Heart–lung transplantation is still occasionally needed for patients with advanced congenital heart disease such as Eisenmenger's syndrome, and is preferred by some surgeons for the treatment of primary pulmonary hypertension unresponsive to medical therapy.

The prognosis following lung transplantation is improving steadily. Modern immunosuppressive drugs yield over 50% 10-yr survival in some UK centres. However, chronic rejection resulting in obliterative bronchiolitis continues to afflict some recipients.

The major factor limiting the availability of lung transplantation is the shortage of donor lungs. To improve organ availability, techniques to recondition the lungs in vitro after removal from the donor are being developed.

OBSTRUCTIVE PULMONARY DISEASES

Asthma

Asthma is characterised by chronic airway inflammation and increased airway hyper-responsiveness leading to wheeze, cough, chest tightness and dyspnoea. Airflow obstruction in asthma is variable over time and reversible with treatment. Around 300 million people worldwide suffer from asthma and the prevalence is increasing.

The relationship between atopy (the propensity to produce IgE in response to allergens) and asthma is well established. Common allergens include house dust mites, cats, dogs, cockroaches and fungi. Allergy is also implicated in some cases of occupational asthma (p. 310).

Aspirin can cause asthma through the production of cysteinyl leukotrienes. In exercise-induced asthma, hyperventilation results in water and heat loss from the airway lining fluid, triggering mediator release.

In persistent asthma, there is a chronic influx of inflammatory cells interacting with airway structural cells, and the secretion of cytokines, chemokines and growth factors. Induced sputum samples demonstrate that, although eosinophils usually dominate, neutrophilic inflammation predominates in some patients, while, in others, scant inflammation is observed: so-called 'pauci-granulocytic' asthma.

With increasing severity and chronicity of asthma, airway remodelling may occur, with fibrosis and fixed narrowing of the airways and a reduced bronchodilator response.

Clinical features

Typical symptoms include recurrent episodes of wheezing, chest tightness, breathlessness and cough. In mild intermittent asthma, patients may be asymptomatic between exacerbations. In persistent asthma, the pattern is one of chronic wheeze and breathlessness.

Symptoms may be precipitated by:
• Exercise. • Cold weather. • Allergen exposure (e.g. pets, occupational). • Viral respiratory tract infections. • Drugs (β-blockers, aspirin and NSAIDs).

There is diurnal variation in symptoms (worse in early morning); sleep is often disturbed by cough and wheeze.

Investigations

Pulmonary function tests: Diagnosis is based on a compatible history and an increase in FEV_1 of ≥15% and at least 200 mL following bronchodilator/trial of corticosteroids; or >20% diurnal variation on ≥3 days in a week for 2 wks on peak expiratory flow (PEF) diary; or a decrease in FEV_1 of ≥15% after 6 mins of exercise. In patients with normal FEV_1, bronchial challenge testing (e.g. with mannitol) is a sensitive though not specific way to demonstrate airway hyperreactivity.

CXR: This is often normal. There is lobar collapse if mucus has occluded a large bronchus. Hyperinflation is present in acute asthma. Flitting infiltrates may be seen in allergic bronchopulmonary aspergillosis (ABPA).

Measurement of allergic status: Total IgE ± allergen-specific IgE and/or skin prick tests are carried out. Sputum or blood eosinophilia may be present.

Management

The goal of asthma therapy is to maintain complete control:
• No daytime symptoms. • No limitation of activities. • No nocturnal symptoms/wakening. • No need for 'rescue' medication. • Normal lung function. • No exacerbations.

Patients who have symptoms requiring rescue medication more than twice a week have partial control, and those with >3 of the above features in any week are termed uncontrolled.

Patient education: Patients should be taught about the importance of key symptoms (e.g. nocturnal waking), different types of medication and the use of PEF to guide management. Written action plans may be helpful.

Avoidance of aggravating factors: Asthma control may be improved by reducing exposure to antigens, e.g. household pets. In occupational asthma, removal from the offending agent may lead to cure. Many patients are sensitised to several antigens, making avoidance almost impossible. Patients should be advised not to smoke.

Pharmacological treatment

Step 1 – Occasional use of inhaled short-acting β_2-adrenoreceptor agonist bronchodilators: This is used for patients with mild intermittent asthma (symptoms <once/wk for 3 mths and <2 nocturnal episodes/mth). Patients often underestimate the severity of asthma.

Step 2 – Regular preventer therapy: Regular inhaled corticosteroids (ICS) are used for any patient who has experienced an exacerbation in the last 2 yrs, uses inhaled β_2-agonists >3 times/wk, reports symptoms >3 times/wk, or is awakened by asthma 1 night/wk.

Step 3 – Add-on therapy: If poor control remains, despite regular ICS up to a dose of 800 µg/day beclometasone dipropionate (BDP) or equivalent, add-on therapy should be considered. Long-acting β_2-agonists (LABAs, e.g. salmeterol, formoterol) are first choice, and combination ICS/LABA inhalers may increase compliance. LABAs have consistently been demonstrated to improve asthma control and reduce exacerbations compared to increased doses of ICS alone. Leukotriene receptor antagonists (e.g. montelukast 10 mg daily) are a less effective add-on therapy.

Step 4 – Poor control on a moderate dose of inhaled steroid and add-on therapy: The ICS dose may be increased to 2000 µg BDP or equivalent daily. A nasal corticosteroid should be used if upper airway symptoms are prominent. Consider trials of leukotriene receptor antagonists, theophyllines or slow-release β_2-agonists and stop if ineffective.

Step 5 – Continuous or frequent use of oral steroids: Prednisolone should be prescribed in the lowest amount necessary to control symptoms. Patients receiving more than three or four courses/yr or long-term corticosteroids (>3 mths) are at risk of systemic side-effects. Osteoporosis should be prevented using bisphosphonates. In atopic patients, omalizumab, a monoclonal anti-IgE antibody, may help to limit steroid dose and improve symptoms.

Step-down therapy: Once asthma control is established, inhaled (or oral) corticosteroid dose should be titrated to the lowest dose at which effective control of asthma is maintained.

Exacerbations of asthma

Asthma exacerbations are characterised by increased symptoms, deterioration in PEF and an increase in airway inflammation. They may be precipitated by infections (most commonly viral), moulds

9.6 Immediate assessment of acute severe asthma

Acute severe asthma

- PEF 33–50% predicted (<200 L/min)
- Inability to complete sentences in 1 breath
- Heart rate ≥110/min
- Respiratory rate ≥25/min

Life-threatening features

- PEF <33% predicted (<100 L/min)
- SpO_2 <92% or PaO_2 <8 kPa (60 mmHg)
- Normal or raised $PaCO_2$
- Silent chest/feeble respiratory effort
- Cyanosis
- Hypotension
- Exhaustion
- Confusion
- Coma
- Bradycardia or arrhythmias

Near-fatal asthma

- ↑$PaCO_2$ and/or requiring mechanical ventilation with raised inflation pressures

(*Alternaria* and *Cladosporium*) and, on occasion, pollen (particularly following thunderstorms). Most attacks are characterised by a gradual deterioration over several hours to days, but some appear to occur with little or no warning: so-called brittle asthma.

Management of mild to moderate exacerbations

Doubling the dose of ICS does not prevent an impending exacerbation. Short courses of 'rescue' oral corticosteroids (prednisolone 30–60 mg daily) are often required where there are worsening symptoms (morning symptoms persisting until midday, nocturnal wakening or diminishing response to bronchodilator) and a fall of PEF to <60% of best recording. Tapering of the dose is not necessary unless given for >3 wks.

Management of acute severe asthma

This is covered in Box 9.6 and Figure 9.1.

Chronic obstructive pulmonary disease

Chronic obstructive pulmonary disease (COPD) is a preventable and treatable disease characterised by persistent progressive airflow limitation associated with chronic inflammation in response to noxious particles or gases. Related diagnoses include chronic bronchitis (cough and sputum on most days for at least 3 mths, in 2 consecutive yrs) and emphysema (abnormal permanent enlargement of the distal air spaces, with destruction of alveolar walls). Extrapulmonary manifestations include weight loss and skeletal muscle dysfunction, and COPD is associated with cardiovascular

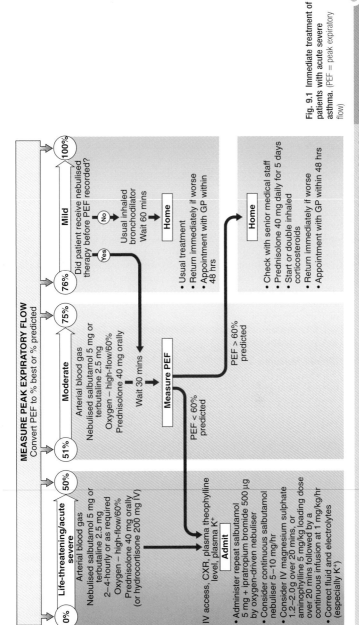

MEASURE PEAK EXPIRATORY FLOW
Convert PEF to % best or % predicted

| 0% | 50% | 51% | 75% | 76% | 100% |

Life-threatening/acute severe

Arterial blood gas
Nebulised salbutamol 5 mg or terbutaline 2.5 mg
2–4-hourly or as required
Oxygen – high-flow/60%
Prednisolone 40 mg orally (or hydrocortisone 200 mg IV)

IV access, CXR, plasma theophylline level, plasma K⁺

Admit

- Administer repeat salbutamol 5 mg + ipratropium bromide 500 μg by oxygen-driven nebuliser
- Consider continuous salbutamol nebuliser 5–10 mg/hr
- Consider IV magnesium sulphate 1.2–2.0 g over 20 mins, or aminophylline 5 mg/kg loading dose over 20 mins followed by a continuous infusion at 1 mg/kg/hr
- Correct fluid and electrolytes (especially K⁺)

Moderate

Arterial blood gas
Nebulised salbutamol 5 mg or terbutaline 2.5 mg
Oxygen – high-flow/60%
Prednisolone 40 mg orally

Wait 30 mins

Measure PEF

PEF < 60% predicted

PEF > 60% predicted

Mild

Did patient receive nebulised therapy before PEF recorded?

No → Usual inhaled bronchodilator
Wait 60 mins

Home
- Usual treatment
- Return immediately if worse
- Appointment with GP within 48 hrs

Yes →

Home
- Check with senior medical staff
- Prednisolone 40 mg daily for 5 days
- Start or double inhaled corticosteroids
- Return immediately if worse
- Appointment with GP within 48 hrs

Fig. 9.1 Immediate treatment of patients with acute severe asthma. (PEF = peak expiratory flow)

RESPIRATORY DISEASE · **9**

281

9.7 Modified MRC dyspnoea scale	
Grade	**Degree of breathlessness related to activities**
0	No breathlessness except with strenuous exercise
1	Breathlessness when hurrying on the level or walking up a slight hill
2	Walks slower than contemporaries on level ground because of breathlessness or has to stop for breath when walking at own pace
3	Stops for breath after walking ~100 m or after a few mins on level ground
4	Too breathless to leave the house, or breathless when dressing or undressing

disease, cerebrovascular disease, the metabolic syndrome, osteoporosis and depression.

The prevalence of COPD is related to the prevalence of tobacco smoking and, in low- and middle-income countries, exposure to biomass fuel smoke. Approximately 80 million people worldwide suffer from moderate to severe disease. In 2005, COPD contributed to over 3 million (5%) deaths globally but it is forecast to become the third most important cause of death worldwide by 2020. This rise will be greatest in Asian and African countries because of increasing tobacco consumption there. Not all smokers develop COPD, and it is unusual in smokers of <10 pack yrs (1 pack yr = 20 cigarettes/day for 1 yr). Other risk factors include air pollution (especially biomass fuels), occupational exposure (coal dust, silica) and inherited deficiency of α_1-antitrypsin.

Clinical features

COPD should be suspected in any patient over the age of 40 yrs with persistent cough and sputum and/or breathlessness. The level of breathlessness should be quantified (e.g. MRC dyspnoea scale, Box 9.7). In advanced disease there may be oedema or morning headaches (hypercapnia). Physical signs (Fig. 9.2) may help to indicate disease severity.

Two classical phenotypes have been described:

• 'Pink puffers': thin and breathless, and maintain a normal $PaCO_2$.
• 'Blue bloaters': develop hypercapnia, oedema and secondary polycythaemia.

In practice, these phenotypes often overlap.

Investigations

• CXR: may reveal hyperinflation, bullae or other complications of smoking (lung cancer). • FBC: may demonstrate polycythaemia. • α_1-antitrypsin level: should be checked in younger patients with emphysema. • Spirometry (% of predicted value): used to classify disease severity (e.g. UK NICE guidelines):

Stage 1 (mild) – FEV_1 >80%, FEV_1/FVC <0.7 plus symptoms;
Stage II (moderate) – FEV_1 50–79%, FEV_1/FVC <0.7;

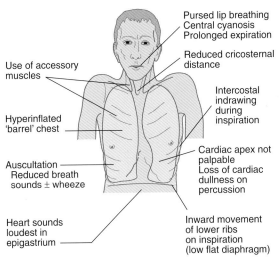

Fig. 9.2 Key features on examination in COPD.

Stage III (severe) – FEV_1 30–49%, FEV_1/FVC <0.7;
Stage IV (very severe) – FEV_1 <30%, FEV_1/FVC <0.7.

• Lung volume measurements: quantify hyperinflation. • Carbon monoxide transfer factor: low in emphysema. • Exercise tests: an objective assessment of exercise tolerance. • Pulse oximetry: may prompt referral for a domiciliary oxygen assessment if <93%. • CT: likely to play an increasing role in the assessment of COPD, as it allows the detection, characterisation and quantification of emphysema.

Management

Pessimism is unjustified, as it is usually possible to improve breathlessness, reduce the frequency and severity of exacerbations, and improve health status and prognosis.

Reduce smoke exposure: Always offer the patient help to stop smoking, combining pharmacotherapy with appropriate support as part of a programme. Cessation is proven to decelerate the decline in FEV_1 (Fig. 9.3). Smokeless alternatives to biofuels should be promoted wherever possible.

Bronchodilators: Short-acting bronchodilators are given for mild disease (β_2-agonist or anticholinergic). Longer-acting bronchodilators are more appropriate for patients with moderate to severe disease. From the wide range available, select a device that the patient can use effectively. Significant improvements in breathlessness may be reported despite minimal changes in FEV_1,

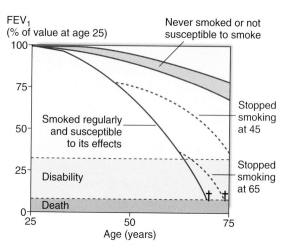

Fig. 9.3 Model of annual decline in FEV_1 with accelerated decline in susceptible smokers. When smoking is stopped, subsequent loss is similar to that in healthy non-smokers.

probably reflecting reduced hyperinflation. Theophylline preparations improve breathlessness but use is limited by side-effects. Oral β_2-agonists and selective phosphodiesterase inhibitors have a limited role.

Inhaled corticosteroids: These reduce the frequency and severity of exacerbations; they are recommended in patients with severe disease (FEV_1 <50%) who report ≥2 exacerbations/yr requiring antibiotics or oral steroids. Regular use leads to a small improvement in FEV_1 but no change in the rate of decline of lung function. ICS/LABA combinations produce further improvements in breathlessness and exacerbation rate. Oral corticosteroids are useful during exacerbations, but maintenance therapy contributes to osteoporosis and impaired muscle function and should be avoided.

Pulmonary rehabilitation: Encourage exercise. Multidisciplinary programmes (usually 6–12 wks' duration) incorporating physical training, education and nutritional counselling reduce symptoms, improve health status and enhance confidence.

Oxygen therapy: Long-term domiciliary oxygen therapy (LTOT) improves survival in selected patients with COPD and hypoxia (PaO_2 <7.3kPa (55 mmHg)). A minimum of 15 hrs/day is recommended, keeping PaO_2 >8 kPa (60 mmHg) or SaO_2 >90%. Ambulatory oxygen should be considered in patients who desaturate on exercise and show objective improved exercise capacity and/or dyspnoea with oxygen. Short-burst oxygen therapy is of no benefit and should be avoided.

Surgical intervention: In highly selected patients, lung volume reduction surgery (removing non-functioning emphysematous lung tissue) reduces hyperinflation and decreases work of breathing.

Bullectomy is occasionally performed for large bullae that compress surrounding lung tissue. Lung transplantation may benefit selected patients.

Other measures: Give influenza vaccination and pneumococcal vaccination; treat depression and cachexia.

COPD has a variable natural history. Prognosis is inversely related to age and directly related to FEV_1. Poor prognostic indicators include weight loss and pulmonary hypertension.

Acute exacerbations of COPD

These are characterised by an increase in symptoms and deterioration in lung function. They are more common in severe disease and may be caused by bacteria, viruses or a change in air quality. Respiratory failure and/or fluid retention may be present. Many patients can be managed at home with the use of increased bronchodilator therapy, a short course of oral corticosteroids and, if appropriate, antibiotics. Cyanosis, peripheral oedema or altered conscious level should prompt hospital referral.

Oxygen therapy: High concentrations of oxygen may cause respiratory depression and worsening acidosis (p. 276). Controlled oxygen at 24% or 28% should be used, aiming for PaO_2 >8 kPa (60 mmHg) (or SaO_2 88–92%) without worsening acidosis.

Bronchodilators: Nebulised short-acting β_2-agonists and anticholinergics are used. If concern exists regarding oxygen sensitivity, nebulisers may be driven by compressed air.

Corticosteroids: Oral prednisolone (usually 30 mg for 5–10 days) reduces symptoms, improves lung function and shortens hospital stay. Prophylaxis against osteoporosis should be considered if frequent courses are needed.

Antibiotics: These are recommended for an increase in sputum purulence, sputum volume or breathlessness. An aminopenicillin or a macrolide should be used. Co-amoxiclav is only required in regions where β-lactamase-producing organisms are known to be common.

Ventilatory support: In patients with persistent tachypnoea and respiratory acidosis (H^+ ≥45 nmol/L (pH <7.35)), NIV is associated with reduced need for intubation and reduced mortality. Consider intubation and ventilation where there is a reversible cause for deterioration (e.g. pneumonia); the evidence for NIV with pneumonia is much weaker.

Additional therapy: Evidence for IV aminophylline is limited and there is a risk of arrhythmias and drug interactions. The respiratory stimulant doxapram has been superseded by NIV. Diuretics should be administered if peripheral oedema has developed.

Bronchiectasis

Bronchiectasis means abnormal dilatation of the bronchi due to chronic airway inflammation and infection. It is usually acquired, but may result from an underlying genetic or congenital defect of airway defences (Box 9.8).

9.8 Causes of bronchiectasis

Congenital

- Cystic fibrosis
- Primary ciliary dyskinesia
- Kartagener's syndrome (sinusitis and transposition of the viscera)
- Primary hypogammaglobulinaemia

Acquired

- Pneumonia (complicating whooping cough or measles)
- Inhaled foreign body
- Suppurative pneumonia
- Pulmonary TB
- Allergic bronchopulmonary aspergillosis complicating asthma
- Bronchial tumours

Clinical features

• Chronic cough productive of purulent sputum. • Pleuritic pain. • Haemoptysis. • Halitosis.

Acute exacerbations may cause fever and increase these symptoms. Examination reveals coarse crackles caused by sputum in bronchiectatic spaces. Diminished breath sounds may indicate lobar collapse. Bronchial breathing due to scarring may be heard in advanced disease.

Investigations

Sputum: Testing may reveal common respiratory pathogens. As disease progresses, *Pseudomonas aeruginosa* or fungi such as *Aspergillus* and various mycobacteria may be seen. Frequent cultures assist appropriate antibiotic selection.

Radiology: CXR may be normal in mild disease. In advanced disease, thickened airway walls, cystic bronchiectatic spaces, and associated areas of pneumonic consolidation or collapse may be seen. CT is much more sensitive and shows thickened dilated airways.

Assessment of ciliary function: Saccharin test or nasal biopsy may be used.

Management and prognosis

In patients with airflow obstruction, inhaled bronchodilators and corticosteroids may enhance airway patency.

Physiotherapy: Patients should perform regular daily physiotherapy to keep the dilated bronchi empty of secretions. Deep breathing followed by forced expiratory manoeuvres ('active cycle of breathing' technique), and devices that generate positive expiratory pressure (PEP mask or flutter valve) can assist with sputum clearance.

Antibiotics: In most patients with bronchiectasis, the same antibiotics are used as in COPD, although higher doses are needed. In patients colonised with staphylococci and Gram-negative bacilli, especially *Pseudomonas* spp., antibiotic therapy should be guided by microbiology results. Regular macrolides help reduce exacerbations in some patients with bronchiectasis, but their use is not yet supported by large trials (except in cystic fibrosis).

Surgical treatment: Surgery is only indicated in a few cases where bronchiectasis is unilateral and confined to a single lobe/segment on CT.

The disease is progressive when associated with ciliary dysfunction and cystic fibrosis, and eventually causes respiratory failure. In other patients, the prognosis can be good with regular physiotherapy and judicious use of antibiotics. Bronchiectasis may be prevented by prophylaxis or treatment of common causes, e.g. measles, whooping cough, TB.

Cystic fibrosis

Cystic fibrosis (CF) is the most common lethal genetic disease in Caucasians, affecting 1 in 2500 births. It is caused by mutations of a gene (on chromosome 7) coding for a chloride channel – cystic fibrosis transmembrane conductance regulator (*CFTR*). The carrier rate of CF mutations is 1 in 25 and inheritance is autosomal recessive. The most common mutation is *ΔF508* but >1000 mutations have been identified. The genetic defect causes increased sodium and chloride in sweat, and depletion of airway lining fluid, leading to chronic bacterial infection in the airways. The gut epithelium, pancreas, liver and reproductive tract are also affected. Neonatal screening for CF is now routine in the UK. The diagnosis is confirmed by genetic testing and sweat electrolyte measurements.

Clinical features

The lungs are normal at birth, but bronchiectasis develops in childhood. *Staph. aureus* is the most common childhood organism; however, in adulthood, increasing numbers are colonised with *Pseudomonas aeruginosa*. Recurrent exacerbations of bronchiectasis cause progressive lung damage, resulting ultimately in death from respiratory failure. Other clinical manifestations of the gene defect include intestinal obstruction, exocrine pancreatic insufficiency with malabsorption, diabetes and hepatic cirrhosis. Men with CF are infertile due to failure of development of the vas deferens.

Management and prognosis

Regular chest physiotherapy is recommended. For exacerbations, *Staph. aureus* infection is often managed with oral antibiotics; IV treatment is usually needed for *Pseudomonas* spp. Resistant strains of *Ps. aeruginosa*, *Stenotrophomonas maltophilia* and *Burkholderia cepacia* are a major problem. *Aspergillus* and 'atypical mycobacteria' are also frequently found (may be benign 'colonisers'). Nebulised antibiotic therapy (Colomycin or tobramycin) is used to suppress chronic *Pseudomonas* infection. Nebulised recombinant human deoxyribonuclease (DNase) liquefies sputum, reduces exacerbations and improves pulmonary function in some patients. Regular macrolides (e.g. azithromycin) reduce exacerbations and improve lung function in patients with *Pseudomonas* colonisation. In advanced disease, home oxygen and NIV may be necessary to treat respiratory failure. Ultimately, lung transplantation can produce dramatic improvements but is limited by donor organ availability.

Treatment of non-respiratory manifestations of CF: Malabsorption is treated with oral pancreatic enzymes and vitamin supplements. Increased calorie requirements of CF patients are met by supplemental feeding, including nasogastric or gastrostomy tube feeding if required. Diabetes eventually appears in ~25% of patients and often requires insulin. Osteoporosis should be sought and treated.

The prognosis of CF has improved greatly in recent decades, mainly because of better nutrition and control of bronchial sepsis. The median survival of patients with CF born in the 21st century is now predicted to be over 40 yrs.

INFECTIONS OF THE RESPIRATORY SYSTEM

Upper respiratory tract infections

Acute coryza (common cold): Sore throat and blocked nose with watery discharge. There is usually a viral cause, but disease may be complicated by lower respiratory tract infection, sinusitis, acute laryngitis or otitis media. Antibiotics are not necessary in uncomplicated coryza.

Acute bronchitis and tracheitis: Often follow acute coryza. Cough is productive of mucoid/mucopurulent sputum. Patients have pyrexia, chest tightness, wheeze and breathlessness. Tracheitis causes pain on coughing. Disease is usually self-limiting, but may lead to bronchopneumonia or an exacerbation of COPD/asthma.

Bordetella pertussis: The cause of whooping cough; an important source of upper respiratory tract infection. It is highly contagious and is notifiable in the UK. Vaccination confers protection and is usually offered in infancy, but efficacy wanes in adult life. Adults usually experience mild coryza, but some develop paroxysms of coughing that can persist for weeks to months. The diagnosis may be confirmed by PCR from a nasopharyngeal swab or serological testing. If recognised early, macrolide antibiotics may ameliorate the course.

Rhinosinusitis: Typically causes nasal congestion, blockage or discharge, and may be accompanied by facial pain or loss of smell. Examination reveals erythematous swollen nasal mucosa with pus. Nasal polyps should be sought and dental infection excluded. Treatment with topical corticosteroids, nasal decongestants and regular nasal douching are usually sufficient and, although bacterial infection is often present, antibiotics are only indicated if symptoms persist for >5 days. Persistent or recurrent episodes should prompt a referral to an ear, nose and throat specialist.

Influenza: Discussed on page 68.

Pneumonia

Pneumonia is defined as an acute respiratory illness associated with recently developed segmental, lobar or multilobar radiological shadowing. It is classified as community-acquired pneumonia, hospital-acquired (nosocomial) pneumonia, or pneumonia occurring in immunocompromised hosts. 'Lobar pneumonia' is a radiological and pathological term referring to homogeneous consolidation of one or more lung lobes, often with pleural inflammation; bronchopneumonia refers to more patchy alveolar consolidation with bronchial and bronchiolar inflammation, often affecting both lower lobes.

Community-acquired pneumonia

In the UK, 5–11/1000 adults contract community-acquired pneumonia (CAP) each year. The incidence is higher in the very young and the elderly. Some 20% of childhood deaths worldwide are due to pneumonia. Most patients may be safely managed at home but hospital admission is necessary in 20–40%. In hospital, death rates are typically 5–10%, rising to 50% in severe illness. The most common organism is *Streptococcus pneumoniae*. *Haemophilus influenzae* should be considered in elderly patients, while *Mycoplasma* and *Chlamydia pneumoniae* are more often seen in the young. Recent influenza may predispose to *Staph. aureus* (although most cases of post-influenza pneumonia are caused by *Strep. pneumoniae*). Rarer causes of severe pneumonia include *Legionella* (from infected warm water – ask about foreign travel) and psittacosis (from birds infected with *Chlamydia psittaci*). Recent foreign travel also increases the chances of pneumonia due to rarer causes such as *Burkholderia pseudomallei* from Southeast Asia and coronavirus, which caused the outbreak of severe acute respiratory syndrome (SARS) in China and Vietnam in 2002.

Clinical features

Fever, rigors, shivering and vomiting often predominate. Cough is followed by mucopurulent sputum (rust-coloured sputum may be seen in patients with *Strep. pneumoniae* infection). Patients have poor appetite and a headache. Pleuritic chest pain is common and may be the presenting feature. Haemoptysis occasionally occurs. Examination may reveal crepitations or bronchial breathing, suggesting underlying consolidation.

Investigations

CXR: In lobar pneumonia, CXR reveals a homogeneous opacity localised to the affected lobe or segment (Fig. 9.4). CXR may also identify complications such as a parapneumonic effusion, intrapulmonary abscess formation, or empyema.

Microbiological investigations: Sputum is sent for microscopy (Gram and Ziehl–Neelsen stains), culture and sensitivity testing. Blood culture is frequently positive in pneumococcal pneumonia. Acute and convalescent samples for *Mycoplasma*, *Chlamydia*, *Legionella* and viral serology should be sent. *Legionella* antigen can

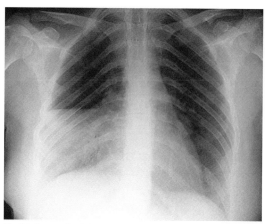

Fig. 9.4 Pneumonia of the right middle lobe.

be detected in urine and pneumococcal antigen can be detected in blood or sputum. Throat/nasopharyngeal swabs may be helpful during an influenza epidemic. Many cases of CAP are managed successfully without identification of the organism.

Blood investigations: ABGs should be done if SaO_2 is <93% or if clinical features suggest severe pneumonia. WCC is often marginally raised or even normal in patients with pneumonia caused by atypical organisms. A very high (>20 × 10⁹/L) or low (<4 × 10⁹/L) WCC may be seen in severe pneumonia. U&Es and LFTs should be checked. CRP is typically elevated.

Management

A scoring system to assess disease severity helps to guide antibiotic and admission policies (Fig. 9.5).

High concentrations (>35%) of oxygen (preferably humidified) should be administered to all patients with tachypnoea, hypoxaemia, hypotension or acidosis, aiming to keep PaO_2 ≥8 kPa (60 mmHg) or SaO_2 ≥92% (except in hypercapnia associated with COPD). IV fluids are given in severe disease, and in elderly or vomiting patients. If possible, take blood cultures prior to starting antibiotics (Box 9.9) but do not delay treatment in severe pneumonia. Consider analgesia for pleural pain, and physiotherapy if cough is suppressed, e.g. due to pain. Refer to ICU for consideration of continuous positive airways pressure (CPAP) or intubation if there is: a CURB score of 4–5 and the patient is failing to respond to treatment; persistent hypoxia despite high inspired O_2; progressive hypercapnia; severe acidosis; shock; or depressed conscious level.

Complications

• Parapneumonic effusion. • Empyema. • Lobar collapse. • Thromboembolic disease. • Pneumothorax. • Lung abscess (*Staph. aureus*).

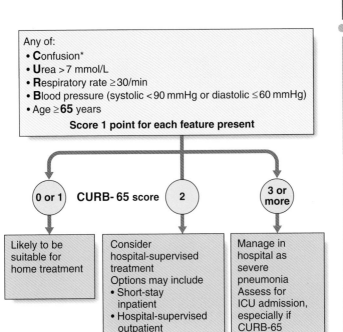

Fig. 9.5 **Hospital CURB-65.** *Defined as an abbreviated mental test score ≤8, or new disorientation in person, place or time. (A urea of 7 mmol/L ≡ 20 mg/dL.)

• Renal failure, ARDS, multi-organ failure. • Ectopic abscess formation (*Staph. aureus*). • Hepatitis, pericarditis, myocarditis, meningoencephalitis. • Pyrexia due to drug hypersensitivity.

Follow-up and prevention

Improvement in the CXR typically lags behind clinical recovery. Review should be arranged at ~6 wks and a CXR obtained if there are persistent symptoms, physical signs or reasons to suspect underlying malignancy.

Influenza vaccination and pneumococcal vaccination are recommended for selected high-risk patients.

Hospital-acquired pneumonia

Hospital-acquired pneumonia (HAP) is defined as a new episode of pneumonia occurring at least 2 days after admission to hospital. The most important distinction between HAP and CAP lies in the spectrum of organisms, with the majority of hospital-acquired infections caused by Gram-negative bacteria, including *Escherichia*, *Pseudomonas* and *Klebsiella* spp. *Staph. aureus*/MRSA are also common. The clinical features and investigation of patients with HAP are very similar to those of CAP.

9.9 Antibiotic treatment for community-acquired pneumonia

Uncomplicated CAP

- Amoxicillin 500 mg 3 times daily orally for 7–10 days
- If penicillin allergy, clarithromycin 500 mg twice daily *or* erythromycin 500 mg 4 times daily

If *Staphylococcus* is cultured or suspected

- Flucloxacillin 1–2 g IV 4 times daily *plus* clarithromycin 500 mg IV twice daily

If *Mycoplasma* or *Legionella* is suspected

- Clarithromycin 500 mg twice daily *or* erythromycin 500 mg–1 g 4 times daily *plus*
- Rifampicin 600 mg IV twice daily in severe cases

Severe CAP

- Clarithromycin 500 mg IV twice daily *or* erythromycin 500 mg–1 g IV 4 times daily *plus*
- Co-amoxiclav 1.2 g IV 3 times daily *or* ceftriaxone 1–2 g daily *or* cefuroxime 1.5 g 3 times daily

Adapted from British Thoracic Society guidelines.

Management and prognosis

Patients who have received no previous antibiotics can be treated with co-amoxiclav or cefuroxime. If the individual has received a course of recent antibiotics, then piperacillin/tazobactam or a third-generation cephalosporin should be considered.

In late-onset HAP, the choice of antibiotics must cover the Gram-negative bacteria (see above), *Staph. aureus* (including MRSA) and anaerobes. Antipseudomonal cover may be provided by mero-penem or a third-generation cephalosporin combined with an aminoglycoside. MRSA cover may be provided using vancomycin or linezolid. The choice of agents is most appropriately guided by local patterns of microbiology and antibiotic resistance. It is usual to commence broad-based cover, discontinuing less appropriate antibiotics as culture results become available.

Physiotherapy is important to aid expectoration in the immobile and elderly, and nutritional support is often required. The mortality from HAP is high (~30%).

Suppurative and aspiration pneumonia (including pulmonary abscess)

In suppurative pneumonia there is destruction of the lung paren-chyma by the inflammatory process. Microabscess formation is a characteristic histological feature of suppurative pneumonia; the term 'pulmonary abscess' refers to large localised collections of pus. Organisms include *Staph. aureus* and *Klebsiella pneumoniae*. Suppu-rative pneumonia may be produced by primary infection, inhalation of septic material from the oropharynx or haematogenous spread (e.g. in IV drug abusers). Bacterial infection of a pulmonary infarct or of a collapsed lobe may also produce suppurative pneumonia or lung abscess.

CXR characteristically demonstrates a dense opacity with cavitation and/or a fluid level. Treatment with co-amoxiclav may be effective. If anaerobes are suspected, oral metronidazole should be added. Prolonged treatment for 4–6 wks may be required.

Pneumonia in the immunocompromised patient

Pulmonary infection is common in patients receiving immunosuppressive drugs and in diseases causing defects of cellular or humoral immune mechanisms. Most infections are caused by the same common pathogens that cause CAP. Gram-negative bacteria, especially *Ps. aeruginosa*, are more of a problem than Gram-positive organisms, however, and unusual organisms or those normally considered to be non-pathogenic may become 'opportunistic' pathogens. More than one organism may be present.

Clinical features and investigations

Patients may have non-specific symptoms and the onset tends to be less rapid in those with opportunistic organisms such as *Pneumocystis jirovecii* and mycobacterial infections. In *P. jirovecii* pneumonia, cough and breathlessness can precede the appearance of CXR abnormality by several days. At presentation the patient is usually pyrexial and hypoxic with normal breath sounds. Induced sputum or bronchoscopy with bronchoalveolar lavage or bronchial brushings may help to establish a diagnosis.

Management

Whenever possible, treatment should be directed against an identified organism. Frequently, the cause is not known and broad-spectrum antibiotic therapy is required (e.g. a third-generation cephalosporin, or a quinolone, + an antistaphylococcal antibiotic, or an antipseudomonal penicillin + an aminoglycoside); treatment is thereafter tailored according to the results of investigations and the clinical response. The investigation and management of *P. jirovecii* infection is detailed on page 134.

Tuberculosis

TB is caused by infection with *Mycobacterium tuberculosis* (MTB), which is part of a complex of organisms that also includes *M. bovis* (reservoir cattle) and *M. africanum* (reservoir human).

Recent figures suggest a decline in the incidence of TB but, despite this, an estimated 8.8 million incident cases occurred in 2010 and TB accounted for nearly 1.5 million deaths. One-third of the world's population has latent TB. The majority of cases occur in the poorest nations, who struggle to cover the costs of management and control programmes. In Africa, the resurgence of TB has been driven largely by HIV disease. Drug resistance is an increasing problem, especially

9.10 Factors increasing the risk of TB

Patient-related

- Age (children > young adults < elderly)
- First-generation immigrants from high-prevalence countries
- Close contacts of smear-positive patients; worse in overcrowding, e.g. prisons, dormitories
- CXR evidence of self-healed TB
- Primary infection < 1 yr previously
- Tobacco use

Associated diseases

- Immunosuppression: HIV, anti-tumour necrosis factor (TNF) therapy, high-dose corticosteroids, cytotoxic agents
- Malignancy (especially lymphoma and leukaemia)
- Type 1 diabetes mellitus
- Chronic kidney disease
- Silicosis
- GI disease with malnutrition (gastrectomy, bypass, pancreatic cancer, malabsorption)
- Deficiency of vitamin D or A
- Recent measles in children

in Africa, the former Soviet states and the Baltic, caused by incomplete treatment of cases.

The formation of a mass of granulomas surrounding an area of caseation leads to the appearance of the primary lesion in the lung, referred to as the 'Ghon focus'. The combination of a primary lesion and regional lymph node involvement is termed the 'Ghon complex'. If the bacilli spread (either by lymph or blood) before immunity is established, secondary foci may be established in other organs, including lymph nodes, serous membranes, meninges, bones, liver, kidneys and lungs. These foci resolve once an immune response is mounted and the organisms gradually lose viability. However, 'latent bacilli' may persist for many years. The estimated lifetime risk of developing disease after primary infection is 10%, with roughly half of cases occurring in the first 2 yrs after infection. Factors predisposing to TB are summarised in Box 9.10.

Clinical features

Primary pulmonary TB: This refers to infection of a previously uninfected (tuberculin-negative) individual. In most cases, infection of a healthy individual is subclinical and indicated only by the appearance of a cell-mediated, delayed-type hypersensitivity reaction to tuberculin (demonstrated by tuberculin skin testing). If the organism cannot be contained, primary progressive disease ensues.

Post-primary pulmonary TB: This is the most frequent form of post-primary disease. Onset occurs insidiously over several weeks.

Systemic symptoms include fever, night sweats, malaise, and loss of appetite and weight, and are accompanied by cough, often with haemoptysis. CXR typically shows an ill-defined opacity situated in one of the upper lobes. As disease progresses, consolidation, collapse and cavitation may develop. A miliary pattern or cavitation suggests active disease.

Miliary TB: Blood-borne dissemination gives rise to miliary TB, which may present acutely but is often characterised by 2–3 wks of fever, night sweats, anorexia, weight loss and dry cough. Hepatosplenomegaly may be present and headache may indicate coexistent tuberculous meningitis. Auscultation is frequently normal, although with more advanced disease widespread crackles occur. Fundoscopy may show choroidal tubercles. CXR demonstrates fine 1–2-mm lesions ('millet seed') distributed throughout the lungs. Anaemia and leucopenia may be present.

Extrapulmonary disease (Fig. 9.6): This accounts for ~20% of cases in HIV-negative individuals and is more common in HIV-positive individuals. Cervical or mediastinal lymphadenitis is the most common extrapulmonary presentation. Meningeal disease represents the most important form of CNS TB, as it is rapidly fatal if unrecognised and untreated.

Investigations

Mycobacterial infection is usually confirmed by direct microscopy (Ziehl–Neelsen or auramine staining) and culture of sputum or other samples from the respiratory tract or other infected site. An estimated 5000–10 000 acid-fast bacilli must be present for sputum to be smear-positive, whereas only 10–100 viable organisms are required for sputum to be culture-positive. Standard culture takes up to 8 wks. Liquid culture media (e.g. BACTEC) can expedite growth and drug sensitivity testing (7–21 days). Where multiple drug-resistant TB (MDRTB) is suspected, molecular tools may be employed to test for the presence of the *rpo* (rifampicin resistance) gene.

Chemotherapy

Standard therapy involves 6 mths' treatment with isoniazid and rifampicin, supplemented in the first 2 mths with pyrazinamide and ethambutol. Fixed-dose tablets combining two or three drugs are preferred. Treatment should be commenced immediately in any patient who is smear-positive or smear-negative but with typical CXR changes and no response to standard antibiotics. Six mths of therapy is appropriate for pulmonary TB and most extrapulmonary TB; however, 12 mths of therapy is recommended for meningeal TB, including spinal TB with spinal cord involvement – in these cases, ethambutol may be replaced by streptomycin. Pyridoxine should be prescribed in pregnant women and malnourished patients to reduce the risk of peripheral neuropathy with isoniazid. Where drug resistance is not anticipated, patients can be assumed to be non-infectious after 2 wks of appropriate therapy.

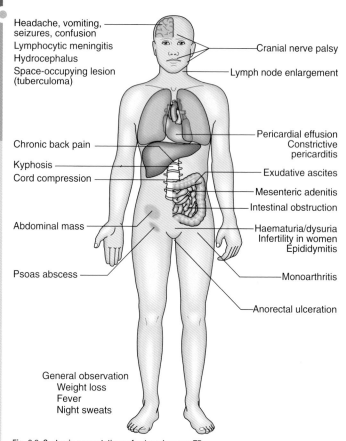

Fig. 9.6 Systemic presentations of extrapulmonary TB.

Regular monitoring of LFTs is important, as several antituberculous drugs are potentially hepatotoxic. Corticosteroids reduce inflammation and limit tissue damage, and are currently recommended when treating pericardial or meningeal disease, and in children with endobronchial disease. They may also be of benefit in pleural effusion, ureteric TB and severe pulmonary TB.

Control and prevention

Detection of latent TB: Contact tracing entails identifying an index case, other persons infected by the index patient, and close contacts who should receive BCG vaccination or chemotherapy. Approximately 10–20% of close contacts of smear-positive patients and 2–5% of those with smear-negative, culture-positive disease have evidence of TB infection.

An otherwise asymptomatic contact with a positive tuberculin skin test but a normal CXR may be treated with chemoprophylaxis (e.g. rifampicin and isoniazid for 3 mths) to prevent progression to clinical disease. Chemoprophylaxis is also recommended for:

• Contacts aged under 16 with a strongly positive tuberculin test. • Children under 2 in close contact with smear-positive disease. • Those with recent confirmed tuberculin conversion. • Babies of mothers with pulmonary TB. • HIV-infected close contacts of a patient with smear-positive disease.

Tuberculin skin testing may be falsely positive in BCG-vaccinated patients and those exposed to non-tuberculous mycobacteria. False-negative skin tests occur with immunosuppression or overwhelming infection. These limitations may be overcome by employing interferon-gamma release assays (IGRAs) that are specific to MTB.

Directly observed therapy (DOT): Poor adherence to therapy causes prolonged illness, risk of relapse, and drug resistance. DOT involves the supervised administration of therapy 3 times weekly. In the UK, it is recommended for at-risk groups, including homeless people, alcohol or drug users, patients with serious mental illness and those with a history of non-adherence.

TB and HIV/AIDS

The close links between HIV and TB, particularly in sub-Saharan Africa, are a major challenge. Programmes that link detection and treatment of TB with detection and treatment of HIV are important, and all patients with TB should be tested for HIV. Mortality is high and TB is a leading cause of death in HIV patients.

Multidrug-resistant TB

There has been a marked increase in drug-resistant strains, particularly in the poorest countries, which is closely linked to inadequate treatment. Cure is possible but prolonged treatment with less effective, more toxic and more expensive therapies is often necessary.

BCG (the Calmette–Guérin bacillus): This is a live attenuated vaccine used to stimulate protective immunity. It prevents disseminated disease in children but efficacy in adults is inconsistent. Vaccination policies vary worldwide; in the UK, vaccination is recommended for infants in high-prevalence communities, health-care workers and selected contacts.

Prognosis

Cure should be anticipated in the majority of patients. There is a small (<5%) risk of relapse and most recurrences occur within 5 mths. Without treatment, a patient with smear-positive TB will remain infectious for ~2 yrs; in 1 yr, 25% of untreated cases will die.

Opportunistic mycobacterial infection

Other species of environmental mycobacteria (often termed 'atypical') may cause human disease. These mycobacteria are low-grade pathogens (with the exception of *M. malmoense* and *M. ulcerans*), tending to cause disease in the setting of immunocompromised or scarred lungs. *M. kansasii, M. avium* complex (MAC), *M. malmoense* and *M. xenopi* are the species that most often cause lung disease. These organisms are not communicable but prolonged treatment is needed.

RESPIRATORY DISEASES CAUSED BY FUNGI

Aspergillus species

Aspergillus spp. may cause allergic bronchopulmonary aspergillosis (ABPA), hypersensitivity pneumonitis (p. 312), intracavitary aspergilloma or invasive pulmonary aspergillosis.

Allergic bronchopulmonary aspergillosis

ABPA is a hypersensitivity reaction to *A. fumigatus*. The diagnosis may be suggested by pulmonary infiltrates on routine CXRs of patients with asthma or cystic fibrosis. A persistent vigorous inflammatory response leads to bronchiectasis.

Investigations

• Proximal bronchiectasis on CT. • High serum total IgE and *Aspergillus*-specific IgE. • Elevated *A. fumigatus* precipitins in serum. • Blood eosinophilia. • *A. fumigatus* in sputum.

Management

• Low-dose regular prednisolone (7.5–10 mg daily) suppresses disease. • Itraconazole may be used as a steroid-sparing agent. • Anti-IgE monoclonal antibodies may be helpful in resistant cases.

Aspergilloma

Inhaled spores may lodge and germinate in cavities in damaged lung tissue, forming a fungal ball (aspergilloma), usually in the upper lobes. Aspergillomas are often asymptomatic, although in some patients they cause recurrent haemoptysis, which can be severe and life-threatening.

Investigations

CXR classically demonstrates a dense rounded shadow in the upper lobe, with the 'crescent sign' (thin rim of air between the fungal ball and the upper wall of the cavity). High-resolution CT (HRCT) provides greater sensitivity. Serum precipitins (IgG) to *A. fumigatus* are usually positive.

Management

Systemic medication is ineffective. Selected patients may benefit from surgery. Bronchial artery embolisation can help control major haemoptysis.

Invasive pulmonary aspergillosis

This serious condition usually occurs in neutropenic patients immunocompromised by either drugs or disease. It should be suspected when such patients develop a severe suppurative pneumonia that has not responded to antibiotics. Demonstration of abundant fungal elements in sputum helps diagnosis. Mortality is high, but treatment with antifungal agents such as voriconazole, amphotericin or caspofungin may be successful.

TUMOURS OF THE BRONCHUS AND LUNG

Lung cancer is the most common cause of cancer death worldwide, accounting for 1.4 million deaths/yr, or 18% of all cancer deaths. Smoking is thought to be directly responsible for at least 90% of lung carcinomas, the risk being directly proportional to the amount smoked and the tar content of cigarettes. Risk falls slowly after smoking cessation, but remains above the risk in non-smokers for many years. Smoking rates and lung cancer incidence are falling in the developed world but rising in developing countries. Exposure to naturally occurring radon is another known risk. The incidence of lung cancer is slightly higher in urban than in rural dwellers; this may reflect differences in atmospheric pollution (including tobacco smoke) or occupation, since a number of industrial materials (e.g. asbestos and silica) are associated with lung cancer.

Bronchial carcinoma

This tumour arises from the bronchial epithelium or mucous glands. The common cell types are squamous (35%), adenocarcinoma (30%), small-cell (20%) and large-cell (15%). Lung cancer presents in many different ways. If the tumour arises in a large bronchus, symptoms arise early, but tumours originating in a peripheral bronchus can grow large without producing symptoms. Peripheral squamous tumours may cavitate. Local spread may occur into the mediastinum and invade or compress the pericardium, oesophagus, superior vena cava, trachea, or phrenic or left recurrent laryngeal nerves. Lymphatic spread to supraclavicular and mediastinal lymph nodes is also frequently observed. Blood-borne metastases most commonly affect liver, bone, brain, adrenals and skin. Even a small primary tumour may cause widespread metastatic deposits; this is a particular characteristic of small-cell lung cancers.

Clinical features

Cough: This is the most common early symptom.

Haemoptysis: This occurs especially with central tumours.

Bronchial obstruction: Complete obstruction causes collapse of a lobe or lung, with breathlessness, mediastinal displacement, dullness to percussion and reduced breath sounds. Partial obstruction may cause unilateral wheeze that fails to clear with coughing, and may also impair the drainage of secretions, causing pneumonia or lung abscess. Persistent pneumonia in a smoker suggests an underlying bronchial carcinoma. Stridor (a harsh inspiratory noise) occurs when the trachea or larynx is narrowed by tumour or nodes.

Breathlessness: Cancer may present with breathlessness by causing collapse, pneumonia or pleural effusion, or by compressing a phrenic nerve and leading to diaphragmatic paralysis.

Pain and nerve entrapment: Pleural pain usually indicates malignant pleural invasion or distal infection. Apical carcinoma may cause Horner's syndrome (ipsilateral partial ptosis, enophthalmos, miosis and hypohidrosis of the face; p. 627) due to involvement of the sympathetic nerves in the neck. Pancoast's syndrome (pain in the inner aspect of the arm, sometimes with weakness or wasting in the hand) indicates involvement of the brachial plexus by an apical tumour.

Mediastinal spread: Involvement of the oesophagus may cause dysphagia. Pericardial involvement may lead to arrhythmia or effusion. Superior vena cava obstruction by malignant nodes causes suffusion and swelling of the neck and face, conjunctival oedema, headache and dilated veins on the chest wall. Involvement of the left recurrent laryngeal nerve by tumours at the left hilum causes voice alteration and a 'bovine' cough. Enlarged supraclavicular lymph nodes may be palpable.

Metastatic spread: This may lead to focal neurological defects, epileptic seizures, personality change, jaundice, bone pain or skin nodules. Lassitude, anorexia and weight loss usually indicate metastatic spread.

Finger clubbing: This is often seen (p. 266).

Hypertrophic pulmonary osteoarthropathy (HPOA): This is a painful periostitis of the distal forearm and leg, most often associated with bronchial carcinoma.

Non-metastatic extrapulmonary effects: These are described in Box 9.11.

9.11 Non-metastatic extrapulmonary manifestations of bronchial carcinoma

- Hyponatraemia (inappropriate ADH secretion)
- Ectopic ACTH secretion
- Hypercalcaemia (PTH-related peptide secretion)
- Myasthenia (Lambert–Eaton syndrome)
- Digital clubbing
- Hypertrophic pulmonary osteoarthropathy
- Polymyositis and dermatomyositis
- Carcinoid syndrome
- Gynaecomastia
- Polyneuropathy
- Myelopathy
- Cerebellar degeneration
- Nephrotic syndrome
- Eosinophilia

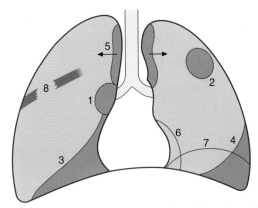

Fig. 9.7 Common radiological presentations of bronchial carcinoma. (1) Hilar mass. (2) Peripheral opacity. (3) Lung, lobe or segmental collapse. (4) Pleural effusion. (5) Broadening of mediastinum. (6) Enlarged cardiac shadow. (7) Elevation of hemidiaphragm. (8) Rib destruction.

Investigations

The main aims of investigation are to:
• Confirm the diagnosis. • Establish the histological cell type.
• Define the extent of the disease.

Common CXR features of bronchial carcinoma are illustrated in Figure 9.7.

Biopsy and histopathology: Central lung tumours can be biopsied at bronchoscopy. For peripheral tumours, percutaneous needle biopsy under CT or USS guidance is the preferred way to obtain tissue. There is a small risk of pneumothorax, which may preclude the procedure if there is extensive COPD. In patients with pleural effusions, pleural aspiration and biopsy is the preferred investigation. Thoracoscopy increases yield by allowing biopsies under direct vision. In patients with metastatic disease, the diagnosis can be confirmed by needle aspiration or biopsy of affected lymph nodes, skin lesions, liver or bone marrow.

Staging to guide treatment: Small-cell lung cancer metastasises early and this normally precludes surgery. In patients with non-small-cell cancer, staging is required to plan treatment. CT scanning is used early to detect local or distant spread. Enlarged upper mediastinal nodes may be sampled using endobronchial ultrasound (EBUS) or mediastinoscopy. Lower mediastinal nodes can be sampled through the oesophageal wall using endoscopic USS. Combined CT and PET is used increasingly to detect metastases. Head CT, radionuclide bone scanning, liver USS and bone marrow biopsy are reserved for patients with clinical or biochemical evidence of spread to these sites. Staging data are used to determine management and prognosis (Fig. 9.8). Physiological testing is also required to assess the patient's fitness for aggressive treatment.

Tumour stage	Lymph node spread			
	N0 (None)	N1 (Ipsilateral hilar)	N2 (Ipsilateral mediastinal or subcarinal)	N3 (Contralateral or supraclavicular)
T1 (< 3 cm)	Ia (50%)	IIa (36%)	IIIa (19%)	IIIb (7%)
T2a (3–5 cm)	Ib (43%)			
T2b (5–7 cm)	IIa (36%)	IIb (25%)		
T3 (> 7 cm)	IIb (25%)	IIIa (19%)		
T4 (Invading heart, vessels, oesophagus, carina, etc.)	IIIa (19%)		IIIb (7%)	
M1 Metastases present	IV (2%)			

Fig. 9.8 Tumour stage and 5-yr survival in lung cancer.

9.12 Contraindications to surgical resection in bronchial carcinoma

- Distant metastasis (M1)
- Malignant pleural effusion (T4)
- Severe/unstable cardiac or other medical condition
- Invasion of mediastinal structures (T4)
- Contralateral mediastinal nodes (N3)
- FEV_1 < 0.8 L

Management and prognosis

Surgical resection carries the best hope of long-term survival. Following resection, 5-yr survival rates are >75% in stage I disease and 55% in stage II disease. Unfortunately, most cases (>85%) have unresectable disease (Box 9.12).

Selected patients treated with radical radiotherapy also achieve prolonged remission or cure. Radiotherapy is, however, used mainly to palliate complications such as large airway obstruction, superior vena cava obstruction, recurrent haemoptysis, and pain from chest wall invasion or skeletal metastases.

The treatment of small-cell carcinoma with chemotherapy, sometimes in combination with radiotherapy, can increase median survival from 3 mths to well over a year. Chemotherapy is generally less effective in non-small-cell bronchial cancers, although platinum-based regimens show some benefit. Malignant pleural effusions should be drained if the patient is symptomatic and pleurodesis performed.

The best outcomes are obtained when lung cancer is managed in specialist centres by multidisciplinary teams including oncologists, thoracic surgeons, respiratory physicians and specialist nurses. Effective communication, pain relief and attention to diet are important.

Overall the prognosis in bronchial carcinoma is very poor, with ~70% of patients dying within 1 yr of diagnosis and <8% of patients surviving 5 yrs after diagnosis.

Carcinoid tumour

This is a low-grade malignant neuro-endocrine tumour. It typically presents with bronchial obstruction or cough. Unlike other primary lung tumours, it carries a good prognosis (95% 5-yr survival with resection).

Secondary tumours of the lung

The most common tumours that metastasise to the lung are those of the breast, kidney, uterus, ovary, testes and thyroid, often with multiple deposits. Lymphatic infiltration (lymphangitis) may develop in patients with carcinoma of the breast, stomach, bowel, pancreas or bronchus. This grave condition causes severe and rapidly progressive breathlessness associated with marked hypoxaemia.

Tumours of the mediastinum

A variety of conditions can present radiologically as a mediastinal mass (Fig. 9.9). Benign tumours and cysts in the mediastinum are often an incidental finding. Malignant mediastinal tumours are distinguished by their power to invade as well as compress structures such as bronchi and lungs. CT (or MRI) is the investigation of choice for mediastinal tumours.

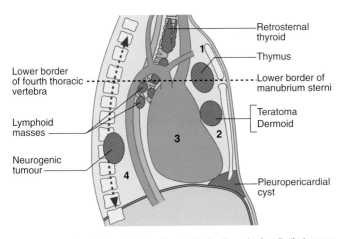

Fig. 9.9 The divisions of the mediastinum described in the diagnosis of mediastinal masses. (1) Superior mediastinum. (2) Anterior mediastinum. (3) Middle mediastinum. (4) Posterior mediastinum. Sites of the more common mediastinal tumours are also illustrated.

RESPIRATORY DISEASE • 9

INTERSTITIAL AND INFILTRATIVE PULMONARY DISEASES

Diffuse parenchymal lung disease

The diffuse parenchymal lung diseases (DPLDs) are a heterogeneous group of conditions affecting the pulmonary parenchyma (interstitium), which share a number of clinical, physiological and radiographic similarities. The current classification is shown in Figure 9.10. They often present with a dry cough and breathlessness that is insidious in onset but relentlessly progressive. Examination reveals fine inspiratory crackles, and in many cases digital clubbing develops. Alternative conditions that may mimic DPLD include diffuse infections (e.g. viral, *Pneumocystis*, TB), malignancy (e.g. lymphoma or bronchoalveolar carcinoma), pulmonary oedema and aspiration.

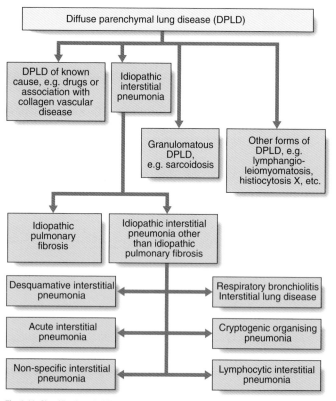

Fig. 9.10 Classification of diffuse parenchymal lung disease.

Investigations

HRCT is central to the evaluation of interstitial lung disease. A pattern typical of usual interstitial pneumonia is normally sufficient to diagnose idiopathic pulmonary fibrosis. Inconsistent clinical or CT findings should prompt consideration of bronchoalveolar lavage or transbronchial or surgical biopsy. CT may also reveal appearances diagnostic of alternative conditions, e.g. sarcoid.

Pulmonary function tests in DPLD typically show a restrictive pattern with diminished lung volumes and a reduced gas transfer (although gas transfer may be elevated in alveolar haemorrhage).

Idiopathic interstitial pneumonias

This is a subgroup of DPLD with unknown aetiology but distinguished by their radiological and histological appearances.

Idiopathic pulmonary fibrosis

Idiopathic pulmonary fibrosis (IPF) is the most common and important of the idiopathic interstitial pneumonias, characterised by pathological (or radiological) evidence of usual interstitial pneumonia (UIP). The aetiology remains unknown; speculation has included exposure to infectious agents (e.g. Epstein–Barr virus) or to occupational dusts (metal or wood), drugs (antidepressants) or chronic gastro-oesophageal reflux. Some cases are familial. A strong association with smoking exists.

Clinical features

• Uncommon before the age of 50 yrs. • Usually presents with progressive breathlessness and a non-productive cough, reduced expansion, tachypnoea and central cyanosis. • May be discovered incidentally on CT scan done for other reasons. • Finger clubbing. • Fine inspiratory crackles likened to the parting of Velcro, classically heard at the lung bases.

Investigations

HRCT may be diagnostic, demonstrating a patchy, predominantly peripheral, subpleural and basal reticular pattern with subpleural cysts (honeycombing) and/or traction bronchiectasis. CXR demonstrates lower-zone bi-basal reticular and reticulonodular opacities. Pulmonary function tests show a restrictive defect with reduced lung volumes and gas transfer. Exercise tests are useful to demonstrate arterial hypoxaemia on exercise, but as IPF advances, hypoxia is present at rest. Blood tests are of little value. Patients with typical clinical features and HRCT appearances consistent with UIP do not require lung biopsy, particularly if other known causes of interstitial lung disease have been excluded.

Management

Treatment is difficult. Large studies suggest that the combination of prednisolone, azathioprine and N-acetylcysteine is ineffective. Disappointing results have also been reported for trials of colchicine, interferon-γ 1b, bosentan and etanercept. In selected cases, pirfenidone may slow the rate of decline of lung function and, by inference, improve mortality. It remains sensible to treat gastro-oesophageal reflux and to look for and treat pulmonary hypertension but experimental agents are best confined to clinical trials. Where appropriate, lung transplantation should be considered. Oxygen may help breathlessness and opiates may be required to relieve severe dyspnoea. The optimum treatment for acute exacerbations is unknown but corticosteroids should probably be used.

A median survival of 3 yrs is widely quoted; however, the rate of progression varies considerably, from death within a few months to survival for many years. Serial lung function may provide useful prognostic information, with relative preservation of lung function suggesting longer survival, and significantly impaired gas transfer and/or desaturation on exercise indicating a poorer prognosis.

Non-specific interstitial pneumonia (NSIP)

The clinical picture of NSIP is similar to that of IPF, although patients tend to be younger and female. It may present as an isolated idiopathic pulmonary condition but is often associated with connective tissue disease, drugs, chronic hypersensitivity pneumonitis and HIV infection, and pulmonary symptoms may precede the appearance of connective tissue disease. HRCT findings are less specific than with IPF and lung biopsy may be required. The prognosis is better than in IPF (5-yr mortality rate of <15%).

Sarcoidosis

Sarcoidosis is a multisystem disorder, characterised by non-caseating epithelioid granulomas; it is more common in colder parts of Northern Europe. It tends to cause more severe disease in people of West Indian and Asian origin, while sparing Inuit, Arab and Chinese populations. The aetiology is unknown, although atypical mycobacteria, viruses and genetic factors have been proposed. Sarcoidosis is less common in smokers.

Clinical features

Any organ may be affected but 90% of cases affect the lungs. Otherwise, lymph glands, liver, spleen, skin, eyes, parotid glands and phalangeal bones are the most frequently involved sites. Löfgren's syndrome – erythema nodosum, peripheral arthropathy, uveitis, bilateral hilar lymphadenopathy (BHL), lethargy and occasionally fever – commonly presents in the third or fourth decade. BHL may be detected in an otherwise asymptomatic individual undergoing CXR. Pulmonary disease may present insidiously with cough, exertional breathlessness and radiographic infiltrates. Fibrosis occurs uncommonly but may cause a silent loss of lung function.

Investigations

• FBC: demonstrates lymphopenia. • LFTs: may be mildly deranged. • Ca^{2+}: may be elevated. • Serum ACE: may provide a non-specific

9.13 CXR stage and outcomes in sarcoidosis	
Stage	**Description**
Stage I: bilateral hilar lymphadenopathy (BHL; usually symmetrical); paratracheal nodes often enlarged	Often asymptomatic but may be associated with erythema nodosum and arthralgia; majority of cases resolve in <1 yr
Stage II: BHL and parenchymal infiltrates	Patients may present with breathlessness or cough; majority of cases resolve spontaneously
Stage III: parenchymal infiltrates without BHL	Disease less likely to resolve spontaneously
Stage IV: pulmonary fibrosis	Can cause progression to ventilatory failure, pulmonary hypertension and cor pulmonale

marker of disease activity. • CXR: used to stage sarcoid (Box 9.13). • HRCT: characteristic appearances include reticulonodular opacities that follow a perilymphatic distribution centred on bronchovascular bundles and the subpleural areas. • Pulmonary function: may show restriction and desaturation on exercise. • Bronchoscopy: may demonstrate a 'cobblestone' appearance of the mucosa, and bronchial and transbronchial biopsies usually show non-caseating granulomas.

The occurrence of erythema nodosum in patients in the second to third decades with BHL on CXR is often sufficient for a confident diagnosis.

Management

The majority of patients enjoy spontaneous remission and, if there is no evidence of organ damage, it is appropriate to withhold therapy for 6 mths. Patients who present with acute illness and erythema nodosum may require NSAIDs and, if systemically unwell, a short course of corticosteroids. Systemic corticosteroids are also indicated in the presence of hypercalcaemia, pulmonary function impairment and renal impairment. Uveitis responds to topical steroids. In patients with severe disease, both methotrexate and azathioprine have been used successfully and selected patients with severe disease may be referred for single lung transplantation.

Lung diseases due to systemic inflammatory disease
Acute respiratory distress syndrome
See page 25.

Respiratory involvement in connective tissue disorders
Pulmonary fibrosis is a recognised complication of many connective tissue diseases. The clinical features are usually indistinguishable

from those of IPF (p. 305) and lung disease may precede the onset of other symptoms. Connective tissue disorders may also cause disease of the pleura, diaphragm and chest wall muscles. Pulmonary hypertension and cor pulmonale may complicate pulmonary fibrosis in connective tissue disorders and is particularly common in systemic sclerosis.

Patients with connective tissue disease may also develop respiratory complications due to pulmonary toxic effects of drugs used to treat the connective tissue disorder (e.g. gold and methotrexate), and secondary infection due to neutropenia or immunosuppressive drug regimens.

Rheumatoid disease: Pulmonary fibrosis is the most common pulmonary manifestation. The clinical features, investigations, treatment and prognosis are usually similar to those of IPF. Pleural effusion is common, especially in men with seropositive disease. Most resolve spontaneously. Biochemical testing shows an exudative effusion with markedly reduced glucose levels and raised LDH. Effusions that fail to resolve spontaneously may respond to prednisolone (30–40 mg daily) but some become chronic. Rheumatoid pulmonary nodules are usually asymptomatic and detected incidentally on CXR. They are usually multiple and subpleural in site, and can mimic cancer. The combination of rheumatoid nodules and pneumoconiosis is known as Caplan's syndrome. Obliterative bronchiolitis and bronchiectasis are also recognised pulmonary complications of rheumatoid arthritis.

Treatments given for rheumatoid arthritis may also be relevant; corticosteroid therapy predisposes to infections, methotrexate may cause pulmonary fibrosis, and anti-TNF therapy has been associated with the reactivation of TB.

Systemic lupus erythematosus (SLE): Recurrent pleurisy is common in SLE, with or without effusions. An acute alveolitis may rarely be associated with diffuse alveolar haemorrhage. This condition is life-threatening and requires immunosuppression. Pulmonary fibrosis is a relatively uncommon manifestation of SLE. Some patients with SLE present with exertional dyspnoea and orthopnoea but without pulmonary fibrosis. Pulmonary function testing shows reduced lung volumes and the CXR reveals elevated diaphragms. This condition ('shrinking lungs') has been attributed to diaphragmatic myopathy. Antiphospholipid syndrome is associated with an increased risk of venous and pulmonary thromboembolism and these patients require lifelong anticoagulation.

Systemic sclerosis: Most patients with systemic sclerosis eventually develop diffuse pulmonary fibrosis (up to 90% at autopsy). In some patients it is indolent, but when progressive, as in IPF, the median survival is ~4 yrs. Pulmonary fibrosis is rare in the CREST variant of progressive systemic sclerosis but isolated pulmonary hypertension may develop. Other pulmonary complications include recurrent aspiration pneumonias secondary to oesophageal disease. Rarely, sclerosis of the skin of the chest wall may be so

i 9.14 Pulmonary eosinophilia

- Helminths, e.g. *Ascaris, Toxocara, Filaria*
- Drugs, e.g. nitrofurantoin, para-aminosalicylic acid (PAS), sulfasalazine, imipramine, chlorpropamide, phenylbutazone
- Fungi, e.g. *Aspergillus fumigatus* causing ABPA (p. 298)
- Cryptogenic eosinophilic pneumonia
- Churg–Strauss syndrome (asthma, blood eosinophilia, neuropathy, pulmonary infiltrates, eosinophilic vasculitis)
- Hypereosinophilic syndrome

extensive as to restrict chest wall movement – the so-called 'hidebound chest'.

Pulmonary eosinophilia and vasculitides

Pulmonary eosinophilia refers to a group of disorders of different aetiology in which lesions in the lungs produce a CXR abnormality associated with pulmonary eosinophilia with or without peripheral blood eosinophilia (Box 9.14). Pulmonary eosinophilias usually respond to withdrawal of the causative agent or to corticosteroids if idiopathic.

Granulomatosis with polyangiitis (formerly Wegener's granulomatosis): This presents with cough, haemoptysis, chest pain and fever. Nasal discharge and crusting, and otitis media also occur. Multiple cavitating nodules are seen on CXR. Nasal or lung biopsies show distinctive necrotising granulomas and vasculitis. Complications include subglottic stenosis and saddle nose deformity. Treatment is with immunosuppression.

Goodpasture's syndrome: IgG antibodies bind to the glomerular or alveolar basement membranes (p. 186), leading to glomerulonephritis and pulmonary haemorrhage. Pulmonary infiltrates, hypoxia and haemoptysis commonly precede renal involvement. It occurs more commonly in men and almost exclusively in smokers.

Lung diseases due to irradiation and drugs

Acute radiation pneumonitis is typically seen within 6–12 wks of lung irradiation, and causes cough and dyspnoea. This may resolve spontaneously but responds to corticosteroid treatment. Chronic interstitial fibrosis may present several months later.

Drugs may cause a number of parenchymal reactions:

ARDS: Hydrochlorothiazide, streptokinase, aspirin and opiates (in overdose).

Pulmonary eosinophilia: See Box 9.14.

Non-eosinophilic alveolitis: Amiodarone, gold, nitrofurantoin, bleomycin, methotrexate.

Pleural disease: Bromocriptine, amiodarone, methotrexate, methysergide, or others via induction of SLE (phenytoin, hydralazine, isoniazid).

Asthma: β-blockers, cholinergic antagonists, aspirin, NSAIDs.

OCCUPATIONAL AND ENVIRONMENTAL LUNG DISEASE

Occupational airway disease

Occupational asthma: This should be considered in any individual of working age who develops new-onset asthma, particularly if the patient reports an improvement in asthma symptoms during absences from work, e.g. at weekends or holidays. Sensitisation to the allergens may be demonstrated by skin testing or measurement of specific IgE. Serial recording of peak flow at work is crucial in confirming causation.

Reactive airways dysfunction syndrome: This is a persistent asthma-like syndrome with airway hyper-reactivity following the inhalation of an airway irritant: typically, a single exposure to a gas, smoke or vapour in very high concentrations. Management is similar to that of asthma.

COPD: Whilst smoking remains the dominant cause of COPD, occupational COPD is seen in workers exposed to coal dust, crystalline silica, cadmium and biomass fuel smoke.

Pneumoconiosis

This means a permanent alteration of lung structure due to the inhalation of mineral dust, excluding bronchitis and emphysema.

Coal worker's pneumoconiosis (CWP): Prolonged inhalation of coal dust overwhelms alveolar macrophages, leading to a fibrotic reaction. Classification is based on the size and extent of radiographic nodularity. Simple coal worker's pneumoconiosis (SCWP) refers to the appearance of small radiographic nodules in an otherwise well individual. Progressive massive fibrosis (PMF) refers to the formation of conglomerate masses (mainly in the upper lobes), which may cavitate, associated with cough, sputum and breathlessness. PMF may progress after coal dust exposure ceases and, in extreme cases, causes respiratory failure.

Silicosis: This occurs in stonemasons who inhale crystalline silica, usually as quartz dust. Classic silicosis develops slowly after years of asymptomatic exposure. Accelerated silicosis is associated with shorter exposure (typically 5–10 yrs) and is more aggressive. Radiological features are similar to those of CWP, with multiple 3–5-mm nodular opacities, in the mid- and upper zones. As the disease progresses, PMF may develop. Enlargement of the hilar glands with an 'egg-shell' calcification is uncommon and non-specific. The patient must be removed from further exposure, but fibrosis progresses even when exposure ceases. Individuals with silicosis are at increased risk of TB, lung cancer and COPD.

Asbestos-related lung and pleural diseases

Asbestos is a naturally occurring silicate, classified into chrysotile (white asbestos: 90% of world production) and serpentine types (crocidolite, blue asbestos, and amosite – brown asbestos). It was used extensively as thermal insulation in industry in the mid-20th

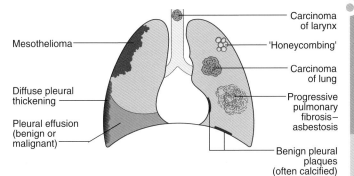

Fig. 9.11 Asbestos: the range of possible effects on the respiratory tract.

Labels in figure:
- Mesothelioma
- Diffuse pleural thickening
- Pleural effusion (benign or malignant)
- Carcinoma of larynx
- 'Honeycombing'
- Carcinoma of lung
- Progressive pulmonary fibrosis—asbestosis
- Benign pleural plaques (often calcified)

century. Asbestos exposure may lead to both pleural and pulmonary disease (Fig. 9.11), after a lengthy latent period.

Pleural plaques: Discrete areas of fibrosis on the parietal pleura, the most common manifestation of past asbestos exposure. They are asymptomatic and are usually identified incidentally on CXR or CT scan, particularly when partially calcified. They do not cause impairment of lung function and are benign.

Acute benign asbestos pleurisy: Estimated to occur in one-fifth of asbestos workers but many episodes are subclinical. When symptomatic, patients present with pleurisy and mild fever. Diagnosis necessitates the exclusion of other known causes of pleurisy and effusion. Repeated episodes may lead to diffuse pleural thickening.

Diffuse pleural thickening (DPT): Affects the visceral pleura and, if extensive, may cause restrictive lung function impairment, exertional breathlessness and, occasionally, persistent chest pain. The CXR shows extensive pleural thickening and obliteration of the costophrenic angles. There is no treatment and the condition may progress in around one-third of individuals. In severe cases, surgical decortication may be considered. Pleural biopsy may be required to exclude mesothelioma.

Asbestosis: A diffuse parenchymal lung disease that occurs after substantial exposure over several years, and is rare with low-level or bystander exposure. It presents with exertional breathlessness and fine, late inspiratory crackles over the lower zones. Finger clubbing may be present. Pulmonary function tests and HRCT appearances are similar to those of UIP. These features, accompanied by a history of substantial asbestos exposure, are generally sufficient to establish the diagnosis; lung biopsy is rarely necessary. Asbestosis is more slowly progressive and carries a better prognosis than UIP. About 40% of patients (usually smokers) develop lung cancer and 10% develop mesothelioma.

Mesothelioma: A malignant tumour affecting the pleura or, rarely, the peritoneum. It almost invariably results from past asbestos exposure, which may be minor. There is a long interval between exposure and disease, so deaths from mesothelioma continue to increase, despite improved asbestos control. Pleural mesothelioma presents with increasing breathlessness resulting from pleural effusion, or unremitting chest pain due to chest wall involvement. As the tumour progresses, it encases the lung and may invade the parenchyma, the mediastinum and the pericardium. Metastatic disease is commonly found at post-mortem. Prognosis is poor. Highly selected patients may benefit from radical surgery, but, in most, therapy aims to palliate symptoms. Chemotherapy may improve quality of life and yield a small survival benefit (~3 mths). Radiotherapy is used to control pain and limit the risk of tumour seeding at biopsy sites. Pleural effusions are managed with drainage and pleurodesis. Survival from onset of symptoms is ~16 mths for epithelioid tumours, 10 mths for sarcomatoid tumours and 15 mths for biphasic tumours.

Lung diseases due to organic dusts
Hypersensitivity pneumonitis

Hypersensitivity pneumonitis (HP; also called extrinsic allergic alveolitis) results from the inhalation of certain types of organic dust that give rise to a diffuse immune complex reaction in the walls of the alveoli and bronchioles. In the UK, 50% of reported cases of HP occur in farm workers; bird fanciers represent another important group.

Clinical features

The acute form of HP should be suspected when anyone exposed to organic dust complains of 'flu'-like symptoms (headache, malaise, myalgia, fever, dry cough, breathlessness) within a few hours of re-exposure to the same dust. Auscultation reveals widespread end-inspiratory crackles and squeaks. Disease onset is more insidious with chronic low-level exposure (e.g. from an indoor pet bird). If unchecked, the disease may progress to cause fibrosis, severe respiratory disability, hypoxaemia, pulmonary hypertension, cor pulmonale and eventually death.

Investigations

• CXR: demonstrates diffuse micronodular shadowing, which is usually more pronounced in the upper zones. • HRCT: in acute disease, shows bilateral areas of ground glass and consolidation with small centrilobar nodules and expiratory air-trapping. In chronic disease, fibrosis may predominate. • Pulmonary function tests: show a restrictive ventilatory defect with reduced lung volumes and gas transfer. • ABGs: may reveal hypoxia in advanced disease. • Serology: shows positive precipitating antibodies to the offending antigen, e.g. *Micropolyspora faeni* (farmer's lung) or avian serum proteins (bird fancier's lung). However, precipitating antibodies may also be present without evidence of HP. • Bronchoalveolar lavage: may show increased CD8+ T lymphocytes. • Lung biopsy: may be necessary for diagnosis.

Management

Whenever possible, the patient should avoid exposure to the inciting agent. This may be difficult, either because of implications for livelihood (e.g. farmers) or addiction to hobbies (e.g. pigeon breeders). Dust masks with appropriate filters may minimise exposure and may be combined with methods of reducing levels of antigen (e.g. drying hay before storage). In acute cases, prednisolone 40 mg/day should be given for 3–4 wks. Most patients recover completely, but the development of interstitial fibrosis causes permanent disability when there has been prolonged exposure to antigen.

PULMONARY VASCULAR DISEASE

Venous thromboembolism

Deep venous thrombosis (DVT) and pulmonary embolism (PE) can be considered under this heading. The majority (80%) of PEs arise from the propagation of lower limb DVT. Rare causes include amniotic fluid, placenta, air, fat, tumour (especially choriocarcinoma) and septic emboli (from endocarditis affecting the tricuspid/pulmonary valves). PE is common, occurring in ~1% of all patients admitted to hospital and accounting for ~5% of in-hospital deaths.

Clinical features

The varied clinical presentation, non-specific nature of the physical signs and the lack of sensitive and specific diagnostic tests can make the diagnosis of PE difficult. It is helpful to consider three questions:

• Is the clinical presentation consistent with PE? • Does the patient have risk factors for PE? • Is there any alternative diagnosis that can explain the patient's presentation?

A recognised risk factor for PE (Box 9.15) is present in 80–90% of patients. The clinical features (Box 9.16) depend largely upon the size of embolism and on comorbidity.

Investigations

CXR: PE may cause a variety of non-specific appearances but most cases have a normal CXR. A normal CXR in an acutely breathless and hypoxaemic patient should raise the suspicion of PE, as should bilateral atelectasis in a patient with unilateral pleuritic chest pain. CXR can also exclude alternatives such as heart failure, pneumonia or pneumothorax.

ECG: ECG is often normal but is helpful in excluding alternatives, e.g. myocardial infarction (MI) or pericarditis. The most common findings in PE are sinus tachycardia and anterior T-wave inversion;

9.15 Risk factors for venous thromboembolism

Surgery	Major abdominal/pelvic surgery; hip/knee surgery; post-operative intensive care
Pregnancy/puerperium	
Cardiorespiratory disease	COPD, congestive cardiac failure or other disabling disease
Lower limb problems	Fracture; varicose veins; stroke/spinal cord injury
Malignant disease	Abdominal/pelvic; advanced/metastatic; concurrent chemotherapy
Miscellaneous	Increasing age, previous proven VTE, immobility, thrombotic disorders (p. 558), trauma

9.16 Categorisation of pulmonary thromboemboli

	Acute massive PE	Acute small/medium PE	Chronic PE
Symptoms	Faintness or collapse, central chest pain, apprehension, severe dyspnoea	Pleuritic chest pain, restricted breathing, haemoptysis	Exertional dyspnoea; late symptoms of pulmonary hypertension or right heart failure
Signs	Major circulatory collapse: tachycardia, hypotension, ↑JVP, right ventricular (RV) gallop rhythm, split P_2; severe cyanosis; ↓urinary output	Tachycardia, pleural rub, raised hemidiaphragm, crackles, effusion (often blood-stained), low-grade fever	Early in disease: may be minimal Later: RV heave, loud, split P_2 Advanced: right heart failure
CXR	Usually normal; may be subtle oligaemia	Pleuropulmonary opacities, pleural effusion, linear shadows, raised hemidiaphragm	Enlarged pulmonary artery trunk, enlarged heart, prominent RV
ECG	$S_1Q_3T_3$, anterior T-wave inversion, right bundle branch block	Sinus tachycardia	RV hypertrophy and strain
ABGs	Markedly abnormal with ↓PaO_2 and ↓$PaCO_2$; metabolic acidosis	May be normal or ↓PaO_2	Exertional ↓PaO_2 or desaturation on exercise testing
Alternative diagnoses	Myocardial infarction, pericardial tamponade, aortic dissection	Pneumonia, pneumothorax, musculoskeletal chest pain	Other causes of pulmonary hypertension

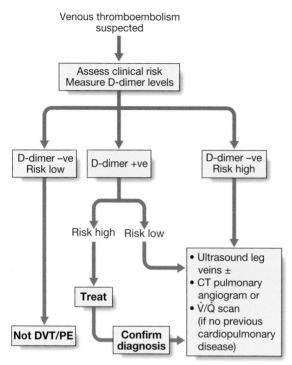

Venous thromboembolism
suspected

Assess clinical risk
Measure D-dimer levels

D-dimer –ve
Risk low

D-dimer +ve

D-dimer –ve
Risk high

Risk high   Risk low

• Ultrasound leg
  veins ±
• CT pulmonary
  angiogram or
• V̇/Q̇ scan
  (if no previous
  cardiopulmonary
  disease)

Treat

Not DVT/PE

**Confirm
diagnosis**

Fig. 9.12 Algorithm for the investigation of patients with suspected pulmonary thromboembolism. Clinical risk is based on the presence of risk factors for VTE and the probability of another diagnosis.

larger emboli may cause right heart strain with an $S_1Q_3T_3$ pattern, ST-segment and T-wave changes, or right bundle branch block.

ABGs: Typically show a reduced PaO_2 and a normal or low $PaCO_2$, but are occasionally normal. Metabolic acidosis may occur in acute massive PE with shock.

D-dimer: A degradation product of fibrin, released into the circulation during endogenous fibrinolysis. A low D-dimer has a high negative predictive value and is a useful screening test (Fig. 9.12). However, a suggestive clinical picture in a high-risk patient must be investigated, even when the D-dimer level is normal. Non-specific elevations of D-dimer are observed in a number of conditions other than PE, including MI, pneumonia and sepsis.

CTPA: This is now the first-line diagnostic test (Fig. 9.13). It may not only exclude PE but also reveal an alternative diagnosis. Contrast media are, however, nephrotoxic and care should be taken in patients with renal impairment.

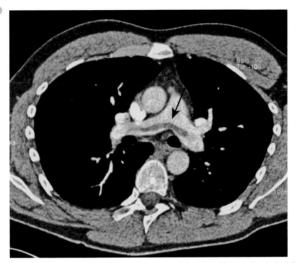

Fig. 9.13 CT pulmonary angiogram. The arrow points to a saddle embolism in the bifurcation of the pulmonary artery.

Ventilation/perfusion scanning: This is seldom used nowadays, although a limited role remains in patients without significant cardiopulmonary disease.

Doppler USS of the leg veins: This remains the investigation of choice in patients with suspected DVT but may also be used in patients with suspected PE, particularly if there are clinical signs in a limb, as many will have identifiable proximal leg vein thrombus.

Echocardiography: This is helpful in the differential diagnosis and assessment of acute circulatory collapse. Acute right heart dilatation is frequently present in massive PE, and thrombus may be visible. Alternative diagnoses, including left ventricular failure, aortic dissection and pericardial tamponade, can also be established.

Pulmonary angiography: This has largely been superseded by CTPA.

Management

Sufficient oxygen should be given to all hypoxaemic patients to restore SpO_2 to >90%. Hypotension should be treated using IV fluid or plasma expander; diuretics and vasodilators should be avoided. Opiates may be necessary to relieve pain and distress but should be used with caution. External cardiac massage may be successful in the moribund patient by dislodging and breaking up a large central embolus.

Anticoagulation: This should be commenced immediately in patients with a high or intermediate probability of PE, but can be safely withheld from patients with a low clinical probability pending investigations. Subcutaneous low molecular weight heparin (LMWH) is as effective as IV unfractionated heparin; the dose is standardised for weight and it does not require monitoring by blood tests. Heparin reduces mortality in PE by reducing clot propagation and the risk of further emboli. It should be administered for at least 5 days and anticoagulation continued using oral anticoagulants, usually warfarin. Heparin should not be discontinued until the INR is >2 for at least 24 hrs. Newer oral alternatives to warfarin offer the chance to avoid blood monitoring, but are harder to reverse in emergencies. The optimum duration of warfarin therapy is not clear but current guidelines suggest:

• Patients with persistent risk factors or previous VTE: should be anticoagulated for life. • Patients with a reversible risk factor: 3 mths of therapy. • Patients with cancer-associated VTE: LMWH is more effective than warfarin. • Patients with unprovoked VTE: prolonged therapy should be considered, particularly in males, those in whom the D-dimer remains elevated 1 mth after stopping warfarin, and those in whom recurrent PE may be fatal.

The balance between risk of recurrence and risk of haemorrhage should be discussed with the patient.

Thrombolytic therapy: Thrombolysis improves outcome when acute massive PE is accompanied by shock (systolic BP <90 mmHg) but shows no advantage over heparin in normotensive patients. Treatment carries a risk of intracranial haemorrhage and patients must be screened carefully for haemorrhagic risk.

Caval filters: Selected patients with recurrent PE despite adequate anticoagulation or those in whom anticoagulation is contraindicated may benefit from insertion of a filter in the inferior vena cava below the origin of the renal veins.

Prognosis

Immediate mortality is greatest in those with echocardiographic evidence of right ventricular dysfunction or cardiogenic shock. Once anticoagulation is commenced, however, the risk of mortality falls rapidly. The risk of recurrence is highest in the first 6–12 mths after the initial event, and at 10 yrs around one-third of individuals will have suffered a further event.

Pulmonary hypertension

Pulmonary hypertension is defined as a mean pulmonary artery pressure of >25 mmHg at rest. The causes are listed in Box 9.17. Further classification is based on the degree of functional disturbance using the New York Heart Association (NYHA) grades I–IV. Respiratory failure due to intrinsic pulmonary disease is the most common cause of pulmonary hypertension.

Primary pulmonary hypertension (PPH) is a rare but important disease that predominantly affects women, aged 20–30 yrs. It is usually sporadic but rarely is associated with an inherited mutation.

9.17 Classification of pulmonary hypertension

Pulmonary arterial hypertension	Primary: sporadic and familial Secondary: collagen vascular disease (limited cutaneous systemic sclerosis), congenital systemic to pulmonary shunts, portal hypertension, HIV infection, exposure to various drugs or toxins, persistent pulmonary hypertension of the newborn
Pulmonary venous hypertension	Left-sided valvular or ventricular disease, pulmonary veno-occlusive disease
Pulmonary hypertension associated with parenchymal lung disease and/or hypoxaemia	COPD; DPLD; sleep-disordered breathing; chronic high-altitude exposure, severe kyphoscoliosis
Chronic thromboembolic disease	

Adapted from Dana Point 2008. Simmoneau G, et al. Updated clinical classification of pulmonary hypertension. J Am Coll Cardiol 2009; 54:S43–554.

Presentation is with exertional breathlessness and syncope. Radiology shows enlarged pulmonary arteries and echocardiography shows an enlarged right ventricle; pulmonary artery pressure can be estimated from the velocity of tricuspid regurgitation on Doppler echo.

The median survival from time of diagnosis (without heart–lung transplantation) is 2–3 yrs. Management should be guided by specialists and includes diuretics, oxygen, anticoagulation and vaccination against infection. Specific treatments include iloprost, epoprostenol, sildenafil and the oral endothelin receptor antagonist bosentan; these can dramatically improve exercise performance symptoms and prognosis in selected cases. Pulmonary thromboendarterectomy should be contemplated in patients with chronic proximal pulmonary thromboembolism and heart–lung transplantation may be considered in selected patients.

DISEASES OF THE UPPER AIRWAY

Diseases of the nasopharynx
Allergic rhinitis

In this disorder there are episodes of nasal congestion, watery nasal discharge and sneezing. It may be seasonal or perennial (continuous symptoms). It is due to an immediate hypersensitivity reaction to antigens including pollens from grasses (hay fever), flowers, weeds or trees. Perennial allergic rhinitis may be a reaction to antigens from house dust, fungal spores or animal dander, or to physical or chemical irritants. Skin hypersensitivity tests with the relevant antigen are

RESPIRATORY DISEASE · 9

usually positive in seasonal allergic rhinitis but less useful in perennial rhinitis.

Management

Exposure to trigger antigens (e.g. pollen) should be minimised. The following medications may be used singly or in combination: an oral antihistamine, a topical steroid nasal spray and/or sodium cromoglicate nasal spray. When severe symptoms interfere with daily activities, oral corticosteroids are occasionally indicated.

Sleep-disordered breathing

A variety of respiratory disorders manifest themselves during sleep, e.g. nocturnal cough and wheeze in asthma. Nocturnal hypoventilation may exacerbate respiratory failure in patients with restrictive lung disease such as that due to kyphoscoliosis, diaphragmatic palsy, or muscle weakness (e.g. muscular dystrophy). In contrast, a small but important group of disorders cause problems only during sleep due to upper airway obstruction (obstructive sleep apnoea) or abnormalities of ventilatory drive (central sleep apnoea).

The sleep apnoea/hypopnoea syndrome

It is now recognised that 2–4% of the middle-aged population suffers from recurrent upper airway obstruction during sleep, which causes sleep fragmentation leading to daytime sleepiness. This results in a threefold increased risk of road traffic accidents.

A reduction in upper airway muscle tone during sleep results in pharyngeal narrowing, which often manifests as snoring. Negative pharyngeal pressure during inspiration can then cause complete upper airway occlusion, usually at the level of the soft palate. This leads to transient wakefulness and recovery of upper airway muscle tone. The subject rapidly returns to sleep, snores and becomes apnoeic once more. This cycle repeats itself many times, causing severe sleep fragmentation (the sleep apnoea/hypopnoea syndrome; SAHS). Predisposing factors include:
• Obesity. • Male gender. • Nasal obstruction. • Acromegaly.
• Hypothyroidism. • Familial causes (back-set mandible and maxilla).
• Alcohol and sedatives (relaxation of the upper airway dilating muscles).

Clinical features

Excessive daytime sleepiness is the principal symptom. Snoring is virtually universal; bed partners report loud snoring in all body positions and often notice multiple breathing pauses (apnoeas). Sleep is unrefreshing. Patients have difficulty with concentration, impaired cognitive function and work performance, depression, irritability and nocturia.

Investigations

A quantitative assessment of daytime sleepiness can be obtained by questionnaire (e.g. Epworth Sleepiness Scale). Overnight studies of breathing, oxygenation and sleep quality are diagnostic (SAHS defined as >15 apnoeas/hypopnoeas per hr of sleep).

Differential diagnosis

Narcolepsy is a rare cause of sleepiness, occurring in 0.05% of the population, and is associated with cataplexy (when muscle tone is lost in fully conscious people in response to emotional triggers), hypnagogic hallucinations (hallucinations at sleep onset) and sleep paralysis.

Idiopathic hypersomnolence occurs in younger individuals and is characterised by long nocturnal sleeps.

Management

The major risk is traffic accidents and all drivers must be advised not to drive until treatment has relieved their sleepiness. Weight reduction and avoidance of alcohol and sedatives is beneficial. Most patients need overnight CPAP by nasal/face mask, which prevents upper airway collapse during sleep. CPAP often leads to dramatic improvements in symptoms, daytime performance and quality of life. Unfortunately, 30–50% of patients are poorly compliant or intolerant of CPAP. Mandibular advancement devices are an alternative approach. There is no evidence that palatal surgery is of benefit.

Laryngeal disorders

The most common symptom of laryngeal disorders is hoarseness. The differential diagnosis of hoarseness that persists beyond a few days is:

• Laryngeal tumour. • Vocal cord paralysis. • Inhaled corticosteroid treatment. • Chronic laryngitis due to excessive use of the voice (particularly in dusty atmospheres). • Heavy smoking. • Chronic infection of nasal sinuses.

Laryngeal paralysis

Disease affecting the motor nerve supply of the larynx is nearly always unilateral and, because of the intrathoracic course of the left recurrent laryngeal nerve, usually left-sided. One or both recurrent laryngeal nerves may be damaged at thyroidectomy or by thyroid carcinoma. Symptoms are hoarseness, a 'bovine cough' and stridor, which may be severe if both vocal cords are affected. In some patients, a CXR may bring to light an unsuspected bronchial carcinoma or pulmonary TB. If no such abnormality is found, laryngoscopy should be performed. In unilateral paralysis, the voice may be improved by injection of Teflon into the affected cord. In bilateral paralysis, tracheal intubation, tracheostomy or laryngeal surgery may be necessary.

Laryngeal obstruction

Laryngeal obstruction is more liable to occur in children than in adults because of the smaller size of the glottis. Sudden complete laryngeal obstruction by a foreign body causes acute asphyxia

– violent but ineffective inspiratory efforts with indrawing of the intercostal spaces and the unsupported lower ribs, accompanied by cyanosis. Unrelieved, the condition is rapidly fatal. When, as in most cases, the obstruction is incomplete at first, the clinical features are progressive breathlessness accompanied by stridor and cyanosis.

Management

Urgent treatment to relieve obstruction is needed:

• When a foreign body causes laryngeal obstruction in children, it can often be dislodged by turning the patient head downwards and squeezing the chest vigorously. • In adults this is often impossible, but a sudden forceful compression of the upper abdomen (Heimlich manœuvre) may be effective. • In other circumstances, the cause should be investigated by direct laryngoscopy, which may also permit the removal of an unsuspected foreign body or the insertion of a tube past the obstruction into the trachea. • Tracheostomy must be performed without delay if these procedures fail to relieve obstruction, but except in dire emergencies this operation should be performed in an operating theatre by a surgeon. • In angioedema, complete laryngeal occlusion can usually be prevented by treatment with adrenaline (epinephrine) 0.5–1 mg (0.5–1 mL of 1:1000) IM, chlorphenamine maleate 10–20 mg by slow IV injection, and IV hydrocortisone sodium succinate 200 mg.

Tracheal disorders
Tracheal obstruction

External compression by enlarged mediastinal lymph nodes containing metastatic deposits, usually from a bronchial carcinoma, is a more frequent cause of tracheal obstruction than the uncommon primary benign or malignant tumours. Rarely, the trachea may be compressed by an aneurysm of the aortic arch, by a retrosternal goitre, or in children by tuberculous mediastinal lymph nodes. Tracheal stenosis is an occasional complication of tracheostomy, prolonged intubation, granulomatosis with polyangiitis or trauma.

Clinical features

Stridor can be detected in every patient with severe tracheal narrowing. Bronchoscopy should be undertaken without delay to determine the site, degree and nature of the obstruction.

Management

Localised tumours of the trachea can be resected but reconstruction after resection may be technically difficult. Endobronchial laser therapy, bronchoscopically placed tracheal stents, chemotherapy and radiotherapy are alternatives to surgery.

Tracheo-oesophageal fistula

This may be a congenital abnormality in newborn infants. In adults, it is usually due to malignant lesions in the mediastinum, such as carcinoma or lymphoma, eroding both the trachea and oesophagus to produce a communication between them. Swallowed liquids enter the trachea and bronchi through the fistula and provoke coughing.

Management

Surgical closure of a congenital fistula, if undertaken promptly, is usually successful. There is usually no curative treatment for malignant fistulae, and death from overwhelming pulmonary infection rapidly supervenes.

PLEURAL DISEASE

Pleurisy, pleural effusion and empyema are described under presenting problems above.

Pneumothorax

Pneumothorax is the presence of air in the pleural space, which can either occur spontaneously, or result from iatrogenic injury or trauma to the lung or chest wall. Primary spontaneous pneumothorax occurs in patients with no history of lung disease. Smoking, tall stature and the presence of apical subpleural blebs are known risk factors. Secondary pneumothorax affects patients with pre-existing lung disease, especially COPD, bullous emphysema and asthma. It is most common in older patients and is associated with the highest mortality rates.

Clinical features

There is sudden-onset unilateral pleuritic chest pain or breathlessness (those with underlying chest disease may have severe breathlessness). With a small pneumothorax the physical examination may be normal; a larger pneumothorax (>15% of the hemithorax) results in decreased or absent breath sounds and a resonant percussion note. A tension pneumothorax occurs when a small communication acts as a one-way valve, allowing air to enter the pleural space from the lung during inspiration but not to escape on expiration; this causes raised intrapleural pressure, which leads to mediastinal displacement, compression of the opposite lung, impaired systemic venous return and cardiovascular compromise.

Investigations

CXR shows the sharply defined edge of the deflated lung with a complete lack of lung markings between this and the chest wall. CXR also shows any mediastinal displacement and gives information regarding the presence or absence of pleural fluid and underlying pulmonary disease. Care must be taken to differentiate between a large pre-existing emphysematous bulla and a pneumothorax to avoid misdirected attempts at aspiration; where doubt exists, CT is useful in distinguishing bullae from pleural air.

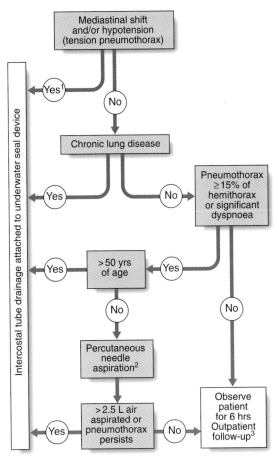

Fig. 9.14 Management of spontaneous pneumothorax. (1) Immediate decompression is required prior to insertion of an intercostal drain. (2) Aspirate in the 2nd intercostal space anteriorly in the mid-clavicular line; discontinue if resistance is felt, the patient coughs excessively, or >2.5 L are aspirated. (3) All patients should be told to attend again immediately in the event of noticeable deterioration.

Management (Fig. 9.14)

Primary pneumothorax, where the lung edge is <2 cm from the chest wall and the patient is not breathless, normally resolves without intervention. In young patients presenting with a moderate or large spontaneous primary pneumothorax, an attempt at percutaneous needle aspiration of air should be made in the first instance, with a 60–80% chance of avoiding the need for a chest drain. Patients with chronic lung disease usually require a chest tube and inpatient observation, as even a small pneumothorax may cause respiratory failure.

Intercostal drains should be inserted in the 4th, 5th or 6th intercostal space in the mid-axillary line, following blunt dissection through to the parietal pleura, or by using a guidewire and dilator ('Seldinger' technique). The tube should be advanced in an apical direction, connected to an underwater seal or one-way Heimlich valve, and secured firmly to the chest wall. Clamping of the drain is potentially dangerous and never indicated. The drain should be removed 24 hrs after the lung has fully re-inflated and bubbling stopped. Continued bubbling after 5–7 days is an indication for surgery.

Supplemental oxygen is given, as this accelerates the rate at which air is reabsorbed by the pleura. Patients with an unresolved pneumothorax should not fly until the pleural air is gone, as the trapped gas expands at altitude. Patients should be advised to stop smoking and informed about the risks of a recurrent pneumothorax (25% after primary spontaneous pneumothorax).

Recurrent spontaneous pneumothorax: Surgical pleurodesis, with thoracoscopic pleural abrasion or pleurectomy, is recommended in all patients following a second pneumothorax (even if ipsilateral), and should be considered following the first episode of secondary pneumothorax if low respiratory reserve makes recurrence hazardous. Patients who plan to continue activities where pneumothorax would be particularly dangerous (e.g. diving) should also undergo definitive treatment after the first episode of a primary spontaneous pneumothorax.

DISEASES OF THE DIAPHRAGM

Congenital disorders: Congenital defects of the diaphragm (foramina of Bochdalek and Morgagni) can allow herniation of abdominal viscera. Abnormal elevation or bulging of one hemidiaphragm (eventration of the diaphragm), more often the left, may result from total or partial absence of muscular development of the septum transversum.

Acquired disorders: Phrenic nerve damage leading to diaphragmatic paralysis may be idiopathic but is most often due to bronchial carcinoma. Other causes include disease of cervical vertebrae, tumours of the cervical cord, shingles, trauma including road traffic and birth injuries, surgery, and stretching of the nerve by mediastinal masses and aortic aneurysms. CXR demonstrates elevation of the hemidiaphragm. Screening USS can demonstrate paradoxical upward movement of the paralysed hemidiaphragm on sniffing. Bilateral diaphragmatic weakness occurs in neuromuscular disease of any type including Guillain–Barré syndrome, poliomyelitis, muscular dystrophies, motor neuron disease and connective tissue disorders, such as SLE and polymyositis.

DEFORMITIES OF THE CHEST WALL

Thoracic kyphoscoliosis: Abnormalities of alignment of the dorsal spine and their consequent effects on thoracic shape may be congenital or caused by:
• Vertebral disease, including TB. • Osteoporosis. • Ankylosing spondylitis. • Trauma. • Previous lung surgery. • Neuromuscular disease such as poliomyelitis.

Kyphoscoliosis, if severe, restricts and distorts expansion of the chest wall. Patients with severe deformity may develop type II respiratory failure.

Pectus excavatum: In pectus excavatum (funnel chest), the body of the sternum, usually only the lower end, is curved backwards. This is rarely of any clinical consequence. Operative correction is usually only indicated for cosmetic reasons.

Pectus carinatum: Pectus carinatum (pigeon chest) is frequently caused by severe asthma during childhood.

Endocrine disease

Endocrinology concerns the synthesis, secretion and action of hormones. These are chemical messengers released from endocrine glands that coordinate the activities of many different cells. Endocrine disease, therefore, has a wide range of manifestations in many organs.

MAJOR ENDOCRINE FUNCTIONS AND ANATOMY

Although some endocrine glands (e.g. the parathyroids and pancreas) respond directly to metabolic signals, most are controlled by hormones released from the pituitary gland. Anterior pituitary hormone secretion is controlled in turn by substances produced in the hypothalamus and released into portal blood, which flows down the pituitary stalk. Posterior pituitary hormones are synthesised in the hypothalamus and transported down nerve axons to be released from the posterior pituitary. Hormone release in the hypothalamus and pituitary is regulated by numerous nervous, metabolic, physical or hormonal stimuli: in particular, feedback control by hormones produced by target glands (thyroid, adrenal cortex and gonads). These integrated endocrine systems are called 'axes' (Figs 10.1 and 10.2).

Some hormones (e.g. insulin, adrenaline (epinephrine)) act on specific cell surface receptors. Other hormones (e.g. steroids, triiodothyronine, vitamin D) bind to specific intracellular receptors, which in turn bind to response elements on DNA to regulate gene transcription.

The classical model of endocrine function involves hormones that are synthesised in endocrine glands and are released into the circulation, acting at sites distant from those of secretion. However, many other organs also secrete hormones or contribute to the metabolism and activation of pro-hormones; many hormones act on adjacent cells (paracrine system, e.g. neurotransmitters) or even act back on the cell of origin (autocrine system); and the sensitivity of target tissues is regulated in a tissue-specific fashion.

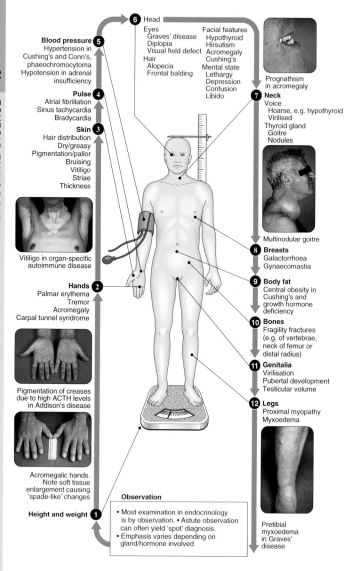

6 Head
Eyes
  Graves' disease
  Diplopia
  Visual field defect
Hair
  Alopecia
  Frontal balding

Facial features
  Hypothyroid
  Hirsutism
  Acromegaly
  Cushing's
Mental state
  Lethargy
  Depression
  Confusion
  Libido

5 Blood pressure
Hypertension in
Cushing's and Conn's,
phaeochromocytoma
Hypotension in adrenal
insufficiency

4 Pulse
Atrial fibrillation
Sinus tachycardia
Bradycardia

3 Skin
Hair distribution
Dry/greasy
Pigmentation/pallor
Bruising
Vitiligo
Striae
Thickness

Vitiligo in organ-specific
autoimmune disease

2 Hands
Palmar erythema
Tremor
Acromegaly
Carpal tunnel syndrome

Pigmentation of creases
due to high ACTH levels
in Addison's disease

Acromegalic hands.
Note soft tissue
enlargement causing
'spade-like' changes

Height and weight **1**

Prognathism
in acromegaly

7 Neck
Voice
  Hoarse, e.g. hypothyroid
  Virilised
Thyroid gland
  Goitre
  Nodules

Multinodular goitre

8 Breasts
Galactorrhoea
Gynaecomastia

9 Body fat
Central obesity in
Cushing's and
growth hormone
deficiency

10 Bones
Fragility fractures
(e.g. of vertebrae,
neck of femur or
distal radius)

11 Genitalia
Virilisation
Pubertal development
Testicular volume

12 Legs
Proximal myopathy
Myxoedema

Pretibial
myxoedema
in Graves'
disease

Observation
• Most examination in endocrinology
  is by observation. • Astute observation
  can often yield 'spot' diagnosis.
• Emphasis varies depending on
  gland/hormone involved

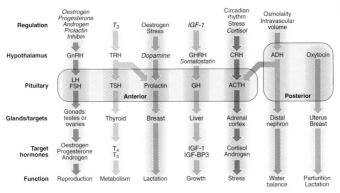

Fig. 10.1 The principal endocrine 'axes' and glands. Parathyroid glands, adrenal zona glomerulosa and endocrine pancreas are not controlled by the pituitary. Italics show negative regulation. (GnRH = gonadotrophin-releasing hormone. For other abbreviations see text.)

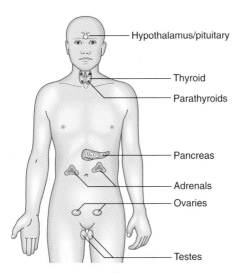

Fig. 10.2 The principal endocrine glands.

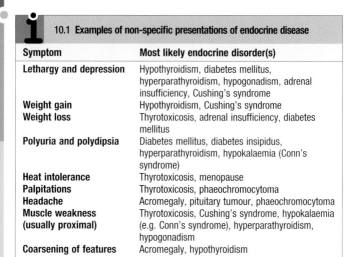

i 10.1 Examples of non-specific presentations of endocrine disease

Symptom	Most likely endocrine disorder(s)
Lethargy and depression	Hypothyroidism, diabetes mellitus, hyperparathyroidism, hypogonadism, adrenal insufficiency, Cushing's syndrome
Weight gain	Hypothyroidism, Cushing's syndrome
Weight loss	Thyrotoxicosis, adrenal insufficiency, diabetes mellitus
Polyuria and polydipsia	Diabetes mellitus, diabetes insipidus, hyperparathyroidism, hypokalaemia (Conn's syndrome)
Heat intolerance	Thyrotoxicosis, menopause
Palpitations	Thyrotoxicosis, phaeochromocytoma
Headache	Acromegaly, pituitary tumour, phaeochromocytoma
Muscle weakness (usually proximal)	Thyrotoxicosis, Cushing's syndrome, hypokalaemia (e.g. Conn's syndrome), hyperparathyroidism, hypogonadism
Coarsening of features	Acromegaly, hypothyroidism

Pathology arising within an endocrine gland is often called 'primary' disease (e.g. primary hypothyroidism in Hashimoto's thyroiditis), while abnormal stimulation of the gland is often called 'secondary' disease (e.g. secondary hypothyroidism in patients with thyroid-stimulating hormone (TSH) deficiency).

PRESENTING PROBLEMS IN ENDOCRINE DISEASE

Patients with endocrine disease present in many ways, to many different specialists, reflecting the diverse effects of hormone deficiency and excess. Presenting symptoms are often non-specific and long-standing (Box 10.1). In many patients, endocrine disease is asymptomatic and detected by routine biochemical testing. The most common classical presentations are of thyroid disease, reproductive disorders and hypercalcaemia. In addition, endocrine diseases are often part of the differential diagnosis of other disorders, including electrolyte abnormalities, hypertension, obesity and osteoporosis. Although diseases of the adrenal glands, hypothalamus and pituitary are relatively rare, their diagnosis often relies on astute clinical observation in a patient with non-specific complaints, so it is important that clinicians are familiar with their key features.

THE THYROID GLAND

Diseases of the thyroid affect 5% of the population, predominantly females. The thyroid axis is involved in the regulation of cellular differentiation and metabolism in virtually all nucleated cells, so that disorders of thyroid function have diverse manifestations. Follicular epithelial cells synthesise thyroid hormones by incorporating iodine into the amino acid tyrosine. The thyroid secretes predominantly thyroxine (T_4) and only a small amount of triiodothyronine (T_3), the more active hormone; ~85% of T_3 in blood is produced from peripheral conversion of T_4. They both circulate in plasma almost entirely (>99%) bound to transport proteins, mainly thyroxine-binding globulin (TBG). The unbound hormones diffuse into tissues and exert diverse metabolic actions. The advantage of measuring free over total hormone is that the former is not influenced by changes in TBG concentrations; in pregnancy, for example, TBG rise and total T_3/T_4 may be raised, but free thyroid hormone levels are normal.

Production of T_3 and T_4 in the thyroid is stimulated by thyroid-stimulating hormone (TSH), a glycoprotein released from the thyrotroph cells of the anterior pituitary in response to the hypothalamic tripeptide thyrotrophin-releasing hormone (TRH). There is a negative feedback of thyroid hormones on the hypothalamus and pituitary such that in thyrotoxicosis, when plasma concentrations of T_3 and T_4 are raised, TSH secretion is suppressed. Conversely, in primary hypothyroidism, low T_3 and T_4 are associated with high circulating TSH levels. TSH is, therefore, regarded as the most useful investigation of thyroid function. However, TSH may take several weeks to 'catch up' with T_4/T_3 levels, e.g. after prolonged suppression of TSH in thyrotoxicosis is relieved by antithyroid therapy. Common patterns of abnormal thyroid function tests (TFTs) are shown in Box 10.2.

Presenting problems in thyroid disease

Thyrotoxicosis

Approximately 76% of cases are due to Graves' disease, 14% to multinodular goitre and 5% to toxic adenoma. Less common causes include transient thyroiditis (de Quervain's, post-partum), iodide-induced (drugs, supplementation), factitious and TSH-secreting pituitary tumour.

Clinical assessment

Manifestations of thyrotoxicosis are shown in Box 10.3. The most common symptoms are:

• Weight loss with a normal appetite. • Heat intolerance.
• Palpitations. • Tremor. • Irritability.

All causes of thyrotoxicosis can cause lid retraction and lid lag, but only Graves' disease causes exophthalmos, ophthalmoplegia and papilloedema.

Investigations

Figure 10.3 summarises the approach to establishing the diagnosis.

TFTs: T_3 and T_4 are elevated in most patients, but T_4 is normal and T_3 raised (T_3 toxicosis) in 5%. In primary thyrotoxicosis, serum TSH is undetectable (<0.05 mU/L).

10.2 How to interpret thyroid function tests

TSH	T$_4$	T$_3$	Most likely interpretation(s)
U.D.	Raised	Raised	Primary thyrotoxicosis
U.D.	Normal[1]	Raised	Primary T$_3$-toxicosis
U.D.	Normal[1]	Normal[1]	Subclinical thyrotoxicosis
U.D. or low	Raised	Low or normal	Non-thyroidal illness, amiodarone therapy
U.D.	Low	Low	Secondary hypothyroidism[4] Transient thyroiditis in evolution
Normal	Low	Low[2]	Secondary hypothyroidism[4]
Mildly elevated 5–20 mU/L	Low	Low[2]	Primary hypothyroidism Secondary hypothyroidism[4]
Elevated >20 mU/L	Low	Low[2]	Primary hypothyroidism
Mildly elevated 5–20 mU/L	Normal[3]	Normal[2]	Subclinical hypothyroidism
Elevated 20–500 mU/L	Normal	Normal	Artefact Endogenous IgG interfering with TSH assay
Elevated	Raised	Raised	Non-compliance with T$_4$ replacement – recent 'loading' dose Secondary thyrotoxicosis[4] Thyroid hormone resistance

(U.D. = undetectable). [1]Usually upper part of reference range. [2]T$_3$ is not a sensitive indicator of hypothyroidism and should not be requested. [3]Usually lower part of reference range. [4]i.e. Secondary to pituitary or hypothalamic disease. Note TSH assays may report detectable TSH.

Antibodies: TSH receptor antibodies (TRAb) are elevated in 80–95% of patients with Graves' disease. Other thyroid antibodies are non-specific, as they are present in many healthy people.

Imaging: ^{99m}Technetium scintigraphy scans indicate trapping of isotope in the gland (see Fig. 10.3).

• In Graves' disease there is diffuse uptake. • In multinodular goitre, there is low, patchy uptake within the nodules. • A hot spot is seen in toxic adenoma, with no uptake in the dormant gland tissue. • In low-uptake thyrotoxicosis, the cause is usually a transient thyroiditis, although rarely patients may induce 'factitious thyrotoxicosis' by consuming thyroxine.

Management

Definitive treatment of thyrotoxicosis depends on the underlying cause (p. 340) and may include antithyroid drugs, radioactive iodine or surgery. A non-selective β-blocker (propranolol 160 mg daily) will alleviate symptoms within 24–48 hrs.

Atrial fibrillation (AF) in thyrotoxicosis: AF is present in ~10% of all patients with thyrotoxicosis (more in the elderly). Subclinical thyrotoxicosis is also a risk factor for AF. Ventricular rate responds

10.3 Clinical features of thyrotoxicosis

Symptoms	Signs
Common	
Weight loss despite normal or increased appetite	Weight loss
Heat intolerance, sweating	Tremor
Palpitations, tremor	Palmar erythema
Dyspnoea, fatigue	Sinus tachycardia
Irritability, emotional lability	Lid retraction, lid lag
Less common	
Osteoporosis (fracture, loss of height)	Goitre with bruit[1]
Diarrhoea, steatorrhoea	Atrial fibrillation[2]
Angina	Systolic hypertension/
Ankle swelling	increased pulse
Anxiety, psychosis	pressure
Muscle weakness	Cardiac failure[2]
Periodic paralysis (predominantly in Chinese)	Hyper-reflexia
Pruritus, alopecia	Ill-sustained clonus
Amenorrhoea/oligomenorrhoea	Proximal myopathy
Infertility, spontaneous abortion	Bulbar myopathy[2]
Loss of libido, impotence	
Excessive lacrimation	
Rare	
Vomiting	Gynaecomastia
Apathy	Spider naevi
Anorexia	Onycholysis
Exacerbation of asthma	Pigmentation

[1]In Graves' disease only.
[2]Features found particularly in elderly patients.

better to β-blockade than digoxin. Thromboembolic complications are particularly common, so anticoagulation with warfarin is indicated. Once the patient is biochemically euthyroid, AF reverts to sinus rhythm spontaneously in ~50% of patients.

Thyrotoxic crisis ('thyroid storm'): This is a medical emergency with a mortality of 10%. The most prominent signs are fever, agitation, confusion, tachycardia or AF, and cardiac failure. It is precipitated by infection in patients with unrecognised thyrotoxicosis and may develop after subtotal thyroidectomy or ^{131}I therapy. Patients should be rehydrated and given propranolol orally (80 mg 4 times daily) or intravenously (1–5 mg 4 times daily). Sodium ipodate (500 mg daily orally) restores serum T_3 levels to normal in 48–72 hrs by inhibiting release of hormones and conversion of T_4 to T_3. Oral carbimazole 40–60 mg daily inhibits the synthesis of new thyroid hormone. In the unconscious patient, carbimazole can be administered rectally. After 10–14 days, maintenance with carbimazole alone is possible.

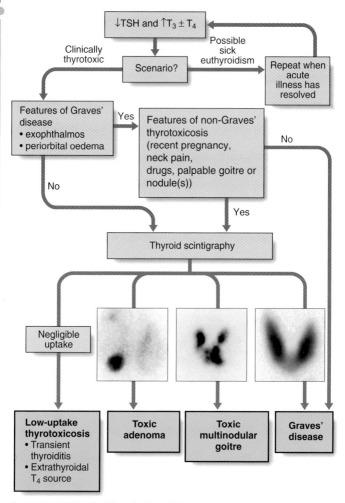

Fig. 10.3 Establishing the differential diagnosis in thyrotoxicosis. Scintigraphy is not necessary in most cases of drug-induced thyrotoxicosis.

Hypothyroidism

Hypothyroidism is a common condition, with a female:male ratio of 6:1.

Autoimmune disease (Hashimoto's thyroiditis) and thyroid failure following ^{131}I or surgical treatment of thyrotoxicosis account for >90% of cases in regions where the population is not iodine-deficient. Less common causes include secondary hypothyroidism, transient thyroiditis, inducement by amiodarone and dyshormonogenesis.

10.4 Clinical features of hypothyroidism	
Symptoms	**Signs**
Common	
Weight gain	Weight gain
Cold intolerance	
Fatigue, somnolence	
Dry skin	
Dry hair	
Menorrhagia	
Less common	
Constipation	Hoarse voice
Hoarseness	Facial features:
Carpal tunnel syndrome	Purplish lips
Alopecia	Malar flush
Aches and pains	Periorbital oedema
Muscle stiffness	Loss of lateral eyebrows
Deafness	Anaemia
Depression	Carotenaemia
Infertility	Erythema ab igne
	Bradycardia hypertension
	Delayed relaxation of reflexes
	Dermal myxoedema
Rare	
Psychosis (myxoedema madness)	Ileus, ascites
Galactorrhoea	Pericardial and pleural effusions
Impotence	Cerebellar ataxia
	Myotonia

Clinical assessment

Clinical features depend on the duration and severity of the hypothyroidism. The classical clinical features listed in Box 10.4 occur when deficiency develops insidiously over months/years.

Investigations

In primary hypothyroidism, T_4 is low and TSH elevated (>20 mU/L) (Fig. 10.4). T_3 is not a sensitive indicator of hypothyroidism and should not be measured. Secondary hypothyroidism is rare and is caused by failure of TSH secretion due to hypothalamic or anterior pituitary disease, e.g. pituitary macroadenoma. T_4 is low and TSH is usually low but sometimes paradoxically detectable. Other biochemical abnormalities associated with hypothyroidism include ↑CK, ↑LDH, ↑AST, ↑cholesterol, ↓Na^+ and anaemia (macrocytic or normocytic). ECG may show sinus bradycardia with small complexes and ST–T abnormalities. Thyroid peroxidase antibodies are usually elevated in autoimmune causes but are also common in the healthy population.

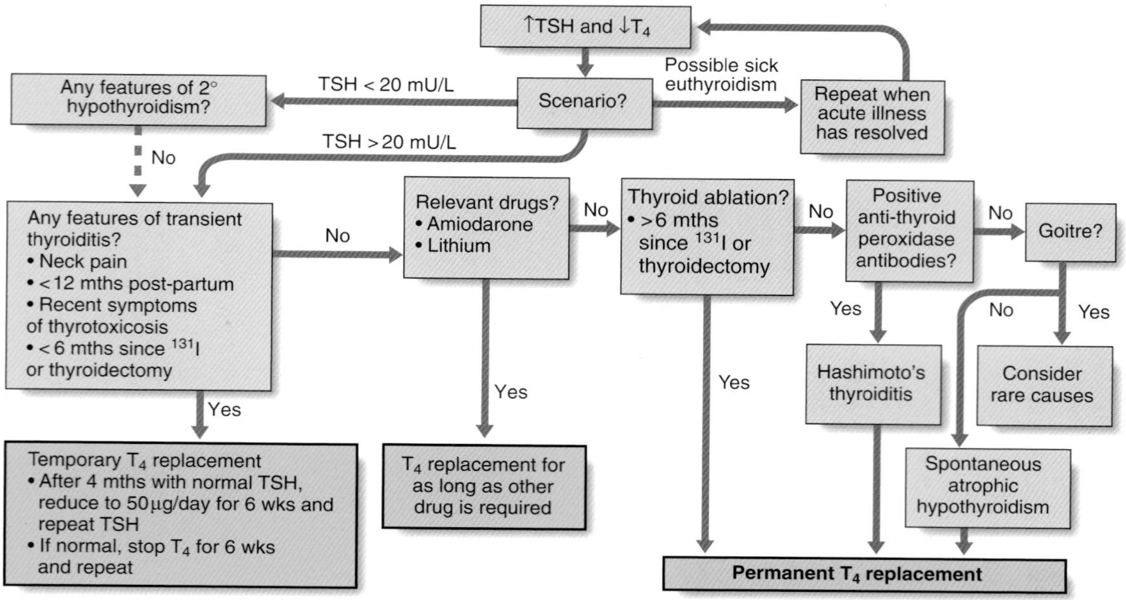

Fig. 10.4 Diagnostic approach to adults with suspected hypothyroidism.
This scheme ignores congenital causes of hypothyroidism, such as thyroid aplasia and dyshormonogenesis. Rare causes of hypothyroidism with goitre include amyloidosis and sarcoidosis.

Management

Most patients require lifelong levothyroxine therapy. A replacement regimen is:

• Levothyroxine 50 µg daily for 3 wks. • Then 100 µg daily for 3 wks. • Then maintenance 100–150 µg daily.

Levothyroxine has a half-life of 7 days, and so 6 wks should pass before repeating TFTs following a dose change. Patients feel better within 2–3 wks; resolution of skin and hair texture and effusions may take 3–6 mths.

The dose of levothyroxine should be adjusted to maintain TSH within the reference range. This usually requires a T_4 level in the upper reference range because the more active T_3 is derived exclusively from peripheral conversion of T_4 without the usual contribution from thyroid secretion. Some physicians advocate combined T_4/T_3 replacement but this approach remains controversial. TFTs should be checked every 1–2 yrs once the dose of thyroxine is stabilised.

Levothyroxine requirements may increase with co-administration of other drugs (e.g. phenytoin, ferrous sulphate, rifampicin) and during pregnancy. In non-compliance, if levothyroxine is taken just prior to clinic, the anomalous combination of a high T_4 and high TSH may result.

Levothyroxine replacement in ischaemic heart disease: Around 40% of patients with angina cannot tolerate full replacement levothyroxine, despite the use of β-blockers. Exacerbation of myocardial ischaemia, infarction and sudden death are well-recognised complications. In known ischaemic heart disease, levothyroxine should be introduced at low dose and increased under specialist supervision. Coronary intervention may be required to allow full replacement dosage.

Pregnancy: Most pregnant women with primary hypothyroidism require a 25–50 µg increase in levothyroxine dose. This is due to increased TBG. Inadequate maternal T_4 therapy may be associated with impaired cognitive development in offspring.

Myxoedema coma: This is a rare presentation of hypothyroidism in which there is depressed consciousness, usually in an elderly patient who appears myxoedematous. Body temperature may be low, convulsions are not uncommon, and CSF pressure and protein content are raised. The mortality rate is 50% and survival depends on early recognition and treatment.

Myxoedema coma is an emergency and treatment must begin before biochemical confirmation of diagnosis. Triiodothyronine is given as an IV bolus of 20 µg, followed by 20 µg 3 times daily until there is sustained clinical improvement. After 48–72 hrs, oral levothyroxine (50 µg daily) may be substituted. Unless it is clear the patient has primary hypothyroidism, thyroid failure should be assumed to be secondary to hypothalamic or pituitary disease and treatment given with hydrocortisone 100 mg 3 times daily, pending T_4 TSH and cortisol results. Other measures include slow rewarming, cautious IV fluids, broad-spectrum antibiotics, and high-flow oxygen and assisted ventilation if required.

Asymptomatic abnormal thyroid function tests

Subclinical thyrotoxicosis: TSH is undetectable, while T_3/T_4 is in the upper reference range. This condition is usually found in older patients with multinodular goitre. There is an increased risk of AF and osteoporosis; hence the consensus view is that such patients require therapy (usually ^{131}I). Otherwise, annual follow-up is required, as overt thyrotoxicosis occurs in 5% annually.

Subclinical hypothyroidism: TSH is raised, while T_3/T_4 is in the lower reference range. Progression to overt thyroid failure is highest in those with antithyroid peroxidase antibodies or TSH >10 mU/L. This group should be treated with levothyroxine to normalise TSH.

Non-thyroidal illness ('sick euthyroidism'): TSH is low, T_4 raised and T_3 normal or low. Other patterns are also seen. During illness, there is decreased conversion of T_4 to T_3 and alterations in affinity to binding proteins. TSH may be low as a result of the illness itself or drug treatments (e.g. corticosteroids). During convalescence, TSH may increase to levels found in primary hypothyroidism. TFTs should therefore not be checked during an acute illness in the absence of clear signs of thyroid disease. If an abnormal result is found, tests should be repeated after recovery.

Thyroid lump or swelling

A lump or swelling in the thyroid has many possible causes (Box 10.5). Most swellings are either a solitary nodule, a multinodular goitre or a diffuse goitre. Nodular thyroid disease is common in adult women. Most thyroid nodules are impalpable but are found incidentally on neck imaging, e.g. Doppler USS of the carotid arteries or CT pulmonary angiography, or during staging of patients with cancer.

Palpable thyroid nodules present as lumps in the neck in 4–8% of adult women and 1–2% of adult men. Multinodular goitres and solitary nodules sometimes present with acute painful swelling due to haemorrhage into a nodule.

Patients with thyroid nodules often worry about cancer, although in reality only 5–10% are malignant. Primary thyroid malignancy (p. 346) is more likely in:

• A solitary nodule in childhood or adolescence, particularly with a past history of local irradiation. • A nodule presenting in an elderly patient. • Patients with cervical lymphadenopathy.

Rarely, a metastasis from renal, breast or lung carcinoma presents as a painful, enlarging thyroid nodule. Thyroid nodules identified on PET scanning have a ~33% chance of being malignant.

Clinical assessment and investigations

On examination, thyroid swellings move during swallowing, and palpation can often distinguish between the three main causes of

10.5 Causes of thyroid enlargement

Diffuse goitre

- Simple goitre[1]
- Hashimoto's thyroiditis[1]
- Graves' disease
- Drugs: iodine, amiodarone
- Transient thyroiditis[2]
- Riedel's thyroiditis[2]
- Iodine deficiency (endemic goitre)[1]

Solitary nodule

- Simple cyst
- Colloid nodule
- Primary thyroid cancer (see Box 10.7 below)
- Follicular adenoma
- Metastasis

Multinodular goitre

[1]May shrink with thyroxine therapy. [2]Usually tender.

thyroid swelling. The differential diagnosis includes lymphadenopathy, branchial cysts, dermoid cysts and thyroglossal duct cysts. USS should be performed urgently, if there is any doubt about an anterior neck swelling.

T_3, T_4 and TSH should be measured and hyper- or hypothyroidism treated as described above.

Thyroid scintigraphy: Scintigraphy with ^{99m}technetium should be performed in patients with low serum TSH and a nodular thyroid to confirm the presence of an autonomously functioning ('hot') nodule (see Fig. 10.3), for which fine needle aspiration is not necessary. 'Cold' nodules on scintigraphy are more likely to prove malignant; however, most are benign and so scintigraphy is not routinely used to investigate thyroid nodules when TSH is normal.

Thyroid USS: If thyroid function is normal, USS is used to distinguish generalised from localised thyroid swelling. Inflammatory disorders causing diffuse goitre (e.g. Graves' disease and Hashimoto's thyroiditis) cause diffuse hypoechogenicity and (in Graves' disease) increased thyroid blood flow on Doppler. Thyroid autoantibodies occur in both disorders, while their absence in younger patients with diffuse goitre and normal function suggests 'simple goitre' (p. 345). USS also reveals the size and number of thyroid nodules and can distinguish solid from cystic nodules. It cannot reliably differentiate between benign and malignant nodules but features suggesting malignancy include hypervascularity, microcalcification and irregular, infiltrative margins. A pure cystic nodule and a 'spongiform' appearance both predict a benign aetiology.

Fine needle aspiration: Cytology of fine needle aspirate is recommended for most thyroid nodules >1 cm in diameter. Smaller nodules suspected of malignancy should also be aspirated, while some clinicians choose to observe spongiform nodules up to 2 cm in size. Patients with a multinodular goitre have the same risk of malignancy as those with a solitary nodule. The choice of nodule to biopsy should be based on USS characteristics. Palpable nodules can be aspirated in clinic, but USS guidance is necessary for impalpable nodules and to sample the solid component of mixed cystic/solid nodules. Aspiration may be therapeutic with cysts, although repeated recurrence is an indication for surgery. Cytology differentiates benign (80%) from definitely malignant or indeterminate nodules (20%), of which 25–50% are confirmed as cancers at surgery.

Management

Solitary nodules with a solid component and inconclusive or malignant cytology are treated by surgical excision. Treatment for histologically confirmed malignancies is described on page 346. Those with benign cytology and a reassuring USS may by observed by interval USS scans.

A diffuse or multinodular goitre may also require surgery for cosmetic reasons or to relieve compression of adjacent structures (resulting in stridor or dysphagia). Levothyroxine may shrink the goitre of Hashimoto's disease, particularly if TSH is elevated.

Autoimmune thyroid disease

Graves' disease

Graves' disease most commonly affects women aged 30–50 yrs. The most common manifestation is thyrotoxicosis (see Box 10.3) with or without a diffuse goitre. Graves' disease also causes ophthalmopathy and, rarely, pretibial myxoedema. These features can occur in the absence of thyroid dysfunction.

Graves' thyrotoxicosis

IgG antibodies are directed against the TSH receptors on follicular cells, stimulating hormone production and goitre formation. These TSH receptor antibodies (TRAb) can be detected in 80–95% of patients. The natural history of the disease follows one of three patterns:
• A prolonged period of hyperthyroidism of fluctuating severity. • Alternating relapse and remission. • A single, short-lived episode of hyperthyroidism, followed by prolonged remission and sometimes hypothyroidism.

There is a strong genetic component in Graves' disease, with 50% concordance between monozygotic twins. Smoking is weakly associated with Graves' thyrotoxicosis but strongly linked with the development of ophthalmopathy.

Management

Symptoms respond to β-blockade but definitive treatment requires control of thyroid hormone secretion. The different options

10.6 Comparison of treatments for the thyrotoxicosis of Graves' disease

Management	Common indications	Contraindications	Disadvantages/ complications
Antithyroid drugs (carbimazole, propylthiouracil)	First episode in patients <40 yrs	Breastfeeding (propylthiouracil suitable)	Hypersensitivity rash 2% Agranulocytosis 0.2% Relapse (>50%)
Subtotal thyroidectomy	Large goitre Poor drug adherence Recurrence after drug treatment	Previous thyroid surgery Dependence on voice, e.g. opera singer, lecturer	Hypothyroidism ~25% Transient hypocalcaemia 10% Hypoparathyroidism 1% Recurrent laryngeal nerve palsy 1%
Radio-iodine	Patients >40 yrs Recurrence following surgery	Pregnancy Active Graves' eye disease	Hypothyroidism: 40% in 1st yr, 80% by 15 yrs Exacerbates ophthalmopathy

are compared in Box 10.6. For patients <40 yrs old, many centres prescribe a course of carbimazole and recommend surgery if relapse occurs, while ^{131}I is employed as first- or second-line treatment in older patients. It is unclear whether ^{131}I increases the incidence of some malignancies; the association may be with Graves' disease rather than its therapy. In many centres, however, ^{131}I is used more extensively, even in young patients.

Antithyroid drugs: The most commonly used are carbimazole and propylthiouracil. These drugs reduce thyroid hormone synthesis by inhibiting tyrosine iodination. Antithyroid drugs are introduced at high doses (carbimazole 40–60 mg daily, propylthiouracil 400–600 mg daily). There is subjective improvement within 2 wks and the patient is biochemically euthyroid at 4 wks, when the dose can be reduced. The maintenance dose is determined by measurement of T_4 and TSH. Carbimazole is continued for 12–18 mths in the hope that permanent remission will occur. Unfortunately, thyrotoxicosis recurs in at least 50% within 2 yrs of stopping treatment. Adverse effects of antithyroid drugs include rash and idiosyncratic but reversible agranulocytosis.

Thyroid surgery: Patients must be rendered euthyroid before operation. Potassium iodide, 60 mg 3 times daily orally, given for 2 wks before surgery, inhibits thyroid hormone release and reduces the size and vascularity of the gland, making surgery easier. Complications are uncommon (see Box 10.6). One yr post-surgery, 80% of patients are euthyroid, 15% are hypothyroid and 5% remain thyrotoxic. Hypothyroidism within 6 mths of operation may be temporary. Long-term follow-up is necessary, as the late development of hypothyroidism and recurrence of thyrotoxicosis are well recognised.

Radioactive iodine: ^{131}I is administered as a single dose (~400 MBq, 10 mCi) and is trapped and organified in the thyroid. It is effective in 75% of patients within 4–12 wks. Symptoms can initially be controlled by β-blockade or with carbimazole. However, carbimazole reduces the efficacy of ^{131}I therapy and should be avoided for 48 hrs after radio-iodine. If thyrotoxicosis persists after 6 mths, a further dose of ^{131}I is indicated. Most patients eventually develop hypothyroidism, necessitating long-term follow-up.

Thyrotoxicosis in pregnancy

TFTs must be interpreted with caution in pregnancy. Thyroid-binding globulin, and hence total T_4/T_3 levels, are increased and TSH reference ranges are lower; a fully suppressed TSH with elevated free hormone levels indicates thyrotoxicosis. The thyrotoxicosis is almost always caused by Graves' disease. Maternal thyroid hormones, TRAb and antithyroid drugs can all cross the placenta.

Propylthiouracil is the preferred treatment in the first trimester, as carbimazole is associated rarely with embryopathy, particularly a skin defect, aplasia cutis. The smallest dose of propylthiouracil (<150 mg/day) is used that maintains maternal TFTs within their reference ranges, thereby minimising fetal hypothyroidism and goitre. TRAb levels in the third trimester predict the likelihood of neonatal thyrotoxicosis; if they are not elevated, antithyroid drugs can be discontinued 4 wks before delivery to avoid fetal hypothyroidism at the time of maximum brain development. During breast-feeding, propylthiouracil is used, as it is minimally excreted in the milk.

Graves' ophthalmopathy

Within the orbit, there is cytokine-mediated fibroblast proliferation, increased interstitial fluid and a chronic inflammatory cell infiltrate. This causes swelling and ultimately fibrosis of the extraocular muscles and a rise in retrobulbar pressure. The eye is displaced forwards (proptosis, exophthalmos) with optic nerve compression in severe cases.

Ophthalmopathy is typically episodic. It is detectable in ~50% of thyrotoxic patients at presentation, more commonly smokers, but may occur long before or after thyrotoxic episodes (exophthalmic Graves' disease). Presenting symptoms are related to increased corneal exposure due to proptosis and lid retraction:

• Excessive lacrimation worsened by wind and sun. • 'Gritty' sensations. • Pain due to corneal ulceration. • Reduced visual acuity/fields or colour vision due to optic nerve compression. • Diplopia resulting from extraocular muscle involvement.

Most patients require no treatment. Methylcellulose eye drops are used for dry eyes and sunglasses reduce the excessive lacrimation. Severe inflammatory episodes are treated with glucocorticoids (prednisolone 60 mg daily) and sometimes orbital irradiation. Loss of visual acuity requires urgent surgical decompression of the orbit. Surgery to ocular muscles may improve diplopia.

Pretibial myxoedema

This infiltrative dermopathy occurs in <10% of patients with Graves' disease.

Pink–purple plaques on the anterior leg and foot are seen. Lesions are itchy and the skin may have a 'peau d'orange' appearance with coarse hair. In severe cases, topical glucocorticoids may be helpful.

Hashimoto's thyroiditis

Hashimoto's thyroiditis increases in incidence with age. It is characterised by destructive lymphoid infiltration leading to a varying degree of fibrosis and thus a varying degree of thyroid enlargement. There is a slightly increased risk of thyroid lymphoma. The term 'Hashimoto's thyroiditis' has been reserved for patients with antithyroid peroxidase autoantibodies and a goitre (with or without hypothyroidism), whilst 'spontaneous atrophic hypothyroidism' has been used in hypothyroid patients without a goitre with TSH receptor-blocking antibodies. However, these syndromes are both variants of Hashimoto's.

At presentation, a small or moderately sized firm diffuse goitre may be palpable. Some 25% of patients are hypothyroid and the remainder are at risk of developing hypothyroidism in future years. Antithyroid peroxidase antibodies are present in >90%. Levothyroxine therapy is given.

Transient thyroiditis
Subacute (de Quervain's) thyroiditis

Subacute thyroiditis is a virus-induced (e.g. Coxsackie, mumps) transient inflammation of the thyroid usually affecting 20–40-yr-old females.

There is classically pain around the thyroid radiating to the jaw and ears, which is worsened by swallowing and coughing. The thyroid is enlarged and tender. Painless transient thyroiditis also occurs. Systemic upset is common. Inflammation in the thyroid causes release of colloid and stored hormones, and damages follicular cells. As a result, T_4/T_3 levels are raised for 4–6 wks until depletion of colloid. A period of hypothyroidism follows, during which follicular cells recover, restoring thyroid function within 4–6 mths. In the thyrotoxic phase, iodine uptake and technetium trapping are low due to follicular cell damage and TSH suppression. Pain and systemic upset respond to NSAIDs. Occasionally, prednisolone 40 mg daily for 3–4 wks is required. Mild thyrotoxicosis is treated with propranolol. Monitoring of thyroid function is required so that levothyroxine can be prescribed temporarily in the hypothyroid phase.

Post-partum thyroiditis

The maternal immune response is enhanced after delivery and may unmask subclinical autoimmune thyroid disease. Transient asymptomatic disturbances of thyroid function occur in 5–10% of women post-partum. However, symptomatic thyrotoxicosis presenting within 6 mths of childbirth is likely to be due to post-partum thyroiditis and the diagnosis is confirmed by negligible radioisotope uptake. The clinical course is similar to that of painless subacute thyroiditis. Post-partum thyroiditis can recur after subsequent pregnancies and may progress to hypothyroidism.

Iodine-associated thyroid disease

Iodine deficiency

In mountainous areas (e.g. Andes, Himalayas), dietary iodine deficiency causes thyroid enlargement (endemic goitre). Most patients are euthyroid and have normal or raised TSH levels.

Iodine-induced dysfunction

Chronic excess of iodine inhibits thyroid hormone release; this is the basis for its utility in the treatment of thyroid storm and prior to subtotal thyroidectomy. Transient thyrotoxicosis may be precipitated in iodine deficiency following prophylactic iodinisation programmes. In individuals who have underlying thyroid disease predisposing to thyrotoxicosis (e.g. multinodular goitre or Graves' disease), thyrotoxicosis can be induced by iodine administration (e.g. radiocontrast media).

Amiodarone

The anti-arrhythmic agent amiodarone contains large amounts of iodine. Amiodarone also has a cytotoxic effect on thyroid follicular cells and inhibits T_4 to T_3 conversion. Around 20% of patients develop hypothyroidism or thyrotoxicosis. TSH provides the best indicator of thyroid function.

Amiodarone-related thyrotoxicosis has been classified as:
• Type I: iodine-induced excess thyroid hormone synthesis. • Type II: transient thyrotoxicosis due to cytotoxic thyroiditis.

Treatment of thyrotoxicosis is difficult. Excess iodine renders the gland resistant to radio-iodine. Antithyroid drugs may be effective in patients with type I thyrotoxicosis but not in type II. If the cardiac state allows, amiodarone should be discontinued. Prior to amiodarone therapy, thyroid function should be measured and amiodarone avoided if TSH is suppressed. Thyroid function should be monitored regularly.

In hypothyroid patients, levothyroxine can be given while amiodarone is continued.

Simple and multinodular goitre
Simple diffuse goitre
This presents in 15–25-yr-olds, often during pregnancy. The goitre is visible, soft and symmetrical and the thyroid is 2–3 times its normal size. There is no tenderness, lymphadenopathy or bruit, and TFTs are normal. The goitre may regress without treatment or may progress to multinodular goitre.

Multinodular goitre
Occasionally, simple goitres become multinodular over 10–20 yrs. These nodules grow at varying rates and secrete thyroid hormone 'autonomously', thereby suppressing TSH-dependent growth and function in the remaining gland. Ultimately, complete TSH suppression occurs in ~25% of cases, with T_4/T_3 levels often within the reference range (subclinical thyrotoxicosis) but sometimes elevated (toxic multinodular goitre). The nodules may represent multiple adenomas or focal hyperplasia.

Clinical features and investigations
Patients present with thyrotoxicosis, a large goitre or sudden painful swelling caused by haemorrhage into a nodule. The goitre is nodular or lobulated on palpation and may extend retrosternally. Very large goitres may cause stridor, dysphagia and superior vena cava obstruction. Hoarseness due to recurrent laryngeal nerve palsy is more suggestive of thyroid carcinoma. The diagnosis is confirmed by USS and/or thyroid scintigraphy. A flow-volume loop is a good screening test for tracheal compression. CT/MRI of the thoracic inlet can quantify the degree of tracheal compression and retrosternal extension. Nodules should be evaluated for neoplasia as described above (p. 338).

Management
Small goitre: Annual thyroid function is required, as progression to toxic multinodular goitre can occur.

Large goitre: Thyroid surgery is indicated for mediastinal compression or cosmetically unattractive goitres. [131]I is used in the elderly to reduce thyroid size but recurrence is common after 10–20 yrs.

Toxic multinodular goitre: [131]I is used; hypothyroidism is less common than in Graves' disease. Partial thyroidectomy may be required for a large goitre. Antithyroid drugs are not usually used, as drug withdrawal invariably leads to relapse.

Subclinical thyrotoxicosis: This is increasingly being treated with ^{131}I, as a suppressed TSH is a risk factor for AF and osteoporosis.

Thyroid neoplasia
Patients with thyroid tumours usually present with a solitary nodule (p. 339). Most are benign and a few (toxic adenomas) secrete excess thyroid hormones. Primary thyroid malignancy is rare (<1% of all

10.7 Malignant thyroid tumours

Origin of tumour	Type of tumour	Frequency (%)	Age at presentation (yrs)	10-yr survival (%)
Follicular cells	Papillary	75–85	20–40	98
	Follicular	10–20	40–60	94
	Anaplastic	<5	>60	9
Parafollicular C cells	Medullary carcinoma	5–8	Childhood or >40	78
Lymphocytes	Lymphoma	<5	>60	45

carcinomas). As shown in Box 10.7, it can be classified according to the cell type of origin. With the exception of medullary carcinoma, thyroid cancer is more common in females.

Toxic adenoma

The presence of a toxic solitary nodule is the cause of <5% of cases of thyrotoxicosis. The nodule is a follicular adenoma, usually >3 cm, which secretes excess thyroid hormones. The remaining gland atrophies following TSH suppression. Most patients are female and >40 yrs old.

The diagnosis is made by thyroid scintigraphy. Thyrotoxicosis is mild, and in 50% of patients T_3 alone is elevated (T_3 thyrotoxicosis). ^{131}I is highly effective and is an ideal treatment, since the atrophic cells surrounding the nodule do not take up iodine, making permanent hypothyroidism unusual. Hemi-thyroidectomy is an alternative.

Differentiated carcinoma

Papillary carcinoma: The most common thyroid malignancy. It may be multifocal and spread is to regional lymph nodes.

Follicular carcinoma: A single encapsulated lesion. Cervical lymph nodes spread is rare. Metastases are blood-borne and are found in bone, lungs and brain.

Management

Total thyroidectomy is carried out, followed by a large dose of ^{131}I in order to ablate remaining thyroid tissue. Thereafter, long-term treatment with levothyroxine in a dose sufficient to suppress TSH (150–200 µg daily) is important, as differentiated thyroid carcinomas are TSH-dependent. Follow-up is by measurement of serum thyroglobulin, which should be undetectable in patients whose thyroid has been ablated. Detectable thyroglobulin suggests tumour recurrence or metastases, which may respond to further radio-iodine therapy. Most patients have an excellent prognosis. Those <50 yrs with papillary carcinoma have near-normal life expectancy if the tumour is <2 cm in diameter, confined to cervical nodes and of low grade. Radio-iodine is usually effective in treating distant metastases.

Anaplastic carcinoma and lymphoma

These two conditions are difficult to distinguish clinically. Patients are usually over 60 and have rapid thyroid enlargement over 2–3 mths. The goitre is hard and symmetrical, and may cause stridor (tracheal compression) and hoarseness (recurrent laryngeal nerve palsy). There is no effective treatment of anaplastic carcinoma, although surgery and radiotherapy are sometimes used.

The prognosis for lymphoma, which may arise from Hashimoto's thyroiditis, is better. External irradiation dramatically shrinks the goitre and, with chemotherapy, results in a median survival of 9 yrs.

Medullary carcinoma

This tumour arises from the parafollicular C cells of the thyroid. The tumour may secrete calcitonin, 5-HT (serotonin) and adrenocortico-trophic hormone (ACTH). As a consequence, carcinoid syndrome and Cushing's syndrome may occur.

Patients present with a firm thyroid mass and cervical lymphad-enopathy. Distant metastases are rare. Serum calcitonin is raised and useful in monitoring response to treatment. Hypocalcaemia is rare. Treatment is by total thyroidectomy with removal of cervical nodes. Medullary carcinoma may occur in childhood in families, as part of the multiple endocrine neoplasia (MEN) type 2 syndrome (p. 378).

Riedel's thyroiditis

This rare, non-malignant condition has a similar presentation to thyroid cancer, with a slow-growing goitre which is irregular and hard. Diagnosis is by biopsy. The thyroid and surrounding struc-tures are infiltrated with fibrous tissue. There may be mediastinal and retroperitoneal fibrosis. Tracheal and oesophageal compression necessitate thyroidectomy. Complications include recurrent laryn-geal nerve palsy, hypoparathyroidism and hypothyroidism.

THE REPRODUCTIVE SYSTEM

In the male, the testis has two principal functions:
• Synthesis of testosterone by the interstitial Leydig cells controlled by luteinising hormone (LH). • Spermatogenesis by Sertoli cells under the control of follicle-stimulating hormone (FSH).

Negative feedback suppression of LH is mediated principally by testosterone, while inhibin suppresses FSH.

In the female, sex hormones vary during the menstrual cycle. FSH produces growth and development of ovarian follicles during the first 14 days. This leads to a gradual increase in oestradiol produc-tion, which initially suppresses FSH secretion (negative feedback) but then, above a certain level, stimulates an increase in the fre-quency and amplitude of gonadotrophin-releasing hormone (GnRH) pulses, resulting in a marked increase in LH secretion (positive feedback). This LH surge induces ovulation. The follicle then differentiates into a corpus luteum, which secretes progesterone. Withdrawal of progesterone results in menstrual bleeding.

The cessation of menstruation (the menopause) occurs in developed countries at an average age of 50 yrs. In the 5 yrs before, there is an increase in the number of anovulatory cycles, referred to as the climacteric. Oestrogen and inhibin secretion falls, resulting in increased pituitary secretion of LH and FSH.

Presenting problems in reproductive disease
Delayed puberty

Genetic factors influence the timing of the onset of puberty, although body weight acts as a trigger. Puberty may be considered delayed if it has not begun by a chronological age >2.5 standard deviations (SD) above the national average (>14 in boys, >13 in girls in the UK).

The differential diagnosis is considered in Box 10.8. The key distinction is between the 'clock running slow' (constitutional delay) and pathology in the hypothalamus/pituitary (hypogonadotrophic hypogonadism) or the gonads (hypergonadotrophic hypogonadism).

Constitutional delay of puberty: This should be considered a normal variant and is the most common cause of delayed puberty. Affected children are typically shorter than their peers throughout

---

10.8 Causes of delayed puberty and hypogonadism

Constitutional delay

Hypogonadotrophic hypogonadism
- Structural hypothalamic/pituitary disease – see Box 10.16
- Functional gonadotrophin deficiency
    Chronic systemic illness (e.g. asthma, coeliac disease, cystic fibrosis)
    Psychological stress, anorexia nervosa, excessive exercise
    Endocrine disease: hyperprolactinaemia, Cushing's, hypothyroidism
- Isolated gonadotrophin deficiency (Kallmann's)

Hypergonadotrophic hypogonadism
- Acquired damage to gonads
    Chemotherapy /radiotherapy
    Trauma/surgery
    Autoimmune gonadal failure
    Mumps, TB
    Haemochromatosis
- Developmental/congenital disorders
    Klinefelter's/Turner's syndrome
    Anorchidism/cryptorchidism

childhood. There is often a family history and bone age is lower than chronological age. Puberty will start spontaneously, but prolonged delay can have significant psychological consequences.

Hypogonadotrophic hypogonadism: This may be due to structural, inflammatory or infiltrative disorders of the pituitary/hypothalamus (p. 370). Other pituitary hormones are likely to be deficient. 'Functional' gonadotrophin deficiency is caused by a variety of factors (see Box 10.8). Isolated gonadotrophin deficiency is due to a genetic abnormality affecting GnRH or gonadotrophin synthesis. The most common form is Kallmann's syndrome, which is also associated with olfactory bulb agenesis, resulting in anosmia. If left untreated, the epiphyses fail to fuse, resulting in tall stature with disproportionately long arms and legs (eunuchoid habitus). Cryptorchidism (undescended testes) and gynaecomastia are seen in all forms of hypogonadotrophic hypogonadism.

Hypergonadotrophic hypogonadism: Hypergonadotrophic hypogonadism associated with delayed puberty is usually due to sex chromosome abnormalities (Klinefelter's/Turner's syndromes, p. 354). Other causes of primary gonadal failure are shown in Box 10.8.

Investigations

• LH/FSH, testosterone, oestradiol, FBC, renal, liver and thyroid function, and coeliac disease autoantibodies: key measurements.
• Elevated gonadotrophin concentrations: chromosome analysis.
• Low gonadotrophin concentrations: differential diagnosis lies between constitutional delay and hypogonadotrophic hypogonadism. • X-ray of the wrist and hand: allows estimation of bone age.
• Neuroimaging: required in hypogonadotrophic hypogonadism.

Management

Puberty can be induced using low doses of oestrogen (in girls) or testosterone (in boys). Higher doses carry a risk of early fusion of epiphyses and therefore therapy should be administered and monitored by a specialist. In constitutional delay, therapy is withdrawn once endogenous puberty is established. In other cases, hormone doses are gradually increased during puberty and full adult replacement doses given when development is complete.

Amenorrhoea

Primary amenorrhoea describes a patient who has never menstruated. This is usually due to delayed puberty but may be a consequence of anatomical defects, e.g. endometrial hypoplasia, vaginal agenesis.

Secondary amenorrhoea describes the cessation of menstruation. The causes of this are:
• Physiological (pregnancy, menopause). • Hypogonadotrophic hypogonadism (see Box 10.8). • Ovarian dysfunction (hypergonadotrophic hypogonadism; see Box 10.8). • Polycystic ovarian syndrome

(PCOS), androgen-secreting tumours. • Uterine dysfunction (Asherman's syndrome).

Premature ovarian failure (premature menopause) is defined as occurring before 40 yrs of age.

Clinical assessment

Hypothalamic/pituitary disease and premature ovarian failure result in oestrogen deficiency, which causes menopausal symptoms: hot flushes, sweating, anxiety, irritability, dyspareunia, vaginal infections. A history of galactorrhoea should be sought. Weight loss for any reason can cause amenorrhoea. Weight gain may suggest hypothyroidism or Cushing's syndrome. Hirsutism and irregular periods suggest PCOS.

Investigations

• Measurement of urinary human chorionic gonadotrophin (hCG): will exclude pregnancy. • LH, FSH, oestradiol, prolactin, testosterone, T_4 and TSH. • ↑LH, ↑FSH and ↓oestradiol: suggest primary ovarian failure. Ovarian autoantibodies may be positive. • ↑LH, ↑prolactin and ↑testosterone with normal oestradiol: common in PCOS. • ↓LH, ↓FSH and ↓oestradiol: suggest hypothalamic/pituitary disease (pituitary MRI indicated). • Assessment of bone mineral density: appropriate in patients with low androgen and oestrogen levels.

Management

Where possible, the underlying cause should be treated. The management of structural pituitary/hypothalamic disease and PCOS is described below. In oestrogen deficiency, oestrogen replacement therapy is necessary to treat symptoms and to prevent osteoporosis. Oestrogen should not be given without progesterone to a woman with a uterus due to the risk of endometrial cancer. It is administered most conveniently as an oral contraceptive pill. In post-menopausal females, HRT relieves menopausal symptoms and prevents osteoporotic fractures, but is associated with adverse effects (e.g. stroke, breast cancer, pulmonary embolism). Many authorities recommend that women should take replacement therapy until the age of 50 and only continue if there are unacceptable menopausal symptoms.

Male hypogonadism

The clinical features of both hypo- and hypergonadotrophic hypogonadism in men include:
• Loss of libido. • Lethargy. • Muscle weakness. • Decreased frequency of shaving. • Gynaecomastia. • Infertility. • Delayed puberty. • Erectile dysfunction.

The causes of hypogonadism are listed in Box 10.8.

Investigations

Male hypogonadism is confirmed by demonstrating a low serum testosterone level. Hypo- and hypergonadotrophic hypogonadism are distinguished by measurement of random LH and FSH. Patients with hypogonadotrophic hypogonadism should be investigated for pituitary disease (p. 371). Patients with hypergonadotrophic hypogonadism should have the testes examined for cryptorchidism or atrophy, and a karyotype should be performed (Klinefelter's syndrome).

Management

Testosterone replacement is indicated to prevent osteoporosis and to restore muscle power and libido. Testosterone administration should be avoided in prostatic carcinoma. In men over 50, prostate-specific antigen (PSA) should be monitored. Men with hypogonadotrophic hypogonadism who wish fertility are usually given injections of hCG.

Infertility

Infertility affects ~1 in 7 couples of reproductive age. Causes in women include anovulation or structural abnormalities preventing fertilisation or implantation. Male infertility may result from impaired quality or number of sperm. Azoospermia or oligospermia is usually idiopathic, but may result from hypogonadism (see Box 10.8). In many couples no cause is found.

Clinical assessment

• History of previous illness/surgery. • Sensitive sexual history. • Menstrual history. • Scrotal examination for testicular size and varicocele.

Investigations

• Performed after failure to conceive for 12 mths, unless there is an obvious abnormality (e.g. amenorrhoea). • Semen analysis for sperm count and quality. • Women with regular periods: is confirmation of ovulation by elevated serum progesterone on day 21 of the cycle. • Transvaginal USS to assess uterine and ovarian anatomy. • Tubal patency: check using laparoscopy or hysterosalpingography.

Management

General advice: Couples are advised to have intercourse every 2–3 days throughout the menstrual cycle.

Ovulation induction:
• In PCOS with anovulatory cycles: clomifene. • In gonadotrophin deficiency or if clomifene fails: daily FSH injections, then hCG to induce follicular rupture. • In hypothalamic disease: pulsatile infusion of GnRH therapy to stimulate pituitary gonadotrophin secretion.

During ovulation induction, monitoring, including USS, is essential to avoid multiple ovulation and complications such as ovarian hyperstimulation syndrome. Women who fail to respond to induction or who have primary ovarian failure may consider donated eggs or embryos, surrogacy and adoption.

10.9 Causes of gynaecomastia

- Idiopathic
- Physiological
- Drug-induced: cimetidine, digoxin, anti-androgens (cyproterone acetate, spironolactone)
- Hypogonadism (see Box 10.8)
- Androgen resistance syndromes
- Oestrogen excess: liver failure (impaired steroid metabolism), oestrogen-secreting tumour (e.g. testis), hCG-secreting tumour (e.g. testis, lung)

In vitro fertilisation (IVF): IVF is widely used for many causes of idiopathic or prolonged (>3 yrs) infertility. The success rate falls in women >40 yrs.

Male infertility: Infertile men with hypogonadotrophic hypogonadism are usually given injections of hCG. Removal of a varicocele can improve semen quality. Sperm extraction from the epididymis and in vitro injection into oöcytes (intracytoplasmic sperm injection; ICSI) are used in men with oligospermia or poor sperm quality. Donated sperm is another option in azoospermia.

Gynaecomastia

Gynaecomastia is the presence of glandular breast tissue in males, resulting from an imbalance between androgen and oestrogen activity (androgen deficiency or oestrogen excess). Causes are listed in Box 10.9. The most common are physiological, i.e. in the newborn baby (maternal oestrogens), in pubertal boys (oestradiol concentrations reach adult levels before testosterone) and in elderly men (↓testosterone concentrations). Gynaecomastia is often asymmetrical.

Palpation may allow breast tissue to be distinguished from adipose tissue observed in obesity. If a clinical distinction between gynaecomastia and adipose tissue cannot be made, then USS or mammography is required. The testes should be examined for cryptorchidism, atrophy or a tumour. Testosterone, LH, FSH, oestradiol, prolactin and hCG should be measured. Elevated oestrogen concentrations are found in testicular tumours and hCG-producing neoplasms. The underlying cause should be addressed, e.g. change of drug treatment, excision of tumour. In physiological gynaecomastia, reassurance is usually sufficient, but if the condition is associated with significant psychological distress, surgical excision may be justified. Androgen replacement improves gynaecomastia in hypogonadal males.

Hirsutism

Hirsutism refers to the excessive growth of thick terminal hair in an androgen-dependent distribution in women (upper lip, chin, chest, back, lower abdomen, thigh, forearm). It should be distinguished

	10.10 Causes of hirsutism	
Cause	**Investigation findings**	**Treatment**
Idiopathic	Normal	Cosmetic measures Anti-androgens
PCOS	LH:FSH ratio >2.5:1 Mild ↑androgens Mild hyperprolactinaemia	Weight loss Cosmetic measures Anti-androgens
Congenital adrenal hyperplasia (95% 21-hydroxylase deficiency)	↑Androgens that suppress with dexamethasone ACTH test causes ↑17OH-progesterone	Glucocorticoid replacement administered in reverse rhythm to suppress early morning ACTH
Exogenous androgen administration	↓LH/FSH Urinalysis detects drug of misuse	Stop steroid misuse
Androgen-secreting tumour of ovary or adrenal cortex	↑Androgens that do not suppress with dexamethasone/oestrogen ↓LH/FSH CT/MRI demonstrates tumour	Surgical excision
Cushing's syndrome	Normal or mild ↑adrenal androgens	Treat cause

from hypertrichosis, which is generalised excessive growth of vellus hair. Causes and treatment of hirsutism are shown in Box 10.10.

Important observations are a drug and menstrual history, BMI, BP, examination for virilisation (clitoromegaly, deep voice, male-pattern balding, breast atrophy) and associated features, e.g. Cushing's syndrome. Recent hirsutism associated with virilisation is suggestive of an androgen-secreting tumour. Testosterone, prolactin, LH and FSH should be measured. If testosterone levels are over twice the upper limit of the normal female range, especially with ↓LH and ↓FSH, then causes other than idiopathic hirsutism and PCOS are more likely.

Polycystic ovarian syndrome (PCOS)

Polycystic ovarian syndrome (PCOS) affects up to 10% of women of reproductive age. It is associated with obesity and the primary cause remains uncertain. Genetic factors are important, as PCOS often affects several family members.

Clinical features

• Pituitary dysfunction: ↑LH, ↑prolactin. • Anovulatory menstrual cycles: oligomenorrhoea, secondary amenorrhoea, cystic ovaries, infertility. • Androgen excess: hirsutism, acne. • Obesity: hyperglycaemia, ↑oestrogens, dyslipidaemia, hypertension.

Management

Weight loss can improve menstrual irregularity, hirsutism and diabetes risk.

Menses: Metformin reduces insulin resistance and can restore regular cycles. High oestrogen may cause endometrial hyperplasia. Inducing regular withdrawal bleeding using cyclical progestogens can reduce the risk of endometrial neoplasia.

Hirsutism: Many patients use shaving, bleaching and waxing. Electrolysis and laser treatment are effective but expensive. Eflornithine cream may reduce hair growth. Anti-androgen therapy may be employed if other measures have failed. Options include:
• Androgen receptor antagonists (e.g. cyproterone acetate).
• 5α-reductase inhibitors (e.g. finasteride): prevent activation of testosterone. • Exogenous oestrogen: suppresses ovarian hormone production.

Infertility: See above.

Turner's syndrome

Turner's syndrome affects ~1 in 2500 females. The syndrome is classically associated with a 45XO karyotype. The genitals are female in character, although gonadal dysgenesis results in 'streak ovaries'. The lack of oestrogen causes loss of negative feedback and elevation of FSH and LH concentrations. There is a wide variation in the spectrum of associated somatic abnormalities. These include:
• Short stature • Webbing of the neck (25–40%). • Widely spaced nipples. • Shield chest. • Horse-shoe kidney. • Lymphoedema of hands and feet (30%). • Coarctation of the aorta. • Aortic root dilatation. • Psychological problems: low IQ. • Deafness.

Short stature may be helped by high doses of growth hormone. Pubertal development is induced with oestrogen therapy, and long-term oestrogen replacement is required.

Klinefelter's syndrome

Klinefelter's syndrome affects ~1 in 1000 males and is usually associated with a 47XXY karyotype. Leydig cell function is impaired, resulting in hypergonadotrophic hypogonadism. The diagnosis is often made in adolescents with gynaecomastia and delayed puberty. Affected individuals usually have small, firm testes and may have learning difficulties. Tall stature is apparent from early childhood, with a long leg length exacerbated by lack of epiphyseal closure in puberty. Individuals with androgen deficiency require androgen replacement.

THE PARATHYROID GLANDS

The four parathyroid glands lie behind the lobes of the thyroid. Parathyroid hormone (PTH) interacts with vitamin D to control calcium metabolism. Calcium exists in serum as 50% ionised, and 50% complexed with organic ions and proteins. The parathyroid chief cells respond directly to changes in calcium concentrations, secreting PTH in response to a fall in ionised calcium. PTH promotes reabsorption of calcium from renal tubules and bone, stimulating alkaline phosphatase and lowering plasma phosphate. PTH also promotes renal conversion of 25-hydroxycholecalciferol to the active metabolite 1,25-dihydroxycholecalciferol, which enhances calcium absorption from the gut.

To investigate disorders of calcium metabolism, measurement of calcium, phosphate, alkaline phosphatase and PTH should be undertaken. Most laboratories measure total calcium in serum. This needs to be corrected if serum albumin is low, by adjusting the value for calcium upwards by 0.02 mmol/L (0.4 mg/dL) for each 1 g/L reduction in albumin below 40 g/L.

Presenting problems in parathyroid disease
Hypercalcaemia

Causes of hypercalcaemia are listed in Box 10.11. Primary hyperparathyroidism and malignant hypercalcaemia are the most common. Familial hypocalciuric hypercalcaemia (FHH) is a rare disorder that is important, as it may be misdiagnosed as primary hyperparathyroidism.

Clinical assessment

Symptoms and signs of hypercalcaemia include polyuria, polydipsia, renal colic, lethargy, anorexia, nausea, dyspepsia, peptic ulceration, constipation, depression and impaired cognition ('bones, stones and abdominal groans'). Patients with malignant hypercalcaemia can have a rapid onset of symptoms. Currently, >50% of patients are discovered incidentally on biochemical testing and are asymptomatic. Hypertension is common in hyperparathyroidism. Parathyroid tumours are almost never palpable. A family history of hypercalcaemia raises the possibility of FHH or MEN.

Investigations

The most discriminant investigation is serum PTH. If PTH levels are detectable or elevated in the presence of hypercalcaemia, then primary hyperparathyroidism is the most likely diagnosis. High plasma phosphate and alkaline phosphatase with renal impairment suggest tertiary hyperparathyroidism. Hypercalcaemia may cause nephrocalcinosis and renal tubular impairment, resulting in hyperuricaemia and hyperchloraemia.

Low urine calcium excretion indicates likely FHH, confirmed by testing for mutations in the gene coding for the calcium-sensing receptor.

If PTH is low and no other cause is apparent, then malignancy with or without bony metastases is likely. The patient should be screened with a CXR, myeloma screen and CT as appropriate. PTH-related peptide, which causes hypercalcaemia associated with malignancy, can be measured by a specific assay.

Management

Treatment of severe hypercalcaemia involves rehydration with normal saline. Calcitonin acts rapidly and can be added for the first 24–48 hrs in patients with life-threatening hypercalcaemia. Bisphosphonates (e.g. pamidronate 90 mg IV over 4 hrs) reduce serum calcium to normal within 5 days, the effect lasting up to 4 wks. Repeated therapy can be given 3–4-weekly as an outpatient. For management of hyperparathyroidism, see page 358. FHH does not require therapy.

Hypocalcaemia

The differential diagnosis of hypocalcaemia is shown in Box 10.12. The most common cause of hypocalcaemia is a low serum albumin with normal ionised calcium concentration. Ionised calcium may be low with a normal total serum calcium in alkalosis, e.g. hyperventilation. Hypocalcaemia may also develop in magnesium deficiency, as this impairs PTH secretion.

10.12 Differential diagnosis of hypocalcaemia	Total serum calcium	Ionised serum calcium	Serum phosphate	Serum PTH concentration
Hypoalbuminaemia	↓	→	→	→
Alkalosis	→	↓	→	→ or ↑
Vitamin D deficiency	↓	↓	↓	↑
Chronic renal failure	↓	↓	↑	↑
Hypoparathyroidism	↓	↓	↑	↓
Pseudohypoparathyroidism	↓	↓	↑	↑
Acute pancreatitis	↓	↓	→ or ↓	↑
Hypomagnesaemia	↓	↓	Variable	↓ or →

Clinical assessment

Low ionised calcium increases excitability of peripheral nerves. Tetany can occur if total serum calcium is <2.0 mmol/L (8 mg/dL). In children, a characteristic triad of carpopedal spasm, stridor and convulsions occurs. Adults complain of tingling in the hands and feet and around the mouth. When overt signs are lacking, latent tetany may be revealed by Trousseau's sign (inflation of a sphygmomanometer cuff to more than the systolic BP causes carpal spasm) or Chvostek's sign (tapping over the facial nerve produces twitching of the facial muscles). Hypocalcaemia causes papilloedema and QT interval prolongation, predisposing to ventricular arrhythmias. Prolonged hypocalcaemia with hyperphosphataemia may cause calcification of the basal ganglia, epilepsy, psychosis and cataracts. Hypocalcaemia with hypophosphataemia (vitamin D deficiency) causes rickets in children and osteomalacia in adults.

Management

To control tetany, alkalosis can be reversed by rebreathing expired air in a bag ($\uparrow Pa\text{CO}_2$). Injection of 20 mL of 10% calcium gluconate slowly into a vein will raise the serum calcium concentration immediately. IV magnesium is required to correct hypocalcaemia associated with hypomagnesaemia.

Hyperparathyroidism

The three categories of hyperparathyroidism are shown in Box 10.13.

Primary hyperparathyroidism: There is autonomous secretion of PTH, usually by a single parathyroid adenoma.

Secondary hyperparathyroidism: There is increased PTH secretion to compensate for prolonged hypocalcaemia, thus increasing serum calcium levels by bone resorption. It is associated with hyperplasia of all parathyroid tissue.

Tertiary hyperparathyroidism: Continuous stimulation of the parathyroids, in secondary hyperparathyroidism, occasionally results in adenoma formation and autonomous PTH secretion. This is called tertiary hyperparathyroidism.

10.13 Hyperparathyroidism		
Type	**Serum calcium**	**PTH**
Primary Single adenoma (90%), multiple adenomas (4%), nodular hyperplasia (5%), carcinoma (1%)	Raised	Not suppressed
Secondary Chronic renal failure, malabsorption, osteomalacia and rickets	Low	Raised
Tertiary	Raised	Not suppressed

Primary hyperparathyroidism

This has a prevalence of 1 in 800 and is 2–3 times more common in women; 90% of patients are over 50. It also occurs in MEN syndromes. Clinical presentation is described under hypercalcaemia (p. 355).

Skeletal and radiological changes include:
• Osteoporosis-reduced bone mineral density on DEXA scanning.
• Osteitis fibrosa resulting from increased bone resorption by osteoclasts with fibrous replacement. It presents as bone pain, fracture and deformity. • Chondrocalcinosis due to deposition of calcium pyrophosphate crystals within articular cartilage, typically the knee, leading to osteoarthritis or acute pseudogout. • X-ray changes: subperiosteal erosions, terminal resorption in the phalanges, 'pepper-pot' skull and renal calcification.

^{99m}Tc-sestamibi scintigraphy or USS can be performed prior to surgery to localise the adenoma but may be negative.

Management

The treatment of choice for primary hyperparathyroidism is surgical excision of a solitary parathyroid adenoma or hyperplastic glands. Experienced surgeons will identify solitary tumours in >90% of cases. Patients with parathyroid bone disease run a significant risk of developing hypocalcaemia post-operatively, but this risk can be reduced by correcting vitamin D deficiency pre-operatively.

Surgery is indicated for patients under 50 and for those with symptoms or complications, e.g. peptic ulceration, renal stones, renal impairment or osteopenia. The remainder can be reviewed annually, with assessment of symptoms, renal function, serum calcium and bone mineral density.

Treatment of severe hypercalcaemia is described above (p. 356).

Cinacalcet is a calcimimetic that enhances the sensitivity of the calcium-sensing receptor, so reducing PTH levels, and is licensed for tertiary hyperparathyroidism and for patients with primary hyperparathyroidism who are unwilling or unfit to have surgery.

Hypoparathyroidism

Causes of hypoparathyroidism include:
• Parathyroid gland damage during thyroid surgery (transient hypocalcaemia in 10%, permanent in 1%). • Infiltration of the glands, e.g. haemochromatosis, Wilson's disease. • Congenital/inherited (rare), e.g. autoimmune polyendocrine syndrome (APS) type I, autosomal dominant hypoparathyroidism.

In pseudohypoparathyroidism there is tissue resistance to PTH. Clinical features include:
• Short stature. • Short 4th metacarpals and metatarsals. • Rounded face. • Obesity. • Subcutaneous calcification.

The term 'pseudo-pseudohypoparathyroidism' describes the condition of individuals with these clinical features in whom serum calcium and PTH concentrations are normal. Due to genomic imprinting, pseudohypoparathyroidism results from inheritance of the gene defect from the mother, but inheritance from the father results in pseudo-pseudohypoparathyroidism.

Persistent hypoparathyroidism and pseudohypoparathyroidism are treated with oral calcium salts and vitamin D analogues (alfacalcidol, calcitriol). Monitoring of therapy is required because of the risks of iatrogenic hypercalcaemia, hypercalciuria and nephrocalcinosis.

THE ADRENAL GLANDS

The adrenals comprise separate endocrine glands within one anatomical structure.

The adrenal medulla is an extension of the sympathetic nervous system that secretes catecholamines. Most of the adrenal cortex is made up of cells that secrete cortisol and adrenal androgens, and form part of the hypothalamic–pituitary–adrenal (HPA) axis. The small outer glomerulosa of the cortex secretes aldosterone under the control of the renin–angiotensin system.

Adrenal anatomy and function are shown in Figure 10.5.

Glucocorticoids: Cortisol is the major glucocorticoid in humans. Levels are highest in the morning and lowest in the middle of the night. Cortisol rises dramatically during stress, including any illness. This elevation protects key metabolic functions and cortisol deficiency is, therefore, most obvious at times of stress.

Mineralocorticoids: Aldosterone is the most important mineralocorticoid. It binds to renal mineralocorticoid receptors, causing sodium retention and increased excretion of potassium and protons. The principal stimulus to aldosterone secretion is angiotensin II, a peptide produced by activation of the renin–angiotensin system (see Fig. 10.5). Renin secretion from the juxtaglomerular apparatus in the kidney is stimulated by low perfusion pressure in the afferent arteriole, low sodium filtration or increased sympathetic nerve activity.

Catecholamines: In humans, most circulating noradrenaline (norepinephrine) is derived from sympathetic nerve endings. However, noradrenaline is converted to adrenaline (epinephrine) in the adrenal medulla. The medulla is thus the major source of circulating adrenaline.

Adrenal androgens: Adrenal androgens are secreted in response to ACTH. They are probably important in the initiation of puberty (the adrenarche), are the major source of androgens in females and may be important in female libido.

Presenting problems in adrenal disease
Cushing's syndrome

Cushing's syndrome is caused by excessive activation of glucocorticoid receptors. Endogenous causes are shown in Box 10.14; by far

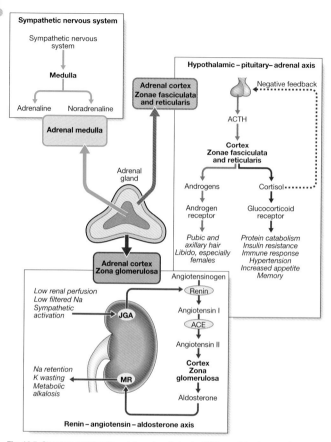

Fig. 10.5 Structure and function of the adrenal glands. (ACE = angiotensin-converting enzyme; JGA = juxtaglomerular apparatus; MR = mineralocorticoid receptor)

the most common cause is iatrogenic, however, due to prolonged administration of synthetic glucocorticoids such as prednisolone.

Clinical assessment

The diverse manifestations of glucocorticoid excess are indicated in Figure 10.6. Some common disorders can be confused with Cushing's syndrome because they are associated with alterations in cortisol secretion, e.g. obesity and depression.

A careful drug history is vital to exclude iatrogenic causes; even inhaled or topical glucocorticoids can induce Cushing's syndrome. Some clinical features are more common in ectopic ACTH syndrome. Ectopic tumours have no negative feedback sensitivity to cortisol. Very high ACTH levels are associated with marked

ACTH-dependent – 80%

- Pituitary adenoma secreting ACTH (Cushing's disease) – 70%
- Ectopic ACTH syndrome (e.g. bronchial carcinoid, small-cell lung carcinoma) – 10%

Non-ACTH-dependent – 20%

- Adrenal adenoma – 15%
- Adrenal carcinoma – 5%

Hypercortisolism due to other causes (pseudo-Cushing's syndrome)

- Alcohol excess (clinical features)
- Major depressive illness (biochemical features)
- Primary obesity (mild biochemical features)

pigmentation with hypokalaemic alkalosis, aggravating both myopathy and hyperglycaemia. When the tumour secreting ACTH is malignant, the onset is usually rapid and may be associated with cachexia. In Cushing's disease, the pituitary tumour is usually a microadenoma (<10 mm diameter); hence other features of a pituitary macroadenoma (hypopituitarism, visual failure or disconnection hyperprolactinaemia) are rare.

Investigations

It is useful to divide investigations into those that establish whether the patient has Cushing's syndrome, and those that are used subsequently to elucidate the aetiology. Additional tests include plasma electrolytes, glucose, glycosylated haemoglobin and bone mineral density measurement. In iatrogenic Cushing's syndrome, cortisol levels are low unless the corticosteroid cross-reacts in immunoassays with cortisol (e.g. prednisolone).

Does the patient have Cushing's syndrome? Cushing's syndrome is confirmed by the demonstration of increased secretion of cortisol (24-hr urinary cortisol) and serum cortisol that fails to suppress either with a 1-mg overnight dexamethasone suppression test or with the 48-hr low-dose dexamethasone suppression test (0.5 mg 4 times daily for 48 hrs). Loss of diurnal variation, with elevated late night salivary or serum cortisol, is also characteristic of Cushing's syndrome.

What is the cause of the Cushing's syndrome? Plasma ACTH <1.1 pmol/L on >2 occasions indicates an adrenal tumour, while ACTH >3.3 pmol/L indicates a pituitary or ectopic source. Tests to discriminate pituitary from ectopic ACTH rely on the fact that pituitary tumours, but not ectopic tumours, retain some features of normal regulation. Thus, in pituitary disease, ACTH and cortisol are stimulated by corticotrophin releasing hormone (CRH) injection and suppressed during a 48-hr high-dose dexamethasone suppression test (2 mg 4 times daily for 48 hrs). CT/MRI detects most adrenal

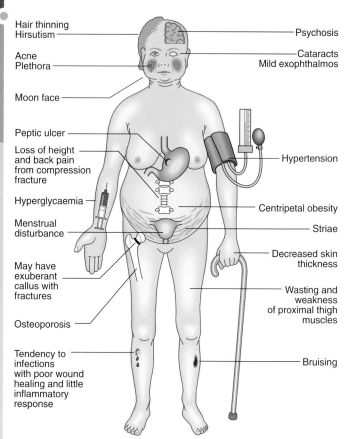

Fig. 10.6 Clinical features of Cushing's syndrome.

adenomas. Adrenal carcinomas are usually large (>5 cm). Tumours
not imaged are localised with selective adrenal vein catheterisation
with cortisol sampling. Pituitary MRI detects ~60% of pituitary
microadenomas. Venous catheterisation with inferior petrosal sinus
ACTH measurement is used if the MRI is non-diagnostic.

Management

Untreated Cushing's syndrome has a 50% 5-yr mortality. Most
patients are treated surgically, and corticosteroid biosynthesis can
be inhibited by metyrapone or ketoconazole pending operation.

Cushing's disease: Trans-sphenoidal surgery with selective
removal of the adenoma is the treatment of choice. Bilateral adrenalectomy is an alternative but there is a risk that the pituitary tumour
will grow in the absence of negative feedback suppression. This can

result in Nelson's syndrome, with an aggressive pituitary macroadenoma and very high ACTH levels causing pigmentation. Nelson's syndrome can be prevented by pituitary irradiation.

Adrenal tumours: Laparoscopic surgery is the treatment of choice for adrenal adenomas. Adrenal carcinomas are resected if possible, then the tumour bed is irradiated and the adrenolytic drug mitotane is given, but recurrence remains common.

Ectopic ACTH syndrome: Localised tumours causing this syndrome should be removed. In unresectable malignancies, the severity of the Cushing's syndrome can be reduced with medical therapy (see above).

Therapeutic use of glucocorticoids

Glucocorticoids are used for many conditions, but even topical preparations (dermal, rectal and inhaled) can cause significant suppression of endogenous ACTH and cortisol secretion. Equivalent doses of 5 mg prednisolone are:

• Hydrocortisone 20 mg. • Cortisone acetate 25 mg. • Dexamethasone 0.5 mg.

Adverse effects of glucocorticoids

The clinical features of glucocorticoid excess are illustrated in Figure 10.6, and are related to dose and duration of therapy.

Diabetes mellitus or glucose intolerance can be worsened. Rapid changes in cortisol can cause marked mood disturbance, either depression or mania, and insomnia Fracture risk is greater in glucocorticoid-induced osteoporosis than in post-menopausal osteoporosis, so when systemic glucocorticoids are prescribed for >3 mths, bone-protective therapy (p. 600) should be considered. Signs of perforation of a viscus may be masked and the patient may show no febrile response to an infection. Glucocorticoids act synergistically with NSAIDs, including aspirin, to increase the risk of gastric erosions and ulceration. Latent TB may be re-activated and patients on corticosteroids should be advised to avoid contact with varicella zoster virus if they are not immune.

Management of glucocorticoid withdrawal

All glucocorticoid therapy can suppress the HPA axis; however, a crisis due to adrenal insufficiency on withdrawal of glucocorticoids occurs only after prolonged (>3 wks) or repeated courses, or doses of prednisolone >7.5 mg/day. In these circumstances, steroid withdrawal must be slow as the HPA axis may take months to recover. Patients must avoid sudden withdrawal, carry a steroid card and/or wear an engraved bracelet.

To confirm that the HPA axis is recovering during glucocorticoid withdrawal, once the dose is down to 4 mg prednisolone, measure plasma cortisol at 0900 hrs before the next dose. If this is detectable, then perform an ACTH stimulation test to confirm that glucocorticoids can be withdrawn completely.

> ### 10.15 Causes of adrenocortical insufficiency
>
> **Secondary (↓ACTH)**
>
> - Withdrawal of glucocorticoid therapy
> - Hypothalamic/pituitary disease
>
> **Primary (↑ACTH)**
>
> - Addison's disease
>   Common: autoimmune, TB, HIV/AIDS, metastatic carcinoma, bilateral adrenalectomy
>   Rare: lymphoma, intra-adrenal haemorrhage (Waterhouse–Friderichsen syndrome in meningococcal septicaemia), amyloidosis, haemochromatosis
> - Corticosteroid biosynthetic enzyme defects
>   Congenital adrenal hyperplasias
>   Drugs: metyrapone, ketoconazole

Adrenal insufficiency

Adrenal insufficiency results from inadequate secretion of cortisol and/or aldosterone. Causes are shown in Box 10.15. The most common is ACTH deficiency (secondary adrenocortical failure), usually because of withdrawal of chronic glucocorticoid therapy or a pituitary tumour. Congenital adrenal hyperplasias and Addison's disease are rare.

Clinical assessment

Patients may present with chronic features or in acute circulatory shock.

With a chronic presentation, initial symptoms are often misdiagnosed (e.g. as depression or chronic fatigue); the diagnosis should be considered in all patients with hyponatraemia. Features of an acute adrenal crisis include circulatory shock with severe hypotension, hyponatraemia, hyperkalaemia and, occasionally, hypoglycaemia and hypercalcaemia. Muscle cramps, vomiting, diarrhoea and fever may be present. The crisis is often precipitated by intercurrent disease, surgery or infection. Pigmentation due to excess ACTH may be prominent, particularly in recent scars and pressure areas. Vitiligo occurs in 10–20% of patients with autoimmune Addison's disease.

Investigations

In an acute crisis, a random blood sample should be stored for measurement of cortisol, but other tests are deferred until treatment has been given. In chronic illness, investigations may be performed before any treatment.

Assessment of glucocorticoids: Random plasma cortisol is usually low in adrenal insufficiency but may be inappropriately within the reference range for a seriously ill patient. The short ACTH stimulation test (tetracosactide, short Synacthen test) requires administration of 250 μg ACTH (Synacthen) IM with serum cortisol measured at 0 and 30 mins. A cortisol >500 nmol/L (>18 μg/dL) at either time excludes adrenal insufficiency. A cortisol level that fails to increase occurs with primary or secondary adrenal insufficiency. These can be distinguished by measurement of ACTH, which is low in ACTH deficiency and high in Addison's disease.

Assessment of mineralocorticoids: Hyponatraemia occurs in both aldosterone and cortisol deficiency. Hyperkalaemia is common in aldosterone deficiency. Plasma renin activity and aldosterone should be measured in the supine position. In mineralocorticoid deficiency, plasma renin activity is high, with a low or low normal plasma aldosterone.

Other tests to establish the cause: Patients with unexplained secondary adrenocortical insufficiency should be investigated as described on page 364. In patients with elevated ACTH, further investigation of the adrenals is required. Adrenal autoantibodies are frequently positive in autoimmune adrenal failure, and other autoimmune diseases may be present. If negative, adrenal imaging with CT or MRI may reveal malignancy, and an AXR may show adrenal calcification in TB. An HIV test should be performed.

Management

Glucocorticoid replacement: Hydrocortisone (i.e. cortisol) is the drug of choice. In the non-critically ill, cortisol is given 10 mg on waking and 5 mg at ~1500 hrs. Replacement doses should not cause Cushingoid side-effects. Excess weight gain usually indicates over-replacement, whilst persistent lethargy or hyperpigmentation may indicate an inadequate dose. Patients on glucocorticoid replacement should be advised to:

• Double the dose of hydrocortisone during intercurrent infection. • Increase the dose peri-operatively (major operation, 100 mg 4 times daily). • Keep parenteral hydrocortisone at home in case of vomiting. • Carry a steroid card and wear a medical bracelet.

An adrenal crisis is a medical emergency and requires IV hydro-cortisone succinate 100 mg IV fluid (normal saline and 10% dextrose for hypoglycaemia). Parenteral hydrocortisone should be continued (100 mg IM 4 times daily) until the patient is able to take oral therapy. The precipitating cause should be treated.

Mineralocorticoid replacement: Fludrocortisone is administered (0.05–0.2 mg daily). Adequacy of replacement can be assessed with measurement of BP, plasma electrolytes and plasma renin activity.

Endocrine hypertension

Investigation and management of hypertension are discussed on page 244. While there is no discernible cause in the majority of patients with hypertension (essential hypertension), a small percentage have an underlying endocrine disorder. Most cases of endocrine hypertension are related to mineralocorticoid excess.

Phaeochromocytoma, Cushing's syndrome, hyperparathyroidism, acromegaly and thyroid dysfunction also raise BP.

Incidental adrenal mass

Adrenal 'incidentalomas' are present in up to 10% of adults. They are identified on abdominal CT or MRI scan that has been performed for another indication. Some 85% are non-functioning adrenal adenomas. The remainder includes functional tumours of the adrenal cortex, phaeochromocytomas, primary/secondary carcinomas or hamartomas.

Investigations should include a 24-hr urine collection for catecholamines and urine free cortisol, plasma renin and aldosterone, and, in women, serum androgens. CT and MRI can be used to assess malignant potential (from size, homogeneity, lipid content and enhancement). Biopsy cannot distinguish adenoma from carcinoma but can help to diagnose metastases. Functional lesions and tumours >4 cm in diameter are removed by laparoscopic adrenalectomy. In non-functioning lesions, <4 cm excision is only required if serial imaging suggests growth.

Mineralocorticoid excess

Indications to test for mineralocorticoid excess in hypertensive patients include:
• Hypokalaemia. • Poor control of BP with conventional therapy.
• Presentation at a young age.

Causes of excessive activation of mineralocorticoid receptors can be differentiated by renin and aldosterone measurement.

High renin and aldosterone (secondary hyperaldosteronism): Renin secretion is increased in response to inadequate renal perfusion and hypotension, e.g. diuretic therapy, cardiac failure, liver failure or renal artery stenosis. Very rarely, renin-secreting renal tumours cause secondary hyperaldosteronism.

Low renin and high aldosterone (primary hyperaldosteronism): A small minority of patients with hypertension will be found to have primary hyperaldosteronism. Most have idiopathic bilateral adrenal hyperplasia and only a minority have an adrenal adenoma secreting aldosterone (Conn's syndrome).

Low renin and aldosterone: The mineralocorticoid receptor pathway in the distal nephron is activated, even though aldosterone levels are low. This can occur with ectopic ACTH syndrome, liquorice misuse, an 11-deoxycorticosterone-secreting adrenal tumour or Liddle's syndrome.

Clinical assessment

Many patients are asymptomatic but they may have features of sodium retention or potassium loss. Sodium retention may cause oedema. Hypokalaemia causes muscle weakness (or even paralysis), polyuria (renal tubular damage producing nephrogenic diabetes insipidus) and occasionally tetany (associated metabolic alkalosis and low ionised calcium). BP is elevated.

Investigations

Biochemical: Plasma electrolytes: hypokalaemia, ↑bicarbonate, sodium upper normal (primary hyperaldosteronism), hyponatraemia (secondary hyperaldosteronism: hypovolaemia stimulates antidiuretic hormone (ADH) release and high angiotensin II levels stimulate thirst). Renin and aldosterone levels distinguish the patterns above.

Localisation: Abdominal CT/MRI can localise an aldosterone-producing adenoma (APA) but non-functioning adrenal adenomas are present in ~20% of patients with essential hypertension. If the scan is inconclusive, adrenal vein catheterisation with measurement of aldosterone may be helpful.

Management

Spironolactone, an aldosterone antagonist, treats both hypokalaemia and hypertension due to mineralocorticoid excess. Spironolactone can be changed to the sodium channel blocker amiloride (10–40 mg/day) if gynaecomastia develops (~20%). In patients with APA, pre-operative therapy to normalise whole-body electrolyte balance should be undertaken before unilateral adrenalectomy. Post-operatively, hypertension remains in as many as 70% of cases.

Phaeochromocytoma and paraganglioma

These rare neuro-endocrine tumours may secrete catecholamines (adrenaline/epinephrine, noradrenaline/norepinephrine). Approximately 80% occur in the adrenal medulla (phaeochromocytomas), while 20% arise in sympathetic ganglia (paragangliomas). Most are benign but ~15% show malignant features. Around 30% are associated with inherited disorders, including neurofibromatosis (p. 672), von Hippel–Lindau syndrome (p. 672) and MEN 2 (p. 378).

Clinical features

These can be paroxysmal and include:
- Hypertension (with postural hypotension). • Palpitations.
- Pallor. • Sweating. • Headache. • Anxiety (with fear of death).
- Abdominal pain. • Glucose intolerance.

Some patients present with a complication of hypertension, e.g. stroke. There may be features of associated familial syndromes (see above).

Investigations

Excessive secretion of catecholamines can be confirmed by measuring metabolites (metanephrine and normetanephrine) in serum and/or urine. False positives occur in stressed patients and with some drugs (e.g. tricyclic antidepressants). False-negative results also occur due to intermittent catecholamine secretion. Phaeochromocytomas are identified by abdominal CT/MRI. To localise paragangliomas, scintigraphy using meta-iodobenzyl guanidine (MIBG) is combined with CT.

Management

Medical therapy is required pre-operatively, preferably for a minimum of 6 wks. The non-competitive α-blocker phenoxybenzamine (10–20 mg orally 3–4 times daily) is used with a β-blocker (e.g. propranolol). Beta-blockers must not be given before the α-blocker, as this may cause a paradoxical rise in BP. Careful pharmacological control of BP is essential during surgery for phaeochromocytoma.

Congenital adrenal hyperplasia

This rare autosomal recessive defect of cortisol biosynthesis causes insufficiency of hormones downstream of the block, with reduced feedback and increased ACTH causing over-production of steroids upstream of the block.

The most common example is 21-hydroxylase deficiency. This causes impaired synthesis of cortisol and aldosterone with accumulation of 17OH-progesterone, which is converted into adrenal androgens. About 30% of cases present in infancy with features of glucocorticoid and mineralocorticoid deficiency and androgen excess, including ambiguous genitalia in girls. The remainder have milder cortisol deficiency and/or ACTH and androgen excess, causing precocious pseudo-puberty. The mildest defects may present in adult females as amenorrhoea and/or hirsutism (p. 352).

Investigations

Circulating 17OH-progesterone levels are raised in 21-hydroxylase deficiency. Assessment is otherwise as described for adrenal insufficiency on page 364. Antenatal diagnosis should be offered to families of affected children.

Management

Replacement of deficient corticosteroids suppresses ACTH-driven adrenal androgen production.

In hirsute women with late-onset 21-hydroxylase deficiency, anti-androgen therapy is equally effective.

THE ENDOCRINE PANCREAS AND GI TRACT

Presenting problems in endocrine pancreas disease
Spontaneous hypoglycaemia

Hypoglycaemia most commonly complicates treatment of diabetes mellitus with insulin or sulphonylureas. Spontaneous hypoglycaemia should only be diagnosed if all three conditions of Whipple's triad are met:

• Symptoms of hypoglycaemia. • Low blood glucose measured at the time of symptoms. • Symptoms resolving on correction of hypoglycaemia.

There is no specific blood glucose at which spontaneous hypoglycaemia occurs, although lower values are more likely to be pathological.

Clinical assessment

Clinical features of hypoglycaemia are described on page 394. Symptoms are episodic and key questions include symptom frequency on fasting/exercise and symptom relief by consumption of sugar. Hypoglycaemia should be considered in all comatose patients, even if there is an apparently obvious cause. In the acute setting, alcohol is the most likely cause.

Investigations

Does the patient have a hypoglycaemic disorder? In an acute presentation, hypoglycaemia is usually tested with capillary blood glucose strips. However, due to their relative inaccuracy, hypoglycaemia should be confirmed by formal laboratory measurement. Establishing the existence of a hypoglycaemic disorder in outpatient clinics requires a prolonged (72-hr) fast:

• Symptoms develop: blood samples are taken to confirm hypoglycaemia and for measurement of insulin and C-peptide. • Symptoms resolve with glucose: Whipple's triad is completed. • Absence of clinical and biochemical hypoglycaemia during the test: excludes the diagnosis of hypoglycaemia.

What is causing the hypoglycaemia? Causes can be classified by the level of insulin and C-peptide measured in serum sampled during hypoglycaemia:

• ↓Insulin and ↓C-peptide: impaired liver glucose release due to alcohol (the most common cause in non-diabetics), drugs, critical illnesses (hepatic or renal failure, malaria), hypopituitarism, adrenocortical failure, non-islet cell tumours. • ↑Insulin and ↓C-peptide: exogenous insulin. • ↑Insulin and ↑C-peptide: insulinoma, drugs (sulphonylureas, pentamidine).

Insulinomas in the pancreas are usually small (<5 mm) and can be identified by CT, MRI or endoscopic/laparoscopic USS. About 10% of insulinomas are malignant. Rarely, sarcomas may cause recurrent hypoglycaemia due to production of insulin-like growth factor-2 (IGF-2).

Management

Acute hypoglycaemia should be treated as soon as blood samples have been taken. IV dextrose (10% or 50%) should be followed with oral carbohydrate. Continuous dextrose infusion may be necessary, especially in sulphonylurea poisoning. IM glucagon (1 mg) stimulates hepatic glucose release but is ineffective when glycogen reserves are depleted (alcohol excess, liver disease). Chronic recurrent hypoglycaemia in insulin-secreting tumours can be treated by regular carbohydrate consumption combined with inhibitors of insulin secretion (diazoxide or somatostatin analogues). Benign insulinomas are usually resected.

Neuro-endocrine tumours

Neuro-endocrine tumours (NETs) are a heterogeneous group derived from neuro-endocrine cells in many organs, including the

GI tract, lung, adrenals (phaeochromocytoma) and thyroid (medullary carcinoma). They range from benign (e.g. most insulinomas) to aggressively malignant. Most GI and pancreatic NETs are non-secretory and grow slowly but can metastasise, e.g. to the liver. NETs may be single or multifocal (typically as part of MEN 1).

GI carcinoid tumours secrete 5-hydroxyindoleacetic acid (5-HIAA) but this only produces carcinoid syndrome (flushing, wheezing and diarrhoea) when hepatic or peritoneal metastases allow vasoactive hormones to reach the systemic circulation. Secretory pancreatic NETs include:

• Gastrinoma: Zollinger–Ellison syndrome. • Insulinoma: recurrent hypoglycaemia. • VIPoma: watery diarrhoea, hypokalaemia. • Glucagonoma: diabetes mellitus, necrolytic migratory erythema. • Somatostatinoma: diabetes mellitus, steatorrhoea.

Investigations

A combination of imaging with USS, CT, MRI and/or radio-labelled somatostatin analogue is used to identify and stage the primary tumour. Biopsy of the primary tumour or metastasis is required to confirm the presence of an NET and the histological type. Carcinoid syndrome is confirmed by elevated concentrations of 5-HIAA in a 24-hr urine collection. False positives can occur after certain foods, e.g. avocado and pineapple. Plasma chromogranin A can be measured in a fasting blood sample, and the pathologically secreted hormones can be useful as tumour markers.

Management

Treatment of solitary tumours is by surgical resection. Diazoxide may reduce insulin secretion in insulinomas and high-dose proton pump inhibitors suppress acid in gastrinomas. Somatostatin analogues reduce the symptoms associated with 5-HT, glucagon and vasoactive intestinal peptide (VIP) excess. Cytotoxic chemotherapy, targeted radionuclide therapy with ^{131}I-MIBG, and resection/embolisation of hepatic metastases have a limited palliative role.

THE HYPOTHALAMUS AND THE PITUITARY GLAND

Diseases of the hypothalamus and pituitary are rare (annual incidence ~3:100 000). The gland is composed of two lobes, anterior and posterior, and is connected to the hypothalamus by the infundibular stalk, which has portal vessels carrying blood from the median eminence of the hypothalamus to the anterior lobe and nerve fibres to the posterior lobe. The functions of the pituitary are summarised in Figure 10.1.

Presenting problems in hypothalamic and pituitary disease

The clinical features of pituitary disease are shown in Figure 10.7. The most common problem is an adenoma of the anterior pituitary.

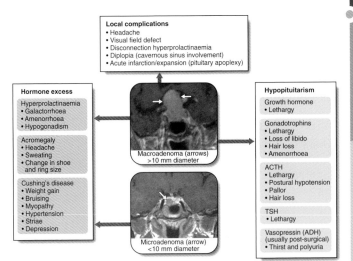

Local complications
• Headache
• Visual field defect
• Disconnection hyperprolactinaemia
• Diplopia (cavernous sinus involvement)
• Acute infarction/expansion (pituitary apoplexy)

Hormone excess

Hyperprolactinaemia
• Galactorrhoea
• Amenorrhoea
• Hypogonadism

Acromegaly
• Headache
• Sweating
• Change in shoe and ring size

Cushing's disease
• Weight gain
• Bruising
• Myopathy
• Hypertension
• Striae
• Depression

Macroadenoma (arrows) >10 mm diameter

Microadenoma (arrow) <10 mm diameter

Hypopituitarism

Growth hormone
• Lethargy

Gonadotrophins
• Lethargy
• Loss of libido
• Hair loss
• Amenorrhoea

ACTH
• Lethargy
• Postural hypotension
• Pallor
• Hair loss

TSH
• Lethargy

Vasopressin (ADH) (usually post-surgical)
• Thirst and polyuria

Fig. 10.7 Clinical effects of large and small pituitary tumours.

Young women with pituitary disease most commonly present with secondary amenorrhoea or galactorrhoea (in hyperprolactinaemia). Men and post-menopausal women are less likely to report symptoms of hypogonadism and so are more likely to present late with larger tumours causing visual field defects. Pituitary tumours are increasingly discovered incidentally on CT/MRI scans.

Size and effect on secretory function determine symptoms:

• Microadenomas (<10 mm diameter) are common incidental findings and should only be treated if they are secreting excess hormones (examples include Cushing's, acromegaly and hyperprolactinaemia). • In addition, macroadenomas may compress adjacent neural tissue and normal pituitary tissue, causing neurological symptoms and hypopituitarism (see Fig. 10.7).

Hypopituitarism

Hypopituitarism means the combined deficiency of any of the anterior pituitary hormones. This most commonly results from the destructive effects of a pituitary macroadenoma, but other causes are shown in Box 10.16.

Clinical assessment

With progressive pituitary lesions, onset of symptoms is insidious. Pituitary functions are lost in a characteristic sequence:

• Growth hormone: lethargy, muscle weakness and increased fat mass. • Gonadotrophins (LH and FSH): loss of libido, gynaecomastia, decreased shaving and, in the female, oligomenorrhoea or amenorrhoea. • ACTH: symptoms of cortisol insufficiency but

10.16 Causes of anterior pituitary hormone deficiency

Structural

- Primary pituitary tumour (adenoma*), craniopharyngioma*, meningioma*, haemorrhage (apoplexy), arachnoid cyst

Inflammatory/infiltrative

- Sarcoidosis, infections (e.g. pituitary abscess, TB, syphilis, encephalitis), haemochromatosis, Langerhans cell histiocytosis

Congenital deficiencies

- GnRH (Kallmann's syndrome)*, TRH, growth hormone releasing hormone (GHRH)*, CRH

Functional*

- Chronic systemic illness, excessive exercise, anorexia nervosa

Other

- Head injury*, (para-)sellar radiotherapy*, (para-)sellar surgery*, post-partum necrosis (Sheehan's syndrome)

*Most common causes of pituitary hormone deficiency.

maintenance of aldosterone secretion. Serum K^+ is normal but postural hypotension and dilutional hyponatraemia may occur. Rather than the pigmentation of Addison's disease, pallor is usually present, due to lack of stimulation of melanocytes by β-lipotrophic hormone (β-LPH, a fragment of the ACTH precursor). • TSH: secondary hypothyroidism contributes further to apathy and cold intolerance.

Investigations

The investigation of pituitary disease is described in Box 10.17. In acutely unwell patients, the priority is to diagnose and treat cortisol deficiency (see above), followed later by other tests. All patients with pituitary hormone deficiency should have an MRI or CT scan to identify pituitary or hypothalamic tumours. If no tumour is identified, further investigations are indicated to exclude infectious or infiltrative causes.

Management

Treatment of acutely ill patients is similar to that described for adrenocortical insufficiency (see above). Once the cause of hypopituitarism is established, specific treatment, e.g. of a pituitary macroadenoma, may be required.

Cortisol replacement: Hydrocortisone is used (p. 365). Mineralocorticoid replacement is not required.

Thyroid hormone replacement: Levothyroxine 50–150 µg once daily should be given. The aim is to maintain serum T_4 in the upper part of the reference range. It is dangerous to give thyroid

| i | 10.17 Investigation of pituitary and hypothalamic disease |

Identify pituitary hormone deficiency

- ACTH deficiency: short ACTH stimulation test; insulin tolerance test (if uncertainty in interpretation of short ACTH stimulation test)
- LH/FSH deficiency: male – random serum testosterone, LH, FSH; pre-menopausal female – ask if menses are regular; post-menopausal female – random serum LH, FSH (usually >30 mU/L)
- TSH deficiency: serum T_4; TSH often detectable in secondary hypothyroidism (inactive circulating TSH isoforms)
- Growth hormone deficiency (only investigate if GH replacement contemplated): measure immediately after exercise; consider other stimulatory tests
- Cranial diabetes insipidus (may be masked by ACTH/TSH deficiency): exclude other causes of polyuria (blood glucose, potassium and calcium measurements); water deprivation test or 5% saline infusion test

Identify hormone excess

- Measure serum prolactin; investigate for acromegaly (glucose tolerance test) or Cushing's syndrome if indicated

Establish the anatomy and diagnosis

- Visual field testing; image pituitary/hypothalamus by MRI/CT

replacement in adrenal insufficiency without first giving glucocorticoid therapy, since this may precipitate adrenal crisis.

Sex hormone replacement: This is indicated for gonadotrophin deficiency in women <50 and in men.

Growth hormone (GH) replacement: GH is administered by daily subcutaneous self-injection to children and adolescents with GH deficiency, and until recently, was discontinued once the epiphyses had fused. There is now evidence that GH improves quality of life and exercise capacity in adults. It also helps young adults to achieve a higher peak bone mineral density. GH replacement is monitored by measurement of serum IGF-1 levels.

Pituitary tumour

Pituitary tumours may produce various local mass effects, or may be discovered incidentally on CT/MRI. A wide variety of disorders can present as a mass in the pituitary/hypothalamus region:

• The majority of intrasellar tumours are pituitary macroadenomas (most commonly non-functioning adenomas). • Most suprasellar masses are craniopharyngiomas. • Parasellar masses are most commonly meningiomas.

A common presentation is headache due to stretching of the dura. Although, classically, compression of the optic chiasm causes bitemporal hemianopia or upper quadrantanopia, any visual field defect can result from suprasellar extension because tumour may compress the optic nerve (scotoma) or tract (homonymous hemianopia). Optic atrophy may be apparent on ophthalmoscopy. Lateral extension may compress the 3rd, 4th or 6th cranial nerve, causing diplopia and strabismus, although this is unusual in anterior pituitary tumours.

Occasionally, pituitary tumours infarct or there is bleeding into cystic lesions. This is termed 'pituitary apoplexy' and may result in sudden localised compression and acute-onset hypopituitarism. Non-haemorrhagic pituitary infarction may occur in obstetric haemorrhage (Sheehan's syndrome), diabetes mellitus and raised intracranial pressure.

Investigations

A precise diagnosis requires surgical biopsy but this is usually performed as part of a therapeutic procedure. All patients should have pituitary function assessed (see Box 10.17).

Management

Specific treatments are described in the sections on hyperprolactinaemia, acromegaly and Cushing's disease. If serum prolactin is raised, dopamine agonists may shrink the lesion, avoiding the need for surgery. Non-functioning pituitary macroadenomas and craniopharyngiomas should be managed surgically, if needed, with radiotherapy reserved for second-line treatment. If there is evidence of pressure on visual pathways, urgent treatment is required. Most operations on the pituitary are performed using the trans-sphenoidal approach, from an incision under the upper lip or through the nose. Transfrontal surgery (craniotomy) is reserved for suprasellar tumours. All operations on the pituitary carry a risk of damaging endocrine function. Associated hypopituitarism should be treated as described above.

Pituitary function (see Box 10.17) should be retested 4–6 wks following surgery to detect the development of new hormone deficits. Imaging is repeated after a few months and, if there is any residual mass, external radiotherapy may reduce the risk of recurrence of radiosensitive tumours. Radiotherapy is not useful in patients requiring urgent therapy because it takes many months to be effective. It carries a lifelong risk of hypopituitarism (first 10 yrs 50–70%) and annual pituitary function tests are obligatory. Non-functioning tumours are followed up by repeated imaging. For smaller lesions, therapeutic surgery may not be indicated and the lesion may be monitored by serial neuroimaging.

Hyperprolactinaemia/galactorrhoea

Hyperprolactinaemia presents with hypogonadism and/or galactorrhoea. Galactorrhoea means lactation without breastfeeding. Prolactin stimulates milk secretion but not breast development; galactorrhoea therefore rarely occurs in men.

The causes of hyperprolactinaemia may be:

Physiological: Pregnancy, lactation, sleep, coitus, stress (e.g. post-seizure).

Drugs: Dopamine antagonists (phenothiazines, antidepressants, metoclopramide); dopamine-depleting drugs (reserpine, methyldopa); oestrogens (contraceptive pill).

Pathological: Pituitary tumours secreting prolactin (prolactinoma), or compressing the infundibular stalk, interrupting the hypothalamic dopaminergic inhibition of prolactin secretion ('disconnection' hyperprolactinaemia).

Other causes of hyperprolactinaemia include primary hypothyroidism, PCOS, hypothalamic disease and macroprolactinaemia. Macroprolactin is prolactin bound to IgG antibodies, which cross-reacts with some prolactin assays. Since macroprolactin cannot cross blood vessel walls to reach prolactin receptors, it is of no pathological significance.

Clinical assessment

In women, in addition to galactorrhoea, the associated hypogonadism causes secondary amenorrhoea and anovulation with infertility. History should include drug use, recent pregnancy and menstrual history. Breast examination is important to exclude malignancy with discharge. In men, there is decreased libido, reduced shaving frequency and lethargy. Further assessment should address the features of any pituitary disease (p. 371).

Investigations

Pregnancy should be excluded. Macroprolactin should be measured and, if present with a normal unbound prolactin concentration, then further investigation is not necessary in the absence of clinical features. Prolactin levels may indicate underlying pathology:

• Normal level: <500 mU/L (~14 ng/mL). • 500–1000 mU/L: stress or drugs most likely in non-pregnant/non-lactating patients. Repeat the measurement. • 1000–5000 mU/L: drugs, microprolactinoma or 'disconnection' hyperprolactinaemia. • >5000 mU/L: suggests a macroadenoma secreting prolactin.

Other investigations include:

• TFTs to exclude primary hypothyroidism (TRH-induced prolactin excess). • MRI/CT of hypothalamus/pituitary if prolactin remains raised after drugs excluded. • Patients with a macroadenoma need tests for hypopituitarism (see Box 10.17).

Management

The underlying cause should be corrected (stop offending drugs; give levothyroxine in primary hypothyroidism). Physiological galactorrhoea can be treated with dopamine agonists. These include bromocriptine 2.5–15 mg/day, cabergoline 250–1000 μg/wk and quinagolide 50–150 μg/day.

Prolactinoma

Most prolactinomas in pre-menopausal women are microadenomas because symptoms trigger early presentation. Occasionally, prolactinomas also secrete GH and cause acromegaly. Prolactin concentration correlates with tumour size: the higher the level, the bigger the tumour.

Management

Dopamine agonists are first-line treatment and shrink most prolactin-secreting macroadenomas, rendering surgery unnecessary. In microprolactinomas, it may be possible to withdraw therapy without recurrence of hyperprolactinaemia after a few years. In macroadenomas, drugs can only be withdrawn after curative surgery or radiotherapy.

If dopamine agonists fail to shrink a prolactinoma, transsphenoidal surgery is effective. It cures 80% of microadenomas, although cure rates in macroadenomas are lower. Radiotherapy may be required for some macroadenomas to prevent regrowth if dopamine agonists are stopped.

Pregnancy

Patients with microadenomas should have dopamine agonist therapy withdrawn as soon as pregnancy is confirmed. In contrast, macroprolactinomas may enlarge rapidly under oestrogen stimulation. Dopamine agonist therapy should be continued with monitoring of prolactin levels and visual fields during pregnancy.

Acromegaly

Acromegaly is caused by GH secretion, usually from a macroadenoma.

Clinical features

If GH hypersecretion occurs before epiphyseal fusion, then gigantism will result. More commonly, GH excess occurs after epiphyseal closure and acromegaly ensues. The most common complaints are headache and sweating. Other clinical features include:

• Skull growth with prominent supraorbital ridges. • Prognathism. • Enlargement of lips, nose and tongue. • Enlargement of hands and feet. • Carpal tunnel syndrome. • Cardiomyopathy. • Increased incidence of diabetes mellitus, hypertension, cardiovascular disease and colonic cancer. Additional features include those of any pituitary tumour (p. 373).

Investigations

An oral glucose tolerance test with GH measurement confirms the diagnosis. In normal subjects, plasma GH suppresses to $<0.5\ \mu g/L$ ($<2\ mU/L$). In acromegaly, it does not suppress, and in ~30% of patients there is a paradoxical rise; IGF-1 is also elevated. Remaining pituitary function should be investigated (see Box 10.17). Prolactin is elevated in ~30% due to tumour co-secretion of prolactin. Screening for colonic neoplasms with colonoscopy may also be undertaken.

Management

Surgical: Trans-sphenoidal surgery is first-line treatment and may result in cure of GH excess, especially in microadenomas. However, surgery usually debulks the tumour and further second-line therapy is required, according to post-operative imaging and glucose tolerance test results.

Radiotherapy: External radiotherapy is usually employed as second-line treatment if acromegaly persists after surgery, to stop tumour growth and lower GH. However, GH falls slowly (over many years) and there is a risk of hypopituitarism.

Medical: Somatostatin analogues (octreotide, lanreotide), administered as slow-release injections, are used to lower GH levels to <1.5 µg/L (<5 mU/L) following surgery. These may be discontinued after several years in patients who have received radiotherapy. Dopamine agonists are less potent in lowering GH but may be helpful in patients with associated hyperprolactinaemia. A GH receptor antagonist (pegvisomant) is available for daily self-injection for patients unresponsive to somatostatin analogue therapy.

Craniopharyngioma

Craniopharyngiomas are benign tumours within the sella or suprasellar space. They usually present because of pressure on the pituitary or adjacent structures and are managed by surgery followed by radiotherapy to reduce relapse rate.

Diabetes insipidus

This uncommon disorder is characterised by the excretion of excessive dilute urine and by thirst. It can be classified as cranial diabetes insipidus (deficient ADH production by hypothalamus) or nephrogenic DI (renal tubules unresponsive to ADH). Causes are listed in Box 10.18. Clinical features include polyuria (5–20 L/24 hrs) and polydipsia. Urine is of low specific gravity and osmolality. Adequate fluid intake can be maintained with an intact thirst mechanism in a conscious individual. However, in unconsciousness or hypothalamic thirst centre damage, DI is potentially lethal. The differential diagnosis includes diabetes mellitus and primary polydipsia (usually in patients with established psychiatric disease).

Investigations

DI is confirmed if, with an elevated plasma osmolality (>300 mOsm/kg), either serum ADH is undetectable or urine is not maximally concentrated (i.e. <600 mOsm/kg). Random simultaneous samples of blood and urine may exclude the diagnosis but, more often, the water deprivation test is required: no fluids are allowed for 8 hrs and body weight, plasma and urine osmolality are measured every 2 hrs; the test is stopped if >3% of body weight is lost. DI is confirmed by plasma osmolality >300 mOsm/kg with urine osmolality <600 mOsm/kg.

10.18 Causes of diabetes insipidus

Cranial

- Structural hypothalamic or high stalk lesion: see Box 10.16
- Idiopathic
- Genetic defect:
    Dominant
    Recessive (DIDMOAD syndrome – diabetes insipidus with diabetes mellitus, optic atrophy, deafness)

Nephrogenic

- Genetic defect: V2 receptor mutation; aquaporin-2 mutation
- Metabolic abnormality: hypercalcaemia; hypokalaemia
- Drug therapy: lithium; demeclocycline
- Poisoning: heavy metals
- Chronic kidney disease: polycystic kidney disease, infiltrative disease, sickle-cell anaemia

---

Desmopressin, an analogue of ADH with a longer half-life (DDAVP) is then given to distinguish cranial and nephrogenic DI:
• Cranial DI: confirmed if urine osmolality rises by >50% after DDAVP. • Nephrogenic DI: DDAVP does not concentrate urine. • Primary polydipsia: suggested by low plasma osmolality at the start of the test.

Anterior pituitary function and suprasellar anatomy should be assessed in patients with cranial diabetes insipidus, as indicated in Box 10.17.

Management

Treatment of cranial DI is with DDAVP, usually administered via the nasal mucous membrane as a spray, although it can be given orally or intramuscularly. The ideal dose prevents nocturia but avoids hyponatraemia, e.g. DDAVP nasal dose 5 μg in the morning and 10 μg at night. Polyuria in nephrogenic DI is improved by thiazide diuretics (bendroflumethiazide 5 mg/day) or amiloride (5–10 mg/day).

DISEASES AFFECTING MULTIPLE ENDOCRINE GLANDS

Multiple endocrine neoplasia

Multiple endocrine neoplasia (MEN) syndromes are rare autosomal dominant syndromes characterised by hyperplasia and tumours in multiple glands.

• MEN 1 (Wermer's syndrome): the association of primary hyper-parathyroidism, pituitary tumours and pancreatic neuro-endocrine tumours. • MEN 2 (Sipple's syndrome): primary hyperparathy-roidism, thyroid medullary carcinoma and phaeochromocytoma.

• MEN 2b: additional phenotypic changes include marfanoid habitus, skeletal abnormalities and mucosal neuromas.

MEN 1 results from inactivating mutations in '*menin*', a tumour suppressor gene on chromosome 11. In MEN 2, mutations are found in the *RET* proto-oncogene on chromosome 10. Genetic testing can be performed on relatives of affected individuals.

Individuals with MEN should have regular surveillance:

• MEN 1: annual measurements of calcium, GI hormones and prolactin; pituitary MRI is performed less frequently. • MEN 2: measurement of calcium and urinary catecholamines. The penetrance of thyroid medullary carcinoma is 100% in individuals with a *RET* mutation. Prophylactic thyroidectomy is therefore performed in childhood.

Autoimmune polyendocrine syndromes

Two distinct autoimmune polyendocrine syndromes are known: APS types 1 and 2.

• APS type 2 (Schmidt's syndrome): more common and observed in women aged 20–60. It is defined as the occurrence of two or more autoimmune endocrine disorders, e.g. Addison's disease, hypoparathyroidism, type 1 diabetes, Graves' disease and coeliac disease. Inheritance is autosomal dominant with incomplete penetrance and there is a strong association with HLA-DR3. • APS type 1 (autoimmune polyendocrinopathy, candidiasis, ectodermal dystrophy – APECED): much rarer and displays autosomal recessive inheritance. In addition to autoimmune diseases, nail dystrophy, dental enamel hypoplasia and mucocutaneous candidiasis are seen.

Diabetes mellitus

11

Diabetes mellitus is a clinical syndrome characterised by hyperglycaemia due to absolute or relative deficiency of insulin. Long-standing metabolic derangement can lead to the development of complications of diabetes, which characteristically affect the eye, kidney and nervous system. Diabetes occurs worldwide and its prevalence is rising; 366 million people had diabetes in 2011, and this is expected to reach 552 million by 2030. Diabetes is a major burden upon health-care facilities in all countries.

FUNCTIONAL ANATOMY, PHYSIOLOGY AND INVESTIGATIONS

Normal glucose and fat metabolism

Blood glucose is maintained within a narrow range by homeostatic mechanisms. The brain relies on glucose for energy as the blood–brain barrier is impermeable to free fatty acids (FFAs). Glucose enters the circulation from the liver and gut and is taken up by peripheral tissues, particularly skeletal muscle.

After ingestion of a carbohydrate meal, insulin, the primary regulator of glucose metabolism, is secreted from pancreatic β cells into the portal circulation in response to a rise in blood glucose. This rise, together with a fall in portal glucagon, suppresses hepatic glucose production, results in net hepatic glucose uptake and stimulates glucose uptake in skeletal muscle and fat.

Between meals, portal vein insulin and glucose concentrations fall while glucagon levels rise, causing increased hepatic glucose output via gluconeogenesis and glycogen breakdown.

Insulin is also the major regulator of fatty acid metabolism. High insulin levels after meals promote triglyceride accumulation, while in the fasting state, low insulin levels permit lipolysis and the release of FFAs and glycerol, which can be oxidised by many tissues. Their partial oxidation in the liver produces ketone bodies, which

CLINICAL EXAMINATION OF THE PATIENT WITH DIABETES

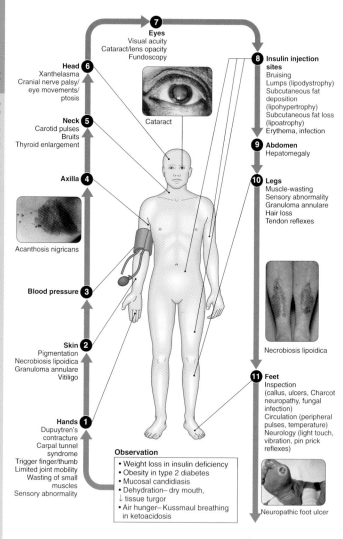

7 Eyes
Visual acuity
Cataract/lens opacity
Fundoscopy

Cataract

6 Head
Xanthelasma
Cranial nerve palsy/
eye movements/
ptosis

5 Neck
Carotid pulses
Bruits
Thyroid enlargement

4 Axilla

Acanthosis nigricans

3 Blood pressure

2 Skin
Pigmentation
Necrobiosis lipoidica
Granuloma annulare
Vitiligo

1 Hands
Dupuytren's
contracture
Carpal tunnel
syndrome
Trigger finger/thumb
Limited joint mobility
Wasting of small
muscles
Sensory abnormality

**8 Insulin injection
sites**
Bruising
Lumps (lipodystrophy)
Subcutaneous fat
deposition
(lipohypertrophy)
Subcutaneous fat loss
(lipoatrophy)
Erythema, infection

9 Abdomen
Hepatomegaly

10 Legs
Muscle-wasting
Sensory abnormality
Granuloma annulare
Hair loss
Tendon reflexes

Necrobiosis lipoidica

11 Feet
Inspection
(callus, ulcers, Charcot
neuropathy, fungal
infection)
Circulation (peripheral
pulses, temperature)
Neurology (light touch,
vibration, pin prick
reflexes)

Neuropathic foot ulcer

Observation
- Weight loss in insulin deficiency
- Obesity in type 2 diabetes
- Mucosal candidiasis
- Dehydration– dry mouth,
  ↓ tissue turgor
- Air hunger– Kussmaul breathing
  in ketoacidosis

can be utilised as metabolic fuel, but may accumulate during starvation.

Aetiology and pathogenesis of diabetes

In both of the common types of diabetes, environmental factors interact with genetic susceptibility to determine which people develop the clinical syndrome, and the timing of its onset. However, the underlying genes, precipitating environmental factors and pathophysiology differ substantially between type 1 and type 2 diabetes.

Type 1 diabetes

Type 1 diabetes is invariably associated with profound insulin deficiency requiring replacement therapy. It is a T-cell-mediated autoimmune disease leading to progressive destruction of the insulin-secreting β cells. Classical symptoms of diabetes occur only when 80–90% of β cells have been destroyed. Pathology shows insulitis (infiltration of the islets with mononuclear cells), in which β cells are destroyed, but cells secreting glucagon and other hormones remain intact. Islet cell antibodies can be detected before clinical diabetes develops and disappear with increasing duration of diabetes; however, they are not suitable for screening or diagnostic purposes. Glutamic acid decarboxylase (GAD) antibodies may have a role in identifying late-onset type 1 autoimmune diabetes in adults (LADA). Type 1 diabetes is associated with other autoimmune disorders, including thyroid disease (p. 339), coeliac disease (p. 438), Addison's disease (p. 364), pernicious anaemia (p. 536) and vitiligo (p. 717).

Genetic predisposition

Genetic factors account for about one-third of the susceptibility to type 1 diabetes, with 35% concordance between monozygotic twins. The human leucocyte antigen (HLA) haplotypes *DR3* and/or *DR4* on chromosome 6 are associated with increased susceptibility to type 1 diabetes.

Environmental factors

Wide geographic and seasonal variations in incidence suggest that environmental factors have an important role in type 1 diabetes. Viral infections implicated in the aetiology include mumps, Coxsackie B4, retroviruses, congenital rubella, cytomegalovirus and Epstein–Barr virus. Various dietary nitrosamines (found in smoked and cured meats) and coffee have been proposed as potentially diabetogenic toxins. Bovine serum albumin (BSA – a constituent of cow's milk) has been implicated in triggering type 1 diabetes, since infants who are given cow's milk are more likely to develop type 1 diabetes in later life than those who are breastfed. Reduced exposure to microorganisms in early childhood may limit maturation of the immune system and increase susceptibility to autoimmune disease (the 'hygiene hypothesis').

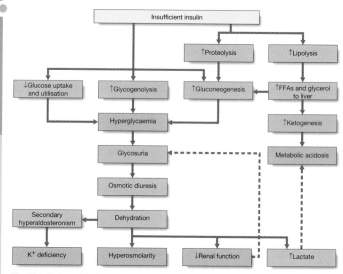

Fig. 11.1 Acute metabolic complications of insulin deficiency. (FFAs = free fatty acids)

Metabolic disturbances in type 1 diabetes

Patients with type 1 diabetes present when adequate insulin secretion can no longer be sustained. High glucose levels may be toxic to the remaining β cells, so that profound insulin deficiency rapidly ensues. Insulin deficiency is associated with the metabolic sequelae shown in Figure 11.1. Hyperglycaemia leads to glycosuria and dehydration, which in turn induces secondary hyperaldosteronism. Unrestrained lipolysis and proteolysis result in weight loss, increased gluconeogenesis and ketogenesis. When generation of ketone bodies exceeds their metabolism, ketoacidosis results. Secondary hyperaldosteronism encourages urinary loss of K⁺. Thus patients usually present with a short history of hyperglycaemic symptoms (thirst, polyuria, fatigue and infections) and weight loss, and may have developed ketoacidosis.

Type 2 diabetes

Type 2 diabetes is only diagnosed after excluding other causes of hyperglycaemia, including type 1 diabetes. Patients retain some capacity to secrete insulin but there is a combination of resistance to the actions of insulin followed by impaired pancreatic β-cell function, leading to 'relative' insulin deficiency.

Insulin resistance: Type 2 diabetes is often associated with other medical disorders; when these coexist, they are termed 'metabolic syndrome' (Box 11.1), with a predisposition to insulin resistance being the primary defect. It is strongly associated with macrovascular disease (coronary, cerebral, peripheral) and an excess mortality.

11.1 Features of the insulin resistance (metabolic) syndrome

- Hyperinsulinaemia
- Type 2 diabetes or impaired glucose tolerance (IGT)
- Hypertension
- Dyslipidaemia ($\uparrow$LDL cholesterol, $\uparrow$triglycerides, $\downarrow$HDL cholesterol)
- Non-alcoholic fatty liver
- Central (visceral) obesity
- Increased fibrinogen, uric acid
- (in women) Polycystic ovarian syndrome

The primary cause of this syndrome remains unclear, and multiple defects in insulin signalling are found. 'Central' adipose tissue may amplify insulin resistance by releasing FFAs and hormones (adipokines). Sedentary people are more insulin-resistant than active people with the same degree of obesity. Inactivity downregulates insulin-sensitive kinases and may also increase the accumulation of FFAs within skeletal muscle. Exercise also allows non-insulin-dependent glucose uptake into muscle, reducing the 'demand' on the pancreatic β cells to produce insulin. Many patients also develop non-alcoholic fatty liver disease.

Pancreatic β-cell failure: In early type 2 diabetes, only around 50% of β-cell function is lost. Amyloid deposits are found around pancreatic islet cells. While β-cell numbers are typically reduced, β-cell mass is unchanged and glucagon secretion is increased, which may contribute to the hyperglycaemia.

Genetic predisposition

Genetic factors are important in type 2 diabetes; different ethnic groups have different susceptibility but monozygotic twins have concordance rates approaching 100%. However, many genes are involved, and individual risk of diabetes is also influenced by environmental factors.

Environmental and other risk factors

Epidemiological studies indicate that type 2 diabetes is associated with overeating, especially when combined with obesity and underactivity. The risk of developing type 2 diabetes increases tenfold in people with a body mass index (BMI) >30 kg/m². However, only a minority of obese people develop diabetes. Obesity probably acts as a diabetogenic factor in those who are genetically predisposed both to insulin resistance and to β-cell failure.

Age: Type 2 diabetes is principally a disease of the middle-aged and elderly. In the UK, it affects 10% of the population >65, and >70% of all cases of diabetes occur after the age of 50 yrs.

Metabolic disturbances in type 2 diabetes

Relatively small amounts of insulin are required to suppress lipolysis, and some glucose uptake is maintained in muscle, so that weight loss and ketoacidosis are rare. Hyperglycaemia develops slowly, so that osmotic symptoms (polyuria and polydipsia) are usually mild. Thus, patients are often asymptomatic but usually present with a long history (typically many months) of fatigue, with or without osmotic symptoms. In some patients, presentation is late and pancreatic β-cell function has declined to the point where there is profound insulin deficiency. These patients may present with weight loss, although ketoacidosis remains uncommon. In some ethnic groups, such as African Americans, however, half of those first presenting with diabetic ketoacidosis have type 2 diabetes.

Intercurrent illness, e.g. infection, increases the production of stress hormones that oppose insulin (cortisol, growth hormone, catecholamines). This can precipitate more severe hyperglycaemia and dehydration (see hyperosmolar non-ketotic coma, p. 393).

Other forms of diabetes

These include:

• Pancreatic disease (e.g. pancreatitis, haemochromatosis, cystic fibrosis). • Excess endogenous production of insulin antagonists (acromegaly, Cushing's disease, thyrotoxicosis). • Genetic defects of β-cell function (e.g. maturity-onset diabetes of the young (MODY), a rare autosomal dominant disease, <5% of diabetes cases). • Genetic defects of insulin action. • Drug-induced diabetes (corticosteroids, thiazides, phenytoin). • Diabetes associated with genetic syndromes (e.g. Down's, DIDMOAD – diabetes insipidus, diabetes mellitus, optic atrophy, deafness).

Investigations

Urine testing

Glucose

Urine dipsticks are used to screen for diabetes. Testing should ideally use urine passed 1–2 hrs after a meal, since this will maximise sensitivity. Glycosuria always warrants further assessment by blood testing; however, glycosuria can be due to a low renal threshold. This is a benign condition unrelated to diabetes, common during pregnancy and in young people. Another disadvantage is that some drugs (such as β-lactam antibiotics, levodopa and salicylates) may interfere with urine glucose tests.

Ketones

Ketonuria may be found in normal people who have been fasting, exercising or vomiting repeatedly, or those on a high-fat, low-carbohydrate diet. Ketonuria is therefore not pathognomonic of diabetes but, if it is associated with glycosuria, diabetes is highly likely. In diabetic ketoacidosis (p. 391), ketones can also be detected in plasma using test sticks (see below).

Protein

Standard dipstick testing will detect urinary albumin >300 mg/L but smaller amounts (microalbuminuria) require specific sticks or laboratory urinalysis. Microalbuminuria or proteinuria, in the absence of urinary tract infection, is an important indicator of diabetic nephropathy and/or increased risk of macrovascular disease (p. 404).

Blood testing

Glucose

Laboratory blood glucose testing is cheap and highly reliable. Capillary blood glucose can also be measured with a portable electronic meter, used to monitor diabetes treatment. Glucose concentrations are lower in venous than in arterial or capillary (fingerprick) blood. Whole blood glucose concentrations are lower than plasma concentrations because red blood cells contain relatively little glucose. Venous plasma values are the most reliable for diagnostic purposes.

Ketones

Whole blood ketone monitoring detects β-hydroxybutyrate and is useful in guiding insulin adjustment during intercurrent illness or sustained hyperglycaemia to prevent or detect DKA. It is also useful in monitoring resolution of DKA in hospitalised patients.

Glycated haemoglobin

Glycated haemoglobin (Hb) provides an accurate and objective measure of glycaemic control over a period of weeks to months.

The non-enzymatic covalent attachment of glucose to Hb (glycation) increases the amount in the HbA_{1c} fraction relative to non-glycated adult Hb (HbA_0). The rate of formation of HbA_{1c} is directly proportional to the blood glucose concentration; a rise of 1% in HbA_{1c} corresponds to an increase of 2 mmol/L (36 mg/dL) in blood glucose. HbA_{1c} concentration reflects blood glucose over the erythrocyte lifespan (120 days); it is most sensitive to glycaemic control in the past month. To enable international comparisons, most countries now report International Federation of Clinical Chemistry and Laboratory Medicine (IFCC)-standardised HbA_{1c} values [IFCC HbA_{1c} (mmol/mol) = (HbA_{1c} (%)–2.15) × 10.929].

HbA_{1c} estimates may be erroneously diminished in anaemia and pregnancy, and may be difficult to interpret in uraemia and haemoglobinopathy.

PRESENTING PROBLEMS IN DIABETES

Newly discovered hyperglycaemia

The key goals are to establish whether the patient has diabetes, what type of diabetes it is and how it should be treated.

Establishing the diagnosis of diabetes

Glycaemia can be classified as either normal, impaired (pre-diabetes) or diabetes. The glucose cut-off that defines diabetes is the level above which there is a significant risk of microvascular

11.2 Diagnosis of diabetes and pre-diabetes

Diabetes is confirmed by either:

- Plasma glucose in random sample or 2 hrs after a 75-g glucose load ≥11.1 (200 mg/dL)
  or
- Fasting plasma glucose ≥7.0 mmol/L (126 mg/dL)

  In asymptomatic patients, two diagnostic tests are required to confirm diabetes.

'Pre-diabetes' is classified as:

- Impaired fasting glucose = fasting plasma glucose ≥6.0 mmol/L (108 mg/dL) and <7.0 mmol/L (126 mg/dL)
- Impaired glucose tolerance = fasting plasma glucose <7.0 mmol/L (126 mg/dL) **and** 2-hr glucose after 75-g oral glucose drink 7.8–11.1 mmol/L (140–200 mg/dL)

complications (retinopathy, nephropathy, neuropathy). Those with pre-diabetes have a negligible risk of microvascular complications but are at increased risk of developing diabetes. Also, because there is a continuous risk of macrovascular disease (atheroma of large blood vessels) with increasing glycaemia in the population, people with pre-diabetes have increased risk of cardiovascular disease (myocardial infarction, stroke and peripheral vascular disease).

In symptomatic patients, diabetes can be confirmed with either a fasting glucose ≥7.0 mmol/L (126 mg/dL) or a random glucose ≥11.1 mmol/L (200 mg/dL) (Box 11.2). Asymptomatic individuals should have a second confirmatory test. Diabetes should not be diagnosed by capillary blood glucose results. The WHO guidelines also include an IFCC HbA_{1c} of >48 mmol/mol as diagnostic of diabetes.

Pre-diabetes can be diagnosed either as 'impaired fasting glucose' (IFG; fasting plasma glucose 6.1–6.9 mmol/L) or 'impaired glucose tolerance' (IGT; glucose 7.8–11 mmol/L 2 hrs after 75-g oral glucose drink). Patients with pre-diabetes should be advised of their risk of progression to diabetes, should be given lifestyle advice to reduce this risk (p. 399), and should receive aggressive management of cardiovascular risk factors such as hypertension and dyslipidaemia.

Stress hyperglycaemia occurs when conditions impose a burden on the pancreatic β cells, e.g. during pregnancy, infection or treatment with corticosteroids. It usually disappears after the acute illness has resolved, but blood glucose should be remeasured.

When diabetes is confirmed, other investigations should include: • U&Es. • Creatinine. • LFTs • TFTs. • Lipids. • Urine: ketones, protein, microalbuminuria.

Clinical assessment

The clinical features of the two main types of diabetes are compared in Box 11.3. Symptoms at presentation include:

11.3 Comparative clinical features of type 1 and type 2 diabetes

	Type 1	Type 2
Typical age at onset	<40 yrs	>50 yrs
Duration of symptoms	Weeks	Months to years
Body weight	Normal or low	Obese
Ketonuria	Yes	No
Rapid death without treatment with insulin	Yes	No
Autoantibodies	+ve in 80–90%	No
Diabetic complications at diagnosis	No	25%
Family history of diabetes	Uncommon	Common
Other autoimmune disease	Common	Uncommon

• Thirst. • Polyuria/nocturia. • Fatigue. • Blurred vision. • Pruritus vulvae/balanitis. • Nausea. • Hyperphagia. • Irritability, poor concentration, headache.

Patients with type 2 diabetes may be asymptomatic or present with chronic fatigue or malaise. Uncontrolled diabetes is associated with increased susceptibility to infection and patients may present with skin infections. A history of pancreatic disease (particularly with alcohol excess) makes insulin deficiency more likely.

Overlap occurs, particularly in age at onset, duration of symptoms and family history. Typical type 2 diabetes occurs increasingly in obese young people. Older adults may have evidence of autoimmune activity against β cells, a slowly evolving variant of type 1 diabetes (LADA). More than 80% of patients with type 2 diabetes are overweight, 50% have hypertension and hyperlipidaemia is common.

Management

Aims are to improve symptoms and minimise complications:

• Type 1 diabetes: urgent therapy with insulin and prompt referral to a specialist. • Type 2 diabetes: advice about dietary and lifestyle modification, followed by initiation of oral antidiabetic drugs if needed. • Hypertension, dyslipidaemia and smoking cessation.

Patient education: This can be achieved by a multidisciplinary team (doctor, dietitian, specialist nurse and podiatrist) in the outpatient setting. Patients requiring insulin need intensive training in how to measure insulin doses, give their own injections, and adjust the dose depending on glucose monitoring, exercise, illness and hypoglycaemia. They must understand the principles of diabetes, recognise the symptoms of hypoglycaemia, and receive advice about the risks of driving with diabetes.

Self-assessment of glycaemic control: Patients with type 2 diabetes do not usually need regular self-assessment of blood glucose, unless they use insulin, or are at risk of hypoglycaemia on sulphonylureas. Insulin-treated patients should be taught to monitor blood

11.4 How to follow up patients with diabetes mellitus	
Lifestyle issues	Smoking, alcohol, stress, sexual health, exercise
Body weight (BMI)	
BP	Individualised target 130–140/70–80 mmHg based on risk
Urinalysis (fasting)	Glucose, ketones, macro- and microalbuminuria
Biochemistry	Renal, liver and thyroid function, lipid profile
Glycaemic control	HbA$_{1c}$, inspection of home blood glucose monitoring record
Hypoglycaemic episodes	Number and cause of severe and mild episodes, nature of symptoms, awareness, driving
Injection sites if on insulin	
Eye examination	Visual acuity, ophthalmoscopy, digital photography
Lower limbs and feet	Signs of peripheral neuropathy, ulceration, deformity, nails

glucose using capillary blood glucose meters, and to use the results to guide insulin dosing and to manage exercise and illness. Pre-meal blood glucose values of 4–7 mmol/L (72–126 mg/dL) and 2-hr post-meal values of 4–8 mmol/L represent optimal control. Urine testing for glucose is not recommended because variability in renal threshold means that some patients with inadequate glycaemic control will not have glycosuria.

Long-term supervision of diabetes

Diabetes is a complex disorder, which progresses in severity with time. Patients with diabetes should therefore be seen at regular intervals for life. A checklist for follow-up visits is given in Box 11.4. The frequency of visits varies from weekly during pregnancy to annually in well-controlled type 2 diabetes.

Therapeutic goals

The target HbA$_{1c}$ depends on the patient. Early on in diabetes (i.e. patients managed by diet or one or two oral agents), a target of 48 mmol/mol (6.5%) or less may be appropriate. However, a higher target of 58 mmol/mol (7.5%) may be more appropriate in older patients with pre-existing cardiovascular disease, or those treated with insulin and therefore at risk of hypoglycaemia. The benefits of lower target HbA$_{1c}$ (primarily a lower risk of microvascular disease) need to be weighed against any increased risks (primarily hypoglycaemia in insulin-treated patients). Type 2 diabetes is usually a progressive condition, so that there is normally a need to increase diabetes medication over time to achieve the individualised target HbA$_{1c}$.

Treatment of hypertension and dyslipidaemia is important to reduce cardiovascular risk. Statins are indicated in those with type

2 diabetes aged >40, regardless of cholesterol level. In all diabetic patients, total cholesterol should be <4 mmol/L (150 mg/dL) and LDL cholesterol <2 mmol/L (75 mg/dL).

Diabetic ketoacidosis

Diabetic ketoacidosis (DKA) is a medical emergency, principally occurring in people with type 1 diabetes. Mortality is low in the UK (~2%), but higher in developing countries and among non-hospitalised patients. It may be the presenting feature of diabetes, or may be precipitated by stress, particularly infection, in those with established diabetes. Sometimes, DKA develops because of errors in self-management. In young patients with recurrent episodes of DKA, up to 20% may have psychological problems complicated by eating disorders.

The cardinal biochemical features of DKA are:
• Hyperglycaemia. • Hyperketonaemia. • Metabolic acidosis.

Hyperglycaemia causes an osmotic diuresis, leading to dehydration and electrolyte loss. Ketosis is caused by insulin deficiency, exacerbated by stress hormones (e.g. catecholamines), resulting in unrestrained lipolysis and supplying FFAs for hepatic ketogenesis. When this exceeds the capacity to metabolise acidic ketones, these accumulate in blood. The resulting acidosis forces hydrogen ions into cells, displacing potassium ions, which are lost in urine or through vomiting. The average loss of fluid and electrolytes in moderately severe DKA in an adult is shown in Box 11.5. Patients with DKA have a total body potassium deficit but this is not reflected by plasma potassium levels, which may initially be raised due to disproportionate water loss. Once insulin is started, however, plasma potassium can fall precipitously due to dilution by IV fluids, potassium movement into cells, and continuing renal loss of potassium.

Clinical assessment

Clinical features of DKA are listed in Box 11.6.

Investigations

The following are important but should not delay IV fluid and insulin replacement:
• U&Es, blood glucose, plasma bicarbonate (<12 mmol/L indicates severe acidosis). • Urine and plasma for ketones. • ECG. • Infection screen: FBC, blood/urine culture, CRP, CXR. Leucocytosis

11.5 Average fluid and electrolyte loss in adult diabetic ketoacidosis of moderate severity

• Water: 6 L	3 L extracellular
• Sodium: 500 mmol	– replace with saline
• Chloride: 400 mmol	3 L intracellular
• Potassium: 350 mmol	– replace with dextrose

11.6 Clinical features of diabetic ketoacidosis

Symptoms

- Polyuria, thirst
- Weight loss
- Weakness
- Nausea, vomiting
- Blurred vision
- Abdominal pain, leg cramps

Signs

- Dehydration
- Hypotension (postural or supine), tachycardia
- Cold extremities/peripheral cyanosis
- Air hunger (Kussmaul breathing)
- Smell of acetone
- Hypothermia
- Confusion, drowsiness, coma (10%)

invariably occurs, representing a stress response rather than infection.

Management

Guidelines for the management of DKA are shown in Box 11.7. Patients should be treated in hospital, preferably in a high-dependency area, and the diabetes specialty team should be involved. Regular clinical and biochemical monitoring is essential, particularly during the first 24 hrs. The principal components of treatment are insulin, fluid and potassium.

Insulin: The preferred route is IV infusion at 0.1 U/kg/hr, but (exceptionally) if this is not possible, 10–20 U can be given IM, followed by 5 U IM hourly thereafter. Blood glucose should ideally fall at 3–6 mmol/L/hr (~55–110 mg/dL/hr); a more rapid fall in blood glucose should be avoided, as it can cause cerebral oedema, particularly in children. Failure of blood glucose to fall within 1 hr of commencing insulin infusion should lead to a re-assessment of insulin dose. When the blood glucose has fallen, 10% dextrose is introduced and insulin infusion continued to encourage glucose uptake into cells and restoration of normal metabolism. SC insulin should be delayed until the patient is eating and drinking normally.

Fluid replacement: Large volumes are required; details are given in Box 11.7.

Potassium: Plasma potassium is often high at presentation; treatment should be started cautiously and carefully monitored. Large amounts may be required (100–300 mmol in the first 24 hrs). Cardiac rhythm should be monitored in severe cases because of the risk of arrhythmia.

Bicarbonate: Adequate fluid and insulin replacement should resolve the acidosis, so IV bicarbonate is currently not recommended.

11.7 Management of diabetic ketoacidosis

First hr

1. Give 0.9% saline IV: 1 L in 60 mins, faster if systolic BP <90 mmHg
2. Give insulin: 50 U human soluble insulin in 50 mL saline IV at 0.1 U/kg/hr
3. Perform initial investigations and treat any precipitating cause – see text
4. Monitor: *hourly* – capillary glucose and ketones, venous bicarbonate and potassium, pulse, BP, O_2 saturation, urine output; *4-hourly* – plasma electrolytes

1–12 hrs

1. Give 0.9% saline IV: 2 L over 4 hrs, then 2 L over 8 hrs; less in elderly, young, renal or cardiac failure; 0.45% saline if Na^+ >155 mmol/L
2. Add potassium chloride according to plasma K^+: >5.5 mmol/L – nil; 3.5–5.5 mmol/L – 40 mmol KCl/L infusion; <3.5 mmol/L – additional KCl required – senior review
3. Add 10% glucose 125 mL/hr IV when glucose <14 mmol/L (250 mg/dL)

12–24 hrs

1. Check that ketonaemia and acidosis have resolved – senior review if not
2. Continue IV fluids and insulin (2–3 U/hr) until patient is eating and drinking
3. If ketonaemia and acidosis have resolved and patient is eating, commence SC insulin with advice from diabetes team

Additional procedures

- Catheterisation if no urine at 3 hrs, CVP line if cardiovascular compromise, ABGs and repeat CXR if O_2 saturation <92%, ECG monitoring if severe, thromboprophylaxis with low molecular weight heparin

Adapted from Joint British Diabetes Society guideline, NHS Diabetes (2010).

Acidosis may reflect an adaptive response, improving oxygen delivery to the tissues, and excessive bicarbonate has been implicated in the pathogenesis of cerebral oedema in children and young adults.

Hyperglycaemic hyperosmolar state

Hyperglycaemic hyperosmolar state (HHS; formerly known as hyperosmolar non-ketotic coma) is characterised by severe hyperglycaemia (>30 mmol/L (600 mg/dL)), hyperosmolality (serum >320 mOsm/kg) and dehydration without significant ketoacidosis. It typically affects elderly patients but is seen increasingly in younger adults. The onset is slow (days to weeks), and dehydration and hyperglycaemia are profound. Plasma osmolality should be measured or osmolarity calculated using the following formula:

$$\text{Plasma osmolarity} = 2[Na^+] + [\text{glucose}] + [\text{urea}] \text{ (all mmol/L)}$$

The normal value is 280–290 mmol/kg and the conscious level is depressed when it is >340 mmol/kg. The patient should be given 0.9% saline, switching to 0.45% if the osmolality is rising, and aiming for a positive fluid balance of 3–6 L in the first 12 hrs. IV insulin

(0.5 U/kg/hr) should only be given if the glucose fails to fall with 0.9% saline or if ketonaemia develops. Give prophylactic heparin (thromboembolic complications).

Mortality is higher than in DKA – up to 20% in the USA.

Hypoglycaemia

Hypoglycaemia (blood glucose <3.5 mmol/L (63 mg/dL)) occurs in a person with diabetes as a result of treatment with insulin and occasionally sulphonylureas. Hypoglycaemia in a non-diabetic person is called 'spontaneous' hypoglycaemia (p. 368). The risk of hypoglycaemia limits the attainment of near-normal glycaemia; fear of hypoglycaemia is common among patients and their relatives.

Clinical assessment

• Symptoms of autonomic nervous system activation: sweating, trembling, palpitation, hunger and anxiety. • Symptoms of glucose deprivation of the brain (neuroglycopenia), including confusion, drowsiness, poor coordination and speech difficulty.

Hypoglycaemia also affects mood, inducing a state of increased tension and low energy. Educating patients to recognise the onset of hypoglycaemia is important in insulin-treated patients. The severity of hypoglycaemia is defined by the ability to self-treat; 'mild' episodes are self-treated, while 'severe' episodes require assistance for recovery.

Circumstances of hypoglycaemia: Risk factors and causes of hypoglycaemia in patients taking insulin or sulphonylurea drugs are listed in Box 11.8. Severe hypoglycaemia can have serious

11.8 Hypoglycaemia: common causes and risk factors

Causes of hypoglycaemia

- Missed/delayed meal
- Unexpected or unusual exercise
- Alcohol
- Error in oral hypoglycaemic or insulin dose/timing
- Lipohypertrophy causing variable insulin absorption
- Gastroparesis due to autonomic neuropathy
- Malabsorption, e.g. coeliac disease
- Unrecognised other endocrine disorder, e.g. Addison's disease
- Factitious (deliberately induced)
- Breastfeeding

Risk factors for severe hypoglycaemia

- Strict glycaemic control
- Impaired awareness of hypoglycaemia
- Extremes of age
- Long duration of diabetes
- History of previous hypoglycaemia
- Renal impairment

morbidity (e.g. convulsions, coma, focal neurological lesions) and has a mortality of up to 4% in insulin-treated patients. Rarely, sudden death during sleep occurs in otherwise healthy young patients with type 1 diabetes. Severe hypoglycaemia is very disruptive and impinges on employment, driving, travel, sport and personal relationships.

Nocturnal hypoglycaemia in type 1 diabetes is common but often undetected, as hypoglycaemia does not usually waken a person. Patients may describe poor sleep quality, morning headaches and vivid dreams or nightmares, or a partner may observe profuse sweating, restlessness, twitching or even seizures. The only reliable way to identify this problem is to measure blood glucose during the night.

Exercise-induced hypoglycaemia occurs in people with well-controlled, insulin-treated diabetes because of hyperinsulinaemia. In health, exercise suppresses endogenous insulin secretion to allow increased hepatic glucose production to meet the increased metabolic demand. In insulin-treated diabetes, insulin levels may increase with exercise because of improved blood flow at injection sites, leading to hypoglycaemia.

Awareness of hypoglycaemia: For most individuals, the glucose threshold at which they become aware of hypoglycaemia varies according to the circumstances (e.g. during the night or during exercise). In addition, with longer duration of disease, and in response to frequent hypoglycaemia, the threshold for symptoms shifts to a lower glucose concentration. This cerebral adaptation has a similar effect on the counter-regulatory hormonal response to hypoglycaemia. Taken together, this means that individuals with type 1 diabetes may have reduced (impaired) awareness of hypoglycaemia. Symptoms can be experienced less intensely, or even be absent, despite blood glucose concentrations <2.5 mmol/L (45 mg/dL). Impaired awareness of hypoglycaemia affects ~20–25% of people with type 1 diabetes and <10% with insulin-treated type 2 diabetes.

Management

Treatment of acute hypoglycaemia depends on severity and on whether the patient is conscious. If hypoglycaemia is recognised early, oral fast-acting carbohydrate, followed by a complex carbohydrate snack, is sufficient. In those unable to swallow, IV glucose (75 mL of 20–50% dextrose, 0.2 g/kg in children) or IM glucagon (1 mg, 0.5 mg in children) should be administered. Viscous glucose gel solution or jam can be applied into the buccal cavity but should not be used if the person is unconscious. Full recovery may not occur immediately and reversal of cognitive impairment may take 60 mins. The possibility of recurrence should be anticipated in those on long-acting insulins or sulphonylureas; a 10% dextrose infusion, titrated to the patient's blood glucose, may be necessary. Cerebral oedema may have developed in patients who fail to regain consciousness after blood glucose is restored to normal. This has a high mortality and morbidity, and requires urgent treatment with mannitol and high-dose oxygen.

Following recovery, it is important to try to identify a cause, make appropriate adjustments to therapy and educate the patient.

The management of self-poisoning with oral antidiabetic agents is given on page 39.

Prevention of hypoglycaemia

Patient education must cover risk factors for, and treatment of hypoglycaemia. The importance of regular blood glucose monitoring and the need to have glucose (and glucagon) readily available should be stressed. A review of insulin and carbohydrate management during exercise is particularly useful.

Relatives and friends also need to be familiar with the symptoms and signs of hypoglycaemia and should be instructed in how to help (including how to inject glucagon).

Diabetes in pregnancy
Gestational diabetes

Glucose metabolism changes during pregnancy. Marked insulin resistance develops, particularly by the second half of pregnancy, due to maternal hormones such as human placental lactogen. Fasting glucose decreases slightly, while blood glucose may be increased post-prandially.

Gestational diabetes is defined as diabetes with first onset or recognition during pregnancy. While this includes a few who develop type 1 or type 2 diabetes during pregnancy, the majority can expect to return to normal glucose tolerance immediately after pregnancy. The definitions of diabetes in pregnancy are based on maternal glucose levels associated with increased fetal growth, and are lower than the definitions for non-gestational diabetes, either:

• Fasting venous plasma glucose >5.1 mmol/L (92 mg/dL) *or*
• >10 mmol/L (>180 mg/dL) at 1 hr or >8.0 mmol/L (144 mg/dL) at 2 hrs after a 75-g glucose load.

Patients at high risk include those with a BMI >30, previous macrosomia or gestational diabetes, family history of type 2 diabetes or a high-risk ethnic group (South Asian, black Caribbean, Middle Eastern).

Management of gestational diabetes

The aim is to normalise maternal blood glucose to prevent excessive fetal growth. Dietary restriction of refined carbohydrate is important. Women with gestational diabetes should regularly check pre- and post-prandial blood glucose, aiming for pre-meal levels <5.5 mmol/L (100 mg/dL) or post-meal levels <7.0 mmol/L (125 mg/dL). If treatment is necessary, metformin or glibenclamide is generally safe in pregnancy, but other therapies should be avoided. Insulin may be required, especially late in pregnancy. If maternal blood glucose is poorly controlled peri-partum, the resulting fetal hyperinsulinaemia leads to neonatal hyperinsulinaemia, which in turn can cause neonatal hypoglycaemia.

After delivery, maternal glucose usually returns rapidly to pre-pregnancy levels. Women should be tested at least 6 wks post-partum with an oral glucose tolerance test. Those who have returned to normal glucose tolerance remain at considerable risk for developing type 2 diabetes (5-yr risk 15–50%), depending on the population, and should be given diet and lifestyle advice (p. 399) to reduce this risk.

Pregnancy in women with established diabetes

Maternal hyperglycaemia early in pregnancy can lead to fetal abnormalities, including cardiac, renal and skeletal malformations, of which the caudal regression syndrome is the most characteristic. Diabetic women should receive pre-pregnancy counselling and be encouraged to achieve excellent glycaemic control before conceiving. High-dose folic acid (5 mg, rather than the usual 400 μg, daily) should be initiated before conception to reduce the risk of neural tube defects.

Good glycaemic control is often difficult to achieve. Pregnancy carries an increased risk of ketosis, which is dangerous for the mother and is associated with a high rate (10–35%) of fetal mortality.

Pregnancy is associated with worsening of diabetic retinopathy and nephropathy. Heavy proteinuria and/or renal dysfunction before pregnancy indicate an increased risk of pre-eclampsia and irreversible loss of renal function. These risks need to be carefully discussed before considering a pregnancy. Diabetes increases perinatal mortality by 3–4 times and congenital malformation 5–6-fold.

Surgery and diabetes

Surgery causes catabolic stress and secretion of counter-regulatory hormones, resulting in increased glycogenolysis, gluconeogenesis, lipolysis, proteolysis and insulin resistance. This normally leads to increased secretion of insulin, which exerts a restraining and controlling influence. In diabetic patients, insulin deficiency leads to increased catabolism and ultimately metabolic decompensation. In addition, hyperglycaemia increases infection risk and impairs wound healing. Hypoglycaemia risk, particularly dangerous in the semiconscious patient, should be minimised.

Pre-operative assessment

This includes assessment of:
• Glycaemic control (HbA$_{1c}$ and pre-prandial glucose). • Cardio-vascular and renal function. • Foot risk (peri-operative pressure relief) • A review of diabetic treatments.

If significant alterations need to be made, patients may need admission prior to surgery. For emergency patients with significant hyperglycaemia or ketoacidosis, this should be corrected first with an IV infusion of saline and/or dextrose plus insulin, 6 U/hr, and potassium as required.

Peri-operative management

The management of patients with diabetes undergoing surgery requiring general anaesthesia is summarised in Figure 11.2. Post-operatively, IV insulin and fluids should be continued (containing appropriate dextrose, sodium and potassium), until the patient's intake of food is adequate, when the normal regimen can be resumed.

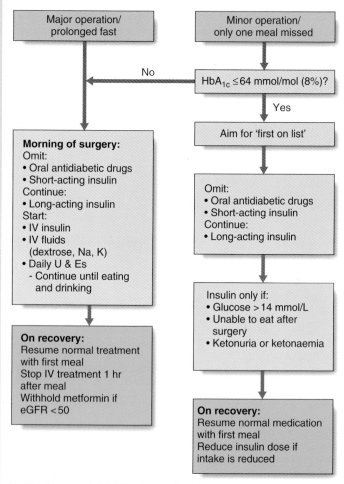

Fig. 11.2 Management of diabetic patients undergoing surgery and general anaesthesia. (Glucose of >14 mmol/L = 250 mg/dL.)

	11.9 Complications of diabetes

Microvascular/neuropathic

Retinopathy, cataract	Impaired vision
Nephropathy	Renal failure
Peripheral neuropathy	Sensory loss, motor weakness
Autonomic neuropathy	Postural hypotension, GI problems
	(gastroparesis; altered bowel habit)
Foot disease	Ulceration, arthropathy

Macrovascular

Coronary circulation	Myocardial ischaemia/infarction
Cerebral circulation	Transient ischaemic attack (TIA), stroke
Peripheral circulation	Claudication, ischaemia

If the infusion is prolonged, urea, electrolytes and urinary ketones should be checked daily.

Diabetes presenting through complications

Diabetic complications (Box 11.9) may be the presenting finding in a patient not known to have diabetes. Around 20% of people with type 2 diabetes have established complications at the time of diagnosis. Patients presenting with hypertension or a vascular event should have coexistent diabetes excluded.

MANAGEMENT OF DIABETES

Of new cases of diabetes, approximately 50% can be controlled adequately by diet alone, 20–30% will need oral antidiabetic medication, and 20–30% will require insulin. Regardless of aetiology, the choice of treatment is determined by the adequacy of residual β-cell function. However, this cannot be determined easily by measurement of plasma insulin concentration because a level that is adequate in one patient may be inadequate in another, depending on sensitivity to insulin. Ideal management allows the patient to lead a completely normal life, to remain symptom-free and to escape the long-term complications of diabetes. The correct treatment may change with time as β-cell function is lost.

Diet and lifestyle

Lifestyle changes, such as taking regular exercise, observing a healthy diet, reducing alcohol consumption and stopping smoking, are important but difficult for many to sustain.

Healthy eating

Dietary measures are required in the treatment of all people with diabetes. People with diabetes should have access to dietitians at diagnosis, at review and at times of treatment change. Nutritional advice should be tailored to individuals and take account of their age and lifestyle. The aims are to improve glycaemic control, manage weight, and avoid both acute and long-term complications.

Carbohydrate

Both the amount and type of carbohydrate determine post-prandial glucose. The effect of a particular ingested carbohydrate on blood glucose relative to the effect of a glucose drink is termed the glycaemic index (GI). Starchy foods, such as rice, porridge and noodles, are favoured, as they have a low GI and produce only a gradual rise in blood glucose. It is now possible to match the amount of carbohydrate in a meal with a dose of short-acting insulin using methods such as DAFNE (dose adjustment for normal eating). This enables motivated individuals with type 1 diabetes to achieve and maintain good glycaemic control, while avoiding post-prandial hyper- and hypoglycaemia. For people with type 2 diabetes, avoidance of refined carbohydrate and restriction of carbohydrate to 45–60% of total energy intake is recommended.

Fat

The intake of total fat should be restricted to <35% of energy intake, with <10% as saturated fat, 10–20% from monounsaturated fat and <10% from polyunsaturated fat.

Salt

People with diabetes should follow the advice given to the general population: namely, to limit sodium intake to no more than 6 g daily.

Weight management

A high percentage of people with type 2 diabetes are overweight or obese, and many antidiabetic medications and insulin encourage weight gain. Abdominal obesity also predicts insulin resistance and cardiovascular risk. Weight loss is achieved through a reduction in energy intake and an increase in energy expenditure through physical activity. In extreme cases, bariatric surgery can induce marked weight loss and improvement in HbA_{1c} in patients with type 2 diabetes, sometimes enabling treatment withdrawal.

Exercise

All patients with diabetes should be advised to achieve a significant level of physical activity (e.g. walking, gardening, swimming or cycling) and to maintain this long term. Supervised exercise programmes may be of particular benefit to people with type 2 diabetes. US guidelines suggest that adults (18–64 yrs) should build up to a weekly minimum of 2.5 hrs of moderate-intensity exercise or 75 mins of vigorous-intensity exercise. The aerobic (moderate-intensity) activity should be performed for at least 10 mins each time and spread throughout the week, with at least 30 mins on at least 5 days of the week. Recently, it has also been suggested that a combination of both aerobic and resistance exercise may lead to greater improvements in glycaemic control.

Alcohol

Alcohol can be consumed in moderation. As alcohol suppresses gluconeogenesis, it can precipitate or prolong hypoglycaemia, particularly in patients taking insulin or sulphonylureas. Drinks containing alcohol can be a substantial source of calories and may have to be reduced to assist weight reduction.

Drugs to reduce hyperglycaemia

Most drugs used to treat type 2 diabetes depend upon a supply of endogenous insulin and therefore have no effect in patients with type 1 diabetes. The sulphonylureas and biguanides have been the mainstay of treatment in the past, but a variety of newer agents are now available and the optimal place for these in treatment is yet to be determined.

Biguanides

In the UK Prospective Diabetes Study, metformin reduced myocardial infarctions, and it is now used widely as first-line therapy in type 2 diabetes. Approximately 25% of patients develop mild gastrointestinal side-effects (diarrhoea, abdominal cramps, bloating and nausea) with metformin, but only 5% are unable to tolerate it even at low dose. It improves insulin sensitivity and peripheral glucose uptake, and impairs both glucose absorption by the gut and hepatic gluconeogenesis. Endogenous insulin is required for its glucose-lowering action, but it does not increase insulin secretion and seldom causes hypoglycaemia. Metformin does not increase body weight and it is therefore preferred for obese patients. It acts synergistically with sulphonylureas, allowing the two to be combined. Metformin is given with food, 2–3 times daily. The usual starting dose is 500 mg twice daily (usual maintenance 1 g twice daily). Its use is contraindicated in alcohol excess and in impaired renal or hepatic function due to the increased risk of lactic acidosis. It should be discontinued temporarily if another serious medical condition develops (especially shock or hypoxaemia).

Sulphonylureas

Sulphonylureas stimulate the release of insulin from the pancreatic β cell (insulin secretagogue). They are best used to treat non-obese people with type 2 diabetes who fail to respond to dietary measures, as treatment is often associated with weight gain. They are known to reduce microvascular complications with long-term use.

Gliclazide and glipizide cause few side-effects, but glibenclamide is long-acting and prone to induce hypoglycaemia so should be avoided in the elderly.

Sulphonylureas are often used as an add-on if metformin fails to produce adequate glycaemic control.

Alpha-glucosidase inhibitors

These delay carbohydrate absorption in the gut by selectively inhibiting disaccharidases. Acarbose or miglitol is taken with each meal and lowers post-prandial blood glucose. Side-effects are flatulence, abdominal bloating and diarrhoea.

Thiazolidinediones

These drugs (TZDs; 'glitazones' or PPARγ agonists) bind and activate peroxisome proliferator-activated receptor-γ found in adipose tissue, and work by enhancing the actions of endogenous insulin. Plasma insulin concentrations are not increased and hypoglycaemia is not a problem.

TZDs have been prescribed widely since the late 1990s, but recently a number of adverse effects have become apparent and their use has declined. Rosiglitazone was reported to increase the risk of myocardial infarction and was withdrawn in 2010. The other TZD in common use, pioglitazone, does not appear to increase the risk of myocardial infarction but it does exacerbate cardiac failure by causing fluid retention, and recent data show that it increases the risk of bone fracture and possibly bladder cancer. These observations have reduced the use of pioglitazone dramatically.

Pioglitazone can be effective in patients with insulin resistance and also has a beneficial effect in reducing fatty liver and non-alcoholic steatohepatitis (NASH; p. 502). Pioglitazone is usually added to metformin with or without sulphonylurea therapy. It may be given with insulin, when it can be very effective, but the combination of insulin and TZDs markedly increases fluid retention and risk of cardiac failure, so should be used with caution.

Incretin-based therapies: DPP-4 inhibitors and GLP-1 analogues

The incretin effect is the augmentation of insulin secretion seen when glucose is given orally rather than intravenously, due to the release of gut peptides (glucagon-like peptide 1 (GLP-1) and gastric inhibitory polypeptide (GIP)). These are broken down by dipeptidyl peptidase 4 (DPP-4).

DPP-4 inhibitors: Prevent breakdown and therefore increase endogenous GLP-1 and GIP levels. Examples include sitagliptin, vildagliptin, saxagliptin and linagliptin. They are well tolerated and are weight-neutral.

GLP-1 receptor agonists: Mimic GLP-1 but are modified to resist DPP-4. They have to be given by SC injection but have a key advantage over DPP-4 inhibitors: they decrease appetite at the level of the hypothalamus. Thus, GLP-1 analogues lower blood glucose and result in weight loss – a major advantage in obese patients with type 2 diabetes. Examples include exenatide (twice daily), exenatide MR (once weekly) and liraglutide (once daily).

Incretin-based therapies do not cause hypoglycaemia.

	11.10 Duration of action (hrs) of insulin preparations			
Insulin		**Onset**	**Peak**	**Duration**
Rapid-acting (insulin analogues – lispro, aspart, glulisine)		<0.5	0.5–2.5	3–4.5
Short-acting (soluble (regular))		0.5–1	1–4	4–8
Intermediate-acting (isophane (NPH), lente)		1–3	3–8	7–14
Long-acting (bovine ultralente)		2–4	6–12	12–30
Long-acting (insulin analogues – glargine, detemir)		1–2	None	18–24

Insulin

The duration of action of the main groups of insulin preparation is given in Box 11.10.

Subcutaneous multiple dose insulin therapy

Insulin is injected subcutaneously into the anterior abdominal wall, upper arms, outer thighs and buttocks. The rate of absorption of insulin may be influenced by the insulin formulation, the site, depth and volume of injection, skin temperature (warming), local massage and exercise. Absorption is delayed from areas of lipohypertrophy at injection sites.

Once absorbed into the blood, insulin has a half-life of just a few minutes. Excretion is hepatic and renal, so insulin levels are elevated in hepatic or renal failure.

Insulin delivered by re-usable syringe has largely been replaced by that delivered by pen injectors containing sufficient insulin for multiple dosing.

Insulin analogues have largely replaced soluble and isophane insulins, especially for type 1 diabetes, because they allow more flexibility and convenience. Unlike soluble insulin, which should be injected 30 mins before eating, rapid-acting insulin analogues can be administered immediately before, during or even after meals. Long-acting insulin analogues are better able than isophane insulin to maintain 'basal' insulin levels for up to 24 hrs, so need only be injected once daily.

The complications of insulin therapy include:

• Hypoglycaemia. • Weight gain. • Peripheral oedema (insulin treatment causes salt and water retention in the short term). • Insulin antibodies (animal insulins). • Local allergy (rare). • Lipodystrophy at injection sites.

A common problem is fasting hyperglycaemia (the 'dawn phenomenon') caused by the release of counter-regulatory hormones during the night, which increases insulin requirement before wakening.

Insulin dosing regimens

The choice of regimen depends on the desired degree of glycaemic control, the severity of insulin deficiency, the patient's lifestyle, and their ability to adjust the insulin dose. Most people with type 1 diabetes require two or more insulin injections daily. In type 2 diabetes, insulin is usually initiated as a once-daily long-acting insulin, with or without oral hypoglycaemic agents.

Twice-daily administration: A short-acting and intermediate-acting insulin (usually soluble and isophane), given before breakfast and the evening meal, is the simplest regimen. Initially, two-thirds of the daily insulin is given in the morning in a ratio of short- to intermediate-acting of 1:2; the remainder is given in the evening. Pre-mixed formulations containing fixed proportions of soluble and isophane insulins are useful if patients have difficulty mixing insulins, but the individual components cannot be adjusted independently. Fixed-mixture insulins also have altered pharmacokinetics, i.e. the peak insulin and time to peak effect are significantly reduced compared with the same insulins injected separately.

Multiple injection regimens: These are popular, with short-acting insulin before each meal, plus intermediate- or long-acting insulin injected once or twice daily (basal-bolus regimen). This regimen allows greater freedom of meal timing and more variable day-to-day physical activity.

Portable pumps: Pumps infusing continuous SC or IV insulin can achieve excellent glycaemic control but will not be widely adopted until they become cheaper and incorporate a miniaturised glucose sensor.

Transplantation

Whole pancreas transplantation presents problems relating to exocrine pancreatic secretions and long-term immunosuppression is necessary. At present, the procedure is usually undertaken only in patients with end-stage renal failure who require a combined pancreas/kidney transplantation and in whom diabetes control is particularly difficult, e.g. because of recurrent hypoglycaemia.

Transplantation of isolated pancreatic islets (usually into the liver via the portal vein) has been achieved safely in an increasing number of centres around the world. Progress is being made towards meeting the needs of supply, purification and storage of islets, but the problems of transplant rejection, and of destruction by the patient's autoantibodies against β cells, remain.

COMPLICATIONS OF DIABETES

People with diabetes have a mortality rate over twice that of age- and sex-matched controls. The range of complications of diabetes is summarised in Box 11.9. Cardiovascular disease accounts for 70% of all deaths. Atherosclerosis in diabetic patients occurs earlier and is more extensive and severe. Diabetes amplifies the effects of the other major cardiovascular risk factors: smoking, hypertension and dyslipidaemia.

Disease of small blood vessels (diabetic microangiopathy) is a specific complication of diabetes. It damages the kidneys, the retina and the peripheral and autonomic nerves, causing substantial morbidity and disability: blindness, difficulty in walking, chronic foot ulceration, and bowel and bladder dysfunction. The risk of microangiopathy is related to the duration and degree of hyperglycaemia.

Preventing diabetes complications

The evidence that improved glycaemic control decreases the risk of microvascular complications of diabetes comes from the Diabetes Control and Complications Trial (DCCT) in type 1 diabetes, and the UK Prospective Diabetes Study (UKPDS) in type 2 diabetes. The DCCT lasted 9 yrs and showed a 60% overall reduction in the risk of diabetic complications in patients with type 1 diabetes on intensive therapy with strict glycaemic control, compared to conventional therapy. However, the intensively treated group had three times the rate of severe hypoglycaemia. The UKPDS showed that, in type 2 diabetes, the frequency of diabetic complications is lower and progression is slower with good glycaemic control and effective treatment of hypertension, irrespective of the type of therapy used. Extrapolation from the UKPDS suggests that, for every 11 mmol/mol (1%) reduction in HbA_{1c}, there is a 21% reduction in deaths related to diabetes, a 14% reduction in myocardial infarction and 30–40% reduction in risk of microvascular complications.

These trials demonstrate that diabetic complications are preventable and that the aim of treatment should be 'near-normal' glycaemia. However, the recent Action to Control Cardiovascular Risk in Diabetes study showed increased mortality in a high-risk subgroup of patients who were treated aggressively to lower HbA_{1c} to <48 mmol/mol (6.5%). Therefore, whilst a low target HbA_{1c} is appropriate in younger patients with earlier diabetes without underlying cardiovascular disease, aggressive glucose-lowering is not beneficial in older patients with long duration of diabetes and multiple comorbidities.

RCTs have also shown that aggressive management of lipids and BP limits complications. ACE inhibitors are valuable in improving outcome in heart disease and in preventing diabetic nephropathy.

Diabetic retinopathy

Diabetic retinopathy (DR) is a common cause of blindness in adults in developed countries. Hyperglycaemia increases retinal blood flow and metabolism, and has direct effects on retinal endothelial cells, resulting in impaired vascular autoregulation. This leads to chronic retinal hypoxia, which stimulates production of growth factors and causes new vessel formation and increased vascular permeability.

Clinical features

The major risk factors for DR are shown in Box 11.11. DR is a progressive condition, comprising non-proliferative ('background') and proliferative stages. The earliest signs of non-proliferative DR are microaneurysms and retinal haemorrhages, sometimes inaccurately called 'dot' and 'blot' haemorrhages (Fig. 11.3A and B). As DR progresses, cotton wool spots, venous beading and intra-retinal microvascular abnormalities appear (Fig. 11.3C–E); this is referred to as pre-proliferative DR. Progression to proliferative DR is characterised by growth of new blood vessels on the retina or optic disc (Fig. 11.3F, G). These vessels are abnormal and often bleed, causing vitreous haemorrhage (Fig. 11.3H), subsequent fibrosis and scarring, and finally tractional retinal detachment.

In addition, patients may also develop clinically significant macular oedema (CSMO; see Fig. 11.3C). This can occur at any stage of DR and is the most common cause of loss of vision in diabetes.

Proliferative retinopathy and severe ocular ischaemia may stimulate new vessels to grow on the anterior surface of the iris: 'rubeosis iridis'. These vessels may obstruct the drainage angle of the eye, causing secondary glaucoma.

Loss of visual acuity: Microaneurysms, abnormalities of the veins, and small haemorrhages and exudates situated in the periphery will not interfere with vision. However, if these changes appear near the macula, and in particular if they are accompanied by loss of visual acuity, CSMO should be suspected. Macular oedema can cause impaired visual acuity, even if only mild peripheral

11.11 Risk factors for diabetic retinopathy

- Long duration of diabetes
- Poor glycaemic control
- Hypertension
- Hyperlipidaemia
- Pregnancy
- Nephropathy/renal disease
- Others: obesity, smoking

Fig. 11.3 Diabetic retinopathy. A *Microaneurysms.* Discrete red dots beside vessels and narrower than the vessels at the disc margin. **B** *Haemorrhages.* Larger than microaneurysms, indistinct margins, wider than vessels at the disc margin, may be flame-shaped. **C** *Hard exudates.* Irregular lesions formed from leaking cholesterol (black arrows). Associated with retinal oedema; if at the macula, can cause sight-threatening clinically significant macular oedema (CSMO, white arrows). **D** *Cotton wool spots.* White, fluffy lesions seen in rapidly advancing retinopathy or with uncontrolled hypertension. **E** *Venous beading.* Saccular bulges in vein walls (black arrow). Intra-retinal microvascular anomalies (IRMA): spidery vessels (white arrow). **F, G** *Neovascularisation.* Fine tufts of vessels forming arcades on the retinal surface, later extending forwards on to the vitreous. Gliosis/fibrosis appears later as a dense white sheet. **H** *Vitreous haemorrhage.* New vessels rupture, causing haemorrhage (arrows) and sudden visual loss.

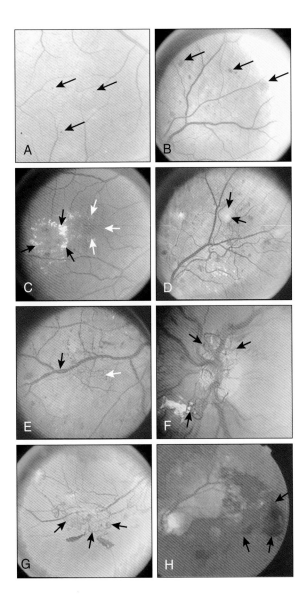

non-proliferative retinopathy is present. Macular oedema can only be confirmed or excluded on slit lamp retinal biomicroscopy.

Sudden visual loss occurs with vitreous haemorrhage or retinal detachment. In pre-proliferative and proliferative retinopathy, with or without visual impairment, prompt laser treatment is important to reduce the risk of haemorrhage, fibrosis/gliosis and irreversible visual impairment.

Prevention

Good glycaemic control reduces the risk of retinopathy. Early diagnosis and treatment is important – in type 2 diabetes, 25% present with established retinopathy. However, rapid reduction in blood glucose may cause an initial deterioration of retinopathy by causing relative ischaemia, so glycaemic control should be improved gradually. Control of hypertension is of proven benefit but intervention for hyperlipidaemia is unproven in DR.

Annual screening for retinopathy is essential in all diabetic patients, especially those with risk factors (see Box 11.11). The preferred method is digital photography, with referral to an ophthalmologist when needed.

Management

Novel agents are emerging, including ranibizumab, a monoclonal antibody fragment that is anti-angiogenic; it is used for diabetic macular oedema.

Severe non-proliferative and proliferative retinopathy is treated with retinal photocoagulation, which has been shown to reduce severe visual loss by 85% (50% in maculopathy). Argon laser photocoagulation is used to:

• Seal leaking microaneurysms. • Destroy areas of retinal ischaemia.
• Reduce macular oedema. • Gliose new vessels on the retinal surface.

Patients must be reviewed regularly to check for recurrence. Extensive bilateral photocoagulation can cause visual field loss, interfering with driving and night vision. Vitrectomy may be used in recurrent vitreous haemorrhage that has failed to clear, or tractional retinal detachment threatening the macula. Rubeosis iridis is managed by early pan-retinal photocoagulation.

Other causes of visual loss in diabetes

Around 50% of visual loss in people with type 2 diabetes is due to causes other than diabetic retinopathy. These include:

• Cataract. • Macular degeneration. • Retinal vein occlusion.
• Retinal arterial occlusion. • Ischaemic optic neuropathy. • Glaucoma.

Cataract occurs prematurely in people with diabetes due to the metabolic insult to the lens.

Diabetic nephropathy

Diabetic nephropathy is among the most common causes of end-stage renal failure (ESRF) in developed countries. About 30% of patients with type 1 diabetes have developed diabetic nephropathy after 20 yrs, but the risk after this time falls to <1%/yr. Risk factors for developing nephropathy include:

• Poor glycaemic control. • Duration of diabetes. • Other microvascular complications. • Ethnicity: Asian, Pima Indians. • Hypertension. • Family history of nephropathy or hypertension.

Pathologically, thickening of the glomerular basement membrane is followed by nodular deposits (Kimmelstiel–Wilson nodules). As glomerulosclerosis worsens, heavy proteinuria develops, sometimes in the nephrotic range, and renal function progressively deteriorates.

Diagnosis and screening

Microalbuminuria (defined as urine albumin:creatinine ratio 2.5–30 mg/mmol creatinine in men, 3.5–30 mg/creatinine mmol in women; undetectable by dipstick) is a risk factor for developing overt diabetic nephropathy, although it is also found in other conditions. Overt nephropathy is defined as the presence of macroalbuminuria (urinary albumin >300 mg/day; detectable on urine dipstick). Patients with type 1 diabetes should be screened annually from 5 yrs after diagnosis; those with type 2 diabetes should be screened annually from the time of diagnosis.

Management

Progression of nephropathy can be reduced by improved glycaemic control and aggressive reduction of BP and other cardiovascular risk factors.

In type 1 diabetes, ACE inhibitors provide greater protection than equal BP reduction achieved with other drugs; similar benefits result from angiotensin II receptor blockers (ARBs) in type 2 diabetes. Non-dihydropyridine calcium antagonists (diltiazem, verapamil) may be suitable alternatives.

Halving the amount of albuminuria with an ACE inhibitor or ARB reduces the risk of progression to end-stage renal disease by nearly 50%. However, in those who do progress, renal replacement therapy is of value at an early stage in diabetes.

Renal transplantation dramatically improves the life of many, and recurrence of diabetic nephropathy in the allograft is rare.

Diabetic neuropathy

This complication affects 50–90% of patients. It is symptomless in the majority and can involve motor, sensory and autonomic nerves. Prevalence is related to the duration of diabetes and the degree of metabolic control.

Clinical features

Symmetrical sensory polyneuropathy: This is commonly asymptomatic. The most common signs are diminished perception of vibration distally, 'glove-and-stocking' impairment of all sensory modalities, and loss of tendon reflexes in the legs. Symptoms may include paraesthesia in the feet or hands, pain on the anterior aspect of the legs (worse at night), burning sensations in the soles of the feet, hyperaesthesia and a wide-based gait. Toes may be clawed with wasting of the interosseous muscles. A diffuse small-fibre neuropathy causes altered pain and temperature sensation and is associated with symptomatic autonomic neuropathy; characteristic features include foot ulcers and Charcot neuroarthropathy.

Asymmetrical motor diabetic neuropathy (diabetic amyotrophy): This presents as severe, progressive weakness and wasting of the proximal muscles of the legs (occasionally arms), accompanied by severe pain, hyperaesthesia and paraesthesia. There may also be marked loss of weight ('neuropathic cachexia') and absent tendon reflexes; the CSF protein is often raised. This condition is thought to involve acute infarction of the lumbosacral plexus. Although recovery usually occurs within 12 mths, some deficits become permanent. Management is mainly supportive.

Mononeuropathy: Either motor or sensory function can be affected within a single peripheral or cranial nerve. Unlike other neuropathies, mononeuropathies are severe and of rapid onset. The patient usually recovers. Most commonly affected are the 3rd and 6th cranial nerves (causing diplopia), and femoral and sciatic nerves. Multiple nerves are affected in mononeuritis multiplex. Nerve compression palsies commonly affect the median nerve and lateral popliteal nerve (foot drop).

Autonomic neuropathy (Box 11.12): This is less clearly related to poor metabolic control, and improved control rarely improves symptoms. Within 10 yrs of developing autonomic neuropathy, 30–50% of patients are dead. Postural hypotension indicates a poor prognosis.

Erectile dysfunction: This affects 30% of diabetic males and is often multifactorial. Psychological problems, depression, alcohol and drug therapy may contribute (p. 163).

Management

See Box 11.12.

The diabetic foot

Tissue necrosis in the feet is a common reason for hospital admission in diabetic patients. Foot ulceration occurs as a result of often trivial trauma in the presence of neuropathy (peripheral and autonomic) and/or peripheral vascular disease; infection occurs as a secondary phenomenon. Most ulcers are neuropathic or neuro-ischaemic in type. They usually develop at the site of a plaque of callus skin, beneath which tissue necrosis occurs, eventually breaking through to the surface. Charcot neuro-arthropathy, with destructive inflammation of neuropathic joints, is usually caused by diabetes.

11.12 Management of peripheral sensorimotor and autonomic neuropathies		
Type of neuropathy	**Symptom/sign**	**Management**
Peripheral somatic neuropathies	Pain and paraesthesiae	Strict glycaemic control
		Anticonvulsants (e.g. gabapentin)
		Antidepressants (e.g. amitriptyline, duloxetine)
		Substance P depleter (capsaicin – topical)
		Opiates (tramadol, oxycodone)
		Membrane stabilisers (mexiletine, IV lidocaine)
		Antioxidant (α-lipoic acid)
Autonomic neuropathy	Postural hypotension	Fludrocortisone, NSAIDs, midodrine
		Support stockings
	Gastroparesis	Metoclopramide, erythromycin
		Gastric pacemaker, enterostomy feeding
	Motility disorders	Diarrhoea: loperamide, octreotide
		Constipation: stimulant laxatives
	Atonic bladder	Intermittent self-catheterisation
	Excessive sweating	Propantheline, clonidine
		Topical antimuscarinics (e.g. glycopyrrolate)
	Erectile dysfunction	Sildenafil
		Prostaglandin injections

Management

Preventative treatment is the most effective method of managing the diabetic foot. Patient education is crucial. Annual screening should include formal testing of sensation and removal of callus (by podiatrist). Further management includes:

• Débridement of dead tissue. • Prompt and prolonged antibiotics in the presence of infection. • Bespoke orthotic footwear (preventing pressure and deformity) • Vascular assessment: angiography/vascular reconstruction if the foot is ischaemic. • Charcot foot: cast immobilisation and avoidance of weight-bearing. • Amputation: if there is extensive tissue/bony destruction, or intractable ischaemic pain when vascular reconstruction is not possible or has failed.

Diseases of the GI tract are a major cause of morbidity and mortality. Approximately 10% of all GP consultations in the UK are for indigestion, and 1 in 14 is for diarrhoea. Infective diarrhoea and malabsorption are responsible for much ill health and many deaths in the developing world.

PRESENTING PROBLEMS IN GASTROINTESTINAL DISEASE

Dysphagia

Dysphagia means difficulty in swallowing, as distinct from globus sensation (a 'lump' in the throat without organic cause) and odynophagia (pain during swallowing). Oropharyngeal dysphagia results from neuromuscular dysfunction that affects swallowing, causing choking, nasal regurgitation or tracheal aspiration. Drooling, dysarthria, hoarseness and other neurological signs may be present. Oesophageal causes include benign or malignant strictures and oesophageal dysmotility. Patients complain of food 'sticking' after swallowing, although swallowing of liquids is normal until strictures become extreme.

Endoscopy is preferred to facilitate biopsy and dilatation of strictures. Videofluoroscopic barium swallow will detect most motility disorders. Oesophageal manometry is occasionally required.

Dyspepsia

Dyspepsia ('indigestion') may arise from within or outside the gut (Box 12.1). Heartburn and other 'reflux' symptoms are separate and are considered elsewhere. Although symptoms correlate poorly with diagnosis, careful history may reveal classical symptoms of peptic ulcer, 'alarm' features requiring urgent investigation (Box 12.2) or symptoms of other disorders. Dyspepsia affects up to 80% of the population at some time, often with no abnormality on investigation, especially in younger patients.

Examination may reveal anaemia, weight loss, lymphadenopathy, abdominal masses or liver disease. Patients with 'alarm' symptoms,

CLINICAL EXAMINATION OF THE GASTROINTESTINAL TRACT

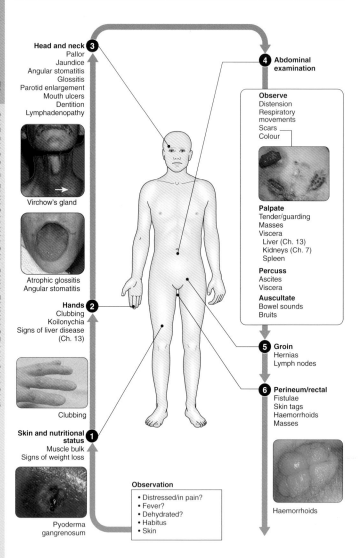

Head and neck ❸
Pallor
Jaundice
Angular stomatitis
Glossitis
Parotid enlargement
Mouth ulcers
Dentition
Lymphadenopathy

Virchow's gland

Atrophic glossitis
Angular stomatitis

Hands ❷
Clubbing
Koilonychia
Signs of liver disease
(Ch. 13)

Clubbing

Skin and nutritional status ❶
Muscle bulk
Signs of weight loss

Pyoderma
gangrenosum

Observation
- Distressed/in pain?
- Fever?
- Dehydrated?
- Habitus
- Skin

❹ **Abdominal examination**

Observe
Distension
Respiratory movements
Scars
Colour

Palpate
Tender/guarding
Masses
Viscera
  Liver (Ch. 13)
  Kidneys (Ch. 7)
  Spleen

Percuss
Ascites
Viscera

Auscultate
Bowel sounds
Bruits

❺ **Groin**
Hernias
Lymph nodes

❻ **Perineum/rectal**
Fistulae
Skin tags
Haemorrhoids
Masses

Haemorrhoids

12.1 Causes of dyspepsia

GI disorders

- Peptic ulcer disease
- Acute gastritis
- Gallstones
- Motility disorders, e.g. oesophageal spasm
- Colonic carcinoma
- 'Functional' (non-ulcer dyspepsia and irritable bowel syndrome)
- Pancreatic disease (cancer, chronic pancreatitis)
- Hepatic disease (hepatitis, metastases)

Systemic disease

- Renal failure
- Hypercalcaemia

Drugs

- NSAIDs
- Iron and potassium supplements
- Corticosteroids
- Digoxin

Others

- Psychological, e.g. anxiety, depression
- Alcohol

12.2 'Alarm' features in dyspepsia

- Weight loss
- Anaemia
- Vomiting
- Haematemesis and/or melaena
- Dysphagia
- Palpable abdominal mass

and those >55 with new dyspepsia require prompt endoscopy. Younger patients should be tested for *Helicobacter pylori*; if symptoms persist after treatment, these patients should have endoscopy.

Vomiting

Vomiting is a complex reflex involving contraction of the diaphragm and intercostal and abdominal muscles, and simultaneous relaxation of the lower oesophageal sphincter, causing forcible ejection of gastric contents.

The history should reveal associated abdominal pain, fever, diarrhoea, relationship to food, drugs, headache, vertigo and weight

> ### 12.3 Common causes of acute upper GI haemorrhage
>
> - Oesophagitis (10%)
> - Mallory–Weiss tear (5%)
> - Varices (2–9%)
> - Peptic ulcer (*H. pylori* or NSAID) (35–50%)
> - Gastric erosions (NSAID or alcohol) (10–20%)
> - Vascular malformation (5%)
> - Carcinoma of stomach or oesophagus (2%)

loss. Pregnancy, alcoholism or bulimia should be considered. Examination may reveal:

• Dehydration. • Fever. • Abdominal masses. • Peritonitis or intestinal obstruction. • Papilloedema. • Nystagmus. • Photophobia. • Neck stiffness.

The diagnostic approach will be dictated by the history and examination.

GI bleeding
Acute upper GI haemorrhage

This is the most common GI emergency, accounting for 50–170 hospital admissions per 100 000 each year in the UK.

Haematemesis may be red with clots when bleeding is profuse, or black ('coffee grounds') when less severe. Syncope may occur with rapid bleeding. Anaemia suggests chronic bleeding. Melaena is the passage of black, tarry stools containing altered blood. This is usually due to upper GI bleeding, although the ascending colon is occasionally responsible. Severe acute upper GI bleeding occasionally causes maroon or bright red stool. Causes of acute upper GI haemorrhage are shown in Box 12.3.

Management

IV access: Access should be secured with a large-bore cannula.

Clinical assessment: Risk of complications is related to circulatory status (tachycardia, hypotension and oliguria indicating severe bleeding), liver disease (jaundice, cutaneous stigmata, hepatosplenomegaly and ascites) and comorbidity (cardiorespiratory, cerebrovascular or renal disease, which increase the hazards of endoscopy and surgery).

Blood tests: These should include FBC (slow bleeding causes anaemia; haemoglobin may be normal after sudden, major bleeding); cross-matching of at least 2 U of blood; U&Es (shock may cause renal failure; the urea also rises as the luminal blood is digested); LFTs and prothrombin time, if there is clinical suggestion of liver disease or in anticoagulated patients.

Resuscitation: Oxygen is given to patients in shock. IV crystalloid infusion restores BP, and blood transfusion is indicated if there is shock and active bleeding. Antibiotics are given in chronic liver disease. CVP monitoring helps to reveal rebleeding and guide fluid replacement, particularly in patients with cardiac disease.

Endoscopy: After resuscitation, this will reveal a diagnosis in 80% of cases. Patients with spurting haemorrhage or a visible vessel can be treated by thermal probe, adrenaline (epinephrine) injection or metal clips. This may stop bleeding and, combined with IV proton pump inhibitor (PPI) therapy, prevent rebleeding, thus avoiding surgery.

Monitoring: Hourly pulse, BP and urine output should be monitored.

Surgery: This is indicated when endoscopic haemostasis fails to stop the bleeding, or rebleeding occurs once in an elderly or frail patient/twice in younger, fitter patients. Following successful surgery for ulcer bleeding, all patients should be treated with *H. pylori* eradication therapy if positive, and should avoid NSAIDs.

Lower GI bleeding

This may be due to haemorrhage from the small bowel, colon or anal canal.

Severe acute lower GI bleeding

Diverticular disease: This is the most common cause. Patients present with profuse, red or maroon diarrhoea and shock. Bleeding almost always stops spontaneously, but if not, the diseased segment is located by angiography or colonoscopy and resected.

Angiodysplasia: Vascular malformations in the proximal colon of elderly patients cause bleeding, which usually stops spontaneously but commonly recurs. Treatment is by colonoscopic thermal ablation, or resection if bleeding continues.

Ischaemia due to inferior mesenteric artery occlusion: Presents with abdominal colic and rectal bleeding. It occurs in elderly patients with atherosclerosis and is diagnosed by colonoscopy. Resection is required only if peritonitis develops.

Meckel's diverticulum: May erode into a major artery and cause profuse lower GI bleeding in children or adolescents. The diagnosis is commonly made only by resection at laparotomy.

Subacute or chronic lower GI bleeding

This is extremely common and is usually due to haemorrhoids or anal fissure. Proctoscopy reveals the diagnosis but if there is altered bowel habit and in all patients presenting at age 40 and over, colonoscopy is necessary to exclude colorectal cancer.

Obscure major GI bleeding

If upper endoscopy and colonoscopy are inconclusive, mesenteric angiography usually identifies the site and embolisation can be used to stop the bleeding. If angiography is negative, double balloon enteroscopy or wireless capsule endoscopy can be employed to identify a bleeding source in the small intestine. When all else fails, laparotomy with on-table endoscopy is indicated.

Occult GI bleeding

Occult bleeding (no visible blood) may reach 200 mL/day, cause iron deficiency anaemia and signify serious disease. The most important cause is colorectal cancer, which may have no GI symptoms. GI investigations should be considered in any patient with unexplained iron deficiency anaemia. A negative faecal occult blood (FOB) test does not exclude important GI disease. FOB is now only used in population screening for bowel cancer.

Diarrhoea

Diarrhoea is defined as the passage of >200 g of stool daily, commonly with increased frequency and loose or watery stools. In severe cases, urgency of defecation and faecal incontinence occur.

Acute diarrhoea

Infective diarrhoea is usually due to faecal–oral transmission of bacteria, viruses or parasites, and is normally short-lived. Diarrhoea lasting >10 days is rarely caused by infection. Drugs, including antibiotics, cytotoxics, PPIs and NSAIDs, may cause acute diarrhoea.

Chronic or relapsing diarrhoea

The most common cause is irritable bowel syndrome, in which diarrhoea is most severe before and after breakfast and rarely occurs at night. At other times the patient is constipated. The stool often contains mucus but never blood, and 24-hr stool volume is <200 g. Chronic diarrhoea can also be due to inflammatory or neoplastic disease of the colon or small bowel, or to malabsorption. Negative investigations suggest irritable bowel syndrome.

Malabsorption

Diarrhoea and weight loss in patients with a normal diet suggest malabsorption. Bulky, pale and offensive stools that float (steatorrhoea) signify fat malabsorption. Abdominal distension, borborygmi, cramps and undigested food in the stool may be present. Malaise, lethargy, peripheral neuropathy and symptoms related to vitamin or mineral deficiencies may occur.

Malabsorption results from abnormalities of the three components of normal digestion.

• Intraluminal maldigestion due to deficiency of bile or pancreatic enzymes. • Mucosal malabsorption from small bowel resection or damage to the small intestinal epithelium. • 'Post-mucosal' lymphatic obstruction preventing the uptake of absorbed lipids into lymphatic vessels.

An approach to investigations is shown in Figure 12.1.

Weight loss

Unplanned weight loss of >3 kg over 6 mths is significant. Previous weight records may be valuable. Pathological weight loss can be

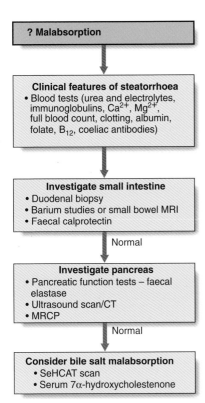

? Malabsorption

Clinical features of steatorrhoea
- Blood tests (urea and electrolytes, immunoglobulins, Ca^{2+}, Mg^{2+}, full blood count, clotting, albumin, folate, B_{12}, coeliac antibodies)

Investigate small intestine
- Duodenal biopsy
- Barium studies or small bowel MRI
- Faecal calprotectin

Normal

Investigate pancreas
- Pancreatic function tests – faecal elastase
- Ultrasound scan/CT
- MRCP

Normal

Consider bile salt malabsorption
- SeHCAT scan
- Serum 7α-hydroxycholestenone

Fig. 12.1 Investigation for suspected malabsorption.

due to psychiatric illness, systemic disease, GI causes or advanced disease of any specific organ system.

History and examination

'Physiological' weight loss: This should be obvious from the history but may be more difficult to determine in older patients when nutritional history may be unreliable; a dietitian's opinion is often valuable.

Psychiatric illness: Features of anorexia nervosa, bulimia and affective disorders may only be apparent after formal psychiatric input. Alcoholic patients lose weight through self-neglect and poor diet.

Systemic diseases: Chronic infections lead to weight loss, and a history of foreign travel, fever, night sweats, rigors, productive cough and dysuria must be sought. Sensitive questions regarding lifestyle (promiscuous sexual activity and drug misuse) may suggest HIV infection. Weight loss is a late feature of disseminated malignancy (carcinoma, lymphoma or other haematological disorders), which may be revealed on examination.

GI disease: Dysphagia and gastric outflow obstruction cause defective intake. Malignancy may cause weight loss by mechanical obstruction, anorexia or systemic effects. Malabsorption from pancreas or small bowel causes profound weight loss and nutritional deficiencies. Crohn's disease and ulcerative colitis cause anorexia, fear of eating, and loss of protein, blood and nutrients from the gut.

Specific diseases of any major organ system: Endocrine disease, including diabetes mellitus, Addison's disease and thyrotoxicosis, may cause weight loss. In patients with disabling end-stage respiratory, cardiac or rheumatological diseases, weight loss occurs from a combination of anorexia, physical disability and the systemic effects of their conditions, often compounded by drug effects (e.g. digoxin), which may cause nausea, dyspepsia, constipation or depression.

Investigations

• Urinalysis for glucose, protein and blood. • Blood tests: LFTs, random blood glucose and TFTs; ESR (often raised in infections, connective tissue disorders and malignancy). • Bone marrow aspiration or liver biopsy: to identify cryptic miliary TB when there is strong clinical suspicion. • Abdominal and pelvic CT: occasionally help, but only after careful history and reweighing.

Constipation

Constipation is the infrequent passage of hard stools, often with straining, a sensation of incomplete evacuation, and perianal or abdominal discomfort. It may be the end result of many disorders.

In the absence of a history suggesting a specific cause (Box 12.4), it is not necessary to investigate every person with constipation. Most respond to dietary fibre supplementation and the judicious use of laxatives. Middle-aged or elderly patients with a short history or worrying symptoms (rectal bleeding, pain or weight loss) must be

---

12.4 Causes of constipation

GI

- Lack of dietary fibre
- Altered motility, e.g. irritable bowel syndrome
- Structural, e.g. colonic carcinoma, diverticular disease, Hirschsprung's disease
- Obstructed defecation, e.g. anal fissure, Crohn's disease

Non-GI

- Drugs, e.g. opiates, anticholinergics
- Neurological, e.g. multiple sclerosis, paraplegia
- Metabolic/endocrine, e.g. hypercalcaemia, hypothyroidism
- Others: any serious illness, especially in the elderly

investigated promptly, by either barium enema or colonoscopy. Others should be investigated as follows:

• Initially, digital rectal examination, proctoscopy and sigmoidoscopy, routine biochemistry, including serum calcium and thyroid function, and an FBC. • If normal: a 1-mth trial of dietary fibre and/or laxatives. • If symptoms persist: examination of the colon by barium enema or colonoscopy to look for structural disease.

Abdominal pain

Abdominal pain may be:
• Visceral: usually midline, due to stretching or torsion of a viscus. • Parietal: usually sharp, lateralised and localised, due to peritoneal irritation. • Referred: e.g. gallbladder pain referred to the back or shoulder tip. • Psychogenic: cultural, emotional and psychosocial factors influence the experience of pain. In some patients, no organic cause is found despite investigation.

The acute abdomen

This accounts for ~50% of all urgent surgical admissions and is a consequence of one or more pathological processes:

Inflammation (e.g. appendicitis, pancreatitis, diverticulitis): Diffuse pain develops gradually, over hours. If the parietal peritoneum is involved, pain becomes localised. Movement exacerbates it; rigidity and guarding occur.

Perforation (e.g. peptic ulcer, ovarian cyst, diverticular disease): Pain starts abruptly, is severe and leads to generalised peritonitis.

Obstruction (intestinal, biliary or ureteric): Pain is colicky, with spasms causing the patient to writhe around. If it does not disappear between spasms, this suggests complicating inflammation.

If there are signs of peritonitis (i.e. guarding and rebound tenderness with rigidity), resuscitation with IV fluids, oxygen and antibiotics is needed. Further investigations should include:

• FBC: may demonstrate leucocytosis. • U&Es: reveal dehydration. • Serum amylase: raised in acute pancreatitis. • Erect CXR: shows air under the diaphragm in perforation; an AXR reveals obstruction. • USS: may help if gallstones, ureteric colic or a soft tissue mass is suspected, and may also reveal free fluid or intra-abdominal abscess. • Contrast studies, by either mouth or anus: useful to evaluate obstruction, and essential to distinguish pseudo-obstruction from mechanical large bowel obstruction. • CT: useful for pancreatitis, retroperitoneal collections or masses, and aortic aneurysm. • Angiography or multi-slice CT angiography: used in mesenteric ischaemia. • Diagnostic laparoscopy: may be useful if the cause remains obscure.

Management

Perforations are closed, inflammatory conditions are treated with antibiotics or resection, and obstructions are relieved. Most but not all patients require surgery. The need for, and urgency of, surgical intervention depend on clinical severity and stability, and the presence or absence of peritonitis.

Acute appendicitis: The risk of perforation or recurrence is high with conservative treatment, so surgery is usually advisable.

Small bowel obstruction: Strangulated hernias require urgent surgery. If the cause is adhesions from previous surgery, only patients who do not settle within 48 hrs with IV fluids, fasting and nasogastric aspiration, or who develop signs of strangulation (colicky pain becoming constant, peritonitis, tachycardia, fever, leucocytosis) require surgery.

Large bowel obstruction: Pseudo-obstruction is treated non-operatively. Some patients benefit from colonoscopic decompression, but mechanical obstruction merits surgery. Differentiation between the two is by a water-soluble contrast enema.

Acute cholecystitis: See page 515.

Acute diverticulitis: See page 470.

Perforated peptic ulcer: See page 436.

Chronic or recurrent abdominal pain

A detailed history, including fever, weight loss and mood, is essential. If abdominal and rectal examination is normal, a careful search should be made for disease affecting the vertebral column, spinal cord, lungs and cardiovascular system.

The choice of investigations depends on the history and examination (Box 12.5). Persistent symptoms require exclusion of colonic or small bowel disease. A history of psychiatric disturbance, repeated negative investigations or vague symptoms not fitting any particular disease or organ pattern may point to a psychological origin.

Constant abdominal pain

Patients with constant abdominal pain usually have features to suggest the underlying diagnosis, e.g. malignancy, chronic

12.5 **Investigation of chronic or recurrent abdominal pain**		
Symptom	**Probable diagnosis**	**Investigation**
Epigastric pain; dyspepsia; relationship to food	Gastroduodenal or biliary disease	Endoscopy and USS
Altered bowel habit; rectal bleeding; features of obstruction	Colonic disease	Barium enema and sigmoidoscopy/ colonoscopy
Pain provoked by food in widespread atherosclerosis	Mesenteric ischaemia	Mesenteric angiography
Upper abdominal pain radiating to the back; history of alcohol misuse; weight loss; diarrhoea	Chronic pancreatitis or pancreatic cancer	USS, CT and pancreatic function tests
Recurrent loin or flank pain with urinary symptoms	Renal or ureteric stones	USS and IV urography

pancreatitis or intra-abdominal abscess. Occasionally no cause will be found, leading to the diagnosis of 'chronic functional abdominal pain'. In these patients a psychological cause is highly likely and treatment is aimed at symptom control, psychological support and minimising disease impact.

DISORDERS OF NUTRITION

Obesity

Obesity is a pandemic with potentially disastrous consequences for health. More than 25% of adults in the UK are obese (BMI >30), compared to 7% in 1980. Over two-thirds of UK adults are overweight (BMI >25).

The pandemic reflects changes in both energy intake and expenditure. The estimated average global daily supply of food energy per person increased from ~2350 kcal in the 1960s to ~2800 kcal in the 1990s. Portion sizes, particularly of sugary drinks and high-fat snacks, have increased. Corresponding changes in energy expenditure are important; obesity is correlated positively with hours spent watching television, and inversely with physical activity.

Although obese people were ridiculed in the past when they bemoaned their inability to control their weight, it is likely that susceptibility does vary between individuals. Twin studies confirm a genetic pattern of inheritance, suggesting a polygenic disorder. In a few cases, specific causal factors can be identified, such as hypothyroidism, Cushing's syndrome or insulinoma. Drugs implicated include: tricyclic antidepressants, sulphonylureas, sodium valproate and β-blockers.

Complications of obesity

Health consequences of obesity include:
• Metabolic syndrome (p. 385). • Non-alcoholic steatohepatitis. • Cirrhosis. • Sleep apnoea. • Osteoarthritis. • Psychosocial disadvantage.

Obesity has adverse effects on both mortality and morbidity; life expectancy is reduced by 13 yrs amongst obese smokers. Coronary artery disease (CAD) is the major cause of death but some cancer rates are also increased.

Clinical features and investigations

Obesity can be quantified using the body mass index (BMI = weight in kilograms divided by the height in metres squared (kg/m^2)):
• Normal 18.5–25. • Overweight 25–30. • Obese >30.

Risk of complications rises steeply to very severe if BMI >40.

A dietary history may be helpful in guiding dietary advice but is susceptible to under-reporting of consumption. Alcohol consumption is an important source of energy intake. All obese patients should have TFTs performed, and an overnight dexamethasone suppression test or 24-hr urine free cortisol if Cushing's syndrome is suspected. Assessment of other cardiovascular risk factors is important. BP should be measured, and type 2 diabetes and dyslipidaemia detected by measuring blood glucose and serum lipids. Elevated transaminases suggest non-alcoholic fatty liver disease.

Management

The health risks of obesity are largely reversible. Interventions that reduce weight in studies in obese patients have also been shown to ameliorate cardiovascular risk factors. Lifestyle advice that lowers body weight and increases physical exercise reduces the incidence of type 2 diabetes.

Most patients seeking assistance will have attempted weight loss previously, sometimes repeatedly. An empathetic explanation of energy balance, recognising that some individuals are more susceptible to obesity, is important. Appropriate weight loss goals (e.g. 10% of body weight) should be agreed.

Lifestyle advice: All patients should be advised to maximise their physical activity by incorporating it into the daily routine (e.g. walking rather than driving to work). Changes in eating behaviour (including portion size control, avoidance of snacking, regular meals to encourage satiety, and use of artificial sweeteners) should be discussed.

Weight loss diets: In overweight people, the lifestyle advice given above may gradually succeed. In obese patients, more active intervention is usually required. Weight loss diets require a reduction in daily total energy intake of ~2.5 MJ (600 kcal) from the patient's normal consumption. The goal is to lose ~0.5 kg/wk. Patient compliance is the major determinant of success. In some patients more rapid weight loss is required, e.g. in preparation for surgery. There is no role for starvation diets, which carry a risk of sudden death from heart disease. Very low calorie diets produce weight loss of 1.5–2.5 kg/wk but require the supervision of a physician and nutritionist.

Drugs: Drug therapy is usually reserved for obese patients with a high risk of complications. Patients who continue to take anti-obesity drugs tend to regain weight with time. This has led to the recommendation that anti-obesity drugs are used short-term to maximise weight loss in patients who are demonstrating their adherence to a low-calorie diet by current weight loss. Several drugs have been withdrawn due to side-effects, and orlistat is the only drug currently licensed for long-term use. Orlistat inhibits pancreatic and gastric lipases, reducing dietary fat absorption by ~30%. Side-effects relate to the resultant fat malabsorption: namely, loose stools, oily spotting, faecal urgency, flatus and malabsorption of fat-soluble vitamins.

Surgery: 'Bariatric' surgery to reduce the size of the stomach is the most effective long-term treatment for obesity. It should be contemplated in motivated patients with a very high risk of developing the complications of obesity, in whom dietary and drug therapy has been ineffective. The mechanism of weight loss may not relate to limiting the stomach capacity per se, but rather in disrupting the release of ghrelin from the stomach, which signals hunger in the hypothalamus. Mortality is low in experienced centres but post-operative complications are common.

Under-nutrition
Starvation and famine
There remain regions of the world, particularly in Africa, where the prevalence of BMI <18.5 in adults remains as high as 20%. In adults, the predominant form of protein–energy malnutrition is under-nutrition, i.e. a sustained negative energy (calorie) balance caused by one of the following:

Decreased energy intake: Causes include:
• Famine. • Persistent regurgitation or vomiting. • Anorexia. • Malabsorption (e.g. small intestinal disease). • Maldigestion (e.g. pancreatic exocrine insufficiency).

Increased energy expenditure: Causes include:
• Increased basal metabolic rate (BMR; thyrotoxicosis, trauma, fever, cancer cachexia). • Excessive physical activity (e.g. marathon runners). • Energy loss (e.g. glycosuria in diabetes). • Impaired energy storage (e.g. Addison's disease, phaeochromocytoma).

Clinical features
The severity of malnutrition can be assessed by measurements of BMI, mid-arm circumference and skinfold thickness. The clinical features of severe under-nutrition in adults include:
• Loss of weight. • Thirst, weakness, a feeling of cold, nocturia, amenorrhoea, impotence. • Lax, pale, dry skin. • Hair thinning or loss. • Cold, cyanosed extremities, pressure sores. • Muscle-wasting. • Loss of subcutaneous fat. • Oedema (even without hypoalbuminaemia). • Subnormal body temperature, slow pulse, low BP. • Distended abdomen, with diarrhoea. • Diminished tendon jerks. • Apathy, loss of initiative, depression, introversion, aggression if food is nearby. • Susceptibility to infections.

Under-nutrition often leads to vitamin deficiencies, especially of thiamin, folate and vitamin C. Diarrhoea causes sodium, potassium and magnesium depletion. The high mortality is often due to infections, e.g. typhus or cholera, but the usual signs may not appear. In advanced starvation, patients become completely inactive and may assume a flexed, fetal position; death comes quietly and often quite suddenly.

Investigations
Plasma free fatty acids are increased, with ketosis and a mild metabolic acidosis. Plasma glucose is low but albumin is often maintained. Insulin secretion is diminished, glucagon and cortisol increase, and reverse T_3 replaces normal triiodothyronine. Resting metabolic rate falls, due to reduced lean body mass and

hypothalamic compensation. There may be mild anaemia, leucopenia and thrombocytopenia.

Management

Patients should be graded according to BMI. Those with moderate starvation need extra feeding, while those who are severely underweight need hospital care. In severe starvation there is atrophy of the intestinal epithelium and the exocrine pancreas.

Small amounts of food should be given at first; it should be palatable and similar to the usual staple meal, e.g. cereal with some sugar, milk powder and oil. Salt should be restricted and micronutrient supplements may be essential (e.g. potassium, magnesium, zinc and multivitamins). Between 6.3 and 8.4 MJ/day (1500–2000 kcal/day) will prevent deterioration, but additional calories are required for regain of weight. During refeeding, a gain of 5% body weight/mth indicates satisfactory progress. Other measures are supportive, and include care for the skin, adequate hydration, treatment of infections, and careful monitoring of body temperature since thermoregulation may be impaired.

Under-nutrition in hospital

One-third of hospital patients in the UK (particularly the elderly) are affected by moderate or severe under-nutrition on admission. Once in hospital, many lose weight due to poor appetite, concurrent illness and being kept 'nil by mouth' for investigations. Under-nutrition leads to impaired immunity and muscle weakness, and to increased morbidity, mortality and length of stay.

Nutritional support of the hospital patient

Normal diet: Inadequate intake may be due to unpalatability of food, cultural and religious factors restricting diet, or simple problems such as difficulty with hand dexterity (arthritis, stroke) or immobility in bed. Patients at risk of malnutrition should have food intake charted.

Dietary supplements: If a patient is unable to achieve sufficient nutritional intake from normal diet alone, then liquid dietary supplements with high energy and protein content should be used.

Enteral tube feeding: Patients who cannot swallow may require artificial nutritional support. The enteral route should be used if possible, as this preserves the integrity of the mucosal barrier, prevents bacteraemia and, in intensive care patients, reduces the risk of multi-organ failure. For short-term support, liquid feeds are given by fine-bore nasogastric tube. Tube position should be checked prior to use; gastric aspirate has a pH < 5. A CXR can confirm tube position if in doubt. A nasojejunal tube can be placed in cases of gastric stasis or outlet obstruction. For long-term enteral feeding, a percutaneous endoscopic gastrostomy (PEG) is more comfortable and less likely to become displaced. However, inserting a gastrostomy is an invasive procedure, and complications include local infection (30%) and perforation of intra-abdominal organs.

Parenteral nutrition: IV feeding is expensive, carries higher risks of complications and should only be used when enteral feeding is impossible. Less than 1 wk of parenteral feeding confers little benefit. There are a number of possible routes:

• Peripheral venous cannula: can only be used for low-osmolality solutions due to the risk of thrombophlebitis. • Peripherally inserted central catheter (PICC): a 60-cm cannula is inserted into a vein in the antecubital fossa. The distal end lies in a central vein, allowing hyperosmolar solutions to be used. • Central line: a single-lumen subclavian catheter in the internal jugular vein is preferred, due to lower infection rates. Hyperosmolar solutions can be used.

The main energy source in total parenteral nutrition (TPN) is provided by carbohydrate, usually as glucose. TPN also contains amino acids, lipid emulsion, electrolytes, trace elements and vitamins, mixed as a large bag in a sterile environment. Constituents are adjusted according to the results of regular blood monitoring. Fever indicates a likely line infection.

Refeeding syndrome

When nutritional support is given to a malnourished patient, anabolic hormones are released. Insulin causes cellular uptake of phosphate, potassium and magnesium. Falling levels can have serious consequences, such as cardiac arrhythmias. Electrolyte levels should be corrected before refeeding is commenced. Wernicke's encephalopathy may be precipitated by refeeding with carbohydrates in thiamin deficiency. This can be countered by giving thiamin before feeding.

Ethical aspects

In severe or terminal disease, the patient and family should be involved in decisions about the extent of invasive nutritional support. Tube feeding is regarded as a medical treatment and all invasive feeding procedures require consent where this is possible, or action in the best interests of the patient where consent is not possible. Teams should formulate, with the patient and family, an agreed nutritional plan for each patient individually.

Vitamin deficiency

Vitamins are categorised as fat-soluble or water-soluble. Deficiency of fat-soluble vitamins occurs in fat malabsorption.

• In developed countries, older people and alcoholic patients are particularly at risk of vitamin deficiency. In developing countries, vitamin deficiency diseases are more prevalent.

Box 12.6 summarises the sources of vitamins and their deficiency states.

Anorexia nervosa

Anorexia nervosa is a well-defined eating disorder, although a much higher prevalence of abnormal eating behaviour in the population

12.6 Clinically important vitamins and vitamin deficiency states

Name	Sources	Deficiency	Investigations
Fat-soluble			
Vitamin A	Liver, milk, butter, fish oils	Xerophthalmia, night blindness, keratomalacia, follicular hyperkeratosis	Serum retinol
Vitamin D	Synthesised in skin	Rickets, osteomalacia	Plasma 25(OH)D/ 1,25(OH)$_2$D
Vitamin E	Vegetables, seed oils	Haemolytic anaemia, ataxia	Plasma vitamin E
Vitamin K	Green vegetables, dairy products	Coagulation disorder	Coagulation assay $\pm$ plasma vitamin K
Water-soluble			
Thiamin (B$_1$)	Cereals, grains, beans, pork	Beri-beri, Wernicke–Korsakoff syndrome	RBC transketolase, whole-blood vitamin B$_1$
Riboflavin (B$_2$)	Milk	Glossitis, stomatitis	RBC glutathione reductase, whole-blood B$_2$
Niacin (B$_3$)	Meat, cereals	Pellagra	Urinary metabolites
Pyridoxine (B$_6$)	Meat, fish, potatoes, bananas	Polyneuropathy	Plasma pyridoxal phosphate or RBC transaminase activation coefficient
Biotin	Liver, egg yolk, cereals	Dermatitis, alopecia, paraesthesiae	Whole-blood or urine biotin
Folate	Liver, milk	Anaemia, neural tube defects during gestation	RBC folate
Vitamin B$_{12}$	Animal products	Anaemia, neurological degeneration	Plasma B$_{12}$
Vitamin C	Fresh fruit, vegetables	Scurvy	Ascorbic acid (plasma: daily intake; leucocyte: tissue stores)

does not meet the diagnostic criteria. There is marked weight loss, arising from food avoidance, in combination with bingeing, purging, excessive exercise, or the use of diuretics and laxatives. Despite their emaciation, patients feel overweight due to body image disturbance. Downy hair (lanugo) develops on the back, forearms and cheeks. Extreme starvation is associated with a range of pathophysiological changes, such as cardiac arrhythmias (prolonged QT and ventricular tachycardia), anaemia and osteoporosis. The condition usually emerges in adolescence, and 90% of cases are female.

Diagnostic criteria are:

• Loss of at least 15% of total body weight. • Avoidance of high-calorie foods. • Distortion of body image. • Amenorrhoea for at least 3 mths.

Differential diagnosis includes:

• Depression. • Inflammatory bowel disease. • Malabsorption. • Hypopituitarism. • Cancer.

Management and prognosis

The aim is to increase weight into the normal range by addressing abnormal beliefs and behaviour. Treatment is given on an outpatient basis, inpatient treatment being indicated only if weight loss is intractable or if there is a risk of death. Measures include cognitive behavioural therapy (CBT) and family therapy. Compulsory admission and tube feeding are resorted to when patients are at risk of death and other measures have failed. About 20% of patients have a good outcome, 20% develop a chronic disorder and the remainder have an intermediate outcome. Long-term mortality is 10–20%.

DISEASES OF THE MOUTH AND SALIVARY GLANDS

Aphthous ulceration: Common, superficial, painful and idiopathic. In severe cases, causes such as infection, drug reaction or Behçet's syndrome must be considered. Topical triamcinolone in Orabase or choline salicylate gel can relieve symptoms.

Squamous carcinoma of the oral cavity: Common worldwide and increasing in the UK. Mortality is ~50%, largely due to late diagnosis. Poor diet, alcohol, smoking or chewing tobacco or areca nuts in betel leaves ('betel nuts') are traditional risk factors, but human papillomaviruses 16 and 18 are also implicated. Suspicious lesions should be biopsied if treatment for local trauma or infection fails to produce improvement after 2 wks. Treatment is by resection, radiotherapy or both.

Candidiasis: Caused by *Candida albicans*, a normal mouth commensal that proliferates to cause thrush in babies, patients receiving corticosteroids, antibiotics or cytotoxic therapy, and people with diabetes or HIV. White patches are seen on the tongue and buccal mucosa. Dysphagia suggests pharyngeal and oesophageal candidiasis. A clinical diagnosis is sufficient to instigate therapy, using nystatin or amphotericin suspensions or lozenges. Oral fluconazole is used in resistant cases.

Parotitis: Due to viral or bacterial infection. Mumps causes a self-limiting acute parotitis. Bacterial parotitis usually occurs as a complication of major surgery and can be avoided by good post-operative care. Broad-spectrum antibiotics are required, whilst surgical drainage is necessary if abscesses are present.

DISEASES OF THE OESOPHAGUS

Gastro-oesophageal reflux disease

Gastro-oesophageal reflux resulting in heartburn affects ~30% of the general population.

Gastro-oesophageal reflux disease (GORD) develops when the oesophageal mucosa is exposed to gastric contents for prolonged periods, resulting in symptoms and, in a proportion of cases, oesophagitis. Reflux may occur if there is reduced oesophageal sphincter tone or frequent inappropriate sphincter relaxation. Herniation of the stomach through the diaphragm (hiatus hernia) occurs in 30% of the population >50 and is often asymptomatic. It causes reflux because of loss of the oblique angle between the cardia and oesophagus. Almost all patients who develop oesophagitis, Barrett's oesophagus or peptic strictures have a hiatus hernia. Defective oesophageal peristaltic activity is common in patients with oesophagitis, and persists after oesophagitis has been healed by acid-suppressing drugs.

Gastric acid is the most important oesophageal irritant and there is a close relationship between acid exposure time and symptoms. Gastric emptying is delayed in patients with GORD. Increased intra-abdominal pressure due to pregnancy and obesity may contribute. Weight loss may improve symptoms. Dietary fat, chocolate, alcohol and coffee relax the lower oesophageal sphincter and may provoke symptoms.

Clinical features

The major symptoms are heartburn and regurgitation, often provoked by bending, straining or lying down. 'Waterbrash', reflex salivation on acid reflux, is often present. Recent weight gain is common. Some patients are woken at night by choking as refluxed fluid irritates the larynx. Others develop odynophagia, dysphagia, chronic cough or atypical chest pain that may mimic angina and is probably due to reflux-induced oesophageal spasm.

Complications

Oesophagitis: Endoscopic findings range from normal through mild redness to severe, bleeding ulceration with stricture formation, with a poor correlation between symptoms and appearances. Normal endoscopy and histology do not exclude significant reflux disease.

Barrett's oesophagus ('columnar lined oesophagus', CLO): This is a pre-malignant condition in which the squamous lining of the lower oesophagus is replaced by columnar mucosa with areas of metaplasia. It occurs in response to chronic reflux and is seen in 10% of endoscopies for reflux. Epidemiology suggests a true prevalence of between 1.5% and 5% of the population, as it is often asymptomatic or first discovered when the patient develops oesophageal cancer. The absolute risk of cancer is low, however, and >95% of patients with CLO die of other causes. Prevalence is increasing, particularly in white men aged >50. Other risk factors include obesity and smoking but not alcohol. Duodenogastro-oesophageal reflux, containing bile, pancreatic enzymes and pepsin in addition to acid, may be important.

Diagnosis requires multiple biopsies to detect intestinal metaplasia and/or dysplasia.

Neither acid suppression nor anti-reflux surgery stops progression of CLO, and treatment is only indicated for symptoms of reflux or complications such as stricture. Endoscopic ablation or photodynamic therapy can induce regression but islands of glandular mucosa remain and cancer risk is not eliminated. Regular endoscopic surveillance is controversial; it can detect dysplasia and early malignancy but, because most CLO is undetected until cancer develops, will not reduce overall oesophageal cancer mortality. Those known to have CLO are recommended to have surveillance endoscopy 2–3-yearly, more often if dysplasia is present.

Those with high-grade dysplasia (HGD) require intense follow-up in specialist centres; treatment options include endoscopic resection or ablation, or oesophagectomy.

Iron deficiency anaemia: This occurs as a consequence of chronic blood loss from oesophagitis. Many such patients have bleeding from erosions in a hiatus hernia. Nevertheless, hiatus hernia is very common and other causes of blood loss, particularly colorectal cancer, must be considered, even when endoscopy reveals oesophagitis and a hiatus hernia.

Benign oesophageal stricture: This develops as a consequence of long-standing oesophagitis, usually in elderly patients presenting with dysphagia for solids. A history of heartburn is common but not invariable in the elderly. Diagnosis is by endoscopy, when biopsies can be taken to exclude malignancy. Endoscopic balloon dilatation or bouginage is helpful, followed by long-term therapy with a PPI, to reduce the risk of recurrence. Dentition should be checked and the patient advised to chew food thoroughly.

Gastric volvulus: Occasionally a massive intrathoracic hiatus hernia twists upon itself (gastric volvulus), causing complete obstruction, severe chest pain, vomiting and dysphagia. The diagnosis is made by CXR and barium swallow. Most resolve spontaneously but then recur and so elective preventive surgery is usually advised.

Investigations

Young patients with typical symptoms of GORD can be treated empirically without investigation.

Endoscopy: Advisable if patients present over the age of 50, if symptoms are atypical or if complications are suspected. A normal endoscopy in a patient with typical symptoms should not preclude treatment for reflux.

24-hr pH monitoring: If the diagnosis is unclear after endoscopy or if surgery is considered. Intraluminal pH and symptoms are recorded during normal activities. A pH of <4 for more than 6–7% of the study is diagnostic of reflux.

Management

Lifestyle advice should cover weight loss, avoidance of dietary triggers, elevation of the bed head, avoidance of late meals and giving up smoking. Antacids, alginates and H_2-receptor antagonists relieve symptoms without healing, while PPIs also heal oesophagitis in the majority, and are the treatment of choice for severe reflux disease. Recurrence is common and some patients require lifelong treatment. Long-term PPI treatment increases the risk of enteric infections and of *H. pylori*-associated gastric mucosal atrophy. Laparoscopic surgery is reserved for patients who fail to respond, are unwilling to take long-term PPIs or have severe regurgitation. Although heartburn and regurgitation are alleviated in most patients, a few develop complications.

Other causes of oesophagitis

Infection: Oesophageal candidiasis is mentioned above (p. 429).

Corrosives: Suicide attempt by bleach or acid causes painful burns of the mouth and pharynx and erosive oesophagitis. Complications include perforation, mediastinitis and stricture. Early treatment is conservative (analgesia and nutritional support); vomiting and endoscopy are avoided to prevent perforation. Later, endoscopic dilatation of strictures is usually necessary, although hazardous.

Drugs: Potassium supplements and NSAIDs may cause oesophageal ulcers if tablets are trapped above a stricture. Bisphosphonates cause oesophageal ulceration and should be used with caution in patients with oesophageal disorders.

Eosinophilic oesophagitis: This may cause dysphagia in children and young adults, and responds to topical corticosteroids.

Motility disorders
Pharyngeal pouch

Incoordination of swallowing leads to herniation of a pouch through the cricopharyngeus muscle. Most patients are elderly and asymptomatic, but regurgitation, halitosis and dysphagia can occur. A barium swallow demonstrates the pouch and may show pulmonary aspiration. Endoscopy may perforate the pouch. Surgical resection is indicated in symptomatic patients.

Achalasia of the oesophagus

Achalasia is characterised by a hypertonic lower oesophageal sphincter that fails to relax during swallowing and by failure of propagated oesophageal contraction, with progressive dilatation. The cause is unknown, although failure of the local nerve supply is implicated. Chagas' disease (infestation with *Trypanosoma cruzi*) is

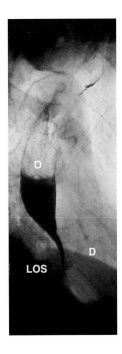

Fig. 12.2 Achalasia. X-ray showing a dilated, barium-filled oesophagus (O) with fluid level and distal tapering, and a closed lower oesophageal sphincter (LOS). (D = diaphragm.)

endemic in South America and causes an indistinguishable clinical syndrome (p. 103).

Clinical features and investigations

Achalasia is rare, affecting 1:100 000 people. It usually develops slowly in middle age with intermittent dysphagia for solids, which is eased by drinking, standing and moving around. Heartburn is absent, but some patients experience severe chest pain due to oesophageal spasm. As dysphagia progresses, nocturnal pulmonary aspiration develops. Achalasia predisposes to squamous carcinoma of the oesophagus.

Endoscopy is essential to rule out carcinoma. Barium swallow (Fig. 12.2) shows tapered narrowing of the lower oesophagus and a dilated, aperistaltic and food-filled oesophageal body. Manometry confirms the non-relaxing lower oesophageal sphincter and poor contractility of the oesophageal body. CXR may show widening of the mediastinum and features of aspiration.

Management

Endoscopic dilatation: Dilatation of the oesophageal sphincter using a fluoroscopically positioned balloon improves symptoms in

80% of patients. Some require repeat dilatation but frequent recurrence is best treated surgically. Endoscopic injection of botulinum toxin into the sphincter induces remission but relapse is common.

Surgical myotomy: Performed either laparoscopically or as an open operation, this is extremely effective. Both dilatation and myotomy may be complicated by gastro-oesophageal reflux, and for this reason myotomy is often augmented by an anti-reflux procedure and a PPI is given.

Other oesophageal motility disorders

Oesophageal spasm or abnormally forceful peristaltic activity: May lead to episodic chest pain mimicking angina. Use of oral or sublingual nitrates or nifedipine is sometimes beneficial.

Systemic sclerosis: Occurs when the oesophageal muscle is replaced by fibrous tissue, leading to heartburn, dysphagia, oesophagitis and benign strictures. Such patients require long-term therapy with PPIs. Dermatomyositis, rheumatoid arthritis and myasthenia gravis may also cause dysphagia.

Rings of submucosal fibrosis at the oesophago-gastric junction: Cause intermittent dysphagia, often in middle age.

Post-cricoid web: A rare complication of iron deficiency anaemia, which may predispose to squamous carcinoma.

Benign strictures: Treated by endoscopic balloon dilatation.

Tumours of the oesophagus
Carcinoma of the oesophagus

Almost all are squamous cancers or adenocarcinomas. Small-cell cancer is a rare third type.

Squamous cancer: Rare in the West (~4:100 000) but common in Iran, parts of Africa and China (200:100 000). Squamous cancer can arise anywhere in the oesophagus but almost all tumours in the upper oesophagus are squamous.

Adenocarcinoma: Arises in the lower third of the oesophagus from Barrett's oesophagus or from the cardia of the stomach. Incidence is increasing in the UK (~5:100 000).

Clinical features and investigations

There is progressive, painless dysphagia for solids. Food bolus obstruction may occur acutely. Chest pain or hoarseness suggests mediastinal invasion. Weight loss is common. Fistulation between the oesophagus and the airway leads to coughing after swallowing, pneumonia and pleural effusion. Physical signs include cachexia and cervical lymphadenopathy but these may be absent.

Endoscopy with biopsy is the investigation of choice. Subsequent investigations are performed to classify the tumour using TNM staging and define operability. Endoscopic ultrasound (EUS) permits nodal sampling and assessment of the depth of tumour penetration. Thoracic and abdominal CT defines metastatic spread and local invasion, which may preclude surgery.

Management and prognosis

Approximately 70% of patients have extensive disease at presentation. In these, treatment is palliative and based upon relief of dysphagia and pain. Endoscopic laser ablation or stenting may improve swallowing, while palliative radiotherapy may shrink both squamous cancers and adenocarcinomas.

Despite treatment, the 5-yr survival of patients with oesophageal cancer is 9–13%. Tumours that have breached the oesophageal wall or involve lymph nodes (T3, N1) have a 5-yr survival of ~10% after surgery. This figure improves significantly for less extensive disease. Five-yr survival following 'potentially curative' surgery (all visible tumour removed) is 30%, and this may be further improved by preoperative chemotherapy. Although squamous carcinomas are radiosensitive, radiotherapy alone is associated with a 5-yr survival of only 5%; with chemoradiotherapy this can rise to 25–30%.

Perforation of the oesophagus

The most common cause is endoscopic perforation complicating dilatation or intubation. A perforated peptic stricture is usually managed conservatively using broad-spectrum antibiotics and parenteral nutrition; most heal within days. Malignant, caustic and radiotherapy stricture perforations require surgery.

Spontaneous oesophageal perforation results from forceful vomiting. Patients present with severe chest pain, shock, subcutaneous emphysema, pleural effusions and pneumothorax. The diagnosis is made using a water-soluble contrast swallow. Treatment is surgical and mortality is high.

DISEASES OF THE STOMACH AND DUODENUM

Gastritis

Acute gastritis: Most commonly results from alcohol, aspirin or NSAID ingestion. It is often asymptomatic and self-limiting, but may cause dyspepsia, anorexia, nausea, vomiting, haematemesis or melaena. In persistent cases, endoscopy is necessary to exclude peptic ulcer or cancer. Treatment involves avoiding the cause; symptomatic therapy with antacids, and acid suppression using PPIs or antiemetics may also be necessary.

Chronic gastritis: Most commonly caused by *H. pylori* infection. Correlation between symptoms and endoscopic and pathological findings is poor. Most patients are asymptomatic and do not require treatment, but patients with dyspepsia may benefit from *H. pylori* eradication.

Autoimmune chronic gastritis: Usually asymptomatic and results from autoimmune activity against parietal cells in the body of the stomach. Circulating parietal cell and intrinsic factor antibodies may be present. In some patients, gastric atrophy leads to loss of intrinsic factor secretion and pernicious anaemia. Other autoimmune conditions, particularly thyroid disease, may be present. There is a fourfold increase in gastric cancer.

Peptic ulcer disease

'Peptic ulcer' means an ulcer in the lower oesophagus, stomach or duodenum, in the jejunum after gastrojejunostomy or, rarely, in the ileum adjacent to a Meckel's diverticulum. Ulcers in the stomach or duodenum may be acute or chronic; both penetrate the muscularis mucosae but acute ulcers show no evidence of fibrosis. Erosions do not penetrate the muscularis mucosae.

Gastric and duodenal ulcer

The prevalence of peptic ulcer is decreasing in many Western communities as a result of *H. pylori* eradication therapy but it remains high in developing countries. The male to female ratio for duodenal ulcer varies from 5:1 to 2:1, whilst that for gastric ulcer is ≤2:1.

Chronic gastric ulcer is usually single; most are situated on the lesser curve within the antrum. Duodenal ulcer usually occurs in the first part of the duodenum just distal to the junction of pyloric and duodenal mucosa. Gastric and duodenal ulcers coexist in 10% of patients and multiple ulcers occur in 10–15%.

H. pylori: In the UK, the prevalence of *H. pylori* infection rises with age (reaching 50% in those aged >50); in the developing world, it affects up to 90%. Infections are probably acquired in childhood by person-to-person contact. Most colonised people remain healthy and asymptomatic. Around 90% of duodenal ulcer patients and 70% of gastric ulcer patients are infected with *H. pylori*; the remaining 30% of gastric ulcers are due to NSAIDs.

H. pylori is a motile Gram-negative organism that uses multiple flagellae to burrow beneath the epithelial mucus layer. Here the pH is nearly neutral and any acidity is buffered by the organism's production of ammonia from urea. *H. pylori* exclusively colonises gastric-type epithelium and is only found in the duodenum at patches of gastric metaplasia. It stimulates chronic gastritis by provoking an inflammatory response in the epithelium.

In most people, *H. pylori* causes antral gastritis with depletion of somatostatin. The subsequent hypergastrinaemia stimulates parietal cell acid production, but usually without clinical consequences. In a few patients, particularly smokers, this process is exaggerated, leading to duodenal ulceration. The pathogenesis of gastric ulcer is less clear but *H. pylori* probably acts by reducing gastric mucosal resistance to acid and pepsin. Occasionally, *H. pylori* causes a pan-gastritis, leading to gastric atrophy and hypochlorhydria, with bacterial proliferation in the stomach, predisposing to gastric cancer.

NSAIDs: See page 789.

Smoking: This increases the risk of gastric and, to a lesser extent, duodenal ulcer. Once the ulcer has formed, it is more likely to cause complications and less likely to heal if the patient smokes.

Clinical features and investigations

Peptic ulcer disease is a chronic condition with spontaneous relapse and remission extending over decades. Duodenal and gastric ulcers share common symptoms:

• Recurrent episodes of epigastric pain in relation to meals.
• Occasionally, vomiting; persistent daily vomiting suggests gastric outlet obstruction.

In one-third of patients, especially elderly subjects taking NSAIDs, the history is less characteristic. Pain may be absent or experienced only as vague epigastric unease. Occasionally, the only symptoms are anorexia and nausea, or a sense of undue repletion after meals. The ulcer may even be 'silent', presenting with anaemia from chronic undetected blood loss, haematemesis or acute perforation. The diagnostic value of individual symptoms of ulcer disease is poor.

Endoscopy is the preferred investigation. Gastric ulcers may occasionally be malignant and therefore must always be biopsied and followed up to ensure healing.

Patients should be screened for *H. pylori* infection (Box 12.7). Some tests require endoscopy; others are non-invasive. Overall, breath or faecal antigen tests are best because of their accuracy, simplicity and non-invasiveness.

Management

The aims of management are to relieve symptoms, induce healing and prevent recurrence.

***H. pylori* eradication:** All patients with acute or chronic duodenal ulcer disease and those with gastric ulcers who are *H. pylori*-positive should receive eradication therapy. This heals ulcers, prevents

12.7 Methods for the diagnosis of *H. pylori* infection		
Test	**Advantages**	**Disadvantages**
Non-invasive		
Serology	Rapid office kits available; good for population studies	Lacks sensitivity and specificity; cannot differentiate current from past infection
^{13}C urea breath tests	High sensitivity and specificity	Requires expensive mass spectrometer
Faecal antigen test	Cheap, >95% specificity	Acceptability
Invasive (antral biopsy)		
Histology	Sensitivity and specificity	False negatives occur; takes several days to process
Rapid urease tests	Cheap, quick; >95% specificity	85% sensitivity
Microbiological culture	'Gold standard'; defines antibiotic sensitivity	Slow and laborious; lacks sensitivity

relapse and eliminates the need for long-term treatment in >90% of patients. A PPI is taken with two antibiotics (from amoxicillin, clarithromycin and metronidazole) for 7 days. First-line therapy is a PPI (twice daily), clarithromycin 500 mg twice daily, and amoxicillin 1 g twice daily or metronidazole 400 mg twice daily, for 7 days. Compliance, side-effects (usually diarrhoea, nausea, vomiting) and metronidazole resistance influence success rates.

Patients who remain infected after initial therapy should be offered second-line therapy. For those who are still colonised after two treatments, the choice lies between a third attempt (guided by antibiotic sensitivity testing) and long-term acid suppression.

H. pylori and NSAIDs are independent risk factors for ulcers, and patients requiring long-term NSAID therapy should first undergo eradication therapy to reduce ulcer risk. Subsequent co-prescription of a PPI with the NSAID is advised but is not always necessary for patients being given low-dose aspirin.

General measures: Cigarette smoking, aspirin and NSAIDs should be avoided. Alcohol in moderation is not harmful and no special dietary advice is required.

Maintenance treatment: This should not be necessary after successful *H. pylori* eradication.

Surgical treatment: Surgery is now rarely required for peptic ulcer, unless there is perforation, persisting haemorrhage, gastric outflow obstruction or persisting or recurrent ulcer after medical treatment. Non-healing gastric ulcer is treated by partial gastrectomy, in which the ulcer and the ulcer-bearing area of the stomach are resected to exclude an underlying cancer. In the emergency situation, biopsies are taken, and then 'under-running' the ulcer for bleeding or 'oversewing' (patch repair) for perforation is sufficient.

Complications of gastric resection or vagotomy

Although ulcer surgery is now uncommon, many patients underwent operations in the pre-*H. pylori* era and some degree of disability is seen in up to 50% of these.

Dumping: Rapid gastric emptying leads to distension of the proximal small intestine as the hypertonic contents draw fluid into the lumen. This causes abdominal discomfort, flushing, palpitations, sweating, tachycardia, hypotension and diarrhoea after eating. Patients should avoid large meals with high carbohydrate content.

Bile reflux gastropathy: Duodenogastric bile reflux leads to chronic gastropathy, which can cause dyspepsia. Symptomatic treatment with aluminium-containing antacids or sucralfate may be effective. A few patients require revisional surgery.

Diarrhoea and maldigestion: Diarrhoea 1–2 hrs after eating may develop after any peptic ulcer operation. Rapid stomach emptying, inadequate mixing with pancreatic and biliary secretions, reduced small intestinal transit times and bacterial overgrowth may lead to malabsorption. Dietary advice should be given to eat small, dry meals with reduced refined carbohydrates. Drugs such as codeine phosphate or loperamide may also help.

Weight loss: Most patients lose weight after surgery and 30–40% are unable to regain all the lost weight. The usual cause is reduced intake because of a small gastric remnant, but diarrhoea and mild steatorrhoea also contribute.

Anaemia: This is common many years after subtotal gastrectomy. Iron deficiency is the most common cause; folic acid and vitamin B_{12} deficiency are much less frequent. Inadequate dietary iron and folate, lack of acid and intrinsic factor secretion, mild chronic low-grade blood loss from the gastric remnant, and recurrent ulceration are responsible.

Metabolic bone disease: Both osteoporosis and osteomalacia occur as a consequence of calcium and vitamin D malabsorption.

Gastric cancer: An increased risk of gastric cancer has been reported. The risk is highest in those with hypochlorhydria, duodeno-gastric reflux of bile, smoking and *H. pylori* infection. Although the relative risk is increased, the absolute risk of cancer remains low and endoscopic surveillance is not indicated following gastric surgery.

Complications of peptic ulcer

Perforation: This allows stomach contents to escape into the peritoneum, causing peritonitis. It is more common in duodenal than in gastric ulcers. About one-quarter of cases occur in acute ulcers, often with NSAIDs. It causes:

• Sudden, severe pain, often the first sign of ulcer, starting in the upper abdomen and becoming generalised. Shoulder tip pain due to diaphragmatic irritation, shallow respiration due to pain, and shock are common. • Generalised rigidity. • Absent bowel sounds. • Loss of liver dullness due to gas under the diaphragm.

Rigidity persists, and although pain may temporarily improve, the patient's condition later deteriorates with general peritonitis. In at least 50% of cases, an erect CXR shows free air beneath the diaphragm. If not, a water-soluble contrast swallow will confirm perforation.

After resuscitation, the acute perforation is closed surgically. Following surgery, *H. pylori* should be treated (if present) and NSAIDs avoided. The mortality from perforation is 25%, reflecting the age and comorbidity of the population affected.

Gastric outlet obstruction: The most common cause is an ulcer near the pylorus, but occasional cases are due to antral cancer or adult hypertrophic pyloric stenosis. Clinical features include:

• Nausea. • Vomiting of large quantities of gastric content. • Abdominal distension.

Examination reveals wasting, dehydration and a succussion splash persisting 4 hrs or more after the last meal. Visible gastric peristalsis is diagnostic.

Investigations show:

• Low serum chloride and potassium. • Raised bicarbonate and urea: dehydration results in enhanced renal absorption of Na$^+$ in exchange for H$^+$ and paradoxical aciduria. • Nasogastric aspiration of at least 200 mL after an overnight fast: suggests the diagnosis. • Endoscopy: performed after the stomach has been emptied by wide-bore nasogastric tube.

Management includes:

• Nasogastric suction and the administration of large volumes of IV isotonic saline with potassium. • PPIs: may heal ulcers, relieve pyloric oedema and overcome the need for surgery. • Balloon dilatation of benign stenosis: may be possible. • Partial gastrectomy after a 7-day period of nasogastric aspiration: necessary in other patients.

Bleeding: See pages 416–418.

Zollinger–Ellison syndrome

This rare disorder (0.1% of duodenal ulcers) is characterised by the triad of severe peptic ulceration, gastric acid hypersecretion and a non-β-cell islet tumour of the pancreas ('gastrinoma'). It is most common between 30 and 50 yrs of age. The gastrinoma secretes large amounts of gastrin, which stimulates and increases the parietal cell mass. The high acid output inactivates pancreatic lipase and precipitates bile acids. Diarrhoea and steatorrhoea result. Around 90% of tumours occur in the proximal duodenal wall or the pancreatic head. Half are multiple, and over half are malignant but slow-growing. Multiple endocrine neoplasia (MEN) type 1 (p. 378) is present in 20–60%.

Patients present with multiple, severe peptic ulcers unresponsive to standard therapy. The history is usually short; bleeding and perforations are common. Diarrhoea occurs in one-third of patients and can be the presenting feature.

Hypersecretion of acid under basal conditions, with little increase following pentagastrin, may be confirmed by gastric aspiration. Serum gastrin is grossly elevated (10- to 1000-fold). Tumour localisation is by EUS and radio-labelled somatostatin receptor scintigraphy.

Approximately 30% of small and single tumours can be localised and resected. In the majority of patients, continuous therapy with high-dose omeprazole heals ulcers and alleviates diarrhoea. SC octreotide reduces gastrin secretion and is sometimes used. All patients should be monitored for the development of other manifestations of MEN 1.

Functional disorders
Functional dyspepsia

This is defined as chronic dyspepsia (pain or upper abdominal discomfort) in the absence of organic disease. Other commonly reported symptoms include fullness, bloating and nausea. The aetiology covers a spectrum of mucosal, motility and psychiatric disorders. Patients are usually young (<40 yrs) and women are affected twice as commonly as men.

Clinical features and investigations

Abdominal pain is associated with a combination of other 'dyspeptic' symptoms, the most common being nausea, early satiety and bloating after meals. Pain or nausea on waking is characteristic, and direct enquiry may elicit symptoms of irritable bowel syndrome. Peptic ulcer disease and intra-abdominal malignancy must be considered. Patients often appear anxious, but there are no diagnostic signs and no weight loss. A drug history should be taken, depression considered and pregnancy excluded. Alcohol misuse should be suspected when early morning nausea and retching are prominent.

The history will often suggest the diagnosis, but in patients >55 yrs, an endoscopy is necessary to exclude mucosal disease.

Management

The most important elements are explanation and reassurance. Possible psychological factors should be explored and the concept of psychological influences on gut function explained. Idiosyncratic diets are of little benefit but fat restriction may help.

Drug treatment is not especially successful but trials of antacids, metoclopramide, domperidone or H$_2$-receptor antagonists may be useful, according to symptoms. Low-dose amitriptyline sometimes helps. *H. pylori* eradication should be offered to infected patients. Counselling or psychotherapy may be of value in those with major stress.

Functional vomiting

This disorder typically occurs on wakening or immediately after breakfast, and is probably a reaction to facing up to everyday worries; in the young it can be due to school phobia. Early morning vomiting also occurs in pregnancy, alcohol misuse and depression. Cyclical bouts of vomiting are often idiopathic or associated with cannabis use. There is little or no weight loss.

In all patients it is essential to exclude other common causes. Tranquillisers and antiemetic drugs have only a secondary place in management. Antidepressants may be effective.

Gastroparesis

Defective gastric emptying without obstruction can be due to inherited or acquired disorders of the gastric pacemaker, autonomic disorders (particularly diabetic neuropathy), disease of the gastro-duodenal musculature (e.g. systemic sclerosis and amyloidosis) or drugs (e.g. opiates or anticholinergics). Early satiety and vomiting are typical symptoms; abdominal fullness and a succussion splash may be present on examination. Treatment is with metoclopramide and domperidone.

Tumours of the stomach
Gastric carcinoma

Gastric cancer is extremely common in China, Japan and parts of South America, less common in the UK and uncommon in the USA. Second-generation Japanese migrants in the USA have a much lower incidence than recent migrants, confirming the importance of environmental factors. Gastric cancer is more common in men and the incidence rises after 50 yrs of age.

H. pylori infection is associated with gastric cancer and may contribute to 60–70% of cases. Infection at an early age may be important. A few *H. pylori*-infected individuals become hypo- or achlorhydric, and these people are thought to be at greatest risk.

Diets rich in salted, smoked or pickled foods and lacking in fresh fruit and vegetables, as well as vitamins C and A, may predispose. Carcinogenic compounds formed by nitrite-reducing bacteria that colonise the achlorhydric stomach may also contribute. No predominant genetic abnormality has been identified, although cancer risk is increased two- to threefold in first-degree relatives of patients.

Virtually all tumours are adenocarcinomas arising from mucus-secreting cells in the base of the gastric crypts. In the developing world, 50% of gastric cancers develop in the antrum, 20–30% in the gastric body, and 20% in the cardia. In Western populations, however, proximal gastric tumours are becoming more common than those arising in the body and distal stomach. This may reflect changes in lifestyle or the decreasing prevalence of *H. pylori* in the West. Diffuse submucosal infiltration by a scirrhous cancer (linitis plastica) is uncommon. Early gastric cancer is defined as cancer confined to the mucosa or submucosa, regardless of lymph node involvement. It is common in Japan, where widespread screening is practised. Over 80% of patients in the West present with advanced gastric cancer.

Clinical features

Early gastric cancer is usually asymptomatic but may be discovered during endoscopy for dyspepsia. Weight loss occurs in two-thirds of patients with advanced cancers. Ulcer-like pain occurs in 50%. Anaemia from occult bleeding is also common. Anorexia and nausea occur in one-third. Early satiety, haematemesis, melaena and dyspepsia are less common features. Dysphagia occurs in tumours that obstruct the gastro-oesophageal junction.

Examination may reveal no abnormalities, but signs of weight loss, anaemia or a palpable epigastric mass are not infrequent. Jaundice or ascites may signify metastatic spread. Occasionally, tumour spread occurs to the supraclavicular lymph nodes, umbilicus or ovaries. Paraneoplastic phenomena, such as acanthosis nigricans, thrombophlebitis and dermatomyositis, occur rarely. Metastases occur most commonly in the liver, lungs, peritoneum and bone marrow.

Investigations

For diagnosis and staging, endoscopy is the investigation of choice and should be performed promptly in any dyspeptic patient with 'alarm features' (see Box 12.2). Multiple biopsies from the edge and base of a gastric ulcer are required. Once the diagnosis is made, CT is necessary for accurate staging and assessment of resectability, but may miss small involved lymph nodes. Even with these techniques, laparoscopy is required to determine whether the tumour is resectable.

Management and prognosis

Surgery: Resection offers the only hope of cure, which can be achieved in 90% of patients with early gastric cancer. Extensive lymph node resection may increase survival rates but carries greater morbidity. Even for those who cannot be cured, palliative resection may be necessary when presentation is with bleeding or gastric outflow obstruction. Complete removal of all macroscopic tumour, combined with lymphadenectomy, will achieve a 50–60% 5-yr survival. Recent evidence suggests that peri-operative chemotherapy improves survival rates but post-operative radiotherapy has no value.

Unresectable tumours: Modest palliation of symptoms can be achieved in some patients with chemotherapy. Endoscopic insertion of stents or laser ablation of tumour for control of dysphagia or bleeding benefits some patients.

The overall prognosis remains very poor, with <30% surviving 5 yrs. Earlier detection offers the best hope of improved survival.

Gastric lymphoma

Primary gastric lymphoma accounts for <5% of all gastric malignancies, but 60% of primary GI lymphomas occur at this site. Lymphoid tissue is not found in the normal stomach but lymphoid aggregates develop in the presence of *H. pylori* infection.

The clinical presentation is similar to that of gastric cancer and, endoscopically, the tumour appears as a polypoid or ulcerating mass. High-grade B-cell lymphomas are treated by a combination of rituximab, chemotherapy, surgery and radiotherapy. The prognosis depends on the stage at diagnosis. Features predicting a favourable prognosis are:

• Stage I or II disease. • Small, resectable tumours. • Tumours with low-grade histology • Age <60 yrs.

DISEASES OF THE SMALL INTESTINE

Disorders causing malabsorption
Coeliac disease

Coeliac disease is an immunologically mediated inflammatory disorder of the small bowel occurring in genetically susceptible individuals. It is caused by intolerance to wheat gluten and similar

12.8 Disease associations of coeliac disease

- Insulin-dependent diabetes mellitus (2–8%)
- Thyroid disease (5%)
- Primary biliary cirrhosis (3%)
- Sjögren's syndrome (3%)
- IgA deficiency (2%)
- Pernicious anaemia
- Inflammatory bowel disease
- Sarcoidosis
- Neurological complications: encephalopathy, cerebellar atrophy, peripheral neuropathy, epilepsy
- Myasthenia gravis
- Dermatitis herpetiformis
- Down's syndrome
- Enteropathy-associated T-cell lymphoma
- Small bowel carcinoma
- Squamous carcinoma of oesophagus
- Ulcerative jejunitis
- Pancreatic insufficiency
- Microscopic colitis
- Splenic atrophy

proteins in rye, barley and oats. It can result in malabsorption and responds to a gluten-free diet. The condition occurs worldwide but is more common in northern Europe (prevalence in UK is 1%).

The precise pathogenesis is unclear but immunological responses to gluten play a key role. Tissue transglutaminase (tTG) is now recognised as the autoantigen for anti-endomysial antibodies. Coeliac disease is associated with other HLA-linked autoimmune disorders and with certain other diseases (Box 12.8).

Clinical features

• Infants: failure to thrive, malabsorption. • Older children: delayed growth and puberty, malnutrition, mild abdominal distension. • Adults: presents in third or fourth or decade; 2:1 female predominance. • Florid malabsorption in some; others present with tiredness, weight loss, iron or folate deficiency. • Oral ulceration, dyspepsia and bloating.

Investigations

Duodenal or jejunal biopsy: Villous atrophy is characteristic but other causes should also be considered (Box 12.9 and Fig. 12.3).

Antibodies: IgA anti-endomysial antibodies are detectable in most untreated cases and are sensitive and specific. IgG antibodies must be analysed in patients with coexisting IgA deficiency. Tissue transglutaminase (tTG) assays are easier to perform, semi-quantitative and more accurate in patients with IgA deficiency. These antibody

12.9 Important causes of subtotal villous atrophy

- Coeliac disease
- Tropical sprue
- Dermatitis herpetiformis
- Lymphoma
- AIDS enteropathy
- Giardiasis
- Hypogammaglobulinaemia
- Radiation
- Whipple's disease
- Zollinger–Ellison syndrome

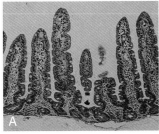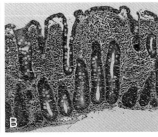

Fig. 12.3 Jejunal mucosa. **A** Normal. **B** Jejunum in coeliac disease, showing subtotal villous atrophy and marked inflammatory infiltrate.

tests are not a substitute for small bowel biopsy; they usually become negative with successful treatment.

Haematology and biochemistry: There is microcytic or macrocytic anaemia from iron or folate deficiency. Target cells, spherocytes and Howell–Jolly bodies are due to hyposplenism. Calcium, magnesium, total protein, albumin and vitamin D are reduced.

Measurement of bone density by DEXA scanning: Osteoporosis is common in older women.

Management

• Lifelong gluten-free diet. • Correction of deficiencies of iron, folate, calcium and vitamin D. • Regular monitoring of symptoms, weight and nutrition. • Repeat jejunal biopsies: should be reserved for patients who do not symptomatically improve or whose tTG antibodies remain high.

Rarely, patients are 'refractory' and require corticosteroids or immunosuppressive drugs to induce remission. Dietary compliance should be carefully assessed, but if this is satisfactory, other conditions such as pancreatic insufficiency or microscopic colitis should be sought, as should complications of coeliac disease such as ulcerative jejunitis or enteropathy-associated T-cell lymphoma.

Complications

There is an increased risk of malignancy, particularly of enteropathy-associated T-cell lymphoma, small bowel carcinoma and squamous carcinoma of the oesophagus.

Ulcerative jejunoileitis may occur; fever, pain, obstruction or perforation may then supervene. The diagnosis is made by laparotomy and full-thickness biopsy. Corticosteroids are used with mixed success and some patients require surgical resection and parenteral nutrition.

Osteoporosis and osteomalacia occur, but are less common in patients who adhere strictly to a gluten-free diet.

Dermatitis herpetiformis

This is characterised by crops of intensely itchy blisters over the elbows, knees, back and buttocks. Almost all patients have partial villous atrophy on jejunal biopsy, even though they usually have no GI symptoms. The rash usually responds to a gluten-free diet but some patients require additional treatment with dapsone.

Tropical sprue

Tropical sprue is a chronic, progressive malabsorption with abnormalities of small intestinal structure and function occurring in patients in or from the tropics. The disease occurs mainly in the West Indies and in Asia, including southern India, Malaysia and Indonesia. It often begins after an acute diarrhoeal illness. Small bowel bacterial overgrowth with *Escherichia coli*, *Enterobacter* and *Klebsiella* is frequently seen. Mucosal pathology closely resembles that of coeliac disease.

Clinical features include:

• Diarrhoea, abdominal distension, anorexia, fatigue and weight loss. • Onset of severe diarrhoea: may be sudden and accompanied by fever.

When chronic:

• Megaloblastic anaemia (folic acid malabsorption). • Ankle oedema, glossitis and stomatitis: common. • Remissions and relapses: may occur.

The differential diagnosis is infective diarrhoea, including giardiasis (p. 111).

Tetracycline (250 mg 4 times daily for 28 days) brings about long-term remission or cure. Folic acid (5 mg daily) improves symptoms and jejunal morphology.

Small bowel bacterial overgrowth ('blind loop syndrome')

The normal duodenum and jejunum contain coliform organisms, but numbers never exceed 10^3/mL. In bacterial overgrowth there may be 10^8–10^{10}/mL organisms, most of which are normally found only in the colon. Disorders that predispose to bacterial overgrowth include hypochlorhydria, impaired motility (e.g.

systemic sclerosis, diabetes), surgical resection, fistulae and hypogammaglobulinaemia.

Clinical features include:

• Watery diarrhoea and/or steatorrhoea. • Anaemia due to vitamin B_{12} deficiency.

There may also be symptoms from the underlying intestinal cause.

Investigations are as follows:

• Serum vitamin B_{12} concentration is low; folate levels are normal or elevated. • Immunoglobulin levels: may exclude hypogammaglobulinaemia. • Barium follow-through or small bowel enema: may reveal blind loops or fistulae. • Endoscopic duodenal biopsies: exclude mucosal disease such as coeliac disease. • Endoscopic aspiration of jejunal contents: for anaerobic and aerobic culture. • Hydrogen breath test: serial breath samples are measured after oral ingestion of glucose or lactulose. Bacteria in the small bowel cause an early rise in breath hydrogen.

Management is of the underlying cause. Tetracycline is the treatment of choice, although up to 50% of patients do not respond. Metronidazole or ciprofloxacin is an alternative. Some patients require up to 4 wks of treatment and a few cases become chronic. IM vitamin B_{12} supplementation is needed in the latter.

Whipple's disease

This rare condition is characterised by infiltration of small intestinal mucosa by 'foamy' macrophages, which stain positive with periodic acid–Schiff (PAS) reagent. The cause is infection of macrophages by Gram-positive bacilli (*Tropheryma whipplei*), detectable in biopsies by PCR.

This is a multisystem disease (Box 12.10). Middle-aged men are most commonly affected and the presentation depends on the pattern of organ involvement. Low-grade fever is common.

Whipple's disease is often fatal if untreated but responds well to 2 wks of IV ceftriaxone followed by co-trimoxazole for at least a year. Relapse occurs in up to one-third of patients, often within the CNS, requiring further prolonged antibiotic treatment.

12.10 Clinical features of Whipple's disease	
GI	Diarrhoea, steatorrhoea, protein-losing enteropathy
Musculoskeletal	Seronegative large joint arthritis, sacroiliitis
Cardiac	Pericarditis, myocarditis, endocarditis
Pulmonary	Pleurisy, cough, infiltrates
Haematological	Anaemia, lymphadenopathy
Neurological	Apathy, fits, dementia, myoclonus
Other	Fever, pigmentation

Ileal resection

Ileal resection is usually performed as treatment for Crohn's disease. The long-term effects depend on the site and the length of intestine resected, and vary from trivial to life-threatening.

Clinical features include:

• Diarrhoea. • Fat malabsorption due to loss of bile salts. • Gallstones due to lithogenic bile. • Oxalate renal calculi. • Vitamin B_{12} deficiency.

Contrast studies of the small bowel and tests of vitamin B_{12} and bile acid absorption are useful.

Parenteral vitamin B_{12} supplementation is necessary. Diarrhoea usually responds well to colestyramine or aluminium hydroxide therapy.

Short bowel syndrome

Short bowel syndrome is defined as malabsorption resulting from extensive small intestinal resection or disease. Loss of surface area for digestion and absorption is the key problem.

Clinical features include:

• Large-volume jejunostomy fluid loss. • If colon is preserved: diarrhoea and steatorrhoea. • Dehydration and signs of hypovolaemia. • Weight loss, loss of muscle bulk and malnutrition.

Management entails:

• TPN: see page 427. • PPI therapy: to reduce gastric secretions. • Enteral feeding: to be cautiously introduced after 1–2 wks and slowly increased as tolerated.

The principles of long-term management are:

• Detailed nutritional assessments at regular intervals. • Monitoring of fluid and electrolyte balance. Patients can usually be taught how to do this for themselves. A readily available supply of oral rehydration solution is useful for intercurrent illness. • Adequate calorie and protein intake. Fats and medium-chain triglyceride supplements should be taken as tolerated. • Replacement of vitamin B_{12}, calcium, vitamin D, magnesium, zinc and folic acid. • Antidiarrhoeal agents, e.g. loperamide or codeine phosphate.

In patients who are unable to maintain positive fluid balance, octreotide to reduce GI secretions is useful, but some individuals require long-term TPN. Small bowel transplantation may be an option.

Radiation enteritis and proctocolitis

Intestinal damage occurs in 10–15% of patients undergoing radiotherapy for abdominal or pelvic malignancy. The risk varies with total dose, dosing schedule and the use of concomitant chemotherapy.

Acutely, there is nausea, vomiting, cramping abdominal pain and diarrhoea. When the rectum and colon are involved, mucus, bleeding and tenesmus occur. The chronic phase develops after 5–10 yrs in some patients and may feature bleeding from telangiectasis, fistulae, adhesions, strictures or malabsorption.

Sigmoidoscopy appearances resemble ulcerative proctitis. Colonoscopy shows the extent of the lesion. Barium follow-through shows small bowel strictures, ulcers and fistulae.

Management entails:
• Acute phase: codeine, loperamide, corticosteroid enemas for proctitis and antibiotics for bacterial overgrowth. • Nutritional supplements for malabsorption; colestyramine for bile salt malabsorption may be necessary. • Endoscopic laser or argon plasma coagulation therapy: may reduce bleeding from proctitis. • Surgery: should be avoided, because the injured intestine is difficult to resect and anastomose, but it may be necessary for obstruction, perforation or fistula.

Miscellaneous disorders of the small intestine
Protein-losing enteropathy

Defined as excessive loss of protein into the gut lumen, sufficient to cause hypoproteinaemia, protein-losing enteropathy occurs in a variety of inflammatory and neoplastic gut disorders but is most common in ulcerating conditions. In other disorders, protein loss results from increased mucosal permeability or obstruction of intestinal lymphatic vessels.

Patients present with peripheral oedema and hypoproteinaemia in the presence of normal liver function and without proteinuria. The diagnosis is confirmed by measurement of faecal clearance of α_1-antitrypsin or ^{51}Cr-labelled albumin after IV injection. Treatment is that of the underlying disorder, with nutritional support and measures to control peripheral oedema.

Meckel's diverticulum

This is the most common congenital anomaly of the GI tract and occurs in 0.3–3% of people. Most patients are asymptomatic. The diverticulum results from failure of closure of the vitelline duct, with persistence of a blind-ending sac, usually within 100 cm of the ileocaecal valve and up to 5 cm long. Approximately 50% contain ectopic gastric mucosa.

Complications usually occur in the first 2 yrs of life but occasionally in young adults. Bleeding results from ulceration of ileal mucosa adjacent to the ectopic parietal cells and presents as recurrent melaena or altered blood per rectum. Diagnosis can be made by gamma scanning following IV ^{99m}Tc-pertechnate, which is concentrated by ectopic parietal cells. Other complications include intestinal obstruction, diverticulitis, intussusception and perforation. Surgery is unnecessary unless complications occur.

Infections of the small intestine
Travellers' diarrhoea, giardiasis and amoebiasis
See pages 87, 111 and 110.

Abdominal tuberculosis

Mycobacterium tuberculosis rarely causes abdominal disease in Caucasians but must be considered in the developing world and in AIDS patients. Gut infection usually results from human *M. tuberculosis* that is swallowed after coughing. Many patients have no pulmonary symptoms and a normal CXR. Infection most commonly affects the ileocaecal region; presentation and radiological findings may resemble those of Crohn's disease. Abdominal pain can be acute or chronic, but diarrhoea is less common in TB than in Crohn's disease. Low-grade fever is common. TB can affect any part of the GI tract, including perianal disease with fistula. Peritoneal TB may result in peritonitis with exudative ascites, abdominal pain and fever. Granulomatous hepatitis also occurs.

Useful investigations include:

• ESR: elevated. • Alkaline phosphatase: raised, suggesting hepatic involvement. • Endoscopy, laparoscopy or liver biopsy: for histological confirmation. • Culture of biopsies: may take 6 wks but faster diagnosis is now possible using rapid PCR techniques.

When the presentation is very suggestive of abdominal TB, chemotherapy with isoniazid, rifampicin, pyrazinamide and ethambutol should be commenced, even if bacteriological or histological proof is lacking.

Tumours of the small intestine

The small intestine is rarely affected by neoplasia and <5% of all GI tumours occur here.

Benign tumours

The most common are peri-ampullary adenomas, GI stromal tumours (GIST), lipomas and hamartomas. Multiple adenomas are common in the duodenum of patients with familial adenomatous polyposis (FAP), who merit regular endoscopic surveillance. Hamartomatous polyps with almost no malignant potential occur in Peutz–Jeghers syndrome (p. 467).

Malignant tumours

These are rare and include adenocarcinoma, carcinoid tumour, malignant GIST and lymphoma. The majority occur in middle age or later. Kaposi's sarcoma is seen in patients with AIDS.

Adenocarcinomas occur with increased frequency in patients with FAP, coeliac disease and Peutz–Jeghers syndrome. Barium follow-through examination or small bowel enema studies will demonstrate most lesions. Enteroscopy, capsule endoscopy, mesenteric angiography and CT are also used. Treatment is by surgical resection.

Carcinoid tumours

These are derived from enterochromaffin cells, and are most common in the ileum, rectum and appendix. Localised spread and the poten-

> **12.11 Clinical features of carcinoid tumours**
>
> - Small bowel obstruction due to the tumour mass
> - Intestinal ischaemia (due to mesenteric infiltration or vasospasm)
> - Hepatic metastases causing pain, hepatomegaly and jaundice
> - Flushing and wheezing
> - Diarrhoea
> - Cardiac involvement (tricuspid regurgitation, pulmonary stenosis, right ventricular endocardial plaques) leading to heart failure
> - Facial telangiectasia
>
> The diagnosis is made by detecting excess levels of the 5-HT metabolite, 5-HIAA, in a 24-hr urine collection.

tial for metastasis to the liver increase with primary lesions >2 cm in diameter. These tumours grow slowly and are less aggressive than carcinomas.

'Carcinoid syndrome': Refers to systemic symptoms produced when secretory products of carcinoid tumours reach the systemic circulation (Box 12.11). Substances produced by the primary tumour are usually metabolised in the liver before reaching the systemic circulation. The syndrome is therefore only seen with hepatic metastases.

Treatment of carcinoid tumour is by surgical resection. The treatment of carcinoid syndrome is palliative because hepatic metastases have occurred, although prolonged survival is common. Removal of the primary tumour is usually attempted and the hepatic metastases can be excised, as reduction of tumour mass improves symptoms. Hepatic artery embolisation retards growth of metastases. Octreotide may reduce tumour release of secretagogues. Chemotherapy has limited benefits.

Lymphoma

Non-Hodgkin lymphoma may involve the GI tract as part of generalised disease or may rarely arise in the gut, most commonly in the small intestine. Lymphomas are more common in patients with coeliac disease, AIDS and other immunodeficiencies.

Colicky abdominal pain, obstruction and weight loss are the usual presenting features, and diagnosis is by small bowel biopsy, contrast studies and CT. After staging, surgical resection is performed where possible, with radiotherapy and chemotherapy reserved for advanced disease.

DISEASES OF THE PANCREAS

Acute pancreatitis

Acute pancreatitis accounts for 3% of all cases of abdominal pain admitted to hospital. It affects 2–28 per 100 000 of the population and may be increasing in incidence.

GASTROINTESTINAL AND NUTRITIONAL DISORDERS • 12

12.12 Causes of acute pancreatitis

Common (90% of cases)

- Gallstones
- Alcohol
- Idiopathic
- Post-ERCP

Rare

- Post-surgical
- Trauma
- Drugs (e.g. azathioprine)
- Infection (e.g. mumps)
- Renal failure
- Hypothermia
- Sphincter of Oddi dysfunction
- Petrochemical exposure

The condition results from premature activation of zymogen granules, releasing proteases that digest the pancreas and surrounding tissue. Causes of acute pancreatitis are given in Box 12.12. It is usually mild and self-limiting, with minimal organ dysfunction and uneventful recovery. In ~20% of patients it is severe, with complications such as necrosis, pseudocyst or abscess, and multi-organ failure.

Clinical features and complications

Severe, constant upper abdominal pain builds up over 15–60 mins, radiating to the back in 65%. There is nausea and vomiting. There is epigastric tenderness, but in the early stages guarding and rebound tenderness are absent because inflammation is mainly retroperitoneal. Bowel sounds become quiet or absent as paralytic ileus develops. There is hypoxia and hypovolaemic shock with oliguria in severe cases. Discoloration of the flanks (Grey Turner's sign) or the periumbilical region (Cullen's sign) is a feature of severe pancreatitis with haemorrhage.

Complications are listed in Box 12.13.

Investigations

Serum amylase or lipase is elevated, although amylase may return to normal in 24–48 hrs. Amylase is also elevated (but less so) in intestinal ischaemia, perforated ulcer and ruptured ovarian cyst, whilst salivary amylase is elevated in parotitis. Persistently elevated serum amylase suggests pseudocyst formation. Peritoneal amylase is massively elevated in pancreatic ascites. An elevated urinary amylase:creatinine ratio is helpful if serum amylase has returned to normal. USS shows evidence of pancreatic swelling and may also show gallstones, biliary obstruction or pseudocyst formation. Plain X-rays help to exclude perforation, obstruction and pulmonary

12.13 Complications of acute pancreatitis	
Complication	**Cause**
Systemic	
Systemic inflammatory response syndrome (SIRS)	Increased vascular permeability from cytokine, platelet aggregating factor and kinin release, paralytic ileus, vomiting; renal failure
Hypoxia	ARDS due to microthrombi in pulmonary vessels
Hyperglycaemia	Disruption of islets of Langerhans with altered insulin/glucagon axis
Hypocalcaemia	Sequestration of calcium in fat necrosis, fall in ionised calcium
Reduced serum albumin	Increased capillary permeability
Pancreatic	
Necrosis	Non-viable pancreatic tissue and peripancreatic tissue death; frequently infected
Abscess	Circumscribed collection of pus close to the pancreas and containing little or no pancreatic necrotic tissue
Pseudocyst	Disruption of pancreatic ducts
Pancreatic ascites or pleural effusion	Disruption of pancreatic ducts
GI	
Upper GI bleeding	Gastric or duodenal erosions
Variceal haemorrhage	Splenic or portal vein thrombosis
Erosion into colon	
Duodenal obstruction	Compression by pancreatic mass
Obstructive jaundice	Compression of common bile duct

complications. CT 6–10 days after admission helps to define the viability of the pancreas; decreased contrast enhancement indicates necrotising pancreatitis. Gas within necrotic material suggests infection and impending abscess formation, in which case percutaneous aspiration for bacterial culture is carried out and appropriate antibiotics prescribed. CT also reveals involvement of the colon, blood vessels and other adjacent structures by the inflammatory process.

Management and prognosis

Adverse prognostic factors are shown in Box 12.14. Serial CRP is a useful indicator of progress. A peak CRP >210 mg/L in the first 4 days predicts severe acute pancreatitis with 80% accuracy. Serum amylase has no prognostic value.

Management comprises diagnosis, resuscitation, detection and treatment of complications, as well as treatment of the underlying cause – specifically, gallstones.

• Analgesia using pethidine. • Correction of hypovolaemia using normal saline or other crystalloids. • Nasogastric aspiration: only necessary if paralytic ileus is present. • Enteral feeding via a

- Age >55 yrs
- PO_2 <8 kPa (60 mmHg)
- WBC >15 × 10^9/L
- Albumin <32 g/L (3.2 g/dL)
- Serum calcium <2 mmol/L (8 mg/dL) (corrected)
- Glucose >10 mmol/L (180 mg/dL)
- Urea >16 mmol/L (45 mg/dL) (after rehydration)
- ALT >200 U/L
- LDH >600 U/L

*Severity and prognosis worsen as the number of these factors increases; >3 implies severe disease.

nasoenteral tube: should be started early in severe pancreatitis. It decreases endotoxaemia and thereby may reduce systemic complications. • Insulin to correct hyperglycaemia. • Oxygen for hypoxic patients; those with systemic inflammatory response syndrome (SIRS) may require ventilatory support. • Calcium: only needed if hypocalcaemic tetany occurs. • Prophylaxis of thromboembolism with low-dose SC heparin: advisable. • Prophylactic broad-spectrum IV antibiotics such as imipenem or cefuroxime: may improve outcome in severe cases.

All severe cases should be managed in HDU/ICU. A central venous catheter and urinary catheter are used to monitor patients with shock.

Patients with cholangitis or jaundice in association with severe acute pancreatitis should undergo urgent ERCP to diagnose and treat choledocholithiasis. In less severe cases of gallstone pancreatitis, biliary imaging (using MRCP) can be carried out after the acute phase has resolved. Cholecystectomy with an on-table cholangiogram should be undertaken within 2 wks of resolution of pancreatitis to prevent further potentially fatal attacks.

Patients with necrotising pancreatitis or pancreatic abscess require urgent endoscopic or minimally invasive débridement of all cavities to remove necrotic material. Pancreatic pseudocysts are treated by delayed drainage into the stomach, duodenum or jejunum.

Mortality is 10–15%. About 80% of all cases are mild with a good prognosis; 98% of deaths occur in the 20% of severe cases. One-third occur within the first week, usually from multi-organ failure.

Chronic pancreatitis

Chronic pancreatitis is a chronic inflammatory disease characterised by fibrosis and destruction of exocrine pancreatic tissue. Diabetes mellitus occurs in advanced cases because the islets of Langerhans are involved. Around 80% of cases in Western countries result from alcohol misuse. Other causes include malnutrition, cassava consumption and recurrent acute pancreatitis, while some cases are idiopathic. Cystic fibrosis causes painless chronic pancreatic destruction (see p. 287). Chronic pancreatitis predominantly affects middle-aged alcoholic men.

Clinical features and complications

• Abdominal pain: in 50% this occurs as episodes of 'acute pancreatitis', although each attack results in further pancreatic damage. Relentless, slowly progressive pain without acute exacerbations affects 35% of patients. Pain may be relieved by leaning forwards or by alcohol. • Diarrhoea without pain: an uncommon presentation. • Weight loss. • Steatorrhoea: indicates that >90% of the exocrine tissue has been destroyed; protein malabsorption develops in the most advanced cases. • Diabetes mellitus in 30%, rising to 70% in those with chronic calcific pancreatitis. • Epigastric tenderness, sometimes with erythema ab igne over the abdomen and back due to chronic use of a hot water bottle. • Features of other alcohol- and smoking-related diseases.

Complications include:

• Pseudocysts and pancreatic ascites: occur in both acute and chronic pancreatitis. • Extrahepatic obstructive jaundice: due to a benign stricture of the common bile duct as it passes through the diseased pancreas. • Duodenal stenosis. • Portal or splenic vein thrombosis leading to segmental portal hypertension and gastric varices. • Peptic ulcer.

Investigations

Investigations are shown in Box 12.15 and Figure 12.4.

Management

Alcohol avoidance: This is crucial in halting disease progression and reducing pain, but advice is frequently ignored.

 12.15 Investigations in chronic pancreatitis

Tests to establish the diagnosis

- USS
- CT (may show atrophy, calcification or ductal dilatation)
- AXR (may show calcification)
- MRCP
- EUS

Tests of pancreatic function

- Collection of pure pancreatic juice after secretin injection (gold standard but invasive and seldom used)
- Pancreolauryl or PABA (para-aminobenzoic acid) test
- Faecal pancreatic chymotrypsin or elastase

Tests of anatomy prior to surgery

- MRCP

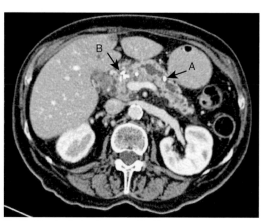

Fig. 12.4 Imaging in chronic pancreatitis. CT scan showing a grossly dilated and irregular duct with a calcified stone (arrow A). Note the calcification in the head of the gland (arrow B).

Pain relief: NSAIDs are valuable but the severe, unremitting pain often leads to opiate use with risk of addiction. Oral pancreatic enzyme supplements suppress pancreatic secretion and reduce analgesic requirement in some patients.

Surgery: Abstinent patients with severe chronic pain resistant to conservative measures may respond to surgical or endoscopic treatment of strictures, calculi and pseudocysts or coeliac plexus neurolysis. Patients without such correctable abnormalities require total pancreatectomy. Unfortunately, even after this, some patients continue to experience pain. Moreover, the procedure causes diabetes, which may be difficult to control.

Fat restriction and oral pancreatic enzyme supplements: These measures are used to treat steatorrhoea. A PPI is added to optimise duodenal pH for pancreatic enzyme activity.

Congenital abnormalities of the pancreas
Annular pancreas

In this congenital anomaly, the pancreas encircles the second/third part of the duodenum, leading to gastric outlet obstruction.

Cystic fibrosis

See page 287.

Tumours of the pancreas

Pancreatic carcinoma affects 10–15 per 100 000 in Western populations, rising to 100 per 100 000 in those over the age of 70. Men are affected twice as often as women. The disease is associated with smoking and chronic pancreatitis. Between 5 and 10% of patients have a genetic predisposition.

Approximately 90% of pancreatic neoplasms are adenocarcinomas, which arise from the pancreatic ducts and spread early to involve local structures and regional lymph nodes.

Clinical features

• Pain: incessant, boring, with radiation to the back; may be eased by bending forward. • Weight loss due to anorexia, steatorrhoea and metabolic effects of the tumour. • Obstructive jaundice: 60% of tumours arise from the head of the pancreas, with obstruction of the common bile duct and associated severe pruritus. • Less common: diarrhoea, vomiting from duodenal obstruction, diabetes mellitus, recurrent venous thrombosis, acute pancreatitis or depression.

Examination reveals evidence of weight loss, abdominal mass due to the tumour itself, a palpable gallbladder or hepatic metastasis. A palpable gallbladder in a jaundiced patient is usually due to biliary obstruction by a pancreatic cancer (Courvoisier's sign).

Investigations

• USS and CT: demonstrate a pancreatic mass. • LFTs: for cholestatic jaundice. • Staging to define operability: entails laparoscopy with laparoscopic EUS to define tumour size, involvement of blood vessels and metastatic spread. • MRCP or ERCP: when diagnosis is in doubt.

In patients unsuitable for surgery because of advanced disease, frailty or comorbidity, USS- or CT-guided cytology or biopsy can be used. EUS with fine needle aspiration is used to define vascular invasion and obtain cytological proof of diagnosis.

Management

Surgical resection: The only curative treatment; 5-yr survival after complete resection is ~20%. Survival may be improved with adjuvant chemotherapy. Only 15% of tumours are amenable to curative resection since most are locally advanced at diagnosis. For the great majority, therapy is based on palliation.

Pain relief: Analgesics with or without coeliac plexus neurolysis by a percutaneous or EUS-guided alcohol injection.

Jaundice: Choledochojejunostomy in fit patients; percutaneous or endoscopic stenting of the common bile duct is useful palliation in the elderly or those with very advanced disease.

Overall survival is only 3–5%; median survival is 3–10 mths, depending on stage.

Pancreatic neuro-endocrine tumours

These may occur in association with parathyroid and pituitary adenomas (p. 378). The majority of endocrine tumours are non-secretory and, although malignant, grow slowly and metastasise late. Other tumours secrete hormones and present because of their endocrine effects.

INFLAMMATORY BOWEL DISEASE

Ulcerative colitis and Crohn's disease are chronic inflammatory bowel diseases that relapse and remit over years. The diseases have many similarities and it is sometimes impossible to distinguish them (Box 12.16). However, ulcerative colitis only involves the colon, while Crohn's disease can involve any part of the GI tract.

The incidence of inflammatory bowel disease (IBD) varies widely between populations. Crohn's disease is rare in the developing world, yet ulcerative colitis is becoming more common. In the West, the prevalence of ulcerative colitis is stable at 100–200 per 100 000, while Crohn's disease is increasing and now affects 50–100 per 100 000. Both diseases most commonly start in young adults.

IBD develops as a response to an environmental trigger in genetically susceptible individuals. There is activation of macrophages, lymphocytes and polymorphonuclear cells with release of inflammatory mediators, events that represent targets for future therapies.

12.16 Comparison of ulcerative colitis and Crohn's disease

	Ulcerative colitis	Crohn's disease
Age group	Any	Any
Gender	M = F	Slight female preponderance
Ethnic group	Any	Any; more common in Ashkenazi Jews
Genetic factors	HLA-DR*103 associated with severe disease	Defective innate immunity: NOD2 mutations predispose
Risk factors	More common in non-/ex-smokers; appendicectomy protects	More common in smokers
Anatomical distribution	Colon only; begins at anorectal margin with variable proximal extension	Any part of GI tract; perianal disease common; patchy distribution – 'skip lesions'
Extra-intestinal manifestations	Common	Common
Presentation	Bloody diarrhoea	Variable; pain, diarrhoea, weight loss all common
Histology	Inflammation limited to mucosa; crypt distortion, cryptitis, crypt abscesses, loss of goblet cells	Submucosal or transmural inflammation common; deep fissuring ulcers, fistulae; patchy changes; granulomas
Management	5-aminosalicylic acid (5-ASA); corticosteroids; azathioprine; anti-TNF; colectomy is curative	Corticosteroids; azathioprine; methotrexate; anti-TNF; nutritional therapy; surgery is not curative; 5-ASA ineffective

Clinical features of ulcerative colitis

These depend upon the site and activity of the disease. The first attack is usually the most severe and thereafter is followed by relapses and remissions; a few have unremitting symptoms. Emotional stress, intercurrent infection, gastroenteritis, antibiotics or NSAIDs may provoke relapse.

Proctitis: Rectal bleeding and mucus discharge, sometimes with tenesmus. Some pass frequent, small-volume fluid stools, while others are constipated. Constitutional symptoms do not occur.

Proctosigmoiditis: Bloody diarrhoea with mucus. Almost all patients are constitutionally well.

Extensive colitis: Bloody diarrhoea with mucus, anorexia, malaise, weight loss and abdominal pain. The patient is toxic with fever, tachycardia and peritoneal inflammation (Box 12.17).

Clinical features of Crohn's disease

Ileal Crohn's disease: The features are:
• Abdominal pain: because of subacute intestinal obstruction, an inflammatory mass, intra-abdominal abscess or acute obstruction.
• Diarrhoea: watery without blood or mucus. • Weight loss: due to anorexia or malabsorption; some patients present with features of fat, protein or vitamin deficiencies.

Crohn's colitis: Presents exactly like ulcerative colitis, with bloody diarrhoea, mucus, lethargy, malaise, anorexia and weight loss. Rectal sparing and perianal disease suggest Crohn's disease rather than ulcerative colitis.

Many patients present with both small bowel and colonic disease. A few have isolated perianal disease, vomiting from jejunal strictures or severe oral ulceration.

Physical examination reveals:
• Weight loss, anaemia, glossitis and angular stomatitis.
• Abdominal tenderness, most marked over the inflamed area.
• Abdominal mass due to matted loops of thickened bowel or an

12.17 Assessment of disease severity in ulcerative colitis		
	Mild	**Severe**
Daily bowel frequency	<4	≥6
Blood in stools	±	+++
Stool volume (g/24 hrs)	<200	>400
Pulse (beats/min)	<90	≥90
Temperature (°C)	Normal	>37.8°C
Hb (g/L)	Normal	<100
ESR (mm/hr)	Normal	>30
Serum albumin (g/L)	>35	<30
AXR	Normal	Dilated bowel and/or mucosal islands
Sigmoidoscopy	Normal or granular mucosa	Blood in lumen

intra-abdominal abscess. • Perianal skin tags, fissures or fistulae in at least 50% of patients.

Complications

Life-threatening inflammation of the colon: This occurs in both ulcerative colitis and Crohn's disease. The colon dilates (toxic megacolon) and bacterial toxins cross the diseased mucosa into the circulation. This occurs most commonly during the first attack of colitis and is associated with the severity indicators in Box 12.17. If an AXR shows the transverse colon is dilated to >6 cm, there is a high risk of perforation. Perforation of the small intestine or colon can occur without the development of toxic megacolon. Life-threatening acute haemorrhage due to erosion of a major artery occurs rarely.

Fistulae and perianal disease: These occur only in Crohn's disease and not in ulcerative colitis. Enteroenteric fistulae cause diarrhoea and malabsorption. Enterovesical fistulation causes recurrent urinary infections and pneumaturia. Enterovaginal fistula causes faeculent vaginal discharge. Fistulation from the bowel may also cause perianal or ischiorectal abscesses, and fissures.

Cancer: Extensive, long-lasting active colitis increases the risk of cancer. The cumulative risk for ulcerative colitis reaches 20% after 30 yrs but is lower for Crohn's colitis. Small bowel adenocarcinoma occasionally complicates long-standing small bowel Crohn's disease. Patients with chronic colitis should start surveillance colonoscopy 10 yrs after diagnosis, with targeted biopsy of areas showing abnormal dye staining (pancolonic chromo-endoscopy). Those with high-grade dysplasia should be considered for panproctocolectomy to prevent cancer.

Extra-intestinal complications: IBD can be considered as a systemic illness and in some patients extra-intestinal complications dominate the clinical picture. Some of these occur during relapse of intestinal disease; others appear unrelated to intestinal disease activity (Box 12.18).

The differential diagnosis is shown in Boxes 12.19 and 12.20.

Investigations

FBC: May show anaemia from bleeding or malabsorption of iron, folic acid or vitamin B_{12}. Serum albumin is low due to protein-losing enteropathy or poor nutrition.

12.18 Systemic manifestations of inflammatory bowel disease	
Eyes	Conjunctivitis, iritis, episcleritis
Mouth	Ulcers
Liver	Abscess, fatty change, hepatitis, sclerosing cholangitis
Vascular	Mesenteric, portal or deep vein thrombosis
Skin	Erythema nodosum, pyoderma gangrenosum (p. 414)
Bone/joint	Metabolic bone disease, sacroiliitis

12.19 Conditions mimicking ulcerative or Crohn's colitis

Infective	For example, *Salmonella*, *Shigella*, *Campylobacter*, *E. coli* 0157, herpes simplex, amoebiasis
Vascular	Radiation proctitis, ischaemic colitis
Neoplastic	Colonic carcinoma
Inflammatory	Behçet's disease
Drugs	NSAIDs

12.20 Differential diagnosis of small bowel Crohn's disease

- Other causes of right iliac fossa mass: caecal carcinoma*, appendix abscess*
- Infection (TB, *Yersinia*, actinomycosis)
- Mesenteric adenitis
- Pelvic inflammatory disease
- Lymphoma

*Common; other causes are rare.

ESR: Raised in exacerbations or because of abscess.

CRP: Helpful in monitoring Crohn's disease activity.

Faecal calprotectin: Sensitive; useful to distinguish from irritable bowel and for monitoring activity.

Stool cultures: Help to exclude superimposed enteric infection in patients with exacerbations.

Blood cultures: Also advisable in febrile patients with known colitis or Crohn's disease.

Sigmoidoscopy: Should be performed in those with diarrhoea. In ulcerative colitis, sigmoidoscopy shows loss of vascular pattern, granularity, friability and ulceration. In Crohn's disease, patchy inflammation with discrete, deep ulcers, perianal disease or rectal sparing occurs.

Endoscopy: Colonoscopy – may show active inflammation with pseudopolyps or a complicating carcinoma. Biopsies are taken to define disease extent and to seek dysplasia in long-standing colitis. In ulcerative colitis, the abnormalities are confluent and most severe in the distal colon and rectum. Stricture formation does not occur in the absence of a carcinoma. In Crohn's colitis, the endoscopic abnormalities are patchy, with intervening normal mucosa, and ulcers and strictures are common. Single or double balloon enteroscopy may be required to make the diagnosis of small bowel Crohn's disease.

Radiology: Barium enema – can show ulcers or strictures but is less sensitive than colonoscopy. If colonoscopy is incomplete, CT colonogram is preferred. Small bowel imaging is essential for staging Crohn's disease, and MRI enterography has replaced barium follow-through, as it can also show extra-intestinal and pelvic manifestations. It can also distinguish inflammatory from fibrotic strictures;

the former respond to anti-inflammatory treatment but the latter require surgery or balloon dilatation.

AXR: May show dilatation of the colon, mucosal oedema or evidence of perforation. In small bowel Crohn's disease, there may be intestinal obstruction or displacement of bowel loops by a mass.

USS: May identify thickened small bowel and stricture in Crohn's disease.

General management

Multidisciplinary management by physicians, surgeons, radiologists and dietitians is advantageous. Ulcerative colitis and Crohn's disease are lifelong conditions and counsellors and patient support groups have important roles. The key aims are to:
• Treat acute attacks. • Prevent bowel damage and relapses.
• Detect carcinoma at an early stage. • Select patients for surgery.

Medical management of ulcerative colitis

Treatment depends upon the extent and activity of colitis. Aminosalicylates (e.g. mesalazine, sulfasalazine, olsalazine) modulate cytokine release from the mucosa and are widely used.

Active proctitis: In mild to moderate disease mesalazine enemas or suppositories, combined with oral mesalazine, are effective. Topical corticosteroids are less effective but are used in patients intolerant of topical mesalazine. Patients who fail to respond are treated with oral prednisolone.

Active left-sided or extensive ulcerative colitis: In mild cases, high-dose aminosalicylates, combined with topical aminosalicylate and corticosteroids, are effective. Oral prednisolone is indicated for severe or unresponsive cases.

Severe ulcerative colitis: Patients with severe colitis (see Box 12.17) unresponsive to maximal oral therapy should be monitored in hospital:

• Clinically, for abdominal pain, temperature, pulse rate, stool blood and frequency. • To check Hb, WCC, albumin, electrolytes, ESR and CRP. • For colonic dilatation on plain AXR.

IV fluids and enteral nutritional support are often needed. IV corticosteroids are given as a constant infusion. Topical and oral aminosalicylates have no role in the acute severe attack. In patients unresponsive to corticosteroids, IV ciclosporin or infliximab avoids the need for colectomy in 60%. Patients who deteriorate, despite 7–10 days' maximal medical therapy, and those with colonic dilatation (>6 cm) require urgent colectomy.

Maintenance of remission: Lifelong maintenance therapy is recommended for all patients with extensive disease and patients with distal disease who relapse more than once a year. Oral 5-aminosalicylates, e.g. mesalazine, are first-line agents. Patients who relapse frequently despite 5-aminosalicylates are treated with thiopurines, e.g. azathioprine.

Medical management of Crohn's disease

Crohn's is a progressive disease with fistula and stricture formation if suboptimally managed. The goal is induction of remission, then maintenance with minimum steroid use.

Active disease: Ileal disease is treated with budesonide, which minimises side-effects. Colitis or resistant ileal disease is treated with oral prednisolone. Patients on steroids should also receive calcium and vitamin D. Nutritional therapy using polymeric or elemental diets can induce remission without steroids, and is a useful option in children and in extensive ileal disease.

Severe colonic disease is treated with IV corticosteroids. Severe ileal or panenteric disease requires anti-TNF therapy (infliximab or adalimubab) with a thiopurine. These are used to induce remission, provided abscess and perforation have been excluded.

Maintenance of remission: A thiopurine (azathioprine or mercaptopurine) or methotrexate is widely used for maintenance. Patients with unresponsive disease are managed with both immunomodulating agents and infliximab. Chronic use of corticosteroids is avoided because of side-effects and because they do not prevent relapse. Smoking cessation is important, as continued smoking predicts relapse.

Fistulating and perianal disease: The site of fistulation is defined using imaging, usually pelvic MRI. Examination under anaesthetic and surgical intervention are usually required, and nutritional support (TPN) is also frequently necessary. For simple perianal disease, metronidazole or ciprofloxacin is used (or both). Thiopurines are given in chronic disease. Anti-TNF therapy helps to heal enterocutaneous fistulae and perianal disease.

Surgical treatment of ulcerative colitis

Up to 60% of patients with extensive ulcerative colitis eventually require surgery. Indications include impaired quality of life, failure of medical therapy, fulminant colitis, cancer or severe dysplasia. Panproctocolectomy with ileostomy or proctocolectomy with ileal–anal pouch anastomosis cures the patient. Before surgery, patients must be counselled both by staff and by patients who have had surgery.

Surgical treatment of Crohn's disease

The indications for surgery are similar to those for ulcerative colitis. Operations are often necessary to deal with fistulae, abscesses and perianal disease, or to relieve small or large bowel obstruction. In contrast to ulcerative colitis, surgery is not curative and disease recurrence is the rule, so a conservative approach is used. Those with extensive colitis require total colectomy but ileal–anal pouch formation should be avoided because of the high risk of recurrence within the pouch with fistulae, abscess formation and pouch failure.

Prognosis

Life expectancy in patients with IBD is now similar to that of the general population and, despite the burden of treatment, the majority are able to work and pursue a normal life.

IRRITABLE BOWEL SYNDROME

Irritable bowel syndrome (IBS) is a common functional bowel disorder in which abdominal pain is associated with defecation or a change in bowel habit in the absence of structural pathology.

Approximately 10–15% of the general population are affected but only 10% of these consult their doctors with symptoms. IBS is the most common cause of GI referral, and causes frequent absence from work and impaired quality of life. Young women are affected 2–3 times more often than men. There is wide overlap with non-ulcer dyspepsia, chronic fatigue syndrome, dysmenorrhoea and urinary frequency. Between 5 and 10% of patients have a history of physical or sexual abuse.

Most patients seen in general practice do not have psychological problems but ~50% of patients referred to hospital have significant anxiety, depression, somatisation, panic attacks and neurosis. Acute psychological stress and overt psychiatric disease alter visceral perception and GI motility. These factors, coupled with abnormal illness behaviour, contribute to but do not cause IBS.

A range of motility disorders from diarrhoea to constipation is found but none is diagnostic. IBS is associated with altered 5-HT release, which is increased in diarrhoea-predominant disease and reduced when constipation occurs.

Some patients develop IBS following an episode of gastroenteritis, more commonly young women and those with existing background psychological problems. Others may be intolerant of specific dietary components, particularly lactose and wheat.

Clinical features and investigations

Recurrent colicky pain in the lower abdomen is relieved by defecation. Abdominal bloating worsens throughout the day; the cause is unknown but it is not excessive intestinal gas. Patients have an abnormal bowel habit. It is useful to classify these as having predominantly constipation or predominantly diarrhoea. The constipated type tends to pass infrequent pellety stools, usually with abdominal pain or proctalgia. Those with diarrhoea have frequent defecation but produce low-volume stools and rarely have nocturnal symptoms. Passage of mucus is common but rectal bleeding does not occur.

Patients do not lose weight and are constitutionally well. Examination does not reveal any abnormalities, although bloating and tenderness to palpation are common.

Investigations are normal. FBC, faecal calprotectin and sigmoidoscopy are usually done routinely, but colonoscopy should only be undertaken in older patients and those with rectal bleeding to exclude colorectal cancer and IBD. Atypical presentations require investigations to exclude organic GI disease. In diarrhoea-predominant cases, coeliac disease, lactose intolerance, thyrotoxicosis and parasitic infection should be excluded.

Management

Many patients are concerned that they have developed cancer, and a cycle of anxiety leading to colonic symptoms, which further heighten anxiety, can be broken by explanation that symptoms are not due to organic disease but are the result of altered bowel motility and sensation. In patients who fail to respond to reassurance, symptomatic treatment should be tried. Elimination diets are generally unhelpful but some may benefit from exclusion of wheat, lactose, excess caffeine or artificial sweeteners such as sorbitol. Probiotics can be effective in some.

Patients with intractable symptoms sometimes benefit from several months of therapy with low-dose amitriptyline. Anxiety or affective disorders should be separately treated. Psychological interventions, such as cognitive behavioural therapy, relaxation and gut-directed hypnotherapy, are reserved for the most difficult cases. Most patients have a relapsing and remitting course.

ISCHAEMIC GUT INJURY

Ischaemic gut injury is usually the result of arterial occlusion. The presentation is variable and the diagnosis is difficult.

Acute small bowel ischaemia

Superior mesenteric blood flow may be compromised by embolism from the heart or aorta (40–50%), thrombosis on underlying atheroma (25%), or hypotension (25%). Vasculitis and venous occlusion are rare causes. Patients usually have evidence of cardiac disease and arrhythmia.

Abdominal pain develops, which is more impressive than the physical findings. In the early stages, the abdomen may be distended, with absent or diminished bowel sounds, and peritonitis is a later feature.

Investigations reveal:
• Leucocytosis. • Metabolic acidosis. • Raised phosphate and amylase. • 'Thumb-printing' on AXR due to mucosal oedema. • An occluded or narrowed major artery on mesenteric or CT angiography.

Management

Resuscitation, management of cardiac disease and IV antibiotic therapy should be followed by laparotomy, embolectomy and vascular reconstruction. In patients at high surgical risk, thrombolysis may sometimes be effective. Survivors often develop short bowel syndrome requiring nutritional support, sometimes including home parenteral nutrition, as well as anticoagulation. Small bowel transplantation is promising in selected patients.

Acute colonic ischaemia

The splenic flexure and descending colon lie in 'watershed' areas of arterial supply. Arterial thromboembolism is usually responsible but colonic ischaemia can also follow severe hypotension, colonic volvulus, strangulated hernia, systemic vasculitis, aortic aneurysm surgery or hypercoagulable states. The patient is usually elderly and presents with sudden cramping left-sided lower abdominal pain and rectal bleeding. The diagnosis is established by colonoscopy within 48 hrs of onset. Symptoms usually resolve spontaneously over 24–48 hrs and healing occurs within 2 wks. Some have a residual fibrous stricture or segment of colitis.

Chronic mesenteric ischaemia

This results from atherosclerotic stenosis affecting at least two of the coeliac axis, superior mesenteric and inferior mesenteric arteries. Patients present with dull but severe mid- or upper abdominal pain ~30 mins after eating, with weight loss and sometimes with diarrhoea. Examination reveals generalised arterial disease and sometimes an audible abdominal bruit. Mesenteric angiography confirms at least two affected arteries. Vascular reconstruction or percutaneous angioplasty is sometimes possible. Left untreated, many patients develop intestinal infarction.

DISORDERS OF THE COLON AND RECTUM

Tumours of the colon and rectum
Polyps and polyposis syndromes

Polyps may be neoplastic or non-neoplastic, single or multiple, and vary from a few mm to several cm in size.

Colorectal adenomas: Extremely common in the Western world; 50% of people >60 yrs of age have adenomas, usually in the rectum and distal colon. Nearly all colorectal carcinomas develop from adenomatous polyps. Large, multiple, villous or dysplastic polyps carry a higher risk of malignancy. Adenomas are usually asymptomatic and discovered incidentally. Occasionally, they cause bleeding and anaemia. Villous adenomas sometimes secrete large amounts of mucus, leading to diarrhoea and hypokalaemia.

Discovery of a polyp at sigmoidoscopy is an indication for colonoscopy and polypectomy, which considerably reduce subsequent cancer risk. Very large or sessile polyps sometimes require surgery. Once all polyps have been removed, patients <75 should undergo surveillance colonoscopy at 3–5-yr intervals, as new polyps develop in 50%.

Between 10 and 20% of polyps show evidence of malignancy. When cancer cells are found within 2 mm of the resection margin, and when the polyp cancer is poorly differentiated or invading lymphatics, segmental colonic resection is recommended. Others can be followed up by surveillance colonoscopy.

The polyposis syndromes are classified by histopathology. They include neoplastic familial adenomatous polyposis and several non-neoplastic syndromes, including Peutz–Jeghers syndrome.

Familial adenomatous polyposis (FAP): An uncommon (1 in 13 000) autosomal dominant disorder. Around 20% are new mutations with no family history. By age 15, 80% of patients will develop up to several thousand adenomatous colonic polyps, with symptoms such as rectal bleeding beginning a few years later. Within 10–15 yrs of the appearance of adenomas, colorectal cancer will develop, affecting 90% by the age of 50. Malignant transformation of duodenal adenomas occurs in 10% and is the leading cause of death after prophylactic colectomy. Extra-intestinal features include subcutaneous epidermoid cysts, benign osteomas, dental abnormalities and lipomas. Dark, round, pigmented retinal lesions (congenital hypertrophy of the retinal pigment epithelium) occur in some patients; in at-risk individuals these are 100% predictive of FAP.

Early identification is essential. Sigmoidoscopy, if normal, excludes the diagnosis. Genetic testing confirms the diagnosis, and first-degree relatives should also be tested. Children of FAP families should undergo mutation testing at 13–14 yrs of age, followed by regular sigmoidoscopy in those carrying the mutation. Affected individuals should undergo colectomy on leaving school or college. Periodic upper GI endoscopy is recommended to detect duodenal adenomas.

Peutz–Jeghers syndrome: Comprises multiple hamartomatous polyps in the small intestine and colon, and melanin pigmentation of the lips, mouth and digits, and is usually asymptomatic. There is a small but significant risk of small bowel or colonic adenocarcinoma and of cancer of the pancreas, lung, ovary, breast and endometrium. Patients should undergo regular upper endoscopy, colonoscopy and imaging of the small bowel and pancreas.

Colorectal cancer

Although relatively rare in the developing world, colorectal cancer is the second most common internal malignancy and the second leading cause of cancer deaths in Western countries. In the UK the incidence is 50–60 per 100 000/yr. The condition becomes increasingly common over the age of 50.

Around 80% are 'sporadic', 5–10% are hereditary non-polyposis colon cancer (HNPCC), 1% are associated with FAP and 1% with inflammatory bowel disease.

Environmental factors account for >80% of all 'sporadic' colorectal cancers. The risk declines in migrants who move from high- to low-risk countries. Dietary factors increasing risk are red meat and saturated fat, while fibre, fruit, vegetables, folic acid and calcium appear to protect.

Colorectal cancer development results from the accumulation of multiple genetic mutations. HNPCC occurs in those with a family history, often having relatives who were affected at a young age. The lifetime risk of colorectal cancer in affected individuals is 80%. Those who fulfil the criteria for diagnosis should be referred for pedigree assessment, genetic testing and colonoscopy, which needs to be repeated every 1–2 yrs, despite which interval cancers still occur. The lifetime risk of developing cancer with one or two affected first-degree relatives is 1 in 12 and 1 in 6, respectively. The risk is even higher if relatives were affected at an early age.

Most tumours arise from malignant transformation of a benign adenomatous polyp. Over 65% occur in the rectosigmoid and a further 15% recur in the caecum or ascending colon. Rectal cancers may invade the pelvic viscera and side walls. Lymphatic invasion is common at presentation, as is hepatic spread. Tumour stage at diagnosis determines prognosis.

Clinical features

In tumours of the left colon, fresh rectal bleeding is common and obstruction occurs early. Tumours of the right colon present with anaemia from occult bleeding or with altered bowel habit, but obstruction is a late feature. Colicky lower abdominal pain is present in two-thirds of patients and rectal bleeding occurs in 50%. A minority present with either obstruction or perforation. Carcinoma of the rectum usually causes early bleeding, mucus discharge or a feeling of incomplete emptying.

On examination there may be a palpable mass, signs of anaemia or hepatomegaly from metastases. Low rectal tumours may be palpable on digital examination.

Investigations and management

• Colonoscopy: more sensitive and specific than barium enema and permits biopsy (Fig. 12.5). • CT colonography: detects tumours and polyps >6 mm diameter and can be used if colonoscopy is incomplete or high risk. • CT: valuable for detecting hepatic metastases. • Pelvic MRI: to stage rectal tumours. • Intraoperative USS: increasingly being used for this purpose. • Carcinoembryonic antigen (CEA): normal in many patients and so of little use in diagnosis, but serial CEA can help to detect early recurrence during follow-up.

Treatment should be discussed and planned at a multidisciplinary meeting.

Neo-adjuvant therapy: Pre-operative radiotherapy or chemoradiotherapy is used to 'down-stage' large rectal cancers, making them resectable.

Surgery: The tumour is removed, along with pericolic lymph nodes. Direct anastomosis is performed wherever possible or colostomy if not. Solitary hepatic or lung metastases are sometimes resected at a later stage. Post-operatively, patients should undergo colonoscopy after 6–12 mths and periodically thereafter to search for

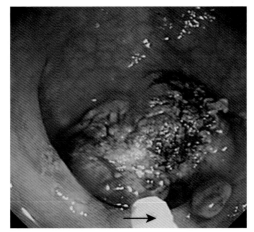

Fig. 12.5 Colonoscopic view of a polypoid rectal carcinoma undergoing laser therapy (arrow) in a patient unfit for surgery.

12.21 Staging and survival in colorectal cancer			
Dukes stage			
	A	**B**	**C**	**D**
Definition	Tumour confined within bowel wall	Extension through bowel wall	Tumour involving lymph nodes	Distant metastases
Prevalence at diagnosis (%)	10	35	30	25
5-yr survival rate (%)	>90	65	30–35	<5

local recurrence or development of new 'metachronous' lesions, which occur in 6% of cases.

Adjuvant therapy: Two-thirds of patients have lymph node or distant spread at presentation and are, therefore, beyond cure with surgery alone (Box 12.21). Most recurrences are within 3 yrs, either at the site of resection or in lymph nodes, liver or peritoneum. Adjuvant chemotherapy reduces recurrence risk in patients with Dukes C colon cancer and some Dukes B tumours. Post-operative radiotherapy is used to reduce the risk of local recurrence if resection margins are involved.

Palliation: Surgical resection of the primary tumour is appropriate for some patients with metastases to treat obstruction, bleeding or pain. Palliative chemotherapy with 5-fluorouracil/folinic acid, oxaliplatin or irinotecan improves survival. Pelvic radiotherapy is sometimes useful for rectal pain, bleeding or severe tenesmus. Endoscopic laser therapy or insertion of an expandable metal stent can be used to relieve obstruction.

Secondary prevention (screening): This aims to detect and remove lesions at an early or pre-malignant stage. Several potential methods exist. Widespread screening by regular FOB testing in those >50 increases early detection and reduces colorectal cancer mortality, and has been adopted in a number of countries. Colonoscopy remains the gold standard but requires expertise, is expensive and carries risks. Flexible sigmoidoscopy has been shown to reduce overall colorectal cancer mortality by ~35% (70% for cases arising in the rectosigmoid). It is recommended in the USA every 5 yrs in all persons over the age of 50.

Diverticulosis

Asymptomatic diverticula ('diverticulosis') occur in the sigmoid and descending colon in >50% of people over 70. Symptomatic ('diverticular disease') occurs in 10–25% of cases, while complicated diverticulosis ('diverticulitis') is uncommon.

Dietary fibre deficiency is thought to be responsible and diverticulosis is rare in populations with a high dietary fibre. Small-volume stools require high intracolonic pressures for propulsion, leading to herniation of mucosa.

Diverticula are protrusions of mucosa covered by peritoneum, which become impacted with faecoliths, then inflamed. This may resolve or progress with haemorrhage, perforation, abscess formation, fistula and peritonitis. Repeated attacks may lead to fibrotic strictures.

Clinical features

• Colicky pain in the suprapubic area or left iliac fossa from associated constipation or spasm. • Palpable sigmoid colon or iliac fossa mass. • Local tenderness, guarding, rigidity ('left-sided appendicitis') with diverticulitis. • Diarrhoea, rectal bleeding or fever. • Complications occur in ~5%; they are more common in patients who take NSAIDs or aspirin.

Investigations and management

• Barium enema: shows diverticula, strictures and fistulae. • Flexible sigmoidoscopy: excludes coexisting neoplasm, easily missed radiologically. • CT: to assess complications.

Asymptomatic diverticulosis requires no treatment. Constipation is relieved by a high-fibre diet with or without a bulking laxative and plenty of fluids. Stimulants should be avoided but antispasmodics sometimes help.

Acute diverticulitis requires 7 days of metronidazole and co-amoxiclav. Trials show no benefit from acute resection compared to conservative management, except for severe haemorrhage or perforation. Percutaneous drainage of acute abscesses can be effective.

Elective resection of the affected segment with primary anastomosis is indicated after repeated acute obstruction.

Constipation and disorders of defecation

Simple constipation: Constipation is extremely common and usually responds to increased dietary fibre or bulking agents with an adequate fluid intake.

Severe idiopathic constipation: This occurs almost exclusively in young women and often begins in childhood or adolescence. The cause is unknown and the condition is often resistant to treatment. Bulking agents may exacerbate symptoms but prokinetic agents or balanced solutions of polyethylene glycol 3350 benefit some patients with slow transit.

Faecal impaction: Impaction tends to occur in frail, disabled, immobile or institutionalised patients. Drugs, autonomic neuropathy and painful anal conditions also contribute. Obstruction, perforation and bleeding may supervene. Treatment involves softening the stool with arachis oil enemas, hydration and careful digital disimpaction.

Melanosis coli and laxative misuse syndromes: Long-term stimulant laxative use causes brown discoloration of the colonic mucosa ('tiger skin'), which is benign and resolves with laxative withdrawal. Surreptitious laxative misuse is a psychiatric condition seen in young women, who may have a history of bulimia or anorexia nervosa. They complain of refractory watery diarrhoea and deny laxative use. Screening of urine for laxatives may be helpful.

Hirschsprung's disease: Congenital absence of ganglion cells causes the internal anal sphincter to fail to relax, leading to constipation and colonic dilatation (megacolon). Constipation, abdominal distension and vomiting usually develop immediately after birth but occasionally in childhood or adolescence. A family history is present in one-third. The rectum is empty on digital examination. Barium enema shows a small rectum and colonic dilatation above the narrowed segment. Full-thickness biopsies confirm the absence of ganglion cells. Treatment involves resection of the affected segment.

Acquired megacolon: In childhood, this is a result of voluntary withholding of stool during toilet training. It presents after the first year and is distinguished from Hirschsprung's disease by the urge to defecate and the presence of stool in the rectum. It usually responds to osmotic laxatives. In adults, acquired megacolon may occur in depressed or demented patients, either as part of the condition or as a side-effect of antidepressant drugs. Prolonged misuse of stimulant laxatives may cause megacolon, as may neurological disorders, scleroderma, hypothyroidism and opioid abuse. Patients are managed by treating the underlying cause, and with high-residue diets, laxatives and enemas.

Acute colonic pseudo-obstruction (Ogilvie's syndrome): This can be caused by trauma, surgery, respiratory or renal failure, or diabetes mellitus. There is sudden, painless, massive enlargement of the proximal colon without features of mechanical obstruction. Bowel sounds are normal or high-pitched rather than absent. The condition may progress to perforation and peritonitis. X-rays show colonic dilatation with air extending to the rectum. A caecal diameter >10–12 cm is associated with a high risk of perforation. Barium enemas demonstrate the absence of mechanical obstruction. Management consists of treating the underlying disorder and correcting any biochemical abnormalities. Neostigmine is used to enhance gut motility. Decompression either with a rectal tube or by careful colonoscopy may be effective.

Colonic infections: These are discussed on pages 85–89.

Anorectal disorders
Faecal incontinence

Common causes include severe diarrhoea, impaction, anorectal or neurological disease and obstetric trauma. A careful history and examination, especially of the anorectum and perineum, may help to establish the underlying cause. Endoanal USS is valuable for defining the integrity of the anal sphincters, while MR proctography, manometry and electrophysiology are also useful.

Management involves treating underlying disorders. Pelvic floor exercises, biofeedback techniques and sphincter repair operations help some patients.

Haemorrhoids ('piles')

Haemorrhoids are extremely common and arise from congestion of the venous plexuses around the anal canal. They are associated with constipation and straining, and may develop during pregnancy. First-degree piles bleed, second-degree piles prolapse but retract spontaneously, and third-degree piles require manual replacement. Symptoms include bright red bleeding after defecation, pain, pruritus ani and mucus discharge. Treatment involves prevention of constipation, injection sclerotherapy or band ligation. A minority require haemorrhoidectomy, which is usually curative.

Pruritus ani

This is common and causes include infections, skin disorders and anal disorders such as haemorrhoids or fissures. These result in contamination of the perianal skin with faecal contents, leading to an itch–scratch–itch cycle that exacerbates the problem. Good personal hygiene is essential, with careful washing after defecation. The perineal area must be kept dry and clean.

Solitary rectal ulcer syndrome

This occurs in young adults who develop an ulcer with mucosal prolapse on the anterior rectal wall. Symptoms include minor bleeding and mucus per rectum, tenesmus and perineal pain. Treatment is often difficult but avoidance of straining at defecation is important.

Anal fissure

This is a superficial tear in the anal mucosa, most commonly in the midline posteriorly, with spasm of the internal anal sphincter. Severe pain occurs on defecation with minor bleeding, mucus discharge and pruritus. The skin may be indurated and an oedematous skin tag, or 'sentinel pile', is common.

Avoidance of constipation with bulk-forming laxatives and increased fluid intake is important. Relaxation of the internal sphincter using glyceryl trinitrate is effective in 60–80% of patients; diltiazem cream is an alternative. Resistant cases may respond to injection of botulinum toxin into the internal anal sphincter to induce sphincter relaxation. Manual dilatation under anaesthesia leads to long-term incontinence and should not be considered.

Anorectal abscesses and fistulae

Perianal abscesses develop between the anal sphincters and may point at the perianal skin. Ischiorectal abscesses occur in the ischiorectal fossa. Crohn's disease is sometimes responsible.

Patients complain of extreme perianal pain, fever and/or discharge of pus. Spontaneous rupture may also lead to the development of fistulae. Abscesses and fistulae are treated surgically.

DISEASES OF THE PERITONEAL CAVITY

Endometriosis

Ectopic endometrial tissue can become embedded on the serosal aspect of the sigmoid and rectum. Cyclical engorgement and inflammation causes low backache, bleeding, diarrhoea, constipation, adhesions or obstruction. It usually affects nulliparous women between 20 and 45 yrs old. Bimanual examination may reveal tender nodules in the pouch of Douglas. Sigmoidoscopy during menstruation reveals a bluish mass with intact overlying mucosa. Treatment options include laparoscopic diathermy and hormonal therapy with progestogens.

Peritonitis

Peritonitis usually occurs as the result of a ruptured viscus, but may also complicate ascites or occur in children without ascites, due to pneumococcal or streptococcal infection. Chlamydial peritonitis is a complication of pelvic inflammatory disease, and presents with right upper quadrant pain, pyrexia and a hepatic rub. TB may cause peritonitis and ascites.

Tumours

The most common is secondary adenocarcinoma from the ovary or GI tract. Mesothelioma is a rare tumour complicating asbestos exposure. The prognosis is extremely poor.

Liver and biliary tract disease

The liver weighs 1–1.8 kg and performs many important functions (Fig. 13.1). In the developed world, the most common cause of liver disease is alcohol abuse, and cirrhosis causes many deaths. In contrast, in the developing world, infections caused by hepatitis viruses and parasites are responsible for most chronic liver disease and hepatobiliary cancer.

PRESENTING PROBLEMS IN LIVER DISEASE

Acute liver failure

Acute liver failure is an uncommon syndrome in which hepatic encephalopathy, characterised by mental changes progressing from confusion to stupor and coma, results from a sudden severe impairment of hepatic function (Box 13.1). In a patient whose liver was previously normal, the level of injury needed to cause liver failure is very high, while in those with pre-existing chronic liver disease, the additional acute insult needed to precipitate liver failure is much less. Although liver biopsy may ultimately be necessary, it is the presence or absence of the clinical features suggesting chronicity that guides the clinician.

Acute viral hepatitis is the most common cause worldwide. Paracetamol toxicity (p. 36) is the most frequent culprit in the UK. Acute liver failure occurs occasionally with other drugs, or from *Amanita phalloides* (mushroom) poisoning, in pregnancy, in Wilson's disease, or following shock (p. 23). The cause remains unknown in others; these patients are often labelled as having non-A–E viral hepatitis or cryptogenic acute liver failure.

Clinical assessment

Cerebral disturbance (hepatic encephalopathy) is the cardinal manifestation of acute liver failure, starting with mild, episodic reduced concentration and alertness, progressing through restlessness and aggressive outbursts to drowsiness and coma. Cerebral oedema may cause increased intracranial pressure, leading to unequal or

CLINICAL EXAMINATION OF THE ABDOMEN FOR LIVER AND BILIARY DISEASE

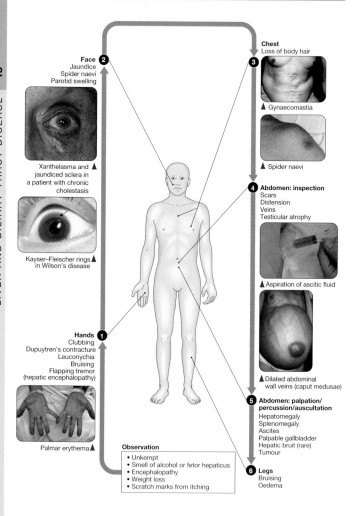

Face ❷
Jaundice
Spider naevi
Parotid swelling

▲ Xanthelasma and jaundiced sclera in a patient with chronic cholestasis

▲ Kayser–Fleischer rings in Wilson's disease

Hands ❶
Clubbing
Dupuytren's contracture
Leuconychia
Bruising
Flapping tremor
(hepatic encephalopathy)

Palmar erythema ▲

Chest ❸
Loss of body hair

▲ Gynaecomastia

▲ Spider naevi

Abdomen: inspection ❹
Scars
Distension
Veins
Testicular atrophy

▲ Aspiration of ascitic fluid

▲ Dilated abdominal wall veins (caput medusae)

Abdomen: palpation/ percussion/auscultation ❺
Hepatomegaly
Splenomegaly
Ascites
Palpable gallbladder
Hepatic bruit (rare)
Tumour

Legs ❻
Bruising
Oedema

Observation
• Unkempt
• Smell of alcohol or fetor hepaticus
• Encephalopathy
• Weight loss
• Scratch marks from itching

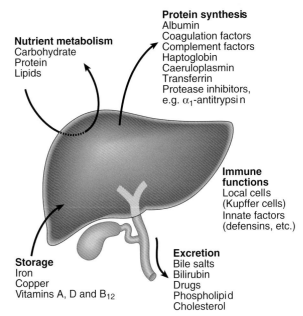

Protein synthesis
Albumin
Coagulation factors
Complement factors
Haptoglobin
Caeruloplasmin
Transferrin
Protease inhibitors,
e.g. α_1-antitrypsin

Nutrient metabolism
Carbohydrate
Protein
Lipids

Immune functions
Local cells
(Kupffer cells)
Innate factors
(defensins, etc.)

Storage
Iron
Copper
Vitamins A, D and B_{12}

Excretion
Bile salts
Bilirubin
Drugs
Phospholipid
Cholesterol

Fig. 13.1 Important liver functions.

i	13.1 Classification of acute liver failure		
Type	**Time: jaundice to encephalopathy**	**Cerebral oedema**	**Common causes**
Hyperacute	<7 days	Common	Viral, paracetamol
Acute	8–28 days	Common	Cryptogenic, drugs
Subacute	29 days to 12 wks	Uncommon	Cryptogenic, drugs

abnormally reacting pupils, fixed pupils, hypertensive episodes, bradycardia, hyperventilation, profuse sweating, local or general myoclonus, focal fits or decerebrate posturing. Papilloedema occurs rarely and is a late sign. More general symptoms include weakness, nausea and vomiting. Right hypochondrial discomfort occasionally occurs.

Examination shows jaundice, which develops rapidly and is usually deep in subsequently fatal cases. However, jaundice is absent in Reye's syndrome, and death occasionally occurs in fulminant acute liver failure before jaundice develops. Hepatomegaly is unusual; if found with sudden-onset ascites, it suggests venous outflow obstruction (Budd–Chiari syndrome). Splenomegaly is

13.2 Investigations to determine the cause of acute liver failure

- Toxicology screen of blood and urine
- IgM anti-HBc, HBsAg
- IgM anti-HAV
- Anti-HEV, HCV, cytomegalovirus, herpes simplex, Epstein–Barr virus
- Caeruloplasmin, serum copper, urinary copper, slit-lamp eye examination
- Autoantibodies: ANF, ASMA, LKM, SLA
- Immunoglobulins
- USS of liver and Doppler of hepatic veins

(ANF = antinuclear factor; anti-HBc = antibody to hepatitis B core antigen; ASMA = anti-smooth muscle antibody; HAV = hepatitis A virus; HBsAg = hepatitis B surface antigen; HCV = hepatitis C virus; HEV = hepatitis E virus; LKM = liver–kidney microsomal antibody; SLA = soluble liver antigen)

13.3 Adverse prognostic criteria in acute liver failure*

Paracetamol overdose

- H^+ >50 nmol/L (pH <7.3) at or beyond 24 hrs following the overdose
  or
- Serum creatinine >300 μmol/L (3.38 mg/dL) + prothrombin time >100 secs + encephalopathy grade 3 or 4

Non-paracetamol cases

- Prothrombin time >100 secs
  or
- Any three of the following: jaundice to encephalopathy time >7 days; age <10 or >40 yrs; indeterminate or drug-induced causes; bilirubin >300 μmol/L (17.6 mg/dL); prothrombin time >50 secs
  or
- Factor V level <15% and encephalopathy grade 3 or 4

*Predict a mortality rate of ≥90%.

uncommon and never prominent. Ascites and oedema are late developments and may be a consequence of fluid therapy.

Investigations

Investigations are used to determine the cause of the liver failure and the prognosis (Boxes 13.2 and 13.3). The prothrombin time rapidly becomes prolonged as coagulation factor synthesis fails; this test is of great prognostic value and should be performed at least twice daily. Plasma aminotransferase activity rises to 100–500 times normal after paracetamol overdose, but falls as liver damage progresses and is not helpful in determining prognosis.

Management

A patient with acute hepatic damage should be treated in an HDU or ICU as soon as progressive prolongation of the prothrombin time or hepatic encephalopathy is identified, so that prompt treatment of complications (hypoglycaemia, infections, renal failure, metabolic acidosis) can be initiated. Treatment is supportive in the hope that hepatic regeneration will occur. *N*-acetylcysteine therapy may improve outcome, particularly in patients with acute liver failure due to paracetamol poisoning. Liver transplantation is an increasingly important treatment option and so, wherever possible, patients should be transferred to a transplant centre early to allow time for assessment of prognosis (see Box 13.3) and to maximise the time for a donor liver to become available. Survival following liver transplantation for acute liver failure is improving and 1-yr survival rates of ~60% can be expected.

Abnormal liver function tests

Abnormal liver function tests (LFTs) are frequently detected on routine testing (e.g. 3.5% of patients measured routinely prior to elective surgery have some elevation of transaminases). The majority of patients with persistently abnormal LFTs have significant liver disease. The most common abnormality is alcoholic or non-alcoholic fatty liver disease (NAFLD; p. 502). An algorithm for investigating abnormal LFTs is shown in Figure 13.2. A full history must include alcohol and drug use (prescribed and otherwise), autoimmune disease, family history, diabetes and features of the metabolic syndrome (p. 385). The presence or absence of stigmata of chronic liver disease (p. 488) does not reliably identify patients with significant chronic liver disease. Also, normal LFTs do not exclude significant chronic liver disease, which might progress to cirrhosis, e.g. primary sclerosing cholangitis, haemochromatosis and chronic hepatitis C.

The pattern of abnormal LFTs (hepatitic or obstructive) indicates the likely causes (Box 13.4).

Jaundice

Jaundice is usually detectable clinically when the plasma bilirubin exceeds 40 μmol/L (~2.5 mg/dL).

Bilirubin metabolism

Bilirubin in the blood is normally almost all unconjugated and, because it is not water-soluble, it is bound to albumin and does not enter the urine. Unconjugated bilirubin is conjugated by glucuronyl transferase into water-soluble conjugates, which are exported into the bile. The excretion pathways for bilirubin are shown in Figure 13.3.

Pre-hepatic jaundice

This is caused either by haemolysis or by congenital hyperbilirubinaemia, and is characterised by an isolated raised bilirubin level.

In haemolysis, destruction of red blood cells or their marrow precursors causes increased bilirubin production. Jaundice due to haemolysis is usually mild because a healthy liver can excrete a

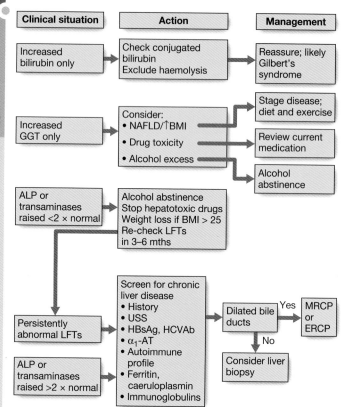

Fig. 13.2 Suggested management of abnormal LFTs in asymptomatic patients.
(α_1-AT = alpha$_1$-antitrypsin; ALP = alkaline phosphatase; ERCP = endoscopic retrograde cholangiopancreatography; GGT = γ-glutamyl transferase; HBsAg = hepatitis B surface antigen; HCVAb = antibody to hepatitis C virus; MRCP = magnetic resonance cholangiopancreatography; NAFLD = non-alcoholic fatty liver disease.)

bilirubin load six times greater than normal before unconjugated bilirubin accumulates in the plasma. This does not apply to newborns, who have less capacity to metabolise bilirubin.

The only common form of non-haemolytic hyperbilirubinaemia is Gilbert's syndrome, a familial autosomal dominant mutation reducing expression of uridine 5′-diphospho(UDP)-glucuronyl transferase. This causes decreased bilirubin conjugation, with isolated accumulation of unconjugated bilirubin in the blood. It has an excellent prognosis and needs no treatment. Other inherited disorders of bilirubin metabolism are very rare.

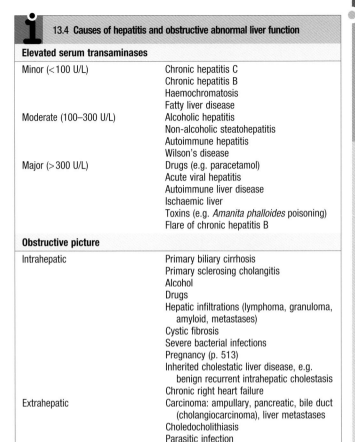

13.4	Causes of hepatitis and obstructive abnormal liver function

Elevated serum transaminases

Minor (<100 U/L)	Chronic hepatitis C
	Chronic hepatitis B
	Haemochromatosis
	Fatty liver disease
Moderate (100–300 U/L)	Alcoholic hepatitis
	Non-alcoholic steatohepatitis
	Autoimmune hepatitis
	Wilson's disease
Major (>300 U/L)	Drugs (e.g. paracetamol)
	Acute viral hepatitis
	Autoimmune liver disease
	Ischaemic liver
	Toxins (e.g. *Amanita phalloides* poisoning)
	Flare of chronic hepatitis B

Obstructive picture

Intrahepatic	Primary biliary cirrhosis
	Primary sclerosing cholangitis
	Alcohol
	Drugs
	Hepatic infiltrations (lymphoma, granuloma, amyloid, metastases)
	Cystic fibrosis
	Severe bacterial infections
	Pregnancy (p. 513)
	Inherited cholestatic liver disease, e.g. benign recurrent intrahepatic cholestasis
	Chronic right heart failure
Extrahepatic	Carcinoma: ampullary, pancreatic, bile duct (cholangiocarcinoma), liver metastases
	Choledocholithiasis
	Parasitic infection
	Traumatic biliary strictures
	Chronic pancreatitis

Hepatocellular jaundice

Hepatocellular jaundice results from an inability of the liver to transport bilirubin into the bile, as a consequence of parenchymal liver disease. In hepatocellular jaundice, the concentrations of both unconjugated and conjugated bilirubin in the blood increase, perhaps because of the variable way in which bilirubin transport is disturbed.

Parenchymal disease causing jaundice usually also elevates transaminase levels. Acute jaundice with an alanine aminotransferase (ALT) >1000 U/L suggests hepatitis A or B, drug toxicity (e.g. paracetamol) or hepatic ischaemia. USS and biopsy are frequently needed for precise diagnosis.

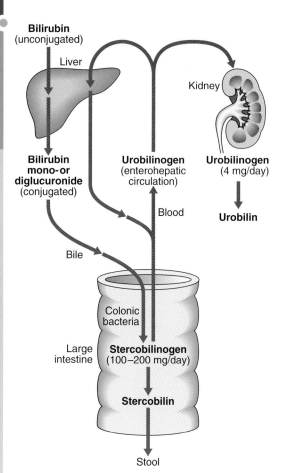

Fig. 13.3 Pathway of bilirubin excretion.

Obstructive (cholestatic) jaundice

Cholestatic jaundice may be caused by:

• Failure of hepatocytes to initiate bile flow. • Obstruction of the bile ducts or portal tracts. • Obstruction of bile flow in the extrahepatic bile ducts between the porta hepatis and the ampulla of Vater.

Without treatment, cholestatic jaundice tends to progress because conjugated bilirubin is unable to enter the bile canaliculi and passes back into the blood, and also because there is a failure of clearance of unconjugated bilirubin arriving at the liver cells. The causes of cholestatic jaundice are listed in Box 13.4. Cholestasis may result from more than one of these defects. Those confined to the extrahepatic bile ducts may be amenable to surgical or endoscopic correction.

Clinical assessment

Abdominal pain suggests choledocholithiasis, pancreatitis or choledochal cyst. Jaundice is progressive in cancer, and fluctuating in sclerosing cholangitis, pancreatitis and stricture. Abdominal examination may reveal irregular hepatomegaly or masses in carcinoma. Faecal occult blood suggests an ampullary tumour.

Hepatomegaly

In Western countries, the most common malignant cause is liver metastasis, whereas primary liver cancer complicating chronic viral hepatitis is more common in the Far East. Cirrhosis can be associated with either hepatomegaly (particularly if due to alcohol or haemochromatosis) or reduced liver size in advanced disease.

Ascites

Ascites means the accumulation of free fluid in the peritoneal cavity and is usually due to malignant disease, cirrhosis or heart failure; however, primary disorders of the peritoneum and visceral organs can produce ascites, and these need to be considered, even in a patient with chronic liver disease (Box 13.5).

Clinical assessment

Small volumes are asymptomatic, but ascites >1 L causes abdominal distension, fullness in the flanks, shifting dullness on percussion and a fluid thrill. Other signs include everted umbilicus, divarication of the recti, scrotal oedema and dilated abdominal veins (with portal hypertension).

Pathophysiology

Splanchnic vasodilatation, mediated mainly by nitric oxide, causes a fall in systemic arterial pressure as cirrhosis advances. This leads

13.5 Causes of ascites

Common causes

- Malignant disease: hepatic, peritoneal
- Cardiac failure
- Hepatic cirrhosis

Other causes

- Hypoproteinaemia: nephrotic syndrome, protein-losing enteropathy, malnutrition
- Pancreatitis
- Lymphatic obstruction
- Infection: TB
- Hepatic venous occlusion: Budd–Chiari syndrome, veno-occlusive disease
- Rare: Meigs' syndrome, hypothyroidism

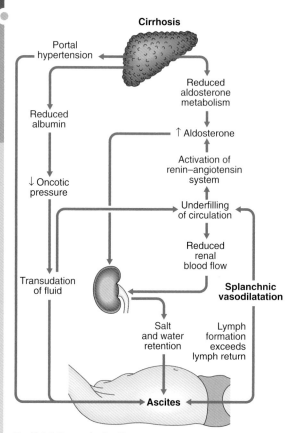

Fig. 13.4 Pathogenesis of ascites.

to activation of the renin–angiotensin system, secondary aldosteronism, increased sympathetic nervous activity, increased atrial natriuretic hormone secretion and altered activity of the kallikrein–kinin system (Fig. 13.4). These systems tend to normalise arterial pressure but produce salt and water retention. The combination of splanchnic vasodilatation and portal hypertension alter intestinal capillary permeability, promoting fluid accumulation within the peritoneum.

Investigations

USS is the best means of detecting ascites. Paracentesis may point to the underlying cause (Box 13.6). Measurement of total protein and serum–ascites albumin gradient (SAAG = serum albumin – ascites albumin) distinguishes transudate from exudate. Cirrhosis typically causes a transudate (total protein <25 g/L with few cells). A SAAG

> ### i 13.6 Ascitic fluid: appearance and analysis
>
> **Cause/appearance**
>
> - Cirrhosis: clear, straw-coloured or light green
> - Malignant disease: bloody
> - Infection: cloudy
> - Biliary communication: heavy bile staining
> - Lymphatic obstruction: milky-white (chylous)
>
> **Useful investigations**
>
> - Total albumin (plus serum albumin)
> - Amylase
> - WCC
> - Cytology
> - Microscopy and culture

>11 g/L is 96% predictive that ascites is due to portal hypertension. Venous outflow obstruction due to cardiac failure or hepatic venous outflow obstruction can also cause transudative ascites (SAAG >11 g/L) but, unlike in cirrhosis, total protein is usually >25 g/L. Exudative ascites (protein >25 g/L or SAAG <11 g/L) suggests infection (especially TB), malignancy, hepatic venous obstruction, pancreatic ascites or, rarely, hypothyroidism. Ascites amylase activity >1000 U/L identifies pancreatic ascites, and low ascites glucose suggests malignancy or TB. Cytology may reveal malignant cells (one-third of cirrhotic patients with a bloody tap have a hepatoma). Polymorphonuclear leucocyte counts $>250 \times 10^6$/L strongly suggest infection (spontaneous bacterial peritonitis – see below).

Management

Successful treatment of ascites relieves discomfort but does not prolong life. If over-vigorous, it can produce serious disorders of fluid and electrolyte balance, and precipitate hepatic encephalopathy (p. 486).

Sodium restriction: Restriction to 100 mmol/day ('no added salt diet') is normally adequate. Avoid sodium-rich drugs (e.g. many antibiotics, antacids) and those promoting sodium retention (e.g. steroids, NSAIDs).

Diuretics: Most patients require diuretics in addition to sodium restriction. Spironolactone (100–400 mg/day) is the drug of choice but may cause gynaecomastia. Some patients will also require loop diuretics, e.g. furosemide.

Paracentesis: Large-volume paracentesis with IV albumin can be used as first-line treatment of refractory ascites or when other treatments fail.

Transjugular intrahepatic portosystemic stent shunt (TIPSS, p. 492): TIPSS can relieve resistant ascites, but does not prolong life and may aggravate encephalopathy.

Hepatorenal syndrome

Around 10% of patients with advanced cirrhosis and ascites develop the hepatorenal syndrome, which is mediated by severe renal vasoconstriction due to underfilling of the arterial circulation.

Type 1 hepatorenal syndrome: Characterised by progressive oliguria, a rapid rise of the serum creatinine and a very poor prognosis. There is usually no proteinuria, urine sodium excretion is <10 mmol/day and urine/plasma osmolarity ratio is >1.5. Treatment consists of albumin infusions in combination with terlipressin and is effective in about two-thirds of patients. Haemodialysis should not be used routinely because it does not improve the outcome.

Type 2 hepatorenal syndrome: Usually occurs in patients with refractory ascites, is characterised by a moderate and stable increase in serum creatinine, and has a better prognosis.

Spontaneous bacterial peritonitis

Spontaneous bacterial peritonitis (SBP) may present with abdominal pain, rebound tenderness, absent bowel sounds and fever in a patient with obvious cirrhosis and ascites. Abdominal signs are mild or absent in about one-third of patients, in whom hepatic encephalopathy and fever dominate. The source of infection cannot usually be determined, but most organisms isolated from ascitic fluid or blood cultures are of enteric origin; *Escherichia coli* is the most frequently found. SBP needs to be differentiated from other intra-abdominal emergencies, and the finding of multiple organisms on culture should arouse suspicion of a perforated viscus.

Treatment should be started immediately with broad-spectrum antibiotics like cefotaxime. Recurrence is common and may be reduced by prophylactic quinolones such as norfloxacin (400 mg daily) or ciprofloxacin (250 mg daily).

Hepatic encephalopathy

Hepatic encephalopathy is a neuropsychiatric syndrome caused by liver disease that progresses from confusion to coma. Confusion needs to be differentiated from delirium tremens and Wernicke's encephalopathy, and coma from subdural haematoma, which can occur in alcoholics after a fall. Liver failure and portosystemic shunting of blood are two important factors underlying hepatic encephalopathy and the balance between these varies in different patients. The 'neurotoxins' causing the encephalopathy are thought to be mainly nitrogenous substances produced by bacterial action in the gut, which are normally metabolised by the healthy liver and excluded from the systemic circulation. Ammonia has long been considered an important factor but much interest has centred recently on γ-aminobutyric acid.

Clinical assessment

The earliest features are very mild and easily overlooked but mental impairment increases as the condition becomes more severe

13.7 Clinical grading of hepatic encephalopathy	
Clinical grade	**Clinical signs**
Grade 1	Poor concentration, slurred speech, slow mentation, disordered sleep rhythm
Grade 2	Drowsy but easily rousable, occasional aggressive behaviour, lethargic
Grade 3	Marked confusion, drowsy, sleepy but responds to pain and voice, gross disorientation
Grade 4	Unresponsive to voice, may or may not respond to painful stimuli, unconscious

(Box 13.7). Precipitating causes include trauma, drugs, infection, protein load (including GI bleeding) and constipation. Convulsions sometimes occur. Examination usually shows:

• A flapping tremor (asterixis). • Inability to perform simple mental arithmetic. • Inability to draw objects such as a star (constructional apraxia). • Hyper-reflexia. • Bilateral extensor plantar responses.

An EEG shows diffuse slowing of the normal alpha waves with eventual development of delta waves.

Management

The principles are to treat or remove precipitating causes and to suppress production of neurotoxins by bacteria in the bowel. Lactulose (15–30 mL 3 times daily) is a disaccharide that is taken orally and produces an osmotic laxative effect. It reduces the colonic pH, thereby limiting colonic ammonia absorption, and promotes the incorporation of nitrogen into bacteria. Rifaximin (400 mg 3 times daily) is a non-absorbed antibiotic that acts by reducing the bacterial content of the bowel. Dietary protein restriction is no longer recommended and can lead to worsening nutritional state in already malnourished patients.

CIRRHOSIS

Cirrhosis is characterised by diffuse hepatic fibrosis and nodule formation, and is an important cause of morbidity and premature death. Worldwide, the most common causes are viral hepatitis, alcohol and NAFLD. Cirrhosis is the most common cause of portal hypertension and its complications.

The causes of cirrhosis are listed in Box 13.8; any condition leading to persistent or recurrent hepatocyte death may result in cirrhosis. It may also occur in prolonged biliary damage or obstruction, as is found in primary biliary cirrhosis (PBC), primary sclerosing cholangitis and post-surgical biliary strictures. Persistent blockage of venous return from the liver, such as occurs in veno-occlusive disease and Budd–Chiari syndrome, can also result in cirrhosis.

13.8 Causes of cirrhosis

- Alcohol
- Chronic viral hepatitis (B or C)
- Non-alcoholic fatty liver disease
- Immune: primary sclerosing cholangitis, autoimmune liver disease
- Biliary: primary or secondary biliary cirrhosis, cystic fibrosis
- Genetic: haemochromatosis, α_1-antitrypsin deficiency, Wilson's disease
- Chronic venous outflow obstruction
- Cryptogenic (unknown)

Clinical features

Cirrhosis may be entirely asymptomatic; in life it may be found incidentally at surgery or may be associated with minimal features such as isolated hepatomegaly. Frequent symptoms include weakness, fatigue, muscle cramps, weight loss and non-specific digestive symptoms such as anorexia, nausea, vomiting and upper abdominal discomfort. Other patients present with clinical features of hepatic insufficiency and portal hypertension.

Hepatomegaly is common in alcoholic liver disease and haemochromatosis. In other causes of cirrhosis (e.g. viral hepatitis or autoimmune liver disease), progressive hepatocyte destruction and fibrosis gradually reduce liver size. The liver is often hard, irregular and non-tender. Jaundice is mild when it first appears and is due primarily to a failure to excrete bilirubin. Palmar erythema can be seen early in the disease but is of limited value, as it occurs in many other conditions and in some healthy people. One or two small spider telangiectasia are found in ~2% of healthy people and can occur transiently in greater numbers in the third trimester of pregnancy, but otherwise they are a strong indicator of liver disease. Endocrine changes are noticed more readily in men, who show loss of male hair distribution and testicular atrophy. Gynaecomastia is common and can be due to drugs such as spironolactone. Easy bruising becomes more frequent as cirrhosis advances. Splenomegaly and collateral vessel formation are features of portal hypertension, which occurs in more advanced disease. Ascites also signifies advanced disease. Evidence of hepatic encephalopathy also becomes increasingly common with advancing disease. Non-specific features include finger and toe clubbing. Dupuytren's contracture is traditionally regarded as being associated with cirrhosis but the evidence for this association is weak.

Chronic liver failure develops when the metabolic capacity of the liver is exceeded. It is characterised by the presence of encephalopathy and/or ascites. The term 'hepatic decompensation' or 'decompensated liver disease' is often used at this stage.

13.9	**Child–Pugh classification of prognosis in cirrhosis**		
Score	1	2	3
Encephalopathy	None	Mild	Marked
Bilirubin (μmol/L)*			
Primary biliary sclerosis/sclerosing cholangitis	<68	68–170	>170
Other causes of cirrhosis	<34	34–50	>50
Albumin (g/L)	>35	28–35	<28
Prothrombin time (secs prolonged)	<4	4–6	>6
Ascites	None	Mild	Marked
Add the individual scores:			
<7 = Child's A; 1-yr survival 82%			
7–9 = Child's B; 1-yr survival 62%			
>9 = Child's C; 1-yr survival 42%			

*To convert bilirubin in mol/L to mg/dL, divide by 17.

Management and prognosis

Management of cirrhosis is by treatment of the underlying cause and its complications, or by liver transplantation in selected cases of advanced cirrhosis. Surveillance should include endoscopy to screen for oesophageal varices every 2 yrs, and USS to detect hepatocellular carcinoma. Prognosis is linked to severity (Box 13.9).

PORTAL HYPERTENSION

Portal hypertension is characterised by prolonged elevation of the portal venous pressure (normally 5–6 mmHg). Clinically significant portal hypertension is present when the gradient exceeds 10 mmHg and risk of variceal bleeding increases over 12 mmHg.

Extrahepatic portal vein obstruction is the usual cause of portal hypertension in childhood and adolescence, while cirrhosis causes 90% or more of portal hypertension in adults in developed countries. Schistosomiasis is a common cause of portal hypertension worldwide but is infrequent outside endemic areas. Causes classified by site of obstruction are shown in Figure 13.5. Increased portal vascular resistance leads to a gradual reduction in the flow of portal blood to the liver and simultaneously to the development of collateral vessels, allowing half or more of the portal blood to bypass the liver and enter the systemic circulation directly.

Clinical features

Splenomegaly is a cardinal finding, and a diagnosis of portal hypertension is unlikely when splenomegaly cannot be detected clinically or by USS. The spleen is rarely enlarged >5 cm below the left costal margin in adults. Collateral vessels may be visible on the anterior abdominal wall and occasionally several radiate from the umbilicus to form a caput medusae. The most important collateral vessels

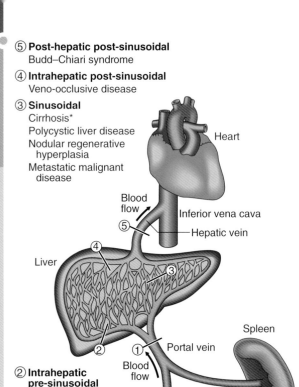

⑤ **Post-hepatic post-sinusoidal**
Budd–Chiari syndrome

④ **Intrahepatic post-sinusoidal**
Veno-occlusive disease

③ **Sinusoidal**
Cirrhosis*
Polycystic liver disease
Nodular regenerative
hyperplasia
Metastatic malignant
disease

② **Intrahepatic
pre-sinusoidal**
Schistosomiasis*
Congenital hepatic
fibrosis
Drugs
Vinyl chloride
Sarcoidosis

① **Prehepatic pre-sinusoidal**
Portal vein thrombosis due to sepsis (umbilical,
portal pyaemia) or procoagulopathy or secondary
to cirrhosis
Abdominal trauma including surgery

Fig. 13.5 Causes of portal hypertension according to site of vascular obstruction. *Most common cause. Note that splenic vein occlusion can also follow pancreatitis, leading to gastric varices.

occur in the oesophagus and stomach, where they can cause severe bleeding. Rectal varices also lead to bleeding and are often mistaken for haemorrhoids. Fetor hepaticus results from portosystemic shunting of blood, which allows mercaptans to pass directly to the lungs. Ascites occurs due to renal sodium retention (p. 484). Bleeding from oesophageal or gastric varices is the most important consequence of portal hypertension.

Investigations

• Endoscopic examination of the upper GI tract: used to detect and to check periodically for varices. • USS: can show splenomegaly and collateral vessels, and may sometimes indicate the cause, such as liver disease or portal vein thrombosis. • CT and MRI angiography: can identify portal vein clot and hepatic vein patency. • Thrombocytopenia: common due to hypersplenism – platelet counts are usually ~100×10^9/L. Leucopenia occurs occasionally but anaemia is more likely to be due to bleeding than hypersplenism. • Portal venous pressure measurements: not routinely needed but can distinguish sinusoidal from pre-sinusoidal forms.

Variceal bleeding

Bleeding usually occurs from varices near the gastro-oesophageal junction or in the stomach. Risk of bleeding within 2 yrs varies from 7% for small varices to 30% for large varices. It is often severe, and recurs if preventative treatment is not given. The mortality from bleeding oesophageal varices has improved to around 15% but remains about 45% in those with advanced liver disease.

Primary prevention of variceal bleeding

If non-bleeding varices are identified at endoscopy, β-blocker therapy with propranolol (80–160 mg/day) or nadolol is effective in reducing portal venous pressure and preventing variceal bleeding. Prophylactic banding is also effective in patients that are unable to tolerate β-blockers.

Management of acute variceal bleeding

See also acute upper GI haemorrhage (p. 416).

The priority in acute bleeding is to restore the circulation with blood and plasma. All patients with cirrhosis and GI bleeding should receive prophylactic broad-spectrum antibiotics such as ciprofloxacin.

Pharmacological reduction of portal venous pressure: Terlipressin is a synthetic vasopressin analogue that can be given by intermittent injection and lowers portal pressure. It reduces mortality in variceal bleeding but should be used with caution in ischaemic heart disease.

Diagnostic endoscopy with banding or sclerotherapy: This is the most widely used initial treatment, which should be undertaken as soon as possible. It stops variceal bleeding in 80% of patients and is repeated at intervals until varices are obliterated. Banding has largely replaced sclerotherapy, as it is less likely to cause perforation and stricture. Active bleeding at endoscopy may make endoscopic therapy difficult, and endotracheal intubation may be required to protect the airway.

Balloon tamponade: This technique employs a Sengstaken–Blakemore tube possessing two balloons that exert pressure in the fundus of the stomach and in the lower oesophagus, respectively. Additional lumens allow aspiration from the stomach and from the oesophagus above the oesophageal balloon. Endotracheal intubation prior to tube insertion reduces the risk of aspiration. Gentle traction is essential to maintain pressure on the varices. Initially, only the gastric balloon should be inflated with 200–250 mL of air, as this will usually control bleeding. Inadvertent inflation of the gastric balloon in the oesophagus causes pain and can lead to oesophageal rupture. If the oesophageal balloon needs to be used because of continued bleeding, it should be deflated for 10 mins every 3 hrs to avoid oesophageal mucosal damage. Pressure in the oesophageal balloon is maintained at <40 mmHg using a sphygmomanometer. Balloon tamponade will almost always stop variceal bleeding, but only creates time for the use of definitive therapy.

TIPSS: This technique uses a stent placed between the portal vein and the hepatic vein within the liver to provide a portosystemic shunt and therefore reduce portal pressure. It is carried out under radiological control via the internal jugular vein; prior patency of the portal vein must be determined angiographically, coagulation deficiencies may require correction with fresh frozen plasma, and antibiotic cover is provided. Successful shunt placement stops and prevents variceal bleeding. Further bleeding necessitates investigation and treatment (e.g. angioplasty) because it is usually associated with shunt narrowing or occlusion. Hepatic encephalopathy may occur following TIPSS and is managed by reducing the shunt diameter. Although TIPSS is associated with less rebleeding than endoscopic therapy, survival is not improved.

Portosystemic shunt surgery: Surgery prevents recurrent bleeding but carries a high mortality and often leads to encephalopathy. In practice, portosystemic shunts are now reserved for situations where other treatments have not been successful and are offered only to those with good liver function.

Oesophageal transection: Rarely, surgical transection of the varices may be performed as a last resort when bleeding cannot be controlled by other means, but operative mortality is high.

Secondary prevention of variceal bleeding

Beta-blockers are used as a secondary measure to prevent recurrent variceal bleeding. Following successful treatment by endoscopic therapy, patients should be entered into an oesophageal banding programme with repeated sessions of therapy at 1- to 2-wk intervals until the varices are obliterated. In selected individuals, TIPSS may also be considered in this setting.

Congestive gastropathy

Long-standing portal hypertension causes chronic gastric congestion, recognisable at endoscopy as multiple areas of punctate erythema. These areas may become eroded, causing bleeding from multiple sites. Acute bleeding can occur, but repeated minor bleeding causing iron-deficiency anaemia is more common. Reduction of the portal pressure using propranolol is the best initial treatment. If this is ineffective, TIPSS can be undertaken.

INFECTIONS AND THE LIVER

Viral hepatitis

This must be considered in anyone presenting with hepatitic liver blood tests (high transaminases). Hepatitis viruses (Box 13.10) are the most common cause, with cytomegalovirus, Epstein–Barr, herpes simplex and yellow fever giving rise to occasional cases. All these viruses cause illnesses with similar clinical and pathological features, which are frequently anicteric or even asymptomatic. They differ in their tendency to cause acute and chronic infections.

i 13.10 **Features of the main hepatitis viruses**

	Hepatitis A	Hepatitis B	Hepatitis C	Hepatitis D	Hepatitis E
Virus					
Group	Enterovirus	Hepadna virus	Flavivirus	Incomplete virus	Calicivirus
Nucleic acid	RNA	DNA	RNA	RNA	RNA
Size (diameter)	27 nm	42 nm	30–38 nm	35 nm	27 nm
Incubation (wks)	2–4	4–20	2–26	6–9	3–8
Spread					
Faeces	Yes	No	No	No	Yes
Blood	Uncommon	Yes	Yes	Yes	No
Saliva	Yes	Yes	Yes	Unknown	Unknown
Sexual	Uncommon	Yes	Uncommon	Yes	Unknown
Vertical	No	Yes	Uncommon	Yes	No
Chronic infection	No	Yes	Yes	Yes	No
Prevention					
Active	Vaccine	Vaccine	No	Prevented by hepatitis B vaccination	No
Passive	Immune serum globulin	Hyper-immune serum globulin	No		No

Note All body fluids are potentially infectious, although some (e.g. urine) are less infectious than others.

Clinical features of acute infection

Prodromal symptoms (headache, myalgia, arthralgia, nausea and anorexia) usually precede jaundice by a few days to 2 wks. Vomiting and diarrhoea may follow and abdominal discomfort is common. Dark urine and pale stools may precede jaundice. There are usually few physical signs. The liver is often tender but only minimally enlarged. Occasionally, mild splenomegaly and cervical lymphad-enopathy are seen. Jaundice may be mild and the diagnosis may be suspected only after finding abnormal liver blood tests in the setting of non-specific symptoms. Symptoms rarely last longer than 3–6 wks, and complications such as liver failure or chronic liver disease are rare.

Investigations

• Serum transaminases: a hepatitic pattern of LFTs develops, with serum transaminases typically between 200 and 2000 U/L. • Plasma bilirubin: reflects the degree of liver damage. • Alkaline phosphatase (ALP): rarely exceeds twice the upper limit of normal. • Prolongation of the prothrombin time: indicates the severity of the hepatitis but rarely exceeds 25 secs. • WCC: usually normal with a relative lymphocytosis. • Serological tests: confirm the aetiology of the infection.

Management

Most individuals do not need hospital care. Drugs such as sedatives and narcotics, which are metabolised in the liver, should be avoided. No specific dietary modifications are needed. Alcohol should be avoided during the acute illness. Elective surgery should be avoided in cases of acute viral hepatitis, as there is a risk of post-operative liver failure.

Hepatitis A

The hepatitis A virus (HAV) is highly infectious and is spread by the faecal–oral route. Infection is common in children but often asymptomatic, and so up to 30% of adults will have serological evidence of past infection but give no history of jaundice. Infection is also more common in areas of overcrowding and poor sanitation. In occasional outbreaks, water and shellfish have been the vehicles of transmission. A chronic carrier state does not occur.

Investigations

Anti-HAV IgM antibodies are diagnostic of acute HAV infection, and are present from the onset of symptoms until up to 3 mths after recovery.

Management

Infection in the community is best prevented by improving over-crowding and poor sanitation. Individuals can be given substantial protection by active immunisation with an inactivated virus vaccine. Immunisation should be considered for individuals with chronic hepatitis B or C infections and for close contacts, the elderly, those with other major disease, people travelling to endemic areas and perhaps pregnant women. Immediate protection can be provided by immune serum globulin if given soon after exposure to the virus.

Acute liver failure complicates acute hepatitis A in only 0.1% of cases; however, HAV infection in patients with chronic liver disease may cause serious or life-threatening disease.

Hepatitis B

The hepatitis B virus (HBV) consists of a core surrounded by surface protein. The virus and an excess of its surface protein (known as hepatitis B surface antigen, HBsAg) circulate in the blood. Humans are the only source of infection. Hepatitis B infection affects 300 million people and is one of the most common causes of chronic liver disease and hepatocellular carcinoma worldwide. The natural history of HBV infection is shown in Figure 13.6. Hepatitis B may cause an acute hepatitis but infection is frequently asymptomatic, particularly neonatal infection. The risk of progression to chronic disease depends on the source and timing of infection, and is greatest with vertical transmission from mother to child. Chronic hepatitis may lead to cirrhosis or hepatocellular carcinoma, after many decades.

Investigations

Serology: In acute infection HBsAg is a reliable marker of HBV infection (Fig. 13.7). Antibody to HBsAg (anti-HBs) appears after about 3–6 mths and persists for many years or even permanently. Anti-HBs implies either a previous infection, in which case anti-HBc (see below) is usually also present; or previous vaccination, when anti-HBc is not present.

The hepatitis B core antigen (HBcAg) is not found in the blood but antibody to it (anti-HBc) appears early in the illness. Anti-HBc is initially of IgM type, with IgG antibody appearing later.

The hepatitis B e antigen (HBeAg) is an indicator of active viral replication. It appears only transiently at the outset of the illness and is followed by the production of antibody (anti-HBe). Chronic HBV infection (see below) is marked by the persistence of HBsAg and anti-HBc (IgG) in the blood. Usually, HBeAg or anti-HBe is also present. Interpretation of serological tests is shown in Box 13.11.

Viral load: HBV-DNA can be measured by PCR in the blood. Viral loads are usually $>10^5$ copies/mL in the presence of active viral replication, as indicated by the presence of e antigen. In contrast, in those with low viral replication, HBsAg- and anti-HBe-positive, viral loads are usually $<10^5$ copies/mL. High viral loads are also found in e antigen-negative chronic hepatitis, which occurs in the Far East and is due to a mutation.

Management

Acute hepatitis B: Treatment is supportive, with monitoring for acute liver failure, which occurs in <1% of cases.

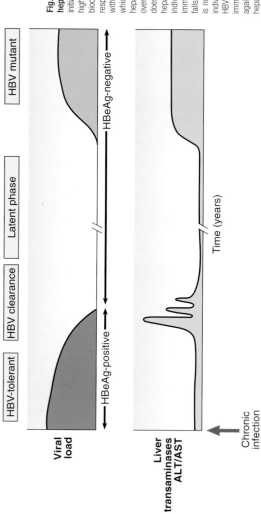

Fig. 13.6 Natural history of chronic hepatitis B infection. There is an initial immunotolerant phase with high levels of virus and normal liver biochemistry. An immunological response to the virus then occurs, with elevation in serum transaminases, which causes liver damage: chronic hepatitis. If this response is sustained over many years and viral clearance does not occur promptly, chronic hepatitis may result in cirrhosis. In individuals who mount a successful immunological response, viral load falls, HBe antibody develops and there is no further liver damage. Some individuals may subsequently develop HBV-DNA mutants, which escape from immune regulation, and viral load again rises with further chronic hepatitis. Mutations in the core protein result in the virus's inability to secrete HBe antigen despite high levels of viral replication; such individuals have HBeAg-negative chronic hepatitis. (ALT = alanine aminotransferase; AST = aspartate aminotransferase.)

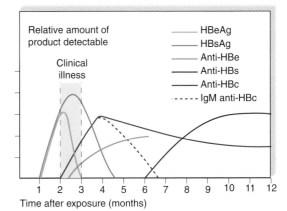

Fig. 13.7 Serological responses to hepatitis B virus infection. (HBsAg = hepatitis B surface antigen; anti-HBs = antibody to HBsAg; HBeAg = hepatitis B e antigen; anti-HBe = antibody to HBeAg; anti-HBc = antibody to hepatitis B core antigen.)

13.11 How to interpret the serological tests of acute hepatitis B virus infection

Interpretation	HBsAg	Anti-HBc IgM	Anti-HBc IgG	Anti-HBs
Incubation period	+	+	−	−
Acute hepatitis				
Early	+	+	−	−
Established	+	+	+	−
Established (occasional)	−	+	+	−
Convalescence				
(3–6 mths)	−	±	+	±
(6–9 mths)	−	−	+	+
Post-infection	−	−	+	±
Immunisation without infection	−	−	−	+
+ positive; − negative; ± present at low titre or absent.				

Chronic hepatitis B: This develops in 5–10% of acute cases and is lifelong. No drug is consistently able to render patients HBsAg-negative.

Lamivudine and tenofovir are both effective, but viral mutations causing resistance commonly develop. Tenofovir also has anti-HIV efficacy, so monotherapy should be avoided in HIV co-infected patients to prevent HIV antiviral drug resistance. Interferon alfa is most effective in patients with low viral load and high transaminases, in whom it acts by augmenting a native immune response. Interferon is contraindicated in the presence of cirrhosis, as it may precipitate liver failure. Longer-acting pegylated interferons, which can be given once weekly, have been evaluated in both HBeAg-positive and HBeAg-negative chronic hepatitis.

The use of post-liver transplant prophylaxis with lamivudine and hepatitis B immunoglobulins has reduced the re-infection rate to 10% and increased 5-yr survival to 80%, making transplantation an acceptable treatment option.

Prevention

Individuals are most infectious when markers of continuing viral replication, such as HBeAg, and high levels of HBV-DNA are present in the blood. HBV-DNA can be found in saliva, urine, semen and vaginal secretions. The virus is about ten times more infectious than hepatitis C, which in turn is about ten times more infectious than HIV. Recombinant hepatitis B vaccines containing HBsAg are available which are capable of producing active immunisation in 95% of normal individuals. Infection can also be prevented or minimised by the IM injection of hyperimmune serum globulin prepared from blood containing anti-HBs. This should be given within 24 hrs, or at most a week, of exposure to infected blood in circumstances likely to cause infection (e.g. needlestick injury, contamination of cuts or mucous membranes).

Neonates born to hepatitis B-infected mothers should be immunised at birth and given immunoglobulin.

Hepatitis D (delta virus)

The hepatitis D virus (HDV) is an RNA-defective virus that has no independent existence; it requires HBV for replication. It can infect individuals simultaneously with HBV, or can superinfect those who are already chronic carriers of HBV. Simultaneous infections give rise to acute hepatitis, which is often severe but is limited by recovery from the HBV infection. Infections in individuals who are chronic carriers of HBV can cause acute hepatitis with spontaneous recovery, and occasionally simultaneous cessation of the chronic HBV infection takes place. Chronic infection with HBV and HDV can also occur, and this frequently causes rapidly progressive chronic hepatitis and eventually cirrhosis.

HDV has a worldwide distribution. It is endemic in parts of the Mediterranean basin, Africa and South America, where transmission is mainly by close personal contact; occasionally, vertical transmission occurs from mothers who also carry HBV. In non-endemic areas, transmission is mainly a consequence of parenteral drug misuse.

HDV contains a single antigen to which infected individuals make an antibody (anti-HDV). Diagnosis depends on detecting anti-HDV. This antibody generally disappears within 2 mths but persists in a few patients.

Hepatitis C

This is caused by an RNA flavivirus. Acute symptomatic infection with hepatitis C virus (HCV) is rare. Infection occurs with IV drug misuse (95% of new UK cases), needlestick injury, unscreened blood products, vertical transmission or through sharing toothbrushes or razors. Most individuals will be unaware of becoming infected and are only identified when they develop chronic liver disease. Eighty per cent of individuals exposed to the virus will become chronically infected. Hepatitis C infection is usually identified in asymptomatic individuals screened because they have risk factors for infection, or incidentally discovered via abnormal liver blood tests.

Investigations

It may take 6–12 wks for antibodies to appear in the blood following acute infection such as a needlestick injury. In these cases, hepatitis C RNA can be identified in the blood as early as 2–4 wks after infection. Active infection is confirmed by the presence of serum hepatitis C RNA in anyone who is antibody-positive. LFTs may be normal or show fluctuating serum transaminases with ALT between 50 and 200 U/L. Jaundice only usually appears in end-stage cirrhosis. Serum transaminase levels in hepatitis C are a poor predictor of the degree of liver fibrosis that has developed as a result of chronic viral hepatitis, and so a liver biopsy is often required to stage the degree of liver damage.

Management

The aim of treatment is to eradicate infection. Until recently, the treatment of choice was dual therapy with pegylated interferon-alfa given weekly SC, together with oral ribavirin, a synthetic nucleotide analogue. The length of treatment and efficacy depend on viral genotype. The main side-effect of ribavirin is haemolytic anaemia. Side-effects of interferon are significant and include flu-like symptoms, irritability and depression. Recently, triple therapy with the addition of protease inhibitors (e.g. telaprevir) has increased the rate of sustained virological response (defined as loss of virus from serum 6 mths after completing therapy). Liver transplantation should be considered when complications of cirrhosis occur. Unfortunately, hepatitis C almost always recurs in the transplanted liver.

Prevention and prognosis

There is no active or passive protection against HCV. Not everyone with hepatitis C infection will necessarily develop cirrhosis but ~20% do so within 20 yrs. Once cirrhosis is present, 2–5%/yr will develop primary hepatocellular carcinoma.

Hepatitis E

Hepatitis E is caused by an RNA virus that is endemic in India and the Middle East, and occurs occasionally in northern Europe. The clinical presentation of hepatitis E is similar to that of hepatitis A. It is spread via the faecal–oral route; in most cases, it presents as a self-limiting acute hepatitis and does not cause chronic liver disease. It differs from hepatitis A in that infection during pregnancy is associated with the development of acute liver failure, which has a high mortality. In acute infection, IgM antibodies to HEV are positive.

Other forms of viral hepatitis

Cytomegalovirus and Epstein–Barr virus infection causes abnormal LFTs in most patients, and occasionally icteric hepatitis occurs. Herpes simplex may cause hepatitis in immunocompromised adults. Abnormal LFTs are also common in chickenpox, measles, rubella and acute HIV infection.

HIV infection and the liver

This is covered on page 127.

Liver abscesses

Liver abscesses can be classified as pyogenic, hydatid or amoebic.

Pyogenic liver abscess

Pyogenic liver abscesses are uncommon but important because they are potentially curable, carry significant risk if untreated, and are easily overlooked.

Infection reaches the liver through the hepatic or portal circulation, up the biliary tree, via injury or by direct spread from adjacent organs. Abscesses most commonly occur in older patients through ascending infection due to biliary obstruction (cholangitis) or contiguous spread from an empyema of the gallbladder. Immunocompromised patients are particularly likely to develop liver abscesses. *E. coli* and various streptococci, particularly *Strep. milleri*, are the most common organisms; anaerobes, including streptococci and *Bacteroides*, may be found when infection has spread from large bowel pathology via the portal vein.

Clinical features

Patients are generally ill with fever, sometimes rigors and weight loss. Abdominal pain in the right upper quadrant, sometimes radiating to the right shoulder, is the most common symptom. The pain may be pleuritic in nature. Hepatomegaly, often with tenderness to percussion, occurs in more than half of patients. Mild jaundice may be present but is severe only when large abscesses cause biliary obstruction. Atypical presentations are common and a gradual onset of pyrexia of unknown origin without localising features may lead to the diagnosis being missed.

Investigations

• USS: reveals 90% or more of symptomatic abscesses and is also used to guide needle aspiration of pus for culture. • Leucocytosis: frequently found. • Plasma ALP activity: usually increased. • Serum albumin: often low. • CXR: may show a raised right diaphragm and lung collapse or an effusion at the base of the right lung. • Blood cultures: positive in 50–80%. • Colonic pathology: should be excluded.

Management and prognosis

Pending the results of culture of blood and pus from the abscess, treatment should commence with a combination of antibiotics such as ampicillin, gentamicin and metronidazole. Aspiration or drainage with a catheter placed in the abscess under USS guidance is required if the abscess is large or if it does not respond to antibiotics. Surgical drainage is rarely required.

The mortality of liver abscesses is 20–40%; failure to make the diagnosis is the most common cause of death. Older patients and those with multiple abscesses also have a higher mortality.

Hydatid cysts and amoebic liver abscesses

These are covered elsewhere (pp. 120 and 111).

ALCOHOLIC LIVER DISEASE

The risk of alcoholic liver disease (ALD) is variable; not everyone who drinks heavily will develop it. A threshold of 14 U/wk in women and 21 U/wk in men is generally considered safe (1 unit = 8 g of ethanol) and risk of ALD begins at around 30 g/day. Although the average alcohol consumption of an individual with cirrhosis is 160 g/day for 8 yrs, there is no clear relationship between dose and liver damage.

Risk factors include:

• Drinking patterns: ALD occurs more in continuous rather than binge drinkers. • Gender: women are at higher risk for a given intake due to their lower volume of distribution. • Genetics: alcoholism is more common in monozygotic than dizygotic twins. • Nutrition: obesity increases the incidence of liver-related death fivefold in heavy drinkers.

Clinical features

Three clinical syndromes occur, with some overlap:

• Alcoholic fatty liver: abnormal liver biochemistry and hepatomegaly. This has a good prognosis; steatosis usually disappears after 3 mths of abstinence. • Alcoholic hepatitis: jaundice, malnutrition, hepatomegaly, portal hypertension. The 5-yr survival is 70% in those who abstain, and 34% in continued drinkers. • Alcoholic cirrhosis: often presents with a serious complication, such as variceal haemorrhage or ascites, and only half of such patients will survive 5 yrs from presentation.

Investigations

A drinking history should be taken from the patient, relatives and friends. Macrocytosis without anaemia may suggest alcohol misuse. Raised γ-glutamyl transferase (GGT) is not specific for alcohol misuse and is also elevated in NAFLD; it may not return to normal with abstinence. Jaundice suggests alcoholic hepatitis. Prothrombin time and bilirubin can be used to give a 'discriminant function' (DF, Maddrey's score), which predicts prognosis in alcoholic hepatitis:

$$DF = [4.6 \times \text{Increase in PT (sec)}] + \text{bilirubin (mg/dL)}$$

A value >32 implies severe liver disease with a poor prognosis. (Divide bilirubin in µmol/L by 17 to convert to mg/dL.)

Management

Cessation of alcohol consumption is the most important treatment; without this, other therapies are of limited value. Abstinence is even effective at preventing progression of liver disease and death when cirrhosis is present. Good nutrition is very important and enteral feeding via a fine-bore nasogastric tube may be needed in severely ill patients. Corticosteroids increase survival in patients with severe alcoholic hepatitis (Maddrey's score >32), but sepsis and varices are contraindications to steroids. Pentoxifylline, which has a weak anti-TNF action, may be beneficial in severe alcoholic hepatitis. It appears to reduce the incidence of hepatorenal failure without increasing sepsis. In many centres, alcoholic liver disease is a common indication for liver transplantation. The challenge is to identify patients with an unacceptable risk of returning to harmful alcohol consumption. Many programmes require 6 mths of abstinence from alcohol before a patient is considered for transplantation. Although this relates poorly to the incidence of alcohol relapse after transplantation, liver function may improve to the extent that transplantation becomes unnecessary. Transplantation for alcoholic hepatitis has a poorer outcome than for complications of alcoholic cirrhosis and is seldom performed.

NON-ALCOHOLIC FATTY LIVER DISEASE

Non-alcoholic fatty liver disease (NAFLD) is a disease of affluent societies and its prevalence is increasing in proportion to the rise in obesity. It can be classified into simple fatty infiltration (steatosis), fat and inflammation (non-alcoholic steatohepatitis, or NASH) and cirrhosis in the absence of excessive alcohol consumption. Simple steatosis does not cause morbidity, while NASH is linked to progressive fibrosis, cirrhosis and liver cancer. NAFLD is strongly associated with obesity, dyslipidaemia, insulin resistance and type 2 diabetes mellitus, and so may be considered to be the hepatic manifestation of the 'metabolic syndrome' (p. 385). It affects 6–15% of apparently healthy living liver-donors in the USA.

Clinical features

Most patients present with asymptomatic abnormal LFTs, particularly elevation of the transaminases or isolated elevation of the GGT. Occasionally, disease presents with a complication of cirrhosis, such as variceal bleeding. Risk factors include:
• Age >45. • Type 2 diabetes. • Obesity (BMI >30). • Hypertension.

Investigations

Alternative causes, including alcohol and viral hepatitis, should first be excluded.

LFTs: Unlike in alcoholic liver disease, alanine aminotransferase (ALT) is normally higher than aspartate aminotransferase (AST) in the early stages. It is important to differentiate simple fatty liver disease, which does not require follow-up, from NASH. Transaminases greater than twice the upper limit of normal and the presence of the metabolic syndrome are useful predictors of NASH. Higher echogenicity on USS indicates raised hepatic fat, but no routine imaging modality can distinguish steatosis from NASH.

Liver biopsy: This remains the gold standard for assessing the degree of inflammation and the extent of liver fibrosis.

Management and prognosis
Current treatment comprises lifestyle interventions to promote weight loss and improve insulin sensitivity through dietary changes and physical exercise. Sustained weight reduction of 7–10% causes significant biochemical and histological improvement in NASH.

No drugs are currently licensed specifically for NASH. Treatment of coexisting metabolic disorders, such as dyslipidaemia and hypertension, should be given. Specific insulin-sensitising agents, in particular glitazones, may help selected patients.

AUTOIMMUNE LIVER DISEASES

Autoimmune hepatitis
Autoimmune hepatitis is a liver disease of unknown aetiology, characterised by autoantibodies, autoimmune T cells, hypergammaglobulinaemia and a strong association with other autoimmune diseases (Box 13.12). It occurs most often in women, particularly in the second and third decades of life, but may develop in either sex at any age.

Clinical features
The onset is usually insidious, with fatigue, anorexia and jaundice. In about one-quarter of patients, the onset is acute, resembling viral

13.12 Conditions associated with autoimmune hepatitis

- Migrating polyarthritis
- Urticarial rashes
- Lymphadenopathy
- Hashimoto's thyroiditis
- Thyrotoxicosis
- Myxoedema
- Ulcerative colitis
- Coombs-positive haemolytic anaemia
- Pleurisy
- Transient pulmonary infiltrates
- Glomerulonephritis
- Nephrotic syndrome

Disease	Antinuclear antibody (%)	Anti-smooth muscle antibody (%)	Antimitochondrial antibody*
Healthy controls	5	1.5	0.01
Autoimmune hepatitis	80	70	15
Primary biliary cirrhosis	25	35	95
Cryptogenic cirrhosis	40	30	15

13.13 Frequency of autoantibodies in chronic non-viral liver diseases and in healthy people

*Patients with antimitochondrial antibody frequently have cholestatic LFTs and may have primary biliary cirrhosis (see text).

hepatitis, but resolution does not occur. This acute presentation can lead to extensive liver necrosis and liver failure. Other features include fever, arthralgia, vitiligo, epistaxis and amenorrhoea. Jaundice is mild to moderate or occasionally absent, but signs of chronic liver disease, especially spider naevi and hepatosplenomegaly, can be present. Associated autoimmune disease, such as Hashimoto's thyroiditis or rheumatoid arthritis, is often present and can modulate the clinical presentation.

Investigations

• Serology: often reveals autoantibodies (Box 13.13) but these are non-specific and occur in health and other diseases. Antimicrosomal antibodies (anti-LKM) occur, particularly in children and adolescents. • Elevated serum IgG: diagnostically helpful but may be absent. • Liver biopsy: typically shows interface hepatitis, with or without cirrhosis.

Management

Treatment with corticosteroids is life-saving in autoimmune hepatitis. Initially, prednisolone 40 mg/day is given orally; the dose is then gradually reduced as the patient and LFTs improve. Maintenance therapy of azathioprine, with or without low-dose prednisolone, is given once LFTs are normal. Exacerbations should be treated with corticosteroids. Although treatment can significantly reduce the rate of progression to cirrhosis, end-stage disease can still occur despite treatment.

Primary biliary cirrhosis

Primary biliary cirrhosis (PBC) is a chronic, progressive cholestatic liver disease of unknown cause, which predominantly affects middle-aged women. It is strongly associated with antimitochondrial antibodies (AMA), which are diagnostic. Granulomatous inflammation of the portal tracts occurs, leading to progressive fibrosis and cirrhosis. It is associated with smoking and occurs in clusters, suggesting an environmental trigger in susceptible individuals.

Clinical features

Non-specific symptoms, such as lethargy and arthralgia, are common and may precede diagnosis for years. Pruritus is the most common initial complaint and may precede jaundice by months or years. Bone pain or fractures can rarely result from osteomalacia (fat-soluble vitamin malabsorption) or from accelerated osteoporosis (hepatic osteodystrophy).

Initially, patients are well nourished but considerable weight loss can occur as the disease progresses. Scratch marks may be found. Jaundice is a late feature and can become intense. Xanthomatous deposits occur in a minority, especially around the eyes, in the hand creases and over the elbows, knees and buttocks. Mild hepatomegaly is common and splenomegaly becomes increasingly common as portal hypertension develops. Liver failure may supervene.

Autoimmune and connective tissue diseases occur with increased frequency in PBC, particularly Sjögren's syndrome (p. 594), systemic sclerosis, coeliac disease (p. 443) and thyroid diseases.

Diagnosis and investigations

• LFTs: show the pattern of cholestasis. • Hypercholesterolaemia: common but non-specific. • AMA: present in >95% of patients; when absent, the diagnosis should not be made without biopsy and cholangiography (MRCP or ERCP) to exclude other biliary disease. • USS: shows no sign of biliary obstruction.

Management

The hydrophilic bile acid, ursodeoxycholic acid (UDCA), improves bile flow, replaces toxic hydrophobic bile acids in the bile acid pool, and reduces apoptosis of the biliary epithelium. It improves LFTs, may slow down histological and clinical progression, and has few side-effects.

Liver transplantation should be considered once liver failure has developed and may be indicated in patients with intractable pruritus. Transplantation is associated with an excellent 5-yr survival of >80%, although late recurrence can occur.

Pruritus: This is best treated with the anion-binding resin colestyramine, which probably acts by binding potential pruritogens in the intestine and increasing their excretion in the stool. Alternative treatments for pruritus include rifampicin, naltrexone (an opioid antagonist), plasmapheresis and a liver support device (e.g. a molecular adsorbent recirculating system (MARS) machine).

Fatigue: This affects about one-third of patients with PBC. Unfortunately, once depression and hypothyroidism have been excluded, there is no treatment.

Malabsorption: Cholestasis is associated with steatorrhoea and malabsorption of fat-soluble vitamins, which should be replaced as necessary.

| 13.14 Diseases associated with primary sclerosing cholangitis |

- Ulcerative colitis
- Crohn's colitis
- Chronic pancreatitis
- Retroperitoneal fibrosis
- Riedel's thyroiditis
- Retro-orbital tumour
- Immune deficiency states
- Sjögren's syndrome
- Angio-immunoplastic lymphadenopathy
- Histiocytosis X
- Autoimmune haemolytic anaemia
- Autoimmune pancreatitis

Osteopenia and osteoporosis: These are common and should be treated with replacement calcium and vitamin D_3. Bisphosphonates should be used if there is evidence of osteoporosis.

Primary sclerosing cholangitis

Primary sclerosing cholangitis (PSC) is a cholestatic liver disease caused by diffuse inflammation and fibrosis that can involve the entire biliary tree. It leads to the gradual obliteration of intrahepatic and extrahepatic bile ducts, and ultimately biliary cirrhosis, portal hypertension and hepatic failure. Cholangiocarcinoma develops in ~10–30% of patients during the course of the disease.

PSC is twice as common in young men. Most patients present at age 25–40 yrs. There is a close association with inflammatory bowel disease, particularly ulcerative colitis (Box 13.14).

The diagnostic criteria are:

• Generalised beading and stenosis of the biliary system on cholangiography. • Absence of choledocholithiasis (or history of bile duct surgery). • Exclusion of bile duct cancer, by prolonged follow-up.

Clinical features

The diagnosis is often made incidentally when persistently raised serum ALP is discovered in an individual with ulcerative colitis. Symptoms include fatigue, intermittent jaundice, weight loss, right upper quadrant abdominal pain and pruritus. Physical signs, most commonly jaundice and hepatomegaly/splenomegaly, are present in only 50% of symptomatic patients.

Investigations

Serum biochemical tests: These usually indicate cholestasis. However, ALP and bilirubin levels vary widely in individual patients during the course of the disease, sometimes spontaneously, sometimes with therapy. In addition to ANCA, low titres of serum ANA and anti-smooth muscle antibodies have been found in PSC but have no diagnostic significance.

Radiology: The key investigation is now MRCP, which is usually diagnostic, revealing multiple irregular stricturing and dilatation. ERCP should be reserved for patients in whom therapeutic intervention is likely to be necessary and should follow MRCP.

Histology: The characteristic early features of PSC are periductal 'onion-skin' fibrosis and inflammation.

Management and prognosis

There is no cure for PSC, but cholestasis and its complications should be treated. UDCA is widely used, although evidence of effect is limited.

The course of PSC is variable. In symptomatic patients, median survival from presentation to death or liver transplantation is ~12 yrs. About 75% of asymptomatic patients survive for more than 15 yrs. Most die from liver failure, ~30% from cholangiocarcinoma, and the remainder from colonic cancer or complications of colitis. Immunosuppressive agents (prednisolone, azathioprine, methotrexate, ciclosporin) have been tried but with generally disappointing results.

Pruritus is treated with colestyramine. Broad-spectrum antibiotics (e.g. ciprofloxacin) should be given for acute cholangitis but do not prevent attacks. If cholangiography shows a well-defined extrahepatic bile duct obstruction, and cholangiocarcinoma has been excluded, balloon dilatation or stenting at ERCP is indicated. Fat-soluble vitamin replacement is necessary in jaundiced patients. Metabolic bone disease (usually osteoporosis) should be treated (p. 599).

Surgical biliary reconstruction has a limited role in non-cirrhotic patients with dominant extrahepatic disease. Transplantation is the only surgical option in patients with advanced liver disease, but is contraindicated if cholangiocarcinoma is present. Colon carcinoma is increased in patients following transplant because of immune suppression, and enhanced surveillance should be instituted.

LIVER TUMOURS

Hepatocellular carcinoma

Hepatocellular carcinoma (HCC) is the most common primary liver tumour. Cirrhosis is present in 75–90% of individuals with HCC and is an important risk factor. The risk is between 1% and 5% in cirrhosis caused by hepatitis B and C. Risk is also increased in cirrhosis due to haemochromatosis, alcohol, NASH and α_1-antitrypsin deficiency. In northern Europe, 90% of HCC patients have underlying cirrhosis, compared with 30% in Taiwan, where hepatitis B is the main cause.

Clinical features

Many tumours are asymptomatic and discovered on screening of high-risk patients. In patients with cirrhosis, HCC may cause variceal haemorrhage, increasing ascites or deterioration in jaundice and LFTs. Other symptoms include weight loss, anorexia and abdominal pain. Examination may reveal hepatomegaly or a right hypochondrial mass.

Investigations

Alpha-fetoprotein (AFP) is produced by 60% of hepatocellular carcinomas, but is also raised in active hepatitis B and C and in acute hepatic necrosis, e.g. paracetamol toxicity. Combinations of USS and CT or MRI are recommended for sizing and staging, as imaging is difficult in cirrhotic liver. Biopsy is advisable to confirm the diagnosis and exclude metastatic tumour in patients with large tumours who do not have cirrhosis or hepatitis B. Biopsy is avoided in patients eligible for transplantation or resection because of a small risk of tumour seeding along the needle tract.

High-risk patients with cirrhosis should be screened 6-monthly with USS and AFP to detect HCC.

Management

Hepatic resection: This is the treatment of choice for non-cirrhotic patients. The 5-yr survival in this group is ~50%. However, there is a 50% recurrence rate at 5 yrs.

Liver transplantation: In the presence of cirrhosis, transplantation has the benefit of curing the cirrhosis and removing the risk of a second de novo tumour.

Percutaneous ablation: Percutaneous ethanol injection into the tumour under USS guidance is efficacious (80% cure rate) for tumours ≤3 cm. Recurrence rates (50% at 3 yrs) are similar to those following surgical resection.

Chemo-embolisation: Hepatic artery embolisation with Gelfoam and doxorubicin yields survival rates of 60% in cirrhotic patients with unresectable HCC and good liver function (compared with 20% in untreated patients) at 2 yrs. Unfortunately, any survival benefit is lost at 4 yrs.

Chemotherapy with sorafenib for advanced disease is under investigation.

Fibrolamellar hepatocellular carcinoma

This rare variant occurs in young adults, in the absence of hepatitis B infection and cirrhosis. The tumours are often large at presentation and the AFP is usually normal. Treatment is by surgical resection.

Secondary malignant tumours

The primary neoplasm (most commonly of the lung, breast or abdomen) is asymptomatic in about half of patients with liver metastases. There is hepatomegaly and weight loss; jaundice may be present. Ascitic fluid, if present, has a high protein content and may be blood-stained; cytology sometimes reveals malignant cells. Hepatic resection can improve survival for slow-growing tumours such as colonic carcinomas.

DRUGS AND THE LIVER

Types of liver injury

Cholestasis: Chlorpromazine, antibiotics (e.g. flucloxacillin) and anabolic steroids cause cholestatic hepatitis, with inflammation and canalicular injury. Co-amoxiclav is the most common antibiotic to cause abnormal LFTs but it may not produce symptoms until 10–42 days after it is stopped.

Hepatocyte necrosis: Paracetamol (p. 36) is the best-known cause. Inflammation is not always present but does accompany necrosis in liver injury due to diclofenac (an NSAID) and isoniazid (an anti-TB drug). Acute hepatocellular necrosis has also been described following the use of cocaine, ecstasy and herbal remedies, including germander, comfrey and jin bu huan.

Steatosis: Tetracyclines and sodium valproate cause microvesicular steatosis; amiodarone toxicity can produce a similar histological picture to NASH.

Hepatic fibrosis: Most drugs cause reversible liver injury, and hepatic fibrosis is very uncommon. Methotrexate, however, as well as causing acute liver injury when it is started, can lead to cirrhosis when used in high doses over a long period of time.

INHERITED LIVER DISEASES

Haemochromatosis

In haemochromatosis, total body iron is increased and excess iron is deposited in and damages several organs, including the liver. It may be primary, or secondary to iatrogenic or dietary iron overload or other rare diseases.

Hereditary haemochromatosis

Hereditary haemochromatosis (HHC) is an autosomal recessive condition that results in increased absorption of dietary iron, such that total body iron may reach 20–60 g (normally 4 g). Approximately 90% of patients have a single-point mutation (C282Y) in a protein (HFE). Iron loss in menstruation and pregnancy may delay the onset in females.

Clinical features

The important organs involved are the liver, pancreatic islets, endocrine glands and heart. Symptomatic disease usually presents in men aged ≥40 yrs with features of hepatic cirrhosis (especially hepatomegaly), diabetes mellitus or heart failure. Fatigue and arthropathy are early symptoms. Leaden-grey skin pigmentation due to excess melanin occurs, especially in exposed parts, axillae, groins and genitalia: 'bronzed diabetes'. Impotence, loss of libido, testicular atrophy and arthritis are common. Cardiac failure or dysrhythmia may complicate heart muscle disease.

Investigations

• Serum ferritin: greatly increased • Plasma iron: also increased, with saturated plasma iron-binding capacity. • Liver biopsy: used to confirm the diagnosis. The iron content of the liver can be measured directly. • Genetic testing: identifies the common mutations.

Management and prognosis

Weekly venesection of 500 mL blood (250 mg iron) is performed until the serum iron is normal; this may take ≥2 yrs. Thereafter, venesection is continued as required to keep the serum ferritin normal. Liver and cardiac problems improve after iron removal but diabetes mellitus does not resolve. First-degree relatives should be screened.

Pre-cirrhotic patients with HHC have a normal life expectancy and three-quarters of cirrhotic patients are alive 5 yrs after diagnosis. Screening for hepatocellular carcinoma (p. 507) is mandatory because this affects about one-third of patients with cirrhosis, irrespective of therapy.

Secondary haemochromatosis

Many conditions, including chronic haemolytic disorders, sideroblastic anaemia, other conditions requiring multiple blood transfusion (generally >50 L), porphyria cutanea tarda, dietary iron overload and occasionally alcoholic cirrhosis, are associated with widespread secondary siderosis.

Wilson's disease

Wilson's disease (hepatolenticular degeneration) is a rare but important autosomal recessive disorder of copper metabolism. Normally, dietary copper is absorbed from the stomach and proximal small intestine, and is rapidly taken into the liver, where it is stored and incorporated into caeruloplasmin, which is secreted into the blood. The accumulation of excessive copper in the body is prevented by its excretion, most importantly via the bile. Wilson's disease is usually caused by a failure of synthesis of caeruloplasmin. The amount of copper in the body at birth is normal, but thereafter it increases steadily; the organs most affected are the liver, basal ganglia of the brain, eyes, kidneys and skeleton.

Clinical features

Symptoms usually appear between the ages of 5 and 45 yrs. Acute hepatitis, sometimes recurrent, can occur, especially in children, and may progress to fulminant liver failure. Chronic hepatitis can develop insidiously and eventually present with established cirrhosis. Neurological effects include extrapyramidal features, particularly tremor, choreoathetosis, dystonia, parkinsonism and dementia (p. 621). Unusual clumsiness for age may be an early symptom. Kayser–Fleischer rings (greenish-brown discoloration of the corneal margin appearing first at the upper periphery, p. 476) are the most important single clinical clue to the diagnosis and are seen in 60% of adults with Wilson's disease. They eventually disappear with treatment.

Investigations
• Low serum caeruloplasmin: the best single laboratory clue to the diagnosis. • High free serum copper concentration. • High urine copper excretion. • Very high hepatic copper content.

Management
The copper-binding agent penicillamine is the drug of choice, given orally for life. Liver transplantation is indicated for fulminant liver failure or for advanced cirrhosis with liver failure. The prognosis is excellent, provided treatment is started before there is irreversible damage. Siblings of patients should be screened.

Alpha₁-antitrypsin deficiency

Alpha₁-antitrypsin (α_1-AT) is a serine protease inhibitor (Pi) produced by the liver. The mutated PiZ protein cannot be secreted into the blood, so PiZZ homozygotes have low plasma α_1-AT concentrations and may develop hepatic and pulmonary disease (p. 280). Liver disease includes cholestatic jaundice in the neonatal period (neonatal hepatitis), which can resolve spontaneously; chronic hepatitis and cirrhosis in adults; and ultimately hepatocellular carcinoma. There are no clinical features to distinguish α_1-AT deficiency from other causes of liver disease, and the diagnosis is made from the low plasma α_1-AT concentration and the genotype. No specific treatment is available; the concurrent risk of severe early-onset emphysema means that all patients must stop smoking.

Gilbert's syndrome

This is covered on page 480.

Cystic fibrosis

Cystic fibrosis (p. 287) is sometimes associated with biliary cirrhosis, which can lead to portal hypertension and varices requiring banding. Liver failure is rare in cystic fibrosis but transplantation is occasionally required.

VASCULAR LIVER DISEASES

Hepatic arterial disease

Liver ischaemic injury is relatively common during hypotensive or hypoxic events and is under-diagnosed. Hepatic artery occlusion may result from inadvertent injury during biliary surgery or may be caused by emboli, neoplasms, polyarteritis nodosa, blunt trauma or radiation. It usually causes severe upper abdominal pain with or without circulatory shock. LFTs show a high transaminase activity. Patients usually survive if the liver and portal blood supply are otherwise normal.

Portal venous disease

Portal venous thrombosis is rare but can occur in any prothrombotic condition. Acute portal venous thrombosis causes abdominal pain and diarrhoea, and may lead to bowel infarction, requiring surgery. Patients need anticoagulation and investigation for underlying thrombophilia. Subacute thrombosis can be asymptomatic but may lead to extrahepatic portal hypertension (p. 489) later on.

Hepatopulmonary syndrome

In this condition, patients with cirrhosis and portal hypertension develop resistant hypoxaemia (PaO_2 <9.3 kPa (70 mmHg)) due to intrapulmonary shunting through direct arteriovenous communications. Clinical features include finger clubbing, spider naevi, cyanosis and a fall in SaO_2 on standing. It resolves following liver transplantation.

Portopulmonary hypertension

This is defined as pulmonary hypertension in a patient with portal hypertension. It is caused by vasoconstriction and obliteration of the pulmonary arterial system, and presents with breathlessness and fatigue.

Hepatic venous disease

Obstruction to hepatic venous blood flow can occur in the small central hepatic veins, the large hepatic veins, the inferior vena cava or the heart.

Budd–Chiari syndrome

This uncommon condition is characterised by thrombosis of the larger hepatic veins and sometimes the inferior vena cava. The cause cannot be found in about half of patients. Some have haematological disorders such as myelofibrosis, primary polycythaemia, paroxysmal nocturnal haemoglobinuria and antithrombin III, protein C or protein S deficiencies (p. 558).

Clinical features

Sudden venous occlusion causes the rapid development of upper abdominal pain, marked ascites and occasionally acute liver failure. More gradual occlusion causes gross ascites and often upper abdominal discomfort. Hepatomegaly, often with tenderness over the liver, is almost always present. Hepatic congestion affecting the centrilobular areas is followed by centrilobular fibrosis, and eventually cirrhosis in those who survive long enough.

Investigations

• LFTs: vary considerably, depending on the presentation, and can show the features of acute hepatitis (p. 494) when the onset is rapid. Ascitic fluid analysis typically shows a protein concentration >25 g/L (exudate) in the early stages. • USS, CT, MRI or venography: may demonstrate occlusion of the hepatic veins and inferior vena cava.

Management

Where recent thrombosis is suspected, thrombolysis with streptokinase followed by heparin and oral anticoagulation should be considered. Short hepatic venous strictures can be treated with angioplasty; more extensive hepatic vein occlusion can be managed by TIPSS.

Veno-occlusive disease

Widespread occlusion of central hepatic veins is the characteristic of this rare condition. Pyrrolizidine alkaloids in *Senecio* and *Heliotropium* plants used to make teas, cytotoxic drugs and hepatic irradiation are all recognised causes. The clinical features are similar to those of the Budd–Chiari syndrome (see above).

Cardiac disease

Hepatic damage due primarily to congestion may develop in all forms of right heart failure (p. 207); the clinical features are predominately cardiac. Very rarely, long-standing cardiac failure and hepatic congestion cause cardiac cirrhosis.

PREGNANCY AND THE LIVER

Acute cholestasis of pregnancy

This usually occurs in the third trimester and is associated with intrauterine growth retardation and premature birth. Presentation is with itching and cholestatic or hepatitic LFTs. Ursodeoxycholic acid (15 mg/kg daily) controls itch and prevents premature birth.

Acute fatty liver of pregnancy

This is more common in twin and first pregnancies. It typically presents between 31 and 38 wks of pregnancy with vomiting and abdominal pain followed by jaundice. In severe cases, lactic acidosis, a coagulopathy, encephalopathy, hypoglycaemia and renal failure may occur. Differentiation from toxaemia of pregnancy (which is more common) can be made by the finding of high serum uric acid levels and the absence of haemolysis. Early diagnosis and delivery of the fetus has led to a fall in maternal and perinatal mortality to 1% and 7%, respectively.

Toxaemia of pregnancy and HELLP

The HELLP syndrome (haemolysis, elevated liver enzymes and low platelets) is a variant of pre-eclampsia affecting mainly multiparous women. It presents with hypertension and proteinuria; complications include disseminated intravascular coagulation, hepatic infarction and rupture. Delivery leads to prompt resolution.

LIVER TRANSPLANTATION

The outcome following liver transplantation has improved significantly over the last decade and it is now an effective treatment for end-stage liver disease.

Indications: 71% of surgery is performed for cirrhosis, 11% for hepatocellular carcinoma, 10% for acute liver failure and 6% for metabolic diseases.

Contraindications: The main contraindications to transplantation are sepsis, extrahepatic malignancy, active alcohol or other substance misuse, and marked cardiorespiratory dysfunction.

Complications: These include primary graft non-function, acute rejection, hepatic artery thrombosis, anastomotic biliary strictures, and infections.

Outcomes: The outcome following transplantation for acute liver failure is worse than for chronic liver disease because most patients have coexisting multi-organ failure. The 1-yr survival is 65%, falling to 59% at 5 yrs. The 1-yr survival for patients with cirrhosis is >90%, falling to 70–75% at 5 yrs.

CHOLESTATIC AND BILIARY DISEASE

Gallstones

Gallstones are conveniently classified into cholesterol or pigment stones, although the majority are of mixed composition. Cholesterol stones are most common in developed countries, whereas pigment stones are more frequent in developing countries.

Cholesterol gallstones: Cholesterol is held in solution in bile by its association with bile acids and phospholipids in the form of micelles and vesicles. In gallstone disease, the liver produces bile that contains a relative excess of cholesterol ('lithogenic bile').

Pigment stones: Brown, crumbly pigment stones are almost always the consequence of bacterial or parasitic infection in the biliary tree. They are common in the Far East, where infection allows bacterial β-glucuronidase to hydrolyse conjugated bilirubin to its free form, which then precipitates as calcium bilirubinate. The mechanism of black pigment gallstone formation in developed countries is not satisfactorily explained but haemolysis is important.

Clinical features

Only 10% of people with gallstones develop clinical evidence of gallstone disease. Symptomatic gallstones (Box 13.15) cause either biliary pain ('biliary colic') or cholecystitis (see below). Typically, the pain occurs suddenly and persists for about 2 hrs; if it continues for >6 hrs, a complication such as cholecystitis or pancreatitis may be present. Pain is usually felt in the epigastrium (70% of patients) or right upper quadrant (20%) and radiates to the interscapular region or the tip of the right scapula.

13.15 Clinical features and complications of gallstones

Clinical features

- Asymptomatic
- Biliary colic
- Acute cholecystitis
- Chronic cholecystitis

Complications

- Empyema of the gallbladder
- Porcelain gallbladder
- Choledocholithiasis
- Pancreatitis
- Fistulae between the gallbladder and duodenum or colon
- Pressure on/inflammation of the common bile duct by a gallstone in the cystic duct (Mirizzi's syndrome)
- Gallstone ileus
- Cancer of the gallbladder

Investigations

• USS: the method of choice for diagnosing gallstones. • CT and MRCP: useful for detecting complications (distal bile duct stone or gallbladder empyema).

Management

Asymptomatic gallstones found incidentally should not be treated because the majority remain asymptomatic. Symptomatic gallstones are best treated by laparoscopic cholecystectomy. Small radiolucent stones causing mild symptoms may alternatively be dissolved by oral administration of ursodeoxycholic acid. Bile duct stones can be treated by shock-wave lithotripsy, endoscopic sphincterotomy with balloon trawl, or surgical exploration.

Cholecystitis
Acute cholecystitis

Acute cholecystitis is almost always associated with obstruction of the gallbladder neck or cystic duct by a gallstone. Occasionally, obstruction may be by mucus, parasitic worms or a tumour. Acalculous cholecystitis can occur in the intensive care setting.

Clinical features

The cardinal feature is severe and prolonged pain in the right upper quadrant but also in the epigastrium, the right shoulder tip or interscapular region. There is usually fever and leucocytosis. Examination shows right hypochondrial tenderness, rigidity worse on inspiration (Murphy's sign) and sometimes a gallbladder mass (in 30%). Jaundice occurs in <10% of patients and is usually due to the passage of stones in the common bile duct.

Investigations

• Leucocytosis: common. • USS: detects gallstones and gallbladder thickening due to cholecystitis. • Plasma amylase: should be measured to detect acute pancreatitis (p. 451). • Plain X-rays of the abdomen and chest: may show radio-opaque gallstones, and rarely intrabiliary gas due to fistulation of a gallstone into the intestine, and are important in excluding lower lobe pneumonia and a perforated viscus.

Management

Medical: This consists of bed rest, pain relief, antibiotics (e.g. cefuroxime and metronidazole) and maintenance of fluid balance.

Surgical: Urgent surgery is required when cholecystitis progresses in spite of medical therapy and when complications such as empyema or perforation develop. Operation should be carried out within 5 days of the onset of symptoms. Delayed surgery after 2–3 mths is no longer favoured. Recurrent biliary colic or cholecystitis is frequent if the gallbladder is not removed.

Chronic cholecystitis

Chronic inflammation of the gallbladder is almost invariably associated with gallstones. The usual symptoms are those of recurrent attacks of upper abdominal pain, often at night and following a heavy meal. The clinical features are similar to those of acute calculous cholecystitis but milder. The patient may recover spontaneously or following analgesia and antibiotics. Patients are usually advised to undergo elective laparoscopic cholecystectomy.

Acute cholangitis

Acute cholangitis is caused by bacterial infection of bile ducts and occurs in patients with other biliary problems such as choledocholithiasis (see below), biliary strictures or tumours, or after ERCP. Jaundice, fever (with or without rigors) and abdominal pain are the main presenting features. Treatment is with antibiotics and removal (if possible) of the underlying cause.

Choledocholithiasis

Stones in the common bile duct (choledocholithiasis) occur in 10–15% of patients with gallstones that have usually migrated from the gallbladder. In Far Eastern countries, primary common bile duct stones are found after bacterial infection secondary to parasitic infections with *Clonorchis sinensis*, *Ascaris lumbricoides* or *Fasciola hepatica* (p. 112). Common bile duct stones can cause partial or complete bile duct obstruction and may be complicated by cholangitis due to secondary bacterial infection, septicaemia, liver abscess and biliary stricture.

Clinical features

Choledocholithiasis may be asymptomatic, may be found incidentally by operative cholangiography at cholecystectomy, or may present with recurrent abdominal pain with or without jaundice. The pain is usually in the right upper quadrant and fever, pruritus and dark urine may be present. Rigors may be a feature; jaundice is common, usually with pain.

Investigations

• Transabdominal USS: shows dilated extrahepatic and intrahepatic bile ducts, but endoscopic USS may be needed to image distal bile duct stones. • LFTs: show a cholestatic pattern with bilirubinuria. • Cholangitis: if present, the patient usually has a leucocytosis.

Management

• Analgesia, IV fluids and broad-spectrum antibiotics, such as cefuroxime and metronidazole. • Urgent ERCP with biliary sphincterotomy and stone extraction: the treatment of choice, successful in ~90% of patients. • Cholangiography: to check clearance of all stones. • Lithotripsy or percutaneous drainage: alternatives if ERCP fails. • Surgery: performed less frequently than ERCP for choledocholithiasis because of higher morbidity and mortality.

Secondary biliary cirrhosis

This develops after prolonged large duct biliary obstruction due to gallstones, benign bile duct strictures or sclerosing cholangitis (p. 506). The clinical features are of chronic cholestasis with episodes of ascending cholangitis or even liver abscess (p. 500). Cirrhosis, ascites and portal hypertension are late features. Cholangitis requires treatment with antibiotics, which can be given continuously if attacks recur frequently.

Tumours of the gallbladder and bile duct
Carcinoma of the gallbladder

This is uncommon, occurring more often in females and usually encountered above the age of 70. More than 90% of such tumours are adenocarcinomas; the remainder are anaplastic or, rarely, squamous tumours. Gallstones are usually present and are thought to be important in the aetiology of the tumour. Local invasion often precludes excision, and treatment is frequently palliative.

Cholangiocarcinoma

This uncommon tumour can arise anywhere in the biliary tree from the small intrahepatic bile ducts to the papilla of Vater. The cause is unknown but the tumour is associated with gallstones, primary and secondary sclerosing cholangitis, and choledochal cysts. In the Far East, chronic liver fluke infection is a major risk factor. The patient presents with obstructive jaundice. The diagnosis is made by a combination of USS and cholangiography, but can be difficult to confirm in patients with sclerosing cholangitis. The prognosis is poor.

Carcinoma at the ampulla of Vater

Nearly 40% of all adenocarcinomas of the small intestine arise in relationship to the ampulla of Vater and present with pain, anaemia, vomiting and weight loss. Jaundice may be intermittent or persistent. Diagnosis is by duodenal endoscopy and biopsy, and staging by CT/MRI. Ampullary carcinoma must be differentiated from carcinoma of the head of the pancreas and cholangiocarcinoma because both have a worse prognosis. Pancreaticoduodenectomy can result in 50% 5-yr survival.

Miscellaneous biliary disorders
Post-cholecystectomy syndrome

Dyspeptic symptoms following cholecystectomy (post-cholecystectomy syndrome) occur in ~30% of patients. The usual complaints include right upper quadrant abdominal pain, flatulence, fatty food intolerance, and occasionally jaundice and cholangitis. USS is used to detect biliary obstruction, and EUS or MRCP to detect common bile duct stones. If retained bile duct stones are excluded, sphincter of Oddi dysfunction should be considered (see below).

Sphincter of Oddi dysfunction

The sphincter of Oddi is a small smooth muscle sphincter situated at the junction of the bile duct and pancreatic duct in the duodenum. Sphincter of Oddi dysfunction (SOD) is characterised by an increase in contractility that produces a benign non-calculous obstruction to the flow of bile or pancreatic juice. This may cause pancreatico-biliary pain, deranged LFTs or recurrent pancreatitis. Patients are predominantly female. Patients with biliary-type SOD experience recurrent episodic biliary-type pain. Patients with pancreatic SOD usually present with unexplained recurrent attacks of pancreatitis. The diagnosis is established by excluding gallstones and demonstrating a dilated or slowly draining bile duct.

Patients with biliary pain, who also have deranged liver enzymes and/or radiological abnormality due to SOD, are treated with endoscopic sphincterotomy. The results are good but patients should be warned that there is a high risk of complications, particularly acute pancreatitis.

Blood disease covers a wide spectrum of illnesses, ranging from common anaemias to rare conditions such as leukaemias and congenital coagulation disorders. Haematological changes occur as a consequence of diseases affecting any system and give important information in the diagnosis and monitoring of many conditions.

PRESENTING PROBLEMS IN BLOOD DISEASE

Anaemia

Anaemia refers to a state in which the level of haemoglobin (Hb) in the blood is below the reference range appropriate for age and sex. Other factors, including pregnancy and altitude, also affect Hb levels. The clinical features of anaemia reflect diminished oxygen supply to the tissues. The symptoms of anaemia will be more severe if the onset is rapid or if there is coexisting cardiorespiratory disease. Many clinical features are non-specific but together they should raise suspicion of anaemia.

Symptoms include:

• Tiredness. • Lightheadedness. • Breathlessness. • Worsening of coexisting disease, e.g. angina.

Signs include:

• Mucous membrane pallor. • Tachypnoea. • Raised JVP. • Flow murmurs. • Ankle oedems. • Postural hypotension. • Tachycardia.

The clinical assessment and investigation of anaemia should gauge its severity and define the underlying cause.

Clinical assessment

Iron deficiency anaemia: This is the most common type of anaemia worldwide. Seek symptoms indicating GI blood loss and menorrhagia in females.

Dietary history: This should assess the intake of iron and folate, which may become deficient in comparison to needs (e.g. in pregnancy or during periods of rapid growth).

CLINICAL EXAMINATION IN BLOOD DISEASE

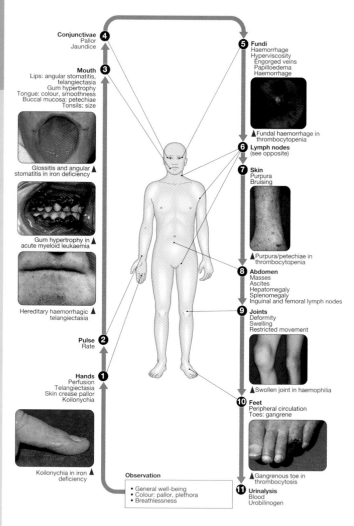

Conjunctivae ❹
Pallor
Jaundice

Mouth ❸
Lips: angular stomatitis,
telangiectasia
Gum hypertrophy
Tongue: colour, smoothness
Buccal mucosa: petechiae
Tonsils: size

Glossitis and angular ▲
stomatitis in iron deficiency

Gum hypertrophy in ▲
acute myeloid leukaemia

Hereditary haemorrhagic ▲
telangiectasia

Pulse ❷
Rate

Hands ❶
Perfusion
Telangiectasia
Skin crease pallor
Koilonychia

Koilonychia in iron ▲
deficiency

Observation
• General well-being
• Colour: pallor, plethora
• Breathlessness

Fundi ❺
Haemorrhage
Hyperviscosity
Engorged veins
Papilloedema
Haemorrhage

▲ Fundal haemorrhage in
thrombocytopenia

Lymph nodes ❻
(see opposite)

Skin ❼
Purpura
Bruising

▲ Purpura/petechiae in
thrombocytopenia

Abdomen ❽
Masses
Ascites
Hepatomegaly
Splenomegaly
Inguinal and femoral lymph nodes

Joints ❾
Deformity
Swelling
Restricted movement

▲ Swollen joint in haemophilia

Feet ❿
Peripheral circulation
Toes: gangrene

▲ Gangrenous toe in
thrombocytosis

⓫ **Urinalysis**
Blood
Urobilinogen

Past medical history: The history may reveal disease known to be associated with anaemia (e.g. rheumatoid arthritis) or previous surgery (e.g. stomach or small bowel resection, which may lead to malabsorption of iron and/or vitamin B_{12}).

Family history: This may be relevant in haemolytic anaemias and pernicious anaemia.

Drug history: Many drugs can be associated with blood loss (e.g. NSAIDs) and others may cause haemolysis or aplasia.

The general physical findings of anaemia (see above) may be accompanied by specific findings related to the underlying aetiology. Examples include a right iliac fossa mass in a patient with caecal carcinoma; jaundice in haemolytic anaemia; and neurological signs, including peripheral neuropathy and subacute combined degeneration of the cord, in patients with vitamin B_{12} deficiency.

Investigations

The investigation of anaemias usually starts with the size of the red cells, most accurately indicated by the mean cell volume (MCV) in the FBC. Commonly:

• A normal MCV (normocytic anaemia) suggests acute blood loss or anaemia of chronic disease (ACD). • A low MCV (microcytic anaemia) suggests iron deficiency or thalassaemia. • A high MCV (macrocytic anaemia) suggests vitamin B_{12} or folate deficiency, or myelodysplasia. • A high MCV (in the absence of anaemia) may be caused by alcohol, liver disease, hypothyroidism, splenectomy, hyperlipidaemia and pregnancy.

Supplementary investigations are often required for a precise diagnosis. A raised reticulocyte count in microcytic anaemia suggests bleeding or haemolysis. A low ferritin indicates iron deficiency. In macrocytic anaemia, the blood film may show typical abnormalities, e.g. a dimorphic picture in sideroblastic anaemia, target cells in liver disease, or hypersegmented neutrophils due to vitamin B_{12} or folate deficiency or drug toxicity.

High haemoglobin

Patients with a raised haematocrit (Hct) (>0.52 males, >0.48 females) for >2 mths should be investigated. 'True' polycythaemia (or absolute erythrocytosis) indicates an excess of red cells, while 'relative' (or 'low-volume') polycythaemia is due to a decreased plasma volume. Causes are shown in Box 14.1.

Clinical assessment and investigations

Males and females with Hct values of >0.60 and >0.56, respectively, can be assumed to have an absolute erythrocytosis. History and examination will identify most patients with polycythaemia secondary to hypoxia. The presence of hypertension, smoking, excess alcohol consumption and/or diuretic use is consistent with low-volume polycythaemia (Gaisbock's syndrome). In polycythaemia rubra vera (PRV), a mutation in a kinase, *JAK-2 V617F*, is found in

	14.1 Causes of erythrocytosis	
	Absolute erythrocytosis	**Relative (low-volume) erythrocytosis**
Haematocrit	High	High
Red cell mass	High	Normal
Plasma volume	Normal	Low
Causes	*Primary*	Diuretics
	Myeloproliferative disorder: Polycythaemia rubra vera	Smoking
	Secondary	Obesity
	↑Epo due to tissue hypoxia: altitude, lung disease, cyanotic heart disease	Alcohol excess
	Inappropriately ↑Epo: renal disease (hydronephrosis, cysts, carcinoma), other tumours (hepatoma, bronchial carcinoma, fibroids, phaeochromocytoma, cerebellar haemangioblastoma)	Gaisbock's syndrome
	Exogenous Epo: drug-taking in athletes	

>90% of cases (p. 554). If the *JAK-2* mutation is absent and there is no obvious secondary cause, a measurement of red cell mass is required to confirm an absolute erythrocytosis, followed by further investigations to exclude hypoxia, and causes of inappropriate erythropoietin secretion. Red cell mass measurement is performed by radiolabelling an aliquot of the patient's red cells, re-injecting them and measuring the dilution of the isotope.

Leucopenia (low white count)

Leucopenia may be due to a reduction in all types of white cell or in individual cell types.

Neutropenia (neutrophil count $<1.5 \times 10^9/L$): Occurs with:

• Infection. • Connective tissue disease. • Alcohol. • Bone marrow infiltration (e.g. leukaemia, myelodysplasia).

A number of drugs can also result in neutropenia, e.g.:

• Antirheumatic drugs (e.g. gold, penicillamine). • Antithyroid drugs (e.g. carbimazole). • Anticonvulsants (e.g. phenytoin, sodium valproate). • Antibiotics (e.g. sulphonamides).

Clinical manifestations of neutropenia range from no symptoms to overwhelming sepsis. Risk increases with lower counts. Fever may be the only manifestation of infection, and immediate antibiotic therapy is required to prevent rapid development of septic shock.

14.2 Causes of lymphadenopathy

Infective	Bacterial, e.g. streptococcal, TB
	Viral, e.g. Epstein–Barr, HIV
	Protozoal, e.g. toxoplasmosis
	Fungal, e.g. histoplasmosis
Neoplastic	Primary, e.g. lymphomas, leukaemias
	Secondary, e.g. lung, breast, thyroid, stomach
Inflammatory	Connective tissue disorders, e.g. rheumatoid arthritis, systemic lupus erythematosus
	Sarcoidosis
Miscellaneous	Amyloidosis

Lymphopenia (lymphocytes $<1 \times 10^9/L$): Occurs in sarcoidosis, lymphoma, renal failure, connective tissue disease and HIV infection.

Leucocytosis (high white count)

Leucocytosis is usually due to an increase in a specific type of white blood cell.

Neutrophilia (increased circulating neutrophils): Occurs with:

• Infection. • Trauma. • Myocardial infarction (MI). • Inflammation. • Malignancy. • Myeloproliferative disorders.

Pregnancy causes physiological neutrophilia.

Lymphocytosis (lymphocyte count $>3.5 \times 10^9/L$): Most commonly due to viral infection.

Eosinophilia (eosinophils $>0.5 \times 10^9/L$): Occurs in:

• Parasitic infections. • Allergy (asthma, drug reactions). • Inflammatory disease (e.g. polyarteritis nodosa). • Malignancy.

Lymphadenopathy

Enlarged lymph nodes may be an indicator of haematological disease but can also occur in reaction to infection or inflammation (Box 14.2). Reactive nodes usually expand rapidly and are painful, whereas those due to haematological disease are frequently painless and may be generalised. Initial investigations in lymphadenopathy should include:

• FBC: to detect neutrophilia in infection or evidence of haematological disease. • ESR. • CXR: to detect mediastinal lymphadenopathy.

If the findings suggest malignancy, lymph node biopsy is required.

Splenomegaly

Causes of splenic enlargement are listed in Box 14.3. Massive splenomegaly occurs in chronic myeloid leukaemia, myelofibrosis, malaria and leishmaniasis. Hepatosplenomegaly is more suggestive of lympho- or myeloproliferative disease or liver disease. The

14.3 Causes of splenomegaly	
Congestive	Portal hypertension, e.g. cirrhosis, portal vein thrombosis
	Cardiac, e.g. congestive cardiac failure
Infective	Bacterial, e.g. endocarditis, septicaemia, TB
	Viral, e.g. hepatitis, Epstein–Barr
	Protozoal, e.g. malaria, leishmaniasis (kala-azar)
	Fungal, e.g. histoplasmosis
Inflammatory/ granulomatous disorders	E.g. Felty's syndrome, SLE, sarcoidosis
Haematological	Red cell disorders, e.g. megaloblastic anaemia, haemoglobinopathies
	Autoimmune haemolytic anaemias
	Myeloproliferative disorders, e.g. chronic myeloid leukaemia, myelofibrosis, polycythaemia rubra vera, essential thrombocythaemia
	Neoplastic, e.g. leukaemias, lymphomas

presence of lymphadenopathy makes a diagnosis of lymphoprolif-erative disease more likely.

An enlarged spleen may cause abdominal discomfort; splenic infarction causes severe pain radiating to the shoulder tip. In rare cases, spontaneous or traumatic rupture may occur.

• USS or CT: show splenic size and texture, and also image the liver and abdominal lymph nodes. • FBC, blood film and CXR: required in all patients. • Further investigations: may include lymph node biopsy and bone marrow examination.

Bleeding

Normal haemostasis

Haemostasis depends upon interactions between the vessel wall, platelets and clotting factors. In the initial phase, the damaged vessel constricts and platelets aggregate to form a plug. This is followed by activation of the coagulation cascade, resulting in the formation of a cross-linked fibrin clot (Fig. 14.1). Clotting factors are synthe-sised by the liver and several are dependent on vitamin K for their activation; activated factors are designated by the suffix 'a'. The extrinsic pathway is the main physiological mechanism in vivo.

Excessive coagulation is prevented by natural inhibitors of the clotting system. Antithrombin is a serine protease inhibitor synthe-sised by the liver, which destroys activated factors XIa and Xa, and thrombin (IIa). Its activity against thrombin and Xa is enhanced by heparin and fondaparinux, explaining their anticoagulant effect. Protein C binds to its co-factor, protein S, and inactivates factors Va and VIIIa. Any reduction in these inhibitors results in a thrombotic tendency.

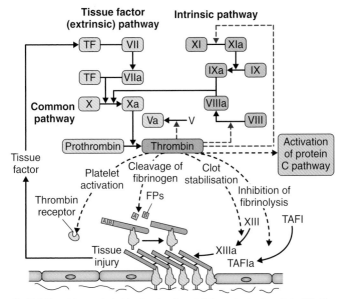

Fig. 14.1 Normal haemostasis. Injury breaches the endothelium, releasing tissue factor (TF); this activates the tissue factor (extrinsic) pathway, generating small amounts of thrombin. Platelets are activated by multiple mechanisms, including thrombin binding. Thrombin from the TF pathway then massively amplifies its own production; the 'intrinsic' pathway becomes activated, generating large amounts of thrombin (dotted red lines represent positive feedback). Thrombin forms clots by cleaving fibrinopeptides (FPs) from fibrinogen to produce fibrin. Fibrin monomers are cross-linked by factor XIII (also activated by thrombin). Thrombin also regulates clot formation via: (a) activation of the protein C pathway, which opposes further coagulation; (b) activation of thrombin-activatable fibrinolysis inhibitor (TAFI).

Clinical assessment

Abnormal bleeding may be due to deficiency of coagulation factors, thrombocytopenia, or occasionally excessive fibrinolysis following therapeutic fibrinolytic therapy.

Muscle and joint bleeds indicate a coagulation defect. Purpura, prolonged bleeding from cuts, epistaxis, GI haemorrhage, excessive post-surgical bleeding and menorrhagia suggest a platelet disorder, thrombocytopenia or von Willebrand disease. Family history and duration of bleeding may indicate whether the disorder is congenital or acquired. Coexisting illness or drug therapy predisposing to bleeding should be sought.

During the examination, check for:
• Bruising. • Purpura. • Telangiectasia on lips (indicates hereditary haemorrhagic telangiectasia). • Swollen joints/haemarthrosis. • Hepatomegaly. • Splenomegaly.

14.4 Causes of thrombocytopenia

Marrow disorders	Hypoplasia
	Infiltration, e.g. leukaemia, myeloma, carcinoma, myelofibrosis
	Vitamin B$_{12}$/folate deficiency
Increased platelet consumption	Disseminated intravascular coagulation (DIC)
	Idiopathic thrombocytopenic purpura (ITP)
	Infections, e.g. Epstein–Barr virus, Gram-negative septicaemia
	Hypersplenism
	Thrombotic thrombocytopenic purpura
	Liver disease
	Haemolytic uraemic syndrome

Investigations

Initial screening tests comprise:

• Platelet count. • Blood film. • Coagulation tests, including the prothrombin time (PT), activated partial thromboplastin time (APTT) and fibrinogen.

PT: Assesses the extrinsic system and is prolonged by deficiencies of factors II, V, VII and X, and by liver disease.

APTT: Assesses the intrinsic system and is sensitive to deficiencies in factors II, V, VIII, IX, X, XI and XII.

International normalised ratio (INR): Used to assess the control of warfarin treatment, and is the ratio of the patient's PT to a normal control using an international reference thromboplastin.

Thrombocytopenia (low platelets)

Causes of thrombocytopenia are listed in Box 14.4. Purpura, bruising and spontaneous oral, nasal, GI or GU bleeding may occur but not usually until the platelet count falls $<20 \times 10^9$/L. Blood film may be diagnostic (e.g. acute leukaemia). Bone marrow examination may reveal:

• A reduced number of megakaryocytes (platelet precursors) in cases of decreased platelet formation (e.g. hypoplastic anaemia).
• An increased number of megakaryocytes, indicating excessive platelet destruction (e.g. idiopathic thrombocytopenic purpura).

Indications for platelet transfusion include:

• A platelet count $<10 \times 10^9$/L. • Troublesome bleeding, such as persistent epistaxis. • Life-threatening bleeding, such as GI haemorrhage.

Transfusions provide only temporary relief because the survival of the platelets in the circulation is a few days at most.

Thrombocytosis (high platelets)

The platelet count may be raised as part of the inflammatory response (reactive thrombocytosis), as with infection, connective tissue disease, malignancy or GI bleeding. Alternatively, it may be a feature of myeloproliferative disorders, such as primary thrombocythaemia, PRV and chronic myeloid leukaemia.

Venous thrombosis

The most common presentation of venous thromboembolism (VTE) is with deep vein thrombosis (DVT) of the leg, with or without pulmonary embolism (PE; p. 313). However, similar principles apply to rarer types of VTE, such as jugular vein thrombosis, upper limb DVT, cerebral sinus thrombosis (p. 640) and intra-abdominal venous thrombosis (e.g. Budd–Chiari syndrome; p. 512).

Risk factors are summarised in Box 14.5.

14.5 Factors predisposing to venous thrombosis

Patient factors

- Increasing age
- Obesity
- Varicose veins
- Family history of unprovoked VTE when young
- Previous DVT
- Pregnancy/puerperium
- Oestrogens: oral contraceptives, HRT
- Immobility
- IV drug use (femoral vein)

Surgical conditions

- Major surgery, especially >30 mins' duration
- Abdominal or pelvic surgery, especially for cancer
- Major lower limb orthopaedic surgery, e.g. joint replacement and hip fracture surgery

Medical conditions

- MI
- Heart failure
- Inflammatory bowel disease
- Malignancy
- Nephrotic syndrome
- Pneumonia
- Neurological conditions causing immobility, e.g. stroke, paraplegia

Haematological disorders

- Polycythaemia rubra vera
- Essential thrombocythaemia
- Deficiency of antithrombin, proteins C and S
- Paroxysmal nocturnal haemoglobinuria
- Prothrombotic mutations: factor V Leiden, prothrombin gene *G20210A*
- Myelofibrosis
- Lupus anticoagulant
- Anticardiolipin antibody

i | 14.6 Predicting the pre-test probability of DVT – Wells score

Clinical characteristic	Score
Active cancer (patient receiving treatment for cancer within previous 6 mths or currently receiving palliative treatment)	1
Paralysis, paresis or recent plaster immobilisation of lower extremities	1
Recently bedridden for ≥3 days, or major surgery within previous 12 wks requiring general or regional anaesthesia	1
Localised tenderness along distribution of deep venous system	1
Entire leg swollen	1
Calf swelling ≥3 cm larger than that on asymptomatic side (measured 10 cm below tibial tuberosity)	1
Pitting oedema confined to symptomatic leg	1
Collateral superficial veins (non-varicose)	1
Previously documented DVT	1
Alternative diagnosis at least as likely as DVT	−2

Clinical probability	Total score
DVT low probability	<1
DVT moderate probability	1–2
DVT high probability	>2

From Wells PS. N Engl J Med 2003; 349:1227; copyright © 2003 Massachusetts Medical Society.

DVT presents with unilateral leg pain, swelling and warmth. Other causes include a calf haematoma, cellulitis and a ruptured Baker's cyst (usually complicating rheumatoid arthritis of the knee). Bilateral leg swelling may result from extensive proximal DVT involving the inferior vena cava, obstructed venous or lymphatic return in the pelvis, right-sided heart failure and hypoalbuminaemia.

Using the patient's symptoms, the probability of DVT can be established using the Wells score (Box 14.6). Those with a low risk should have a D-dimer levels measured – if normal, further investigation is not needed. Those with elevated D-dimer or medium- or high-risk Wells score should undergo further investigation.

Compression USS is the imaging modality of choice. It has a sensitivity for proximal DVT (popliteal vein or above) of 99.5%. In patients with proven DVT, further imaging to diagnose PE is not required unless massive PE is clinically suspected or there is unexplained breathlessness (p. 265).

Predisposing factors (see Box 14.5) should be considered and investigation pursued.

Management

The management of leg DVT includes elevation, analgesia and anticoagulation with low molecular weight heparin (LMWH) for 5 days, followed by a coumarin anticoagulant, such as warfarin. An alternative is the oral Xa inhibitor rivaroxaban, which has a rapid onset of action and can be used immediately from diagnosis without the need for LMWH. Patients with DVT and a strong contraindication to anticoagulation should be considered for an inferior vena cava filter to prevent PE.

Patients with unprovoked thrombosis are usually anticoagulated for 6 mths. However, those with a temporary risk factor that resolves can usually be treated for shorter periods (e.g. 3 mths). In patients with cancer and VTE, there is evidence that LMWH should be continued for 6 mths rather than being replaced by a coumarin. Longer duration of anticoagulation does not alter the rate of recurrence following discontinuation.

BLOOD PRODUCTS AND TRANSFUSION

Blood transfusion from an unrelated donor inevitably carries some risk, including adverse immunological interactions between the host and infused blood, and transmission of infectious agents. Although there are many compelling clinical indications for blood component transfusion, there are also many clinical circumstances in which the evidence for the effectiveness of transfusion is limited. In these settings, transfusion may be avoided by the use of low haemoglobin thresholds for red cell transfusion, peri-operative blood salvage and antifibrinolytic drugs.

Blood products

Red cell concentrate: Used to increase red cell mass in patients with anaemia and in acute blood loss. ABO compatibility with the patient is essential.

Platelet concentrate: Used to treat and prevent bleeding due to thrombocytopenia.

Fresh frozen plasma (FFP): Used to replace coagulation factors.

Cryoprecipitate: Obtained from plasma and contains proteins, including fibrinogen, factor VIII and von Willebrand factor (vWF). It is used to replace fibrinogen.

Coagulation factor concentrates: Used to treat haemophilia and von Willebrand disease (factors VIII and IX). Recombinant manufactured factors are preferred, as they avoid infection risk.

IV immunoglobulin: Used to prevent infection in patients with hypogammaglobulinaemia. It is also used in idiopathic thrombocytopenic purpura and Guillain–Barré syndrome.

Every blood donation must be reliably tested to exclude those containing transmissible agents. In the developed world, this includes:

• Hepatitis B. • Hepatitis C. • HIV. • Human T lymphotrophic virus (HTLV).

Plasma donated in the UK is not used at present for producing pooled plasma derivatives in view of concerns about transmission of variant Creutzfeldt–Jakob disease (vCJD; p. 669).

14.7 The ABO system		
Blood group	**Red cell A or B antigens**	**Antibodies in plasma**
0	None	Anti-A and anti-B
A	A	Anti-B
B	B	Anti-A
AB	A and B	None

Adverse effects of transfusion
Red cell incompatibility

There are four different ABO groups, determined by whether or not an individual's red cells express A or B antigens. Healthy individuals have antibodies directed against the A or B antigens that are not expressed on their own cells (Box 14.7). If red cells of an incompatible ABO group are transfused, the patient's antibodies bind to the transfused cells, leading to red cell haemolysis. This is the main cause of an acute transfusion reaction, and can give rise to disseminated intravascular coagulation (DIC), renal failure and death.

About 15% of Caucasians lack the Rhesus D (RhD) red cell antigen ('Rhesus-negative'). IgG antibodies to RhD-positive red cells are produced if such cells enter the circulation of an RhD-negative individual via fetomaternal haemorrhage during pregnancy. During a subsequent pregnancy with an RhD-positive fetus, these antibodies can cross the placenta and cause haemolytic disease of the newborn and severe neurological damage. Administration of anti-RhD immunoglobulin (anti-D) after delivery blocks the immune response to the RhD antigen and prevents the development of Rhesus antibodies in RhD-negative women.

Transfusion reactions

Temperature rise: A rise of <2°C to ≤38°C in an otherwise well patient indicates a febrile non-haemolytic transfusion reaction. Paracetamol should be given and the transfusion rate slowed.

Urticarial rash or itch: This is treated by giving an antihistamine (e.g. chlorphenamine 10 mg IV) and slowing the transfusion rate.

Severe allergic reactions: These present with bronchospasm, angioedema and hypotension. The transfusion should be stopped and any unused units returned to the blood bank. The patient should be treated with oxygen, IV chlorphenamine, nebulised salbutamol and, in hypotensive patients, IM adrenaline (epinephrine; 0.5 mL of 1 in 1000).

ABO incompatibility: This causes red cell haemolysis, leading to fever, rigors, tachycardia, hypotension, chest and abdominal pain, and shortness of breath. The transfusion is stopped and an IV saline infusion given to maintain urine output >100 mL/hr. DIC should be treated with appropriate blood components.

Bacterial contamination: This should be considered if discoloration or damage of the pack is seen, or if the patient has a temperature >39°C or hyper- or hypotension. The pack should be returned to the blood bank, blood cultures sent, and broad-spectrum antibiotics given if infection seems likely. Transmission of malaria or Chagas' disease by transfusion occasionally occurs in endemic areas.

Breathlessness: This suggests fluid overload and is treated by stopping the transfusion and administering oxygen and IV furosemide.

Safe transfusion procedures

Red cells from the patient's blood sample are tested to determine the ABO and RhD type. The patient's plasma is tested to detect any red cell antibodies that could haemolyse transfused red cells. The transfusion laboratory then performs either a 'group and screen' or a 'cross-match'.

• Group and screen procedure: the sample is held in the laboratory and compatible blood can be prepared rapidly if required. • Cross-matching: involves allocating specific red cell units to a particular patient for transfusion.

It is essential to ensure that no ABO-incompatible red cell transfusion is ever given. Most incompatible transfusions result from:

• Mistakes in taking and labelling the blood sample for pre-transfusion testing. • Failure to perform standard checks before infusion to ensure the correct pack has been selected for the patient.

HAEMATOPOIETIC STEM CELL TRANSPLANTATION

Transplantation of haematopoietic stem cells (HSCT) offers the only hope of 'cure' for many blood diseases. The indications for HSCT are being refined and extended, and currently include:

• Leukaemias (AML, ALL, CML – p. 543). • Myeloma. • Myelodysplastic syndrome. • Non-Hodgkin lymphoma. • Severe aplastic anaemia. • Myelofibrosis. • Severe immune deficiency syndromes.

The type of HSCT is defined according to the donor and source of stem cells.

Allogeneic HSCT

Stem cells from a donor – either related (usually an HLA-identical sibling) or a closely HLA-matched volunteer unrelated donor (VUD) – are infused after planned ablation of the patient's own marrow. In addition to restoring marrow function, donor immune cells can attack recipient malignant cells ('graft versus disease effect').

There is considerable morbidity and mortality associated with HSCT. The best results are obtained in young patients with minimal residual disease. Around 25% die from complications such as graft-versus-host disease (see below), and there remains a significant risk of disease relapse. The long-term survival for patients undergoing allogeneic HSCT in acute leukaemia is ~50%.

Graft-versus-host disease

Graft-versus-host disease (GVHD) is due to the cytotoxic activity of donor T lymphocytes that become sensitised to their new host, regarding it as foreign.

Acute GVHD: This occurs in the first 100 days after transplant in around one-third of patients. It varies from mild to lethal, causing rashes, jaundice and diarrhoea. Prevention includes HLA-matching of the donor and immunosuppressant drugs.

Chronic GVHD: This may follow acute GVHD or arise independently. It often resembles a connective tissue disorder, and is usually treated with corticosteroids and prolonged immunosuppression (e.g. ciclosporin).

Autologous HSCT

Stem cells are harvested from the patient's bone marrow or peripheral blood and frozen until required. After aggressive chemotherapy to treat disease (with associated myeloablation), stem cells are re-infused to restore marrow function. Autologous HSCT is used to allow aggressive chemotherapy for diseases that spare the marrow or those in which very good remission has been achieved.

ANTICOAGULANT AND ANTITHROMBOTIC THERAPY

Broadly speaking, antiplatelet agents (e.g. aspirin, clopidogrel) are more effective in preventing arterial thrombosis than VTE. Antiplatelet agents are therefore the drugs of choice in acute coronary and cerebrovascular disease, while warfarin and other anticoagulants are favoured in VTE. Indications for anticoagulation are given in Box 14.8.

Heparin

Unfractionated heparin (UFH) produces its anticoagulant effect by potentiating the activity of antithrombin. This results in prolongation of the APTT. The low molecular weight heparins (LMWHs) augment antithrombin activity preferentially against factor Xa. LMWHs produce reliable dose-dependent anticoagulation when given as a daily SC injection in a weight-related dose. Blood monitoring is not required.

LMWHs are widely used for the treatment of VTE and have replaced UFH, except where rapid reversibility is important. The short half-life of UFH (~1 hr) makes it useful for those with a predisposition to bleeding (e.g. patients with a peptic ulcer). UFH is started with a loading dose of 80 U/kg IV, followed by a continuous infusion, initially of 18 U/kg/hr, adjusted to maintain the APTT at 1.5–2.5 times control. If a patient bleeds, it is usually sufficient just to discontinue the infusion; however, if bleeding is severe, the excess can be neutralised with IV protamine. It is normally appropriate to start warfarin therapy at the same time as heparin, as it takes several days to decrease the concentration of the vitamin K-dependent clot-

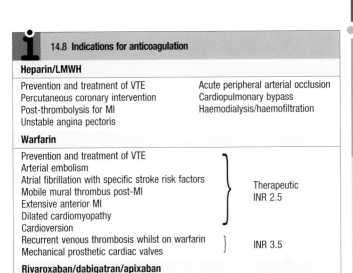

14.8 Indications for anticoagulation		
Heparin/LMWH		
Prevention and treatment of VTE	Acute peripheral arterial occlusion	
Percutaneous coronary intervention	Cardiopulmonary bypass	
Post-thrombolysis for MI	Haemodialysis/haemofiltration	
Unstable angina pectoris		
Warfarin		
Prevention and treatment of VTE		
Arterial embolism		
Atrial fibrillation with specific stroke risk factors		Therapeutic
Mobile mural thrombus post-MI		INR 2.5
Extensive anterior MI		
Dilated cardiomyopathy		
Cardioversion		
Recurrent venous thrombosis whilst on warfarin		INR 3.5
Mechanical prosthetic cardiac valves		
Rivaroxaban/dabigatran/apixaban		
Prevention or treatment (rivaroxaban) of VTE	Atrial fibrillation with stroke risk	

ting factors. Heparin should be continued until the INR is >2.0 for 2 consecutive days.

Heparin-induced thrombocytopenia

In a small proportion of patients treated with heparin, the platelet count declines after 5–14 days due to the development of an antibody directed against a factor on the platelet surface. Heparin should be discontinued immediately and an alternative agent, such as the direct thrombin inhibitor argatroban, given instead.

Warfarin

Warfarin inhibits the vitamin K-dependent carboxylation of factors II, VII, IX and X in the liver. Indications for warfarin and appropriate target INRs are listed in Box 14.8. Warfarin therapy must be initiated with a loading dose (e.g. 10 mg orally) on the first day; subsequent daily doses depend on the INR and can be predicted using an algorithm. The duration of warfarin therapy depends on the clinical indication, and while treatment of DVT or preparation for cardioversion requires a limited duration, anticoagulation to prevent cardioembolic stroke in atrial fibrillation or from heart valve disease is long-term.

Drug interactions are common through protein binding and metabolism by the cytochrome P450 system.

Bleeding is the most common serious side-effect of warfarin. If the INR is above the desired therapeutic level, the warfarin dose should be reduced or withheld. The anticoagulant effect of warfarin may be

14.9 Antithrombotic prophylaxis

Patients in the following categories should be considered for specific antithrombotic prophylaxis:

Moderate risk of DVT

- Major surgery in patients >40 yrs or with other risk factor
- Major medical illness, e.g. heart failure, sepsis, malignancy, inflammatory bowel disease, stroke or other reason for immobility

High risk of DVT

- Major abdominal or pelvic surgery for malignancy or with history of DVT or known thrombophilia
- Specific surgical risk: major hip or knee surgery, neurosurgery

reversed by administering vitamin K but this takes ~6 hrs. If the patient has a serious haemorrhage, reversal can be effected quickly by giving coagulation factor concentrate or fresh frozen plasma.

Prevention of venous thrombosis

All patients admitted to hospital should be assessed for their risk of developing VTE (Box 14.9). Early mobilisation of all patients is important to prevent DVTs. Patients at medium or high risk may require additional antithrombotic measures such as graduated compression stockings and LMWH; those at high risk may need prolonged prophylaxis.

ANAEMIAS

Around 30% of the world population is anaemic; iron deficiency is the cause in half of these.

Iron deficiency anaemia

This occurs when iron losses exceed absorption:

Blood loss: The most common explanation in men and postmenopausal women is GI blood loss. This may result from gastric or colorectal malignancy, peptic ulceration, inflammatory bowel disease, diverticulitis and angiodysplasia. Worldwide, hookworm and schistosomiasis are common causes (pp. 112 and 118). GI bleeding may be exacerbated by the use of aspirin or NSAIDs. In younger women, menstrual bleeding and pregnancy often contribute to iron deficiency.

Malabsorption: Gastric acid is required to release iron from food and helps keep it in the soluble ferrous state. Hypochlorhydria due to proton pump inhibitor (PPI) treatment or previous gastric surgery may contribute to deficiency. Iron is absorbed actively in the upper small intestine and absorption can be affected by coeliac disease.

Physiological demands: Increased demands for iron during puberty and pregnancy can lead to deficiency.

Investigations

Blood film shows microcytic hypochromic red cells (low MCV, low mean cell Hb (MCH)). Iron deficiency is confirmed by a low plasma ferritin level; however, ferritin levels may also be raised (up to 100 µg/L) by liver disease and in the acute phase response, even in the presence of iron deficiency. In these patients, measurement of transferrin saturation (<16%) and soluble transferrin receptor (raised) may be helpful.

The underlying cause of the iron deficiency should be established. Men >40 yrs and post-menopausal women should undergo investigation of the upper and lower GI tract by endoscopy or barium studies. If coeliac disease is suspected, anti-endomysium or anti-transglutaminase antibodies and duodenal biopsy are indicated. In the tropics, stool and urine should be examined for parasites.

Management

Unless the patient has angina, heart failure or evidence of cerebral hypoxia, transfusion is not necessary and oral iron supplementation (ferrous sulphate 200 mg 3 times daily for 3–6 mths) is appropriate, together with treatment of the underlying cause. The Hb should rise by 10 g/L every 7–10 days.

Anaemia of chronic disease

This common type of anaemia occurs in the setting of chronic infections, chronic inflammation and neoplasia. The anaemia is mild and is usually associated with a normal MCV (normocytic, normochromic), though this may be reduced in long-standing inflammation. Hepcidin, a key regulatory protein, inhibits the export of iron from cells, resulting in anaemia despite high iron stores. Raised ferritin and reduced total iron binding capacity (TIBC) and soluble transferrin receptor help to distinguish anaemia of chronic disease from iron deficiency. Measures that reduce the severity of the underlying disorder generally help to improve the anaemia.

Megaloblastic anaemia

This results from deficiency of vitamin B_{12} or folic acid, both of which are required for DNA synthesis. Deficiency leads to red cells with arrested nuclear maturation but normal cytoplasmic development within the bone marrow (megaloblasts). There is a macrocytic anaemia with an MCV often >120 fl, and mature red cells are commonly oval in shape. Involvement of white cells and platelets can lead to neutrophils with hypersegmented nuclei and, in severe cases, pancytopenia. Bone marrow examination reveals hypercellularity and megaloblastic changes.

Vitamin B_{12}

The average diet contains well in excess of the 1 µg daily requirement of vitamin B_{12}, mainly in meat, eggs and milk. In the stomach, gastric enzymes release vitamin B_{12} from food and it binds to a carrier protein called R protein. The gastric parietal cells produce intrinsic factor, a vitamin B_{12}-binding protein. As gastric emptying occurs, vitamin B_{12} released from the diet switches from the R protein to intrinsic factor. Vitamin B_{12} is absorbed in the terminal ileum and is transported in plasma bound to transcobalamin II, a transport protein produced by the liver. The liver stores enough vitamin B_{12} for 3 yrs, and deficiency therefore takes many years to become manifest, even if all dietary intake is stopped.

Vitamin B_{12} deficiency can result in neurological disease, including peripheral neuropathy (glove and stocking paraesthesiae) and subacute combined degeneration of the cord. The latter involves the posterior columns (causing diminished vibration sense and proprioception, leading to sensory ataxia) and corticospinal tracts (resulting in upper motor neuron signs). Dementia and optic atrophy can also occur.

Causes of vitamin B_{12} deficiency

Dietary deficiency: This only occurs in strict vegans.

Gastric factors: Gastric surgery (including gastrectomy) can result in vitamin B_{12} deficiency due to impaired secretion of gastric acid and intrinsic factor.

Pernicious anaemia: This is an autoimmune disorder characterised by atrophy of the gastric mucosa. Loss of the parietal cells causes intrinsic factor deficiency, leading to vitamin B_{12} malabsorption. Pernicious anaemia has an average age of onset of 60 yrs, and is associated with other autoimmune conditions including Hashimoto's thyroiditis, Graves' disease, vitiligo and Addison's disease. Antiparietal cell antibodies are present in 90% of cases but also occur in 20% of normal females >60 yrs. The Schilling test, involving measurement of absorption of radio-labelled vitamin B_{12} after oral administration, before and after replacement of intrinsic factor, has fallen out of favour with the availability of autoantibody tests, greater caution in the use of radioactive tracers and limited availability of intrinsic factor.

Small bowel factors: Terminal ileal disease (e.g. Crohn's disease) and ileal resection result in vitamin B_{12} malabsorption. Motility disorders can cause bacterial overgrowth and the resulting competition for free vitamin B_{12} leads to deficiency.

Folate

Leafy vegetables, fruits, liver and kidney provide rich sources of dietary folate. An average Western diet meets the daily requirement, but total body stores are small and deficiency can develop within weeks. Causes of folate deficiency include:

• Diet, e.g. poor intake of vegetables. • Malabsorption, e.g. coeliac disease. • Increased demand, e.g. pregnancy, haemolysis. • Drugs, e.g. phenytoin, contraceptive pill, methotrexate.

Serum folate is very sensitive to dietary intake, and red cell folate is therefore a more accurate indicator of the body's folate stores.

Management of megaloblastic anaemia

If a patient with severe megaloblastic anaemia requires treatment before vitamin B_{12} and red cell folate results are available, both folic acid and vitamin B_{12} are given. Folic acid therapy alone in the presence of vitamin B_{12} deficiency may result in worsening of neurological defects.

Vitamin B_{12} deficiency: Treated with IM hydroxycobalamin (1000 µg, 6 doses 2 or 3 days apart, followed by lifelong therapy of 1000 µg every 3 mths). Hb should rise by 10 g/L per wk, but neuropathy may take 6–12 mths to correct.

Folate deficiency: Treated with oral folic acid 5 mg daily. Folic acid supplementation in pregnancy may reduce the risk of neural tube defects. Prophylactic folic acid is also given in chronic haematological disease associated with reduced red cell lifespan (e.g. autoimmune haemolytic anaemia or haemoglobinopathies).

Haemolytic anaemia

Normal red cells have a lifespan of 120 days. Increased red cell destruction (haemolysis) leads to increased LDH, a modest increase in unconjugated bilirubin and mild jaundice. Compensatory bone marrow activity results in increased reticulocytes and immature granulocytes in peripheral blood; blood films may also show the reason for haemolysis (e.g. spherocytosis). The erythroid hyperplasia may also cause folate deficiency, leading to megaloblastosis. When destruction exceeds production, haemolytic anaemia results.

Extravascular haemolysis: Occurs in the reticulo-endothelial cells of the liver and spleen, so avoiding free Hb in the plasma. In most haemolytic states, haemolysis is predominantly extravascular.

Intravascular haemolysis: Releases free Hb into the plasma, where it binds to haptoglobin (an α_2 globulin produced by the liver), resulting in a fall in haptoglobin levels. Once haptoglobins are saturated, free Hb is oxidised to form methaemoglobin. Excess free Hb may also be absorbed by renal tubular cells, where it is degraded and the iron stored as haemosiderin. When the tubular cells are subsequently sloughed into the urine, they give rise to haemosiderinuria.

Red cell membrane defects
Hereditary spherocytosis

This is usually inherited as an autosomal dominant condition and has an incidence of 1:5000. The most common abnormalities are deficiencies of the red cell membrane proteins, beta spectrin or ankyrin. The cells lose their normal elasticity and undergo destruction when they pass through the spleen. The severity of spontaneous haemolysis varies. Most cases feature an asymptomatic compensated chronic haemolytic state with spherocytes on the blood film and a reticulocytosis. Pigment gallstones occur in up to 50% of patients and may cause cholecystitis.

The clinical course may be complicated by crises:
• Haemolytic crisis: occurs uncommonly, usually with infection.
• Megaloblastic crisis: follows the development of folate deficiency.
• Aplastic crisis: occurs in association with parvovirus B19 infection; the virus directly invades red cell precursors and switches off red cell production.

Investigations:
• Hb levels: variable, depending on the degree of compensation.
• Blood film: shows spherocytes and reticulocytes. • Direct Coombs test (see Fig. 4.2): negative, excluding immune haemolysis. • Bilirubin and LDH: raised. • Screening of family members.

Management: Folic acid prophylaxis (5 mg weekly) should be given for life. Acute severe haemolytic crises require transfusion. Splenectomy should be considered in moderate to severe cases but only after the age of 6 yrs because of the risk of sepsis. Prior to splenectomy, patients should receive vaccination against pneumococcus, *Haemophilus influenzae* type B, meningococcus group C and influenza. They should undergo regular immunisation against pneumococcus and influenza, and receive lifelong penicillin V.

Hereditary elliptocytosis

This is less common and generally milder than hereditary spherocytosis. The blood film shows elliptocytic red cells and there is variable haemolysis. Most cases are asymptomatic and do not require specific treatment; more severe cases are managed in a similar way to hereditary spherocytosis.

Glucose-6-phosphate dehydrogenase deficiency

Glucose-6-phosphate dehydrogenase deficiency (G6PD) is the most common inherited enzymopathy, affecting 10% of the world's population. G6PD is pivotal in the hexose monophosphate shunt and helps to protect the red cells against oxidative stress. G6PD deficiency is an X-linked condition principally affecting males. It results in acute intravascular haemolysis secondary to infection, drugs (e.g. antimalarials, sulphonamides, nitrofurantoin) and ingestion of fava beans. It can also cause chronic haemolysis and neonatal jaundice. Management involves stopping any precipitant drugs. Transfusion may be required in severe cases.

Acquired haemolytic anaemia
Autoimmune haemolytic anaemia

This results from increased red cell destruction due to red cell autoantibodies. If an antibody avidly fixes complement, it will result in intravascular haemolysis, but if complement activation is weak, the haemolysis will be extravascular. Immune haemolysis is classified according to whether the antibodies bind best at 37°C (warm antibodies, 80% of cases) or 4°C (cold antibodies).

Direct antiglobulin test (DAT) (Coombs test)

Detects the presence of antibody bound to
the red cell surface, e.g.
1. autoimmune haemolytic anaemia
2. haemolytic disease of newborn (HDN)
3. transfusion reactions

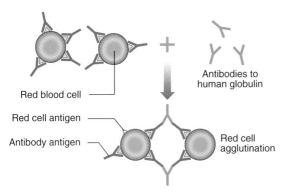

Red blood cell

Antibodies to
human globulin

Red cell antigen

Antibody antigen

Red cell
agglutination

Indirect antiglobulin test (IAT) (indirect Coombs test)

Detects antibodies in the plasma, e.g. antibody screen
in pre-transfusion testing

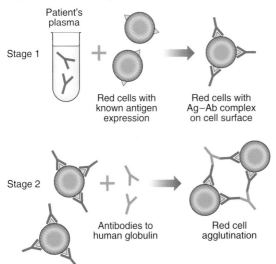

Patient's
plasma

Stage 1

Red cells with
known antigen
expression

Red cells with
Ag–Ab complex
on cell surface

Stage 2

Antibodies to
human globulin

Red cell
agglutination

Fig. 14.2 Direct and indirect antiglobulin tests.

Warm autoimmune haemolysis

Warm autoimmune haemolysis occurs at all ages but is more common in middle age. Antibodies are usually IgG. No underlying cause is identified in up to 50% of cases but known causes include:
• Lymphoid neoplasms, e.g. lymphoma. • Solid tumours, e.g. lung, colon. • Connective tissue disease, e.g. systemic lupus erythematosus, rheumatoid arthritis. • Drugs, e.g. methyldopa.

Investigations: There is evidence of haemolysis and spherocytes on the blood film. The diagnosis is confirmed by the direct Coombs or antiglobulin test (see Fig. 14.2), in which red cells are mixed with Coombs reagent containing antibodies against human IgG/M/complement. If the red cells have been coated by antibody in vivo, agglutination occurs. The test will miss IgA and IgE antibodies.

Management: Any underlying cause must be treated and any implicated drugs stopped. Oral prednisolone (1 mg/kg) is the mainstay of treatment. It works by decreasing macrophage destruction of antibody-coated red cells and reducing antibody production. Transfusion may be required for severe anaemia. Splenectomy should be considered in refractory cases; this removes a main site of red cell destruction and antibody production. Alternative immunosuppressive therapy (e.g. azathioprine, cyclophosphamide) may be required in some patients.

Cold agglutinin disease

This is due to antibodies ('cold agglutinins'), usually IgM, which bind to the red cells at 4°C and cause them to agglutinate. Agglutination may cause intravascular haemolysis if complement fixation occurs. Causes include:
• Lymphoma. • Infections, e.g. *Mycoplasma pneumoniae*, infectious mononucleosis. • Paroxysmal cold haemoglobinuria.

Cold antibodies optimally bind red cells at lower temperatures. Red cell agglutination therefore occurs in small vessels in exposed areas, and patients may experience cold, painful and blue fingers and toes (acrocyanosis).

Management: Any underlying cause must be treated. All patients should receive folate supplements. Patients must keep extremities warm, especially in winter. Corticosteroid therapy and blood transfusion may be required in some patients.

Non-immune haemolytic anaemia
Physical trauma

Physical disruption of red cells may occur in a number of conditions and is characterised by the presence of red cell fragments on the blood film and markers of intravascular haemolysis.

Mechanical heart valves: High flow through incompetent valves results in shear stress damage.

March haemoglobinuria: Prolonged marching or marathon running can cause red cell damage in the capillaries in the feet.

Microangiopathic haemolytic anaemia: Fibrin deposition in capillaries can cause severe red cell disruption. Causes include malignant hypertension, haemolytic uraemic syndrome and DIC.

Infection

Plasmodium falciparum malaria may be associated with intravascular haemolysis; when severe, this is termed blackwater fever due to the associated haemoglobinuria.

Haemoglobinopathies
Sickle-cell anaemia

The normal Hb molecule is composed of two alpha and two non-alpha globin polypeptide chains, each containing a haemoglobin group. Haemoglobin A (HbA-$\alpha_2\beta_2$) is the predominant form in adults. Sickle-cell disease results from a single glutamic acid to valine substitution at position 6 of the beta globin chain. It is inherited as an autosomal recessive trait.

Homozygotes produce only abnormal beta chains that make haemoglobin S (HbS, termed SS), resulting in the clinical syndrome of sickle-cell disease. Heterozygotes produce a mixture of normal and abnormal beta chains that make normal HbA and HbS (termed AS), and this results in the clinically asymptomatic sickle-cell trait.

Individuals with sickle-cell trait are relatively resistant to the lethal effects of *falciparum* malaria, which explains the high incidence of the sickle gene in equatorial Africa, where *falciparum* malaria is endemic.

Clinical features

When HbS is deoxygenated, the Hb molecules polymerise and the red cell membrane becomes distorted, producing characteristic sickle-shaped cells. Sickling is precipitated by hypoxia, dehydration and infection. Sickled cells have a shortened survival and plug vessels in the microcirculation. This results in a number of acute syndromes termed 'crises' and chronic organ damage.

Vaso-occlusive crisis: Plugging of small vessels in the bone results in avascular necrosis, producing acute severe bone pain. Commonly affected sites include the femur, humerus, ribs, pelvis and vertebrae. Vaso-occlusion in the spleen can give rise to recurrent splenic infarction and adults may have no functional spleen. Occlusion at other sites can result in cerebrovascular accidents and proliferative retinopathy.

Sickle chest syndrome: This may follow on from a vaso-occlusive crisis and is the most common cause of death in adult sickle disease. Bone marrow infarction results in fat emboli to the lungs, which cause sickling and infarction, leading to ventilatory failure.

Sequestration crisis: Thrombosis of the venous outflow from an organ causes loss of function and acute painful enlargement. Massive splenic enlargement may result in severe anaemia and circulatory collapse. Sequestration in the liver leads to severe pain due to capsular stretching.

Aplastic crisis: Infection with parvovirus B19 results in severe red cell aplasia, producing a very low Hb.

Investigations

Patients with sickle-cell disease have a compensated anaemia (usually 60–80 g/L) with a reticulocytosis and sickle cells on the blood film. Hb electrophoresis demonstrates a predominance of HbS with absent HbA.

Management and prognosis

Patients with sickle disease should receive prophylaxis with folic acid. Pneumococcal infection may be lethal in the presence of hyposplenism; patients should therefore receive prophylaxis with daily penicillin V and vaccination against pneumococcus. Patients should also be vaccinated against *Haemophilus influenzae* B and hepatitis B.

Vaso-occlusive crises are managed by aggressive rehydration, oxygen therapy and adequate analgesia (which often requires opiates) and antibiotics. Top-up transfusion may be used in sequestration or aplastic crises. Exchange transfusion, where a patient is simultaneously venesected and transfused to replace HbS with HbA, may be used in life-threatening crises. The oral cytotoxic agent hydroxycarbamide induces increased synthesis of fetal Hb (HbF-$\alpha_2\gamma_2$), which in turn inhibits polymerisation of HbS and reduces sickling; this may be helpful in individuals with recurrent severe crises. Allogenic stem cell transplantation is rarely performed but may be potentially curative. Sickle-cell anaemia has mortality of 15% by the age of 20 yrs and 50% by the age of 40 yrs.

The thalassaemias

The thalassaemias are a group of inherited disorders of Hb production in which there is impaired synthesis of alpha or beta globin chains. The resultant imbalance in the ratio of alpha to beta chains leads to precipitation of the excess chains, causing membrane damage and reduced red cell survival.

Beta-thalassaemia

Failure to synthesise beta chains is the most common type of thalassaemia and most frequently occurs in the Mediterranean area.

Heterozygotes have beta-thalassaemia minor, a condition in which there is usually mild anaemia and little or no clinical disability. The anaemia has a microcytic hypochromic pattern but individuals are not iron-deficient. Homozygotes have beta-thalassaemia major and are either unable to synthesise HbA or at best produce very little. After the first 4 mths of life, they develop a profound hypochromic anaemia. Levels of HbF ($\alpha_2\gamma_2$) are raised.

Management:
Cure is now a possibility for selected children, with allogeneic HSCT (p. 531). Blood transfusions maintain the Hb level >100 g/L. Daily folic acid 5 mg is given. Repeated transfusions can lead to iron

overload, which is treated with chelation therapy. Splenectomy is indicated for splenomegaly and excessive transfusion needs.

Alpha-thalassaemia

Reduced or absent alpha-chain synthesis is common in South-east Asia. There are two alpha gene loci on chromosome 16 and therefore four alpha genes.

• If one is deleted: no clinical effect. • If two are deleted: there may be a mild microcytic hypochromic anaemia. • If three are deleted: the patient makes haemoglobin H, a beta tetramer that is functionally useless; treatment is similar to that for beta-thalassaemia of intermediate severity. • If all four alpha genes are deleted: the baby is stillborn (hydrops fetalis).

HAEMATOLOGICAL MALIGNANCIES

Haematological malignancies arise when the processes of proliferation or apoptosis are corrupted in blood cells. If mature differentiated cells are involved, the cells produce indolent neoplasms, such as low-grade lymphomas and chronic leukaemias, where survival for many years is expected. If more primitive stem cells are involved, the cells produce rapidly progressive life-threatening illnesses, such as acute leukaemias and high-grade lymphomas.

Leukaemias

Leukaemias are malignant disorders of haematopoietic stem cells, associated with increased numbers of white cells in the bone marrow and/or peripheral blood. The aetiology is unknown in most patients, but several factors are associated with the development of leukaemia:

Ionising radiation: Both wartime exposure and iatrogenic exposure are known to increase risk.

Cytotoxic chemicals: Alkylating drugs can induce myeloid leukaemia after a latent period of several years. Industrial benzene exposure is associated with leukaemia.

Retroviruses: One rare form of T-cell leukaemia is associated with retroviral infection.

Genetics: Males are affected more than females. There is a greatly increased incidence in identical twins of affected individuals. Incidence is also increased in Down's syndrome. Ethnic variation also occurs; chronic lymphocytic leukaemia is rare in Chinese populations.

Immunology: Immune deficiency states (e.g. hypogammaglobulinaemia) are associated with risk of haematological malignancy.

Leukaemias are traditionally classified into four main groups:
• Acute lymphoblastic leukaemia (ALL). • Acute myeloid leukaemia (AML). • Chronic lymphocytic leukaemia (CLL). • Chronic myeloid leukaemia (CML).

Lymphocytic and lymphoblastic cells are derived from the lymphoid stem cell (B cells and T cells). Myeloid refers to the other lineages: precursors of red cells, granulocytes, monocytes and platelets.

Acute leukaemia

Acute leukaemias occur at all ages, but ALL has a peak incidence in children aged 1–5 yrs. AML occurs mainly over the age of 50. In acute leukaemia there is proliferation of primitive stem cells leading to an accumulation of blast cells in the bone marrow, which causes bone marrow failure. Eventually, this proliferation spills into the blood. The presenting features are usually anaemia, bleeding and infection.

Investigations

FBC usually shows anaemia and thrombocytopenia. The leucocyte count varies from as low as $1 \times 10^9/L$ to as high as $500 \times 10^9/L$ or more. The appearance of blast cells on the blood film is usually diagnostic.

Bone marrow aspiration is the most valuable investigation and provides material for cytology, cytogenetics and immunological phenotyping. The marrow is typically hypercellular, with replacement of normal elements by leukaemic blast cells in varying degrees. The presence of Auer rods in the cytoplasm of blast cells indicates myeloblastic leukaemia. Classification and prognosis are determined by immunophenotyping, chromosome and molecular analysis.

Management

Specific treatment for acute leukaemia is aggressive, has a number of side-effects, and may not be appropriate for very elderly patients or those with significant comorbidity. In these patients, supportive treatment only should be considered.

Specific therapy

Before specific therapy is embarked upon, any underlying infection should be treated. Anaemia and thrombocytopenia should be corrected with red cell and platelet transfusions. The aim of treatment is to destroy the leukaemic clone of cells without destroying the residual normal stem cell compartment. There are three phases:

Remission induction: The bulk of the tumour is destroyed by combination chemotherapy. The patient goes through a period of severe bone marrow hypoplasia, requiring intensive inpatient support.

Remission consolidation: Residual disease is attacked by several courses of chemotherapy during the consolidation phase. This again results in periods of marrow hypoplasia. In poor-prognosis leukaemia, this phase may include stem cell transplantation.

Remission maintenance: If the patient is still in remission after the consolidation phase for ALL, a period of outpatient maintenance therapy is given, consisting of a repeating cycle of drug administration. In ALL, prophylactic cranial irradiation and intrathecal chemotherapy are used to ensure therapy penetrates the CNS.

Supportive therapy

Aggressive chemotherapy involves periods of bone marrow failure and requires adequate supportive care. The following problems are common:

Anaemia: This is treated with red cell transfusion.

Bleeding: Thrombocytopenic bleeding requires platelet transfusions. Prophylactic platelet transfusion should be given to maintain the platelet count $>10 \times 10^9/L$. Coagulation abnormalities should be treated appropriately, usually with fresh frozen plasma.

Infection: Fever ($>38°C$) lasting over 1 hr in a significantly neutropenic patient (neutrophil count $<1.0 \times 10^9/L$) indicates possible septicaemia. IV broad-spectrum antibiotic therapy is essential. Empirical therapy is given with a combination of an aminoglycoside (e.g. gentamicin) and a broad-spectrum penicillin (e.g. piperacillin/tazobactam). This combination is synergistic and bactericidal. The organisms most commonly associated with severe neutropenia are skin-based Gram-positive bacteria such as *Staphylococcus aureus* and *Staph. epidermidis*, which gain entry via cannulae and central lines, and Gram-negative bacteria from the gut.

Patients with ALL are susceptible to infection with *Pneumocystis jirovecii*, which causes severe pneumonia. They should receive prophylactic oral co-trimoxazole during chemotherapy. Diagnosis may require sputum induction, and if negative, bronchoalveolar lavage. Treatment is with high-dose IV co-trimoxazole.

Patients receiving intensive chemotherapy receive prophylaxis against fungal infections with itraconazole or posaconazole. Systemic fungal infection with *Candida* or *Aspergillus* is treated with IV liposomal amphotericin or voriconazole.

Herpes simplex infection frequently occurs around the lips and nose during chemotherapy and is treated with aciclovir. Herpes zoster should be dealt with early using high-dose aciclovir, as it can be fatal in immunocompromised patients.

Metabolic problems: Continuous monitoring of renal and hepatic function is necessary. Renal toxicity occurs with some antibiotics (e.g. aminoglycosides) and antifungal agents (amphotericin). Cellular breakdown during induction therapy increases uric acid production, which may cause renal failure; allopurinol and IV hydration are given as prophylaxis against this.

Psychological support: Support from a trained multidisciplinary team is essential.

Haematopoietic stem cell transplantation

This is described on page 531 and can increase 5-yr survival from 20% to 50% in high-risk acute leukaemia.

Prognosis

Without treatment, the median survival of patients with acute leukaemia is ~5 wks. Around 80% of adult patients <60 yrs of age achieve remission with specific therapy. Remission rates are lower for older patients. However, the relapse rate continues to be high. The introduction of the drug tretinoin for acute promyelocytic leukaemia has greatly reduced the death rate from bleeding.

Chronic myeloid leukaemia

Chronic myeloid leukaemia (CML) is a myeloproliferative stem cell disorder resulting in proliferation of all haematopoietic lineages but predominantly the granulocytic series. Cell maturation proceeds fairly normally. The peak incidence is at the age of 55 yrs. Around 95% of patients with CML have a chromosome abnormality (Philadelphia chromosome, Ph), a shortened chromosome 22 formed by reciprocal translocation with chromosome 9. A resulting chimeric gene (*BCR ABL*) codes for a protein with tyrosine kinase activity, which plays a causative role in the disease, influencing cellular proliferation and differentiation.

Clinical features

The disease has three phases:

Chronic phase: The disease is responsive to treatment and is easily controlled. Formerly, this stage lasted 3–5 yrs, but since the advent of imatinib therapy can be prolonged to >8 yrs in many patients.

Accelerated phase: Disease control becomes more difficult.

Blast crisis: The disease transforms into an acute leukaemia (AML in 70%, ALL in 30%), which is relatively refractory to treatment and often fatal. Imatinib therapy greatly reduces the number of patients per year who transform to blast crisis.

Common symptoms include lethargy, weight loss, abdominal discomfort and sweating. About 25% of patients are asymptomatic at diagnosis. Splenomegaly is characteristic and may be massive; hepatomegaly occurs in 50% of cases.

Investigations

• FBC: usually shows a normocytic, normochromic anaemia. • Leucocyte count: varies from 10 to 600 × 10^9/L. • Platelet count: very high in ~one-third of patients – up to 2000 × 10^9/L. • Blood film: neutrophils are the predominant cell type, although the full range of granulocyte precursors is seen. The number of circulating blasts increases dramatically as the disease enters blast transformation. • Chromosome analysis of bone marrow: reveals the Ph chromosome, and RNA analysis the *BCR ABL* gene defect.

Management

Chronic phase: Imatinib specifically inhibits BCR ABL tyrosine kinase activity and reduces white cell proliferation. It is first-line therapy in chronic phase CML, producing a complete response at

18 mths in 76% of patients. Monitoring is by bone marrow until cytogenetic response occurs, then by measuring BCR ABL mRNA in blood. Alternative agents, such as dasatinib or nilotinib, are used in non-responders. Allogeneic HSCT can provide a cure for younger patients in the chronic phase who are imatinib-resistant.

Accelerated phase and blast crisis: Blast crisis is the main cause of death in patients with CML. Tyrosine kinase inhibitors should be tried if patients have not already had these. Otherwise, blast crisis is treated as acute leukaemia but responds poorly, and supportive therapy alone may be appropriate in elderly patients.

Chronic lymphocytic leukaemia

Chronic lymphocytic leukaemia (CLL) is the most common variety of leukaemia, typically presenting between the ages of 65 and 70 yrs. There is uncontrolled proliferation of immuno-incompetent B lymphocytes, leading to impaired immunity and haematopoiesis.

Clinical features

The onset is very insidious. In ~70% of patients, the diagnosis is made incidentally on a routine FBC. Presenting problems include:
• Anaemia. • Infections. • Lymphadenopathy. • Systemic symptoms, such as night sweats and weight loss.

Investigations

Peripheral blood shows a mature lymphocytosis ($>5 \times 10^9$/L). Immunophenotyping confirms the monoclonal origin of the B cells. Serum immunoglobulins indicate the degree of immunosuppression. Direct Coombs test may show autoimmune haemolytic anaemia. Bone marrow examination may be helpful in difficult cases, to monitor response and to judge prognosis.

The clinical stages of CLL are:
• A (60% of patients): no anaemia or thrombocytopenia; <3 areas of lymphadenopathy. • B (30%): as for A but ≥3 areas of lymphadenopathy. • C (10%): anaemia and/or thrombocytopenia.

Management and prognosis

Most stage A patients do not require treatment.

Treatment is indicated if there is bone marrow failure, massive lymphadenopathy or splenomegaly, systemic symptoms, rapidly increasing lymphocyte count or autoimmune anaemia or thrombocytopenia.

Initial therapy for stages B and C is with the oral alkylating agent chlorambucil or the purine analogue fludarabine. Rituximab may also increase remission rates

Supportive care is required in progressive disease, e.g. transfusions for symptomatic anaemia or thrombocytopenia and prompt treatment of infections.

The main prognostic factor is stage of disease. Older patients with stage A disease have a normal life expectancy. Patients with advanced CLL are more likely to die from their disease or infectious complications. In those treated with chemotherapy and rituximab, 90% are alive 4 yrs later.

Myelodysplastic syndrome

Myelodysplastic syndrome (MDS) predominantly affects elderly patients, and is characterised by peripheral blood cytopenias and abnormal-looking (dysplastic) blood cells. It inevitably progresses to AML.

Bone marrow failure results in symptoms of anaemia, infections or bleeding. Bone marrow is hypercellular with evidence of dysplasia.

MDS is usually incurable. Supportive care with red cell and platelet transfusions is the main treatment. Erythropoietin and granulocyte–colony stimulating factor (G–CSF) may improve Hb and WCC in selected individuals. Allogeneic HSCT may afford a cure in younger patients. In low-risk patients, median survival is 5.7 yrs and time for 25% of patients to develop AML is 9.4 yrs; equivalent figures in high-risk patients are 0.4 and 0.2 yrs, respectively.

Lymphomas

These neoplasms arise from lymphoid tissues, and are classified according to biopsy findings into Hodgkin and non-Hodgkin lymphoma. The majority are of B-cell origin.

Hodgkin lymphoma

Hodgkin lymphoma (HL) typically affects adults aged 20–35, although there is a second peak at 50–70 yrs of age. The condition is more common in individuals with a previous history of infectious mononucleosis, although no causal link has been proved. Reed–Sternberg cells, large malignant lymphoid cells of B-cell origin, are the histological hallmark of HL. Four histological patterns of classical HL are recognised, according to the WHO classification:

• Nodular sclerosing (common in young patients and women).
• Mixed cellularity. • Lymphocyte-rich. • Lymphocyte-depleted.

A nodular lymphocyte-predominant form of HL is also recognised, and carries a good prognosis.

Clinical features

There is painless rubbery lymphadenopathy, usually in the neck or supraclavicular fossae. Some patients have no systemic 'B' symptoms; others have weight loss and drenching sweats. Hepatosplenomegaly may be present. Dry cough and breathlessness may occur in those with mediastinal adenopathy.

Investigations

• FBC: may be normal or show normocytic, normochromic anaemia. Lymphopenia or eosinophilia may be present. • ESR: may be raised. • Liver function: may be abnormal with or without hepatic infiltration. • Raised LDH levels: indicate adverse prognosis. • CXR: may show a mediastinal mass. • CT scanning of chest, abdomen and pelvis: permits staging and guides management (Box 14.10). • Lymph node biopsy: required to confirm the diagnosis.

Management and prognosis

Clinical trials have shown that patients with early-stage disease have better outcomes if treated with chemotherapy and adjunctive radiotherapy. The ABVD regimen (doxorubicin, vinblastine, bleomycin and dacarbazine) is followed by radiotherapy to the involved lymph nodes. Treatment response is assessed clinically and by repeat CT and PET scanning.

Patients with advanced-stage disease are most commonly managed with chemotherapy alone. As with early disease, initial PET-negative remission predicts long-term remission. Cure rates are lower with advanced disease. Patients with resistant disease may be considered for autologous HSCT (p. 532).

Over 90% of patients with early-stage HL achieve complete remission, and the great majority are cured. Between 50 and 70% of those with advanced-stage HL can be cured.

Non-Hodgkin lymphoma

Non-Hodgkin lymphoma (NHL) represents a monoclonal proliferation of lymphoid cells and may be of B-cell (70%) or T-cell (30%) origin. It has a peak incidence between 65 and 70 yrs of age. The most important factor influencing treatment and prognosis is grade.

High-grade NHL: Has high proliferation rates, rapidly produces symptoms and is fatal if untreated, but is potentially curable.

Low-grade NHL: Has low proliferation rates, may be asymptomatic for many months and runs an indolent course, but is not curable by conventional therapy.

Clinical features

• Lymph node enlargement. • Systemic upset, e.g. weight loss, sweats and fever. • Hepatosplenomegaly. • Extranodal disease: more common in NHL, with involvement of the bone marrow, gut, thyroid, lung and skin. • Bone marrow involvement: more common in low-grade than high-grade disease.

The same staging system (see Box 14.10) is used for both HL and NHL, but NHL is more likely to be stage III or IV at presentation.

Investigations

These are as for HL, but in addition patients should undergo:

• Bone marrow aspiration and trephine. • Immunophenotyping of surface antigens to distinguish T- and B-cell tumours. • Cytogenetic analysis for translocations. • Urate levels – can cause renal failure during treatment. • HIV testing – if risk factors are present.

Management

Low-grade NHL: Asymptomatic patients may not require therapy. Indications for treatment include systemic symptoms,

i	14.10 Clinical stages of Hodgkin lymphoma (Ann Arbor classification)
Stage	**Definition**
I	Involvement of a single lymph node region or extralymphatic site
II	Involvement of two or more lymph node regions or an extralymphatic site and lymph node regions on the same side of the diaphragm
III	Involvement of lymph node regions on both sides of the diaphragm with or without localised extralymphatic involvement or involvement of the spleen or both
IV	Diffuse involvement of one or more extralymphatic tissues, e.g. liver or bone marrow
A	No systemic symptoms
B	Weight loss >10%, drenching sweats

lymphadenopathy causing discomfort and bone marrow failure. Radiotherapy can be used for localised disease. Chemotherapy (cyclophosphamide, vincristine and prednisolone), in combination with rituximab, is first-line therapy. This increases survival but is not curative. High-dose chemotherapy with HSTC extends survival in relapsed disease.

High-grade NHL: The most common form, diffuse large B-cell NHL, responds to cyclophosphamide, doxorubicin, vincristine, prednisolone, and rituximab (R-CHOP). Radiotherapy is used for debulking, cord compression or localised stage I disease. Autologous HSTC is used in relapsed disease.

Prognosis

Low-grade NHL runs an indolent remitting and relapsing course, with a median survival of 10 yrs. In diffuse large B-cell high-grade NHL, 75% of patients initially respond to therapy, and 50% are disease-free at 5 yrs.

Paraproteinaemias

Polyclonal gammopathies occur with infection, inflammation or malignancy. A monoclonal increase in a single immunoglobulin class may occur with normal or reduced levels of the other immunoglobulins. Such monoclonal proteins are called paraproteins or M-proteins.

Monoclonal gammopathy of uncertain significance

In monoclonal gammopathy of uncertain significance (MGUS), a paraprotein is present in the blood without any other features of myeloma or related disease. It predominantly affects asymptomatic elderly patients, and blood tests are otherwise normal. No specific treatment is required, but patients should receive annual monitoring to identify progression to myeloma (~1% per annum).

Waldenström macroglobulinaemia

This rare low-grade lymphoma occurs in the elderly and is associated with the production of an IgM paraprotein. Patients present with features of hyperviscosity, such as visual disturbance and confusion. Other features include anaemia, systemic symptoms, splenomegaly and lymphadenopathy. Plasma electrophoresis demonstrates an IgM paraprotein, and bone marrow aspiration shows infiltration of lymphoid cells. Severe hyperviscosity may require plasmapheresis to remove IgM. Treatment with chlorambucil, fludarabine or rituximab may be effective.

Multiple myeloma

This is a malignant proliferation of plasma cells and has a peak incidence between the ages of 60 and 70 yrs. Normal plasma cells are derived from B cells and produce immunoglobulins containing heavy and light chains. In myeloma, plasma cells produce a monoclonal immunoglobulin (paraprotein). Light chains may appear in the urine as Bence Jones proteinuria. IgG is the most common paraprotein type in myeloma.

Clinical features and investigations

The clinical features are shown in Figure 14.3. The diagnosis of myeloma requires two of the following:

- Increased malignant plasma cells on bone marrow aspiration.
- Paraprotein on plasma and/or urinary protein electrophoresis.
- Lytic lesions on skeletal survey.

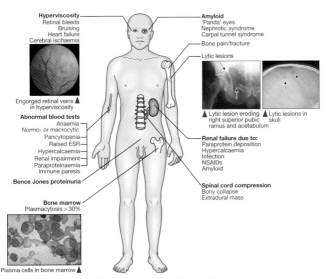

Hyperviscosity
Retinal bleeds
Bruising
Heart failure
Cerebral ischaemia

Engorged retinal veins ▲
in hyperviscosity

Abnormal blood tests
Anaemia
Normo- or macrocytic
Pancytopenia
Raised ESR
Hypercalcaemia
Renal impairment
Paraproteinaemia
Immune paresis

Bence Jones proteinuria

Bone marrow
Plasmacytosis > 30%

Plasma cells in bone marrow ▲

Amyloid
'Panda' eyes
Nephrotic syndrome
Carpal tunnel syndrome

Bone pain/fracture

Lytic lesions

▲ Lytic lesion eroding   ▲ Lytic lesions in
right superior pubic   skull
ramus and acetabulum

Renal failure due to:
Paraprotein deposition
Hypercalcaemia
Infection
NSAIDs
Amyloid

Spinal cord compression
Bony collapse
Extradural mass

Fig. 14.3 Clinical and laboratory features of multiple myeloma.

Other investigations include FBC, U&Es and serum calcium. ESR is usually elevated. Alkaline phosphatase and bone scans are normal in the absence of fractures.

Management

Asymptomatic patients without kidney, marrow or bone damage may not require treatment.

Supportive therapy:
• High fluid intake to treat renal impairment and hypercalcaemia. • Analgesia for bone pain. • Allopurinol to prevent urate nephropathy. • Bisphosphonates for hypercalcaemia and to reduce the incidence of fractures. • Plasmapheresis, as necessary, for hyperviscosity.

Specific therapy: In older patients, thalidomide combined with melphalan and prednisolone has increased the median overall survival to >4 yrs. Thalidomide is both anti-angiogenic and immunomodulatory but is highly teratogenic.

In younger, fitter patients, chemotherapy is followed by autologous HSCT, which improves quality of life and prolongs survival but does not cure myeloma. Bortezomib followed by lenalidomide is used for subsequent progression.

Radiotherapy is used for bone pain and cord compression. Long-term bisphosphonates can reduce bone pain and protect bone.

Prognosis

The median survival of patients receiving standard treatment varies from 29 to 62 mths, depending on disease stage.

APLASTIC ANAEMIA

Primary idiopathic acquired aplastic anaemia

This is a rare disorder in Europe and North America. It is characterised by failure of the pluripotent stem cells, resulting in hypoplasia of the bone marrow with pancytopenia. Usually no cause is found but enquiry should be made into causes of secondary aplasia.

Clinical features and investigations

Patients present with symptoms of bone marrow failure, including anaemia, bleeding and infection. FBC demonstrates pancytopenia with low reticulocytes. Bone marrow aspiration reveals hypercellularity.

Management

Patients require supportive treatment with red cell and platelet transfusions and aggressive management of infection. The curative treatment for patients <30 yrs of age is allogeneic HSCT, which offers a 75–90% chance of long-term cure. Immunosuppressive therapy with ciclosporin and antithymocyte globulin is used in older patients.

14.11 Causes of secondary aplastic anaemia

- Drugs:
  Cytotoxic drugs
  Antibiotics: chloramphenicol, sulphonamides
  Antirheumatic agents: penicillamine, gold
  Antithyroid drugs
  Anticonvulsants
  Immunosuppressives: azathioprine
- Chemicals:
  Benzene toluene solvent misuse: glue-sniffing
  Insecticides: organophosphates
- Radiation
- Viral hepatitis
- Pregnancy
- Paroxysmal nocturnal haemoglobinuria

Secondary aplastic anaemia

Causes of secondary aplastic anaemia are listed in Box 14.11. In some instances, the cytopenia is more selective and affects only one cell line, most often the neutrophils. Clinical features and investigations are the same as for primary aplastic anaemia. Any underlying cause should be addressed.

MYELOPROLIFERATIVE DISORDERS

These chronic conditions are characterised by clonal proliferation of marrow precursor cells, and include polycythaemia rubra vera (PRV), essential thrombocythaemia, myelofibrosis and chronic myeloid leukaemia (p. 546). Although most patients have one of these disorders, some have overlapping features or progress from one to another, e.g. PRV to myelofibrosis. A mutation in the gene encoding the signal transduction molecule *JAK-2* has been found in >90% of PRV cases and 50% of those with essential thrombocythaemia and myelofibrosis.

Myelofibrosis

In myelofibrosis, the marrow is initially hypercellular, with an excess of abnormal megakaryocytes that release growth factors, resulting in fibroblast proliferation. As the disease progresses, the marrow becomes fibrosed.

Clinical features

Most patients present over the age of 50 yrs with fatigue, weight loss and night sweats. The spleen may be massively enlarged due to extramedullary haematopoiesis, and painful splenic infarcts may occur.

Investigations

There is anaemia with a leucoerythroblastic blood picture (circulating immature red cells and granulocyte precursors). WCC and platelet count may be high, normal or low. Increased cell turnover commonly leads to high urate levels and folate deficiency. Bone marrow is often difficult to aspirate; trephine biopsy shows replacement by fibrous tissue. Finding the *JAK-2* mutation supports the diagnosis.

Management

Supportive treatment includes red cell transfusions for anaemia. Folic acid should be given to prevent deficiency. Cytotoxic therapy with hydroxycarbamide may help reduce the WCC and spleen size, but splenectomy may be required for massive splenomegaly. HSCT may be considered in younger patients. Survival is variable, with a median of 4 yrs.

Primary thrombocythaemia

This is characterised by a raised level of circulating platelets that are often dysfunctional. Reactive causes of increased platelets must be excluded before making the diagnosis. The *JAK-2* mutation supports the diagnosis but is not universal. Patients present at a median age of 60 yrs with vascular occlusion or bleeding events. A small percentage may transform to acute leukaemia or myelofibrosis.

Aspirin should be considered for all patients to reduce the risk of thrombosis. Hydroxycarbamide may be used to control high platelet counts.

Polycythaemia rubra vera

PRV occurs mainly in patients over the age of 40 yrs. It is characterised by increased erythropoiesis due to a primary increase in marrow activity.

Clinical features

Patients present with an incidental finding of a high Hb, or with symptoms of hyperviscosity such as lassitude, headaches, dizziness and pruritus. Some present with manifestations of peripheral arterial disease or a cerebrovascular accident. There is an increased risk of VTE. Peptic ulceration is common and is sometimes complicated by bleeding. Patients are often plethoric and have splenomegaly.

Investigations

The investigation of polycythaemia is covered on page 521. High haematocrit plus the *JAK-2* mutation usually makes the diagnosis. In *JAK-2*-negative cases, secondary polycythaemia (see Box 14.1) should be excluded. Neutrophil and platelet counts are often raised.

Management and prognosis

Aspirin reduces the risk of thrombosis. Venesection relieves hyperviscosity symptoms and should be repeated to maintain the haematocrit <45%.

Hydroxycarbamide or interferonalfa can be used to suppress the underlying myeloproliferation. Radioactive phosphorus (^{32}P) is reserved for older patients, as it increases the risk of transformation to acute leukaemia 6–10-fold. Median survival exceeds 10 yrs. Conversion to myelofibrosis or acute leukaemia occurs in 25%.

BLEEDING DISORDERS

Disorders of primary haemostasis

Platelet functional disorders, thrombocytopenia, von Willebrand disease and diseases affecting the vessel wall may all result in failure of platelet plug formation in primary haemostasis.

Vessel wall abnormalities
Hereditary haemorrhagic telangiectasia

Hereditary haemorrhagic telangiectasia (HHT) is a dominantly inherited condition characterised by abnormalities of vascular modelling.

Telangiectasia and small aneurysms occur on the fingertips, on the face, in the nasal passages, on the tongue, in the lung and in the GI tract. Many patients develop larger pulmonary arteriovenous malformations that cause arterial hypoxaemia and are associated with stroke and cerebral abscess due to paradoxical embolism; these should be treated by percutaneous embolisation. Patients present with recurrent bleeds (particularly epistaxis) or with iron deficiency due to occult GI bleeding.

Treatment includes iron therapy and local cautery or laser therapy to prevent lesions from bleeding.

Thrombocytopenia

Causes of thrombocytopenia are listed in Box 14.4 and treatment is discussed on page 526.

Idiopathic thrombocytopenic purpura

The presence of autoantibodies directed against platelets results in platelet destruction. Spontaneous bleeding occurs mainly with platelet counts $<20 \times 10^9$/L. At higher counts, the patient may complain of easy bruising, epistaxis or menorrhagia. Many cases with counts $>50 \times 10^9$/L are discovered by chance.

In adults, idiopathic thrombocytopenic purpura (ITP) more commonly affects females and may have an insidious onset. Unlike ITP in children, there is usually no history of a preceding viral infection. Patients aged >65 yrs should have a bone marrow examination to exclude an accompanying B-cell malignancy and autoantibody testing if connective tissue disease is likely. HIV testing should be considered. There is a greatly reduced platelet count and the bone marrow reveals increased megakaryocytes.

Management

Most cases of childhood ITP are self-limiting and resolve within a few weeks. Indications for oral prednisolone include severe purpura, bruising or epistaxis, and a platelet count $<10 \times 10^9/L$. Adults are also treated with prednisolone, although this is often less effective than in children. Intravenous IgG (IVIgG) raises the platelet count and is indicated if the bleeding is immediately life-threatening. Persistent or potentially life-threatening bleeding should be treated with platelet transfusion. Splenectomy should be considered in patients with relapsing disease.

Coagulation disorders

Coagulation factor disorders can arise from deficiency of a single factor (usually congenital, e.g. haemophilia A) or of multiple factors (often acquired, e.g. liver disease).

Congenital bleeding disorders
Haemophilia A

Factor VIII deficiency (haemophilia A) is the most common congenital coagulation disorder. It affects 1:10000 individuals. Factor VIII is manufactured by liver and endothelial cells; the gene is located on the X chromosome. Haemophilia A is inherited as an X-linked recessive disorder and patients are therefore male. All daughters of haemophiliacs are carriers. If a carrier has a son, he will have a 50% chance of having haemophilia, and a daughter will have a 50% chance of being a carrier. Antenatal screening is possible in affected families.

Clinical features and investigations

The diagnosis is normally made after the age of 6 mths, when babies become more mobile and first experience bruising or haemarthrosis. The features of haemophilia A are related to the plasma factor VIII level (Box 14.12). Individuals with severe haemophilia experience recurrent haemarthroses in large joints, which over time lead to secondary osteoarthrosis. Although joints and muscles are the most common sites for haemorrhage, bleeding can occur at almost any site. Intracranial haemorrhage is often fatal.

Management

Bleeding episodes should be treated early with IV factor VIII concentrate. Freeze-dried factor VIII concentrates can be stored at 4°C

i	**14.12 Severity of haemophilia**	
Degree of severity	**Factor VIII or IX level**	**Clinical presentation**
Severe	<0.01 U/mL	Spontaneous haemarthroses and muscle haematomas
Moderate	0.01–0.05 U/mL	Mild trauma or surgery causes haematomas
Mild	>0.05–0.4 U/mL	Major injury or surgery results in excess bleeding

in domestic refrigerators, and many patients are therefore able to treat themselves at home. The concentrates are prepared from blood donor plasma that has been screened for hepatitis B, C and HIV, and has undergone a viral inactivation process during manufacture. Factor VIII concentrates prepared by recombinant technology are also widely available now and, although more expensive, are perceived as being safer than those derived from plasma. In individuals with mild haemophilia A, IV or intranasal desmopressin can be used to increase factor VIII levels. This is often sufficient to treat a mild bleed or cover minor surgery such as dental extraction.

Complications of therapy

Before 1986, concentrates were not virally inactivated and many patients became infected with hepatitis B, hepatitis C and HIV. All potential recipients of pooled blood products should therefore be offered hepatitis A and B immunisation. There is now concern that variant CJD may be transmissible via pooled plasma products, so these are now prepared from plasma from countries with a low incidence of bovine spongiform encephalopathy.

The other serious consequence of factor VIII infusion is the development of anti-factor VIII antibodies, which arise in ~20–30% of severe haemophiliacs. Such antibodies rapidly neutralise therapeutic infusions, making treatment relatively ineffective. Infusion of factor VIIa may stop bleeding.

Haemophilia B (Christmas disease)

This is caused by deficiency of factor IX and is also an X-linked condition. The disorder is clinically indistinguishable from haemophilia A but is less common. Treatment is with factor IX concentrate.

Von Willebrand disease

Von Willebrand disease is a common but usually mild bleeding disorder with autosomal dominant inheritance. Von Willebrand factor (vWF) is a protein that performs two principal functions:

• It acts as a carrier protein for factor VIII; deficiency of vWF therefore results in a secondary reduction in the plasma factor VIII level.
• It facilitates platelet binding to subendothelial collagen; deficiency therefore also leads to impaired platelet plug formation.

Clinical features

Patients present with haemorrhagic manifestations similar to those in individuals with reduced platelet function. Superficial bruising, epistaxis, menorrhagia and GI haemorrhage are common. Bleeding episodes are usually far less common and severe than in severe haemophilia.

Investigations

There is a reduced level of vWF, with secondary reduction in factor VIII. Mutation analysis is informative in most cases.

Management

- Mild haemorrhage: desmopressin, which raises the vWF level.
- Mucosal bleeding: tranexamic acid. • Severe bleeding: factor VIII concentrates.

Acquired bleeding disorders
Disseminated intravascular coagulation

Disseminated intravascular coagulation (DIC) may cause bleeding, but begins with intravascular coagulation and is considered below.

Liver disease

In severe parenchymal liver disease, bleeding may arise from many different causes. These include reduced synthesis of coagulation factors, DIC and thrombocytopenia secondary to hypersplenism. Cholestatic jaundice reduces vitamin K absorption and leads to deficiency of factors II, VII, IX and X. This deficiency can be treated with parenteral vitamin K.

Renal disease

Advanced renal failure is associated with platelet dysfunction and bleeding, especially GI bleeding.

Thrombotic disorders

Predisposing conditions for VTE are listed in Box 14.5. Clinical features and investigations are described on page 527.

Inherited abnormalities of coagulation

Several inherited conditions predispose to VTE; none of them is strongly associated with arterial thrombosis, however. All carry a slightly increased risk in pregnancy. Apart from antithrombin deficiency and homozygous factor V Leiden, most carriers will never have an episode of VTE. Detection of these abnormalities does not predict recurrence of VTE. None of these conditions per se requires treatment with anticoagulants, unless thrombosis occurs or particular risk factors are also present.

Antithrombin deficiency: Antithrombin is a protein that inactivates factors IIa (thrombin), IXa, Xa and XIa. Its activity is greatly potentiated by heparin. Familial deficiency of antithrombin is an autosomal dominant disorder that is associated with a marked predisposition to VTE.

Protein C and S deficiencies: Protein C and S are natural anticoagulants involved in switching off coagulation factor activation (factors Va and VIIIa) and thrombin generation. Inherited deficiency of either protein C or S therefore results in a prothrombotic state.

Factor V Leiden: Factor V Leiden results from a mutation that prevents the cleavage and hence inactivation of activated factor V. This causes a relative risk of venous thrombosis of 5 in heterozygotes and >50 in rare homozygotes.

Antiphospholipid syndrome (APS): In this syndrome, antiphospholipid antibodies (which include lupus anticoagulant and

| | 14.13 Clinical associations with antiphospholipid syndrome |

Primary antiphospholipid syndrome

- Venous thromboembolic disease
- Arterial thromboembolic disease
- Recurrent pregnancy failure: fetal death, pre-eclampsia

Secondary antiphospholipid syndrome

- Systemic lupus erythematosus
- Rheumatoid arthritis
- Temporal arteritis
- Systemic sclerosis
- Sjögren's syndrome
- Behçet's syndrome

anticardiolipin antibodies) interact with the coagulation cascade, causing arterial and venous thromboembolism. The syndrome sometimes occurs as a complication of rheumatic disease, e.g. systemic lupus erythematosus (secondary APS); when it occurs in the absence of associated disease, it is known as primary APS (Box 14.13).

Disseminated intravascular coagulation

DIC can be initiated by a number of mechanisms. Examples include infections, malignancy, drug toxicity, burns and obstetric problems (e.g. placental abruption, amniotic fluid embolism). Systemic activation of the pathways involved in coagulation and its regulation, either via cytokine pathways or by tissue factor, causes the generation of intravascular fibrin clots leading to multi-organ failure, with simultaneous coagulation factor and platelet consumption causing bleeding. This may be exacerbated by activation of the fibrinolytic system secondary to the deposition of fibrin.

Investigations

• Thrombocytopenia. • Prolonged PT and APTT due to coagulation factor deficiency. • Low fibrinogen. • Increased levels of D-dimer (a fibrin degradation product).

Management

Therapy should be aimed at treating the underlying condition causing DIC (e.g. IV antibiotics for septicaemia). Blood products such as platelets and/or fresh frozen plasma should be given to correct identified abnormalities.

Thrombotic thrombocytopenic purpura

Thrombotic thrombocytopenic purpura (TTP) is a rare autoimmune disorder in which thrombosis is accompanied by paradoxical thrombocytopenia. TTP is characterised by five features:

- Thrombocytopenia. • Microangiopathic haemolytic anaemia.
• Neurological sequelae. • Fever. • Renal impairment.

The features are of microvascular occlusion by platelet thrombi affecting key organs, principally brain and kidneys. It may occur alone or in association with drugs (ticlopidine, ciclosporin), HIV, shiga toxins and malignancy. Treatment is by emergency plasma exchange; corticosteroids, aspirin and rituximab also have a role. Untreated, mortality rates are 90% in the first 10 days.

Rheumatology and bone disease

15

Disorders of the musculoskeletal system affect all ages and ethnic groups, accounting for ~25% of general practice consultations in the UK. Musculoskeletal diseases affect bones, joints, muscles, or connective tissues such as skin and tendon, causing pain and impairment of locomotor function.

Musculoskeletal diseases tend to be more common in women and most increase with age. Osteoarthritis is the most common arthritis, affecting up to 80% of people aged over 75. Osteoporosis is the most common bone disease, affecting 50% of women and 20% of men by their eighth decade. Musculoskeletal diseases are the most common cause of physical disability in older people.

PRESENTING PROBLEMS IN MUSCULOSKELETAL DISEASE

Acute monoarthritis

Causes of acute monoarthritis are listed in Box 15.1. Reactive arthritis (p. 587) is most common in young men, gout in middle-aged men and pseudogout in older women. Gout classically affects the first metatarsophalangeal (MTP) joint, whereas the wrist and shoulder are typical sites for pseudogout. Rapid onset (6–12 hrs) favours gout or pseudogout; joint sepsis develops slowly and progresses until treated. Haemarthrosis typically causes a large effusion in an injured joint. Recent diarrhoeal illness or sexual contact suggests reactive arthritis, whereas intercurrent illness, dehydration or surgery may trigger crystal-induced arthritis.

Joint aspiration is normally required to exclude sepsis and to look for crystals.

Polyarthritis

Polyarthritis is inflammation affecting five or more joints. Inflammatory arthritis causes early morning stiffness and worsening of symptoms with inactivity, along with synovial swelling and tenderness on examination. The pattern of joint involvement and associated features help to determine the underlying cause (Box 15.2).

CLINICAL EXAMINATION OF THE MUSCULOSKELETAL SYSTEM

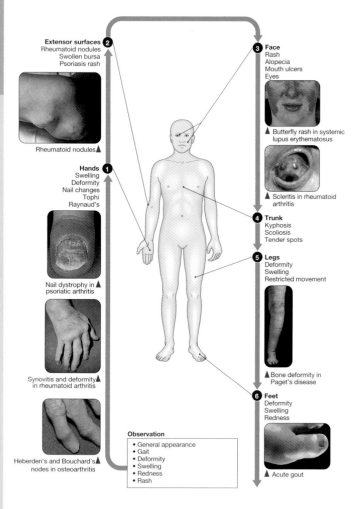

Extensor surfaces ❷
Rheumatoid nodules
Swollen bursa
Psoriasis rash

Rheumatoid nodules ▲

Hands ❶
Swelling
Deformity
Nail changes
Tophi
Raynaud's

Nail dystrophy in ▲
psoriatic arthritis

Synovitis and deformity ▲
in rheumatoid arthritis

Heberden's and Bouchard's
nodes in osteoarthritis ▲

Face ❸
Rash
Alopecia
Mouth ulcers
Eyes

▲ Butterfly rash in systemic
lupus erythematosus

▲ Scleritis in rheumatoid
arthritis

Trunk ❹
Kyphosis
Scoliosis
Tender spots

Legs ❺
Deformity
Swelling
Restricted movement

▲ Bone deformity in
Paget's disease

Feet ❻
Deformity
Swelling
Redness

▲ Acute gout

Observation
• General appearance
• Gait
• Deformity
• Swelling
• Redness
• Rash

15.1 Causes of acute monoarthritis

Common

- Septic arthritis
- Gout
- Pseudogout
- Reactive arthritis
- Trauma
- Haemarthrosis
- Seronegative spondyloarthritis:
  Psoriatic arthritis
  Ankylosing spondylitis
  Enteropathic arthritis

Uncommon

- Erythema nodosum
- Rheumatoid arthritis
- Juvenile idiopathic arthritis
- Pigmented villonodular synovitis
- Foreign body reaction
- Other infection: gonococcal, TB
- Leukaemia
- Osteomyelitis

Asymmetry, lower limb predominance and greater involvement of large joints are characteristic of seronegative spondyloarthritis.

Blood should be checked for inflammatory markers and viral serology. USS or MRI is used to detect synovitis. Treatment is that of the underlying condition.

Generalised musculoskeletal pain

The differential diagnosis includes:

• Malignant disease with bone metastases: relentlessly progressive pain with weight loss. • Paget's disease: usually more focal and localised to the site of involvement. • Osteoarthritis (OA): localised to affected sites, e.g. lumbar spine, hips, knees and hands. • Osteomalacia: generalised bone pain and tenderness with limb girdle weakness. • Fibromyalgia: generalised pain particularly affecting the trunk, back and neck.

Regional musculoskeletal pain

Back pain

Back pain is extremely common. In the UK, 7% of the adult population consult their GP each year with back pain.

Clinical assessment

The aim of history and examination is to distinguish the few patients with serious spinal pathology from the majority who have self-limiting mechanical pain.

i 15.2 Causes of polyarthritis

Cause	Characteristics
Common	
Rheumatoid arthritis	Symmetrical, any joint, upper and lower limbs
Viral arthritis	Symmetrical, small joints; with rash and prodromal illness
Osteoarthritis	Symmetrical, targets DIP joints in hands, knees, hips, back and neck; Heberden's and Bouchard's nodes
Psoriatic arthritis	Asymmetrical, targets PIP and DIP joints of hands and feet, nail pitting, large joints also affected
Ankylosing spondylitis and enteropathic arthritis	Large joints, lower >upper limbs, possible history of back pain
Systemic lupus erythematosus	Symmetrical, small joints, synovitis unusual
Less common	
Juvenile idiopathic arthritis	Symmetrical, any joint, upper and lower limbs
Chronic gout	Distal >proximal joints, acute attacks
Chronic sarcoidosis (p. 306)	Symmetrical, any joint
Polymyalgia rheumatica	Symmetrical, any joint
Rare	
Systemic sclerosis, polymyositis	Any joint
Hypertrophic osteoarthropathy	Small joints, clubbing
Haemochromatosis (p. 509)	Any joint
Acromegaly (p. 376)	Mainly large joints and spine

(DIP/PIP = distal/proximal interphalangeal)

Mechanical pain: This accounts for >90% of back pain episodes, usually affecting patients aged 20–55 yrs. It is more common in heavy manual workers, and often starts suddenly while lifting or bending. Symptoms are worsened by activity and relieved by rest. Pain is typically asymmetrical and is confined to the lumbosacral region, buttock or thigh, with no clear-cut nerve root distribution (unlike radicular pain). Examination may reveal paraspinal muscle spasm with painful restriction of movement. Prognosis is good, with 90% recovery at 6 wks. Psychological factors (e.g. job dissatisfaction, depression) increase the risk of progression to chronic disability.

Pain due to serious pathology: Causes include bony destruction due to malignancy, fracture or infection. 'Red flag' features suggesting serious spinal pathology include:

• Age <20 or >50 yrs. • Constant, progressive pain unrelieved by rest. • Thoracic pain. • History or symptoms of malignancy or TB. • Systemic corticosteroid use. • Constitutional symptoms: sweats, malaise, weight loss.

	15.3 Features of radicular pain

Nerve root pain

- Unilateral leg pain worse than low back pain
- Radiates beyond knee
- Paraesthesia in same distribution
- Nerve irritation signs (reduced straight leg raising, reproduces pain)
- Motor, sensory or reflex signs (limited to one nerve root)

Cauda equina syndrome

- Difficulty with micturition
- Loss of anal sphincter tone or faecal incontinence
- Saddle anaesthesia
- Gait disturbance
- Pain, numbness or weakness affecting one or both legs

Examination may reveal painful spinal deformity with signs at multiple nerve root levels. In all cases it is important to exclude signs of cauda equina syndrome (see below).

Inflammatory pain: Pain due to spondylitis is gradual in onset and often occurs before the age of 40 yrs. It is usually axial, symmetrical and spread over many segments. Sacroiliitis causes maximal pain in the buttock, with radiation down the posterior thigh. Patients often experience morning stiffness that improves with activity.

Degenerative disc disease: This causes nerve root pain (Box 15.3) in young adults, most commonly at L4 or L5. Around 70% of patients improve by 4 wks. Compression of multiple nerve roots in the cauda equina occurs in Paget's disease and spinal OA, and requires urgent treatment.

Investigations

Investigations are not required for mechanical back pain. Those with persistent pain (>6 wks) or 'red flags' should undergo MRI, which can demonstrate spinal stenosis, cord or nerve root compression, inflammatory spondyloarthropathy and infection causing spinal abscess. Plain X-rays can be of value if vertebral compression fractures, OA and degenerative disc disease are suspected. If metastatic disease is suspected, radionuclide bone scan or SPECT is useful. Additional investigations include:

• Biochemistry and haematology, including ESR and CRP (to screen for sepsis and inflammatory disease). • Protein and urinary electrophoresis (for myeloma). • Prostate specific antigen (for prostate carcinoma).

Management

Treatment of mechanical back pain involves reassurance, education, simple analgesia and early mobilisation. Bed rest is not helpful and increases the risk of chronic disability. Physiotherapy may be

15.4 Causes of neck pain	
Mechanical	Postural, 'whiplash', disc prolapse, cervical spondylosis
Inflammatory	Infection, spondylitis, rheumatoid arthritis, polymyalgia rheumatica
Neoplasia	Bony metastases, myeloma, lymphoma
Other	Fibromyalgia, torticollis
Referred pain	Pharynx, teeth, angina, Pancoast tumour, cervical lymph nodes

required in individuals not settling with the above measures. Surgery is required for <1% of patients. The management of serious spinal pathology is dictated by the cause.

Neck pain

Neck pain is a common symptom that can occur following injury (e.g. whiplash), after falling asleep in an awkward position, as a result of stress, or in association with OA of the spine. Common causes are shown in Box 15.4. Most cases resolve spontaneously or with a short course of NSAID or analgesics, and a soft collar. Patients with persistent pain in a nerve root distribution and those with neurological signs and symptoms should be referred for an MRI scan, and if necessary a neurosurgical opinion.

Shoulder pain

Rotator cuff syndrome: In this common condition, tendinitis or bursitis around the glenohumeral joint causes pain that is reproduced by resisted movement. Treatment is by physiotherapy, analgesia and steroid injections.

Adhesive capsulitis ('frozen shoulder'): This presents with upper arm pain that progresses over 4–10 wks before receding over a similar time course. Glenohumeral restriction is present from the outset, but progresses and reaches its maximum as the pain is receding. In the early phase there is marked anterior joint tenderness and pain at extremes of movement; later there is painless restriction, often affecting all movements. Treatment comprises analgesia, local corticosteroid injection and regular 'pendulum' exercises of the arm. The natural history is for slow but complete recovery.

Elbow pain

Common causes are shown in Box 15.5. Olecranon bursitis may also complicate infection, gout and rheumatoid arthritis (RA). Management is by rest, analgesics and topical or systemic NSAIDs. Local steroid injection is used in resistant cases.

Hand and wrist pain

Pain from hand or wrist joints is localised to the affected joint, except for pain from the first metacarpal joint, which often radiates down the thumb and to the radial aspect of the wrist. Non-articular causes of hand pain include:

15.5 Local causes of elbow pain

Lesion	Pain	Examination findings, tests
'Tennis elbow'	Lateral epicondyle Radiation to extensor forearm	Tenderness over epicondyle Pain reproduced by resisted active wrist extension
'Golfer's elbow'	Medial epicondyle Radiation to flexor forearm	Tenderness over epicondyle Pain reproduced by resisted active wrist flexion
Olecranon bursitis	Olecranon	Fluctuant tender swelling over olecranon

15.6 Common causes of lower limb pain

Lesion	Pain	Examination findings
Trochanteric bursitis	Upper lateral thigh, worse on lying on that side at night	Tender over greater trochanter
Adductor tendinitis	Upper inner thigh Usually clearly sports-related	Tender over adductor origin/tendon/muscle Pain reproduced by resisted active hip adduction
Pre-patellar bursitis	Anterior patella	Tender fluctuant swelling in front of patella
Popliteal cyst ('Baker's cyst')	Popliteal fossa	Tender swelling of popliteal fossa, usually reducible by massage with knee in mid-flexion
Plantar fasciitis	Under heel, worse on standing and walking	Tender under distal calcaneus/plantar fascia insertion site
Osteochondritis (Osgood–Schlatter disease)	Anterior upper tibia	Affects adolescents Pain on resisted active knee extension
Achilles tendinitis	Localised to tendon	Tender on squeezing tendon Pain reproduced by standing on toes or resisted plantar flexion

• Tenosynovitis: flexor or extensor; pain and swelling, with or without fine crepitus on volar or extensor aspect. De Quervain's tenosynovitis involves the tendon sheaths of abductor pollicis longus and extensor pollicis brevis, and produces pain and tenderness maximal over the radial aspect of the distal forearm and wrist. It usually occurs as a repetitive strain injury. There is marked pain on forced ulnar deviation of the wrist with the thumb held across the patient's palm. • Raynaud's phenomenon (p. 590). • C8/T1 radiculopathy. • Reflex sympathetic dystrophy: regional sympathetic dysfunction often triggered by fracture.

Lower limb pain

Common causes of lower limb pain are shown in Box 15.6.

15.7 Causes of proximal muscle pain and weakness

Inflammatory	Polymyositis, dermatomyositis, polymyalgia rheumatica
Endocrine	Hypothyroidism, hyperthyroidism, Cushing's syndrome, Addison's disease
Metabolic	Myophosphorylase/phosophofructokinase deficiency, hypokalaemia, osteomalacia
Drugs/toxins	Alcohol, fibrates, statins, cocaine, penicillamine, zidovudine
Infections	HIV, cytomegalovirus, Epstein–Barr virus, staphylococci, TB, schistosomiasis

Muscle pain and weakness

It is important to distinguish between a subjective feeling of generalised weakness or fatigue, and 'true' weakness with objective loss of muscle power. The former is a non-specific manifestation of many diseases, including depression, whereas the latter often indicates intrinsic muscle disease. Proximal muscle weakness causes difficulty in standing from a seated position, squatting and lifting overhead. Causes of proximal myopathy are listed in Box 15.7. Weakness should be graded on the MRC 6-point scale (0 = no power, 5 = full power).

Investigations include biochemistry and haematology, ESR, CRP and CK. Serum 25(OH) vitamin D levels and parathyroid hormone (PTH) should be checked in suspected osteomalacia. Raised CK levels suggest muscle pathology but do not establish the cause. The ESR and CRP may be raised in inflammatory myositis. Muscle biopsy and electromyography (EMG) are usually required to make the diagnosis, but MRI can be used to identify focal areas of muscle abnormality and increase the diagnostic yield from muscle biopsies.

PRINCIPLES OF MANAGEMENT OF MUSCULOSKELETAL DISORDERS

Key aims of management of musculoskeletal conditions are:
• Patient education. • Pain control. • Optimisation of function.
• Beneficial modification of the disease process.

These therapeutic objectives are achieved most effectively via a multidisciplinary team approach.

Education and lifestyle interventions

Patient education has been shown to reduce pain and disability. Local strengthening exercise should be combined with aerobic exercise to maximise benefit. Adverse mechanical factors should be addressed; examples include shock-absorbing footwear, walking aids, and weight loss in obese patients. Tuition in coping strategies (e.g. yoga, relaxation, avoidance of maladaptive pain behaviour) can assist patients with incurable disease.

Pharmacological treatment
Analgesia
Paracetamol is effective for the treatment of mild to moderate pain. It acts by inhibiting central prostaglandin synthesis but has little effect on peripheral prostaglandin production. It is safe, has few contraindications and drug interactions, and is low in cost. It is therefore an appropriate first-line analgesic in most patients. If paracetamol fails to control pain, it can be combined with codeine or dihydrocodeine, as in co-codamol (codeine and paracetamol) or co-dydramol (dihydrocodeine and paracetamol). The centrally acting analgesics tramadol and meptazinol are used for temporary control of unresponsive severe pain. Although these drugs are more effective than paracetamol, side-effects include constipation, headache, confusion, dizziness and somnolence, especially in the elderly. Withdrawal symptoms may occur after chronic use. The non-opioid nefopam (30–90 mg 3 times daily) can help moderate pain, though side-effects (nausea, anxiety, dry mouth) limit its use. Patients with severe pain may require oxycodone and morphine.

Non-steroidal anti-inflammatory drugs
Non-steroidal anti-inflammatory drugs (NSAIDS; e.g. ibuprofen, diclofenac) are effective in combating pain and stiffness associated with inflammatory disease. They also help reduce bone pain due to metastatic deposits. They act by inhibiting cyclo-oxygenase (COX) and thereby reducing prostaglandin synthesis (Fig. 15.1). There are two isoforms of COX, encoded by distinct genes.

Details of the usage, dose and side-effects of NSAIDs are given on page 789.

Topical agents
NSAID and capsaicin (chilli extract) creams provide safe and effective pain relief from arthritis (especially OA) and periarticular lesions. They may be used as monotherapy or as an adjunct to oral analgesics. Topical capsaicin causes pain fibres to discharge substance P. Initial application results in a burning sensation, but continued use reduces substance P activity with consequent pain reduction.

Non-pharmacological interventions
Local heat, ice packs and wax baths can induce muscle relaxation and provide temporary relief of symptoms in a range of rheumatic diseases. Hydrotherapy induces muscle relaxation and facilitates enhanced movement in a warm, pain-relieving environment free from gravity and load-bearing. The combination of these with education and therapist contact enhances their benefits.

Splints can give temporary rest and support for painful joints but prolonged rest must be avoided. Orthoses are more permanent appliances used to reduce instability and excessive abnormal movement. They are particularly suited to severely disabled

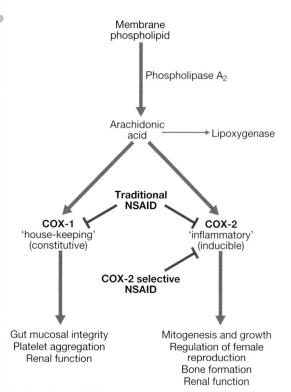

Fig. 15.1 COX-1 and COX-2 pathways.

patients in whom surgery is inappropriate, and often need to be custom-made.

Aids and appliances can provide dignity and independence in activities of daily living. Common examples are a raised toilet seat, raised chair height, extended handles on taps, a shower instead of a bath, thick-handled cutlery, and extended 'hands' to pull on tights and socks. Input from an occupational therapist is essential to maximise benefit.

Surgery

Soft tissue release and tenosynovectomy may reduce inflammatory symptoms and improve function. Synovectomy does not prevent disease progression but may provide pain relief when other measures have failed. Surgery may involve osteotomy (cutting bone to alter joint mechanics), excision arthroplasty (removing part or all of the joint), joint replacement and arthrodesis (joint fusion).

OSTEOARTHRITIS

OA is by far the most common form of arthritis. It is strongly associated with ageing, and is a major cause of pain and disability in older people. Up to 45% of all people develop knee OA and 25% hip OA at some point during life. It is characterised by focal loss of articular cartilage with new bone proliferation and remodelling of the joint contour. Inflammation is not a prominent feature. OA preferentially targets certain small and large joints (Fig. 15.2); the knee and hip are the principal large joints involved.

Repetitive adverse loading of joints during occupation or sports is a predisposing factor in farmers, miners and athletes. For most people, however, sport does not increase the risk of OA, unless there has been significant joint trauma. Congenital joint abnormalities (e.g. slipped femoral epiphysis), Paget's disease and obesity are also associated with OA, presumably due to abnormal load distribution within the joint. In obesity, cytokines released from adipose tissue may also play a role. Genetic factors are also important in OA; there is an increased incidence in women, and family studies show that the heritability of OA ranges from 43% at the knee to 60–65% at the hip and hand.

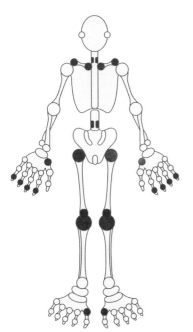

Fig. 15.2 The distribution of osteoarthritis. Although OA can affect any synovial joint, those shown in red are the most commonly targeted.

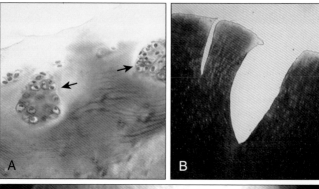

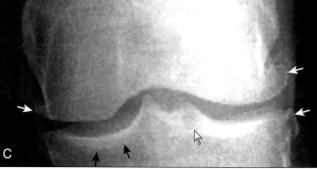

Fig. 15.3 Pathological changes in osteoarthritis. A Abnormal nests of proliferating chondrocytes (arrows) interspersed with matrix devoid of normal chondrocytes. **B** Fibrillation of cartilage. **C** X-ray changes of OA in a knee joint: osteophytes at the joint margin (white arrows), subchondral sclerosis (black arrows) and subchondral cyst (open arrow).

The pathogenesis of OA involves enzymatic degradation of aggrecan and collagen within the articular cartilage, with fissuring and thinning of the cartilage surface (Fig. 15.3). Cysts develop within the subchondral bone, possibly due to osteonecrosis resulting from increased pressure on the bone as the cartilage fails. At the joint margins, new fibrocartilage grows and then ossifies, forming osteophytes. Bone remodelling and cartilage thinning gradually alter the shape of the OA joint. This is accompanied by wasting of the surrounding muscles, synovial hyperplasia and thickening of the joint capsule.

Clinical features

Symptoms:

• Pain and functional restriction. • Insidious onset over months or years. • Pain worsened by movement and relieved by rest. • Only

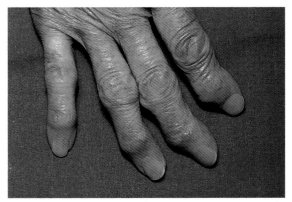

Fig. 15.4 Nodal osteoarthritis. Heberden's nodes and lateral deviation of the distal interphalangeal joints, with mild Bouchard's nodes at the proximal interphalangeal joints.

brief (<15 mins) morning stiffness and brief 'gelling' after rest (in contrast to inflammatory arthritis). • Usually only one or a few painful joints.

Examination:

• Restricted range of movement. • Palpable coarse crepitus. • Bony swelling and deformity around joint margins. • Joint-line or periarticular tenderness. • Muscle wasting. • Synovitis mild or absent.

Generalised nodal OA

This common form of OA has a strong genetic predisposition and is more common in middle-aged women. Patients develop pain, stiffness and swelling affecting the finger interphalangeal joints (IPJs) (distal > proximal). Affected joints develop swellings that harden to become Heberden's (distal IPJ) and Bouchard's (proximal IPJ) nodes (Fig. 15.4). Involvement of the first carpometacarpal joint is also common. The condition is associated with a good functional prognosis. There is, however, an increased risk of OA at other sites ('generalised OA'), especially the knee.

Knee OA

OA of the knee may be primary, or secondary to trauma; the latter is more common in men and is typically unilateral. Pain is usually localised to the anterior and medial aspects of the knee. Functional difficulties include those involved in prolonged walking, rising from a chair and bending to put on shoes. Examination reveals:

• A jerky, asymmetric, 'antalgic' gait (less time weight-bearing on the painful side). • Deformity: varus, less commonly valgus, fixed flexion. • Bony swelling around the joint line. • Wasting of the quadriceps. • Joint line and/or periarticular tenderness. • Restricted flexion/extension with coarse crepitus.

Hip OA

Pain due to hip OA is usually maximal deep in the anterior groin, with variable radiation to the buttock, thigh or knee. Lateral hip pain, worse on lying on that side with tenderness over the greater trochanter, suggests secondary trochanteric bursitis. Functional difficulties are similar to those in knee OA. Examination shows:

• An antalgic gait. • Wasting of quadriceps and gluteal muscles. • Pain and restriction of internal rotation with the hip flexed (the earliest sign of hip OA); other movements may subsequently be affected. • Anterior groin tenderness. • Fixed flexion, external rotation deformity of the hip.

Spine OA

This affects the cervical and lumbar spine (cervical and lumbar spondylosis, respectively), presenting with lower back or neck pain. Radiation of pain to the arms, buttocks and legs also occurs, due to nerve root compression. On examination, the range of movement is limited, loss of lumbar lordosis is typical, and neurological signs may confirm nerve root compression.

Investigations

Plain X-rays may reveal joint space narrowing, subchondral sclerosis, osteophytes and bone cysts. However, correlation between radiographic changes, symptoms and disability is variable. MRI is indicated if nerve root compression is suspected. Routine blood tests are normal in OA.

Management

Treatment follows the principles set out on pages 568–70 and includes:

• Full explanation of the nature of OA. • Local strengthening and aerobic exercises. • Reduction of adverse mechanical factors (e.g. weight loss if obese, shock-absorbing footwear, walking aids). • Analgesia (initially paracetamol, then consider topical NSAID or capsaicin, then paracetamol plus oral NSAIDs, then opioid analgesics). • Intra-articular corticosteroid injection: may provide temporary relief of moderate to severe pain. • Local physical therapies such as heat or cold. • Surgery: should be considered for patients with uncontrolled pain and progressive functional impairment despite medical treatment; options include osteotomy and joint replacement.

CRYSTAL-INDUCED ARTHRITIS

Crystal deposition in and around joints can result in acute and chronic inflammatory arthritis.

Gout

Gout is caused by the deposition of monosodium urate monohydrate (MSUM) crystals at synovial joints. It has a prevalence of 1–2%,

15.8 Causes of hyperuricaemia and gout

Diminished renal excretion (>90% of cases)

- Inherited reduction in renal tubular excretion of urate
- Renal failure
- Drug therapy (e.g. thiazide and loop diuretics, low-dose aspirin, ciclosporin)
- Lead toxicity (e.g. in 'moonshine' drinkers)
- Lactic acidosis (alcohol)

Increased intake

- Red meat, seafood, offal

Over-production of uric acid

- Myeloproliferative or lymphoproliferative disorders, chemotherapy for leukaemias, psoriasis
- Increased de novo synthesis: cause unknown in most, rarely specific enzyme defects, e.g. glucose-6-phosphatase deficiency

and is more common in men, in certain ethnic groups and with increasing age. Uric acid mainly comes from the metabolism of purines within the body but some is ingested with food. Gout is becoming more common with increased longevity and prevalence of metabolic syndrome (p. 385), of which hyperuricaemia is a component. Causes of hyperuricaemia are shown in Box 15.8.

Clinical features

Acute gout: This presents with rapid onset of severe pain in a single distal joint, commonly the first metatarsophalangeal joint (Fig. 15.5A). Other common sites include the ankle, midfoot, knee, hand, wrist and elbow. Examination reveals marked synovitis with swelling, red shiny skin and extreme tenderness. Periarticular swelling and fever may also be present. Symptoms are usually self-limiting over 5–14 days. The differential diagnosis includes septic arthritis, cellulitis and reactive arthritis.

Recurrent and chronic gout: Following an acute attack, many patients go on to experience a second attack within a year. The frequency of attacks increases with time. Involvement of several joints with continued MSUM deposition eventually leads to joint damage and chronic pain.

Chronic tophaceous gout: MSUM crystal deposits produce irregular firm nodules ('tophi') around extensor surfaces of fingers (Fig. 15.5B), forearms, elbows, Achilles tendons and ears. Tophi are usually a late feature of gout.

Renal and urinary tract manifestations: Chronic hyperuricaemia may be complicated by renal stone formation (p. 190) and sometimes renal impairment due to interstitial nephritis caused by urate deposition in the kidney. This particularly affects patients with chronic tophaceous gout who are on diuretics.

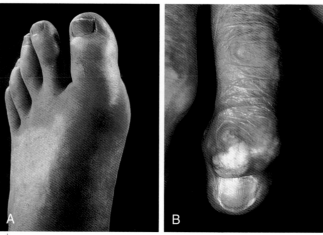

Fig. 15.5 Gout. A Acute gout causing inflammation of the first metatarsophalangeal joint (podagra). **B** Tophus.

Investigations

Joint aspiration reveals long, needle-shaped MSUM crystals, which are negatively birefringent under polarised light. Synovial fluid in acute gout appears turbid due to the high neutrophil count (>90%). Serum uric acid is usually elevated, but hyperuricaemia itself does not confirm gout. Equally, acute inflammation reduces levels, so a normal uric acid level does not exclude gout. Serum creatinine should be checked to exclude renal impairment. There is neutrophilia with a raised CRP in acute gout; FBC and ESR may detect myeloproliferative disorders during remission of the acute episode. Joint X-rays are usually normal in early gout. Changes of secondary OA and gouty erosions may develop with chronic disease.

Management

Acute attacks: Oral NSAIDs are standard treatment. Ice packs provide symptomatic relief. Oral colchicine is also very effective but vomiting and diarrhoea are common side-effects. Joint aspiration and intra-articular corticosteroid injections are effective in more severe cases.

Long-term management: Allopurinol lowers serum uric acid levels by inhibiting xanthine oxidase, which reduces conversion of hypoxanthine and xanthine to uric acid. It is indicated in patients with recurrent attacks of acute gout, tophi, joint damage or renal impairment. Allopurinol initiation can trigger an acute attack; it should therefore be initiated after the acute attack has settled, and should be co-prescribed with an NSAID or colchicine for the first few weeks.

Predisposing factors should be addressed:

• Weight loss: advised in obese patients. • Excess beer: avoid. • Diuretics: stop if possible. • High-purine diet (seafood, red meat and offal): avoid.

Calcium pyrophosphate dihydrate crystal deposition

Calcium pyrophosphate dihydrate (CPPD) crystal deposition within articular cartilage causes chondrocalcinosis. Risk factors include age, OA and primary hyperparathyroidism. Rarely, it is associated with metabolic disease (e.g. haemochromatosis, hypophosphataemia, hypomagnesaemia and Wilson's disease). It is often clinically silent, but can cause episodes of acute synovitis ('pseudogout') or occur as a chronic arthritis that is associated with OA.

Clinical features

Acute synovitis ('pseudogout'): This is the most common cause of acute monoarthritis in the elderly. The knee is the most common site, followed by the wrist, shoulder and ankle. The typical attack resembles acute gout with rapid onset of pain, stiffness and swelling. Examination reveals erythema, marked joint tenderness and signs of synovitis (large effusion, warmth and restricted movement). Fever may be present. Septic arthritis and gout are the main differential diagnoses.

Chronic CPPD arthritis: Chronic symptoms usually occur in elderly women. The distribution is similar to that of pseudogout. Symptoms are chronic pain with variable early morning stiffness. Affected joints show features of OA (bony swelling, crepitus, restriction) with varying degrees of synovitis.

Investigations

Joint fluid aspiration in acute pseudogout reveals small, rhomboid-shaped CPPD crystals that are positively birefringent under polarised light. Gram stain and culture of the fluid will exclude sepsis. X-rays may show chondrocalcinosis within the articular cartilage. Blood tests should be performed to exclude metabolic causes of CPPD crystal deposition in younger patients and in individuals with polyarticular disease.

Management

• Joint aspiration with intra-articular corticosteroid injection: provides rapid pain relief. • Oral NSAIDs and colchicine: effective for acute pseudogout.

FIBROMYALGIA

This is a common cause of generalised regional pain and disability, and is frequently associated with medically unexplained symptoms in other systems. The prevalence in the UK is ~2–3%. It increases in prevalence with age, to reach a peak of 7% in women aged over 70. There is a female predominance of ~10:1. Risk factors include stressful life events, such as marital disharmony, alcoholism in the family, injury or assault, low income and self-reported childhood abuse.

No structural, inflammatory or metabolic abnormality has been identified, although abnormalities of non-rapid eye movement (REM) sleep and of central pain processing have been postulated as potential aetiological factors.

Clinical features and investigations

The main presenting feature is multiple regional pain, affecting the neck, back, both arms and both legs; it is unresponsive to analgesics and NSAIDs. Patients commonly report fatigability, particularly in the morning, and reported disability is often marked. Although people can usually dress and groom themselves, they may struggle with daily tasks such as shopping and housework, and may have given up work because of pain and fatigue. Non-locomotor features include tension headache, irritable bowel syndrome and irritable bladder.

Examination usually reveals hyperalgesia at multiple specific tender sites. Moderate pressure at each site may be uncomfortable in a normal subject but in fibromyalgia it produces a wince/ withdrawal response. Although there are no abnormal investigations associated with fibromyalgia, it is important to screen for alternative musculoskeletal conditions.

Management

The patient should be reassured that the widespread pain does not reflect inflammation, tissue damage or disease. Low-dose amitriptyline with or without fluoxetine may be useful. Graded exercise may improve well-being. Relaxation techniques and coping strategies employing a cognitive behavioural approach should be encouraged. Patient organisations can provide valuable support.

BONE AND JOINT INFECTION

Septic arthritis

Septic arthritis is a medical emergency. It usually arises from haematogenous spread of bacterial infection from another site, commonly the skin or upper respiratory tract. Infection from direct puncture wounds or that secondary to joint aspiration is uncommon. Risk factors for septic arthritis include increasing age, pre-existing joint disease (especially RA), diabetes mellitus, immunosuppression and IV drug misuse.

Clinical features

The usual presentation is with acute or subacute monoarthritis. The joint is usually swollen, hot and red, with pain at rest and on movement. The knee and hip are the most common sites. The usual culprit organism is *Staphylococcus aureus*. Disseminated gonococcal infection is another cause in young, sexually active adults. This presents with migratory arthralgia and low-grade fever, followed by the development of oligo- or monoarthritis. Painful pustular skin lesions may also be present. Lyme disease and brucellosis are less common causes of septic arthritis.

Investigations

Joint fluid aspiration for Gram stain and culture is essential, under image guidance if deep. Aspirated fluid often looks turbid or blood-stained. Blood cultures may be positive due to bacteraemia. Blood tests may reveal leucocytosis with raised ESR and CRP, although these may be absent in elderly or immunocompromised patients. Concurrent cultures from the genital tract are indicated if gonococcal infection is likely.

Management

• Pain relief. • IV antibiotics: IV flucloxacillin 2 g three times daily is first choice until identification of the organism and its sensitivities is possible. IV treatment is usually continued for 2 wks, followed by oral treatment for a further 4 wks. • Daily joint aspiration in the initial stages to minimise the effusion. If this is unsuccessful, surgical drainage may be required. • Early mobilisation.

Viral arthritis

Parvovirus B19 is the most common cause of viral arthritis; other causes include hepatitis B and C, rubella and HIV. The usual presentation is with acute polyarthritis, fever and rash. Symptoms are usually self-limiting. Diagnosis is confirmed by viral serology.

Osteomyelitis

Infection of bone usually arises from haematogenous spread, although directly introduced infection may complicate a compound fracture, penetrating injury or orthopaedic surgery. Organisms most frequently implicated are staphylococci, *Pseudomonas* and *Mycobacterium tuberculosis*. Risk factors include young age, diabetes, immunodeficiency and sickle-cell disease. Infection often results in a florid inflammatory response and localised areas of osteonecrosis.

Clinical features and investigations

Presentation is with localised bone pain and tenderness, fever and night sweats. A discharging sinus may form in advanced cases. X-rays may show osteolysis or osteonecrosis, but MRI is the imaging method of choice as it is much more sensitive. Confirmation of the diagnosis should be obtained by blood culture and culture of a bone aspirate or biopsy.

Management

• Pain relief. • 2 wks of IV antibiotics, followed by 4 wks of oral antibiotics. • Surgical decompression and removal of any dead bone. • Rehabilitation.

Tuberculosis

TB of the musculoskeletal system usually targets the spine (Pott's disease), hip, knee or ankle. The presentation is with pain, swelling and fever. X-rays are non-specific and mycobacteria are seldom identified in the synovial fluid, so tissue biopsy is required for diagnosis. Antituberculous chemotherapy is described on page 295. Occasionally, surgical débridement of joints or stabilisation and decompression of the spine is required.

RHEUMATOID ARTHRITIS

Rheumatoid arthritis (RA) is the most common persistent inflammatory arthritis and occurs throughout the world and in all ethnic groups. The prevalence is lowest in black Africans and Chinese; in Caucasians it is ~1.0–1.5% with a female : male ratio of 3 : 1. The clinical course is usually lifelong, with exacerbations and remissions. Factors that predict poor prognosis are disability at presentation, female gender, involvement of MTP joints, radiographic damage at presentation, smoking and a positive rheumatoid factor (RF) or anti-citrullinated peptide antibodies (ACPA). It is likely that the prognosis will improve as more effective treatment is introduced in patients with early disease.

Concordance rates are higher in monozygotic twins (12–15%) than in dizygotic twins (3%). Up to 50% of the genetic susceptibility is due to genes in the HLA region, particularly HLA-DR4.

RA is an autoimmune condition characterised by chronic inflammation, granuloma formation and joint destruction. The earliest change is swelling and congestion of the synovial membrane and the underlying connective tissues, which become infiltrated with lymphocytes, plasma cells and macrophages. TNF plays a central role in triggering local inflammation and regulating cytokines responsible for the systemic effects of RA. Hypertrophy of the synovial membrane occurs, and inflammatory granulation tissue (pannus) spreads over and under the articular cartilage, causing progressive cartilage destruction. Muscles adjacent to inflamed joints atrophy and there may be focal infiltration with lymphocytes. Subcutaneous rheumatoid nodules are granulomatous lesions consisting of a central area of fibrinoid material surrounded by proliferating mononuclear cells. Similar nodules may occur in the pleura, lung and pericardium.

Clinical features

The most common presentation is with a gradual onset of symmetrical arthralgia and synovitis of small joints of the hands, feet and wrists. Large joint involvement, systemic symptoms and extra-articular features may also occur. Clinical criteria for the diagnosis of RA are shown in Box 15.9.

Sometimes RA has a very acute onset, with florid morning stiffness, polyarthritis and pitting oedema. This occurs more commonly

15.9 Criteria for diagnosis of rheumatoid arthritis*	
Criterion	**Score**
Joints affected	
1 large joint	0
2–10 large joints	1
1–3 small joints	2
4–10 small joints	5
Serology	
Negative RF and ACPA	0
Low positive RF or ACPA	2
High positive RF or ACPA	3
Duration of symptoms	
<6 wks	0
>6 wks	1
Acute phase reactants	
Normal CRP and ESR	0
Abnormal CRP or ESR	1
Patients with a score ≥6 are considered to have definite RA.	

*European League Against Rheumatism/American College of Rheumatology 2010 Criteria. (ACPA = anti-citrullinated peptide antibodies; CRP = C-reactive protein; ESR = erythrocyte sedimentation rate; RF = rheumatoid factor)

in old age. Other patients may present with proximal muscle stiffness mimicking polymyalgia rheumatica (p. 597). Occasionally, the onset is palindromic, with relapsing and remitting episodes of pain, stiffness and swelling that last for only a few hours or days.

Examination reveals typical symmetrical swelling of the metacarpophalangeal (MCP) and PIP joints. The joints are tender on pressure when actively inflamed and have stress pain on passive movement. Erythema is unusual and suggests coexistent sepsis. Characteristic deformities may develop with long-standing uncontrolled disease, including 'swan neck' deformity, the boutonnière ('button hole') deformity, and Z deformity of the thumb (Fig. 15.6). Dorsal subluxation of the ulna at the distal radio-ulnar joint is common and may contribute to rupture of the fourth and fifth extensor tendons. Trigger fingers may occur because of nodules in the flexor tendon sheaths. Hand deformities are becoming less common because of more aggressive treatment.

In the foot, dorsal subluxation of the MTP joints may result in pain on weight-bearing on the exposed metatarsal heads. Popliteal ('Baker's') cysts usually complicate knee synovitis. Cyst rupture, often induced by knee flexion with a large effusion, leads to calf pain and swelling that may mimic DVT.

Extra-articular features: Anorexia, weight loss and fatigue are common and may occur throughout the disease course. Extra-articular features (Box 15.10) are more common in patients with

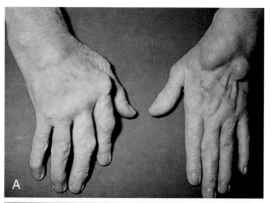

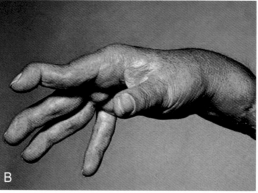

Fig. 15.6 The hand in rheumatoid arthritis. **A** Ulnar deviation of the fingers with wasting of the small muscles of the hands and synovial swelling at the wrists, the extensor tendon sheaths, the metacarpophalangeal and proximal interphalangeal joints. **B** 'Swan neck' deformity of the fingers.

long-standing seropositive erosive disease but may occur at presentation, especially in men.

Rheumatoid nodules occur in seropositive patients, usually at sites of pressure such as the extensor surfaces of the forearm, Achilles tendon and toes. Rheumatoid vasculitis occurs in older seropositive patients and varies from benign nail-fold infarcts to widespread cutaneous ulceration.

The most common ocular symptom is dry eyes (keratoconjunctivitis sicca, secondary Sjögren's syndrome). Painless episcleritis may cause intense redness but sight is unimpaired. Scleritis is more serious and potentially sight-threatening; the eye is red and painful, and vision is impaired. Scleromalacia is painless thinning of the sclera, with the affected area appearing blue or grey (the colour of the underlying choroid). No specific treatment is required.

> **i** 15.10 Extra-articular manifestations of rheumatoid disease
>
> | | |
> |---|---|
> | **Systemic** | Fever, fatigue, weight loss, susceptibility to infection |
> | **Musculoskeletal** | Muscle-wasting, tenosynovitis, bursitis, osteoporosis |
> | **Haematological** | Anaemia, eosinophilia, thrombocytosis |
> | **Lymphatic** | Splenomegaly, Felty's syndrome (RA, splenomegaly and neutropenia) |
> | **Nodules** | Sinuses, fistulae |
> | **Ocular** | Episcleritis, scleritis, scleromalacia, keratoconjunctivitis sicca |
> | **Vasculitis** | Digital arteritis, ulcers, pyoderma gangrenosum, mononeuritis multiplex, visceral arteritis |
> | **Cardiac** | Pericarditis, myocarditis, endocarditis, conduction defects, coronary vasculitis, granulomatous aortitis |
> | **Pulmonary** | Nodules, pleural effusions, pulmonary fibrosis, Caplan's syndrome (RA plus pneumoconiosis), bronchiolitis, bronchiectasis |
> | **Neurological** | Cervical cord compression, compression neuropathies, peripheral neuropathy, mononeuritis multiplex |
> | **Amyloidosis** | |

Cardiac involvement occurs in up to 30% of seropositive patients but is usually asymptomatic. The risk of atheroma and cardiovascular disease is, however, increased in RA. Pulmonary fibrosis can occur in advanced RA and may cause dyspnoea (p. 204).

Median nerve compression in the carpal tunnel is common and bilateral compression can occur as an early presenting feature of RA.

Investigations

Diagnosis is based on clinical criteria (see Box 15.9). ESR and CRP are usually elevated in patients with active disease. ACPA are positive in ~70% of cases and are highly specific for RA, often occurring before clinical onset of disease. RF is positive in ~70%, many of whom also have positive ACPA. Low titres of RF are found in ~10% of the normal population.

USS examination and MRI are mainly used to detect synovitis and early erosions. Plain X-rays are of limited value in early RA but periarticular osteoporosis and marginal joint erosions are characteristic. Patients who are suspected of having atlanto-axial disease should have MRI. In patients with Baker's cyst, USS may be required to establish the diagnosis and exclude DVT.

Management

Disease-modifying antirheumatic drugs (DMARDs): The early use of small-molecule DMARDs is the mainstay of treatment and improves clinical outcome in RA. Corticosteroids are used for induction of remission. Partial or non-response to DMARDs necessitates dose escalation, use of an additional DMARD, or progression to biological drugs if necessary. Regular monitoring of DMARD

15.11 Commonly used disease-modifying antirheumatic drugs*

Drug	Disease indications	Side-effects	Monitoring requirement
Methotrexate	RA, seroneg, SLE, CTD, vasculitis, PMR	GI upset, mouth ulcers, alopecia, hepatotoxicity, hepatic fibrosis, acute pneumonitis	FBC, LFTs: monthly, then 3-monthly
Sulfasalazine	RA, seroneg	GI upset, hepatitis, neutropenia	FBC, LFTs: monthly for 3 mths, then 3-monthly
Hydroxychloroquine	RA, SLE	Diarrhoea, headache, rash, corneal deposits, retinopathy	Visual acuity, fundoscopy: 12-monthly
Leflunomide	RA	Rash, GI upset, alopecia, hepatitis, hypertension	FBC, LFTs, BP: 2–4-weekly
D-Penicillamine	RA	Rash, stomatitis, metallic taste, proteinuria, thrombocytopenia	FBC, urine (protein): initially 1–2-weekly, later 4–6-weekly
Gold	RA	Rash, stomatitis, alopecia, proteinuria, thrombocytopenia	FBC, urine (protein): each injection
Ciclosporin	RA	GI upset, renal impairment, hypertension	

*Most DMARDs can cause a rash, nausea and myelosuppression as well as the listed side-effects.

(CTD = connective tissue disease; PMR = polymyalgia rheumatica; seroneg = peripheral arthritis due to seronegative spondarthritis; SLE = systemic lupus erythematosus)

therapy is essential because of the risk of liver and haematological toxicity. Some DMARDs are contraindicated in pregnancy, especially during the first trimester. Further details of individual DMARDs are given in Box 15.11.

Biological therapies: Biological agents are reserved for patients who have high disease activity despite an adequate trial of traditional DMARDs. Although generally well tolerated, biological therapies are expensive and increase the risk of serious infections due to suppression of the immune response.

Anti-TNF therapy (e.g. infliximab, etanercept, adalimumab): These are the first-line biological drugs in RA. Most are co-prescribed with methotrexate, as this is more efficacious. The main adverse effects are serious infections and reactivation of latent TB. Anti-TNF therapy can increase the risk of some malignancies, but may reduce the risk of vascular disease in RA patients.

Rituximab: This is an anti-CD20 receptor antibody that depletes B lymphocytes. It is mostly used in patients with RA who fail to respond to TNF blockade. Abatacept (T-cell activation inhibitor) and tocilizumab (anti-IL-6) are alternative licensed biological treatments.

Corticosteroids: Glucocorticoids have rapid and dramatic anti-inflammatory actions. However, unacceptable level side-effects, including iatrogenic Cushing's syndrome, steroid-induced diabetes and osteoporosis, limit their use to rapid and short-term control of severe synovitis or systemic inflammation.

Local injections: Intra-articular injection of a long-acting corticosteroid (e.g. triamcinolone) can be a useful adjunctive therapy for controlling synovitis affecting one or a few joints. Symptom relief typically lasts for 2–8 wks. Iatrogenic infection is the most important adverse effect, which can be avoided by proper aseptic technique. Other side-effects include local skin atrophy and temporary symptom exacerbation. Periarticular steroid injections can be used to provide rapid, effective pain relief for conditions such as bursitis, tenosynovitis and lateral epicondylitis. The steroid is sometimes combined with local anaesthetic to provide more rapid analgesia.

Non-pharmacological interventions: These important aspects of treatment are covered on page 569.

Surgery: Synovectomy of wrist or finger tendon sheaths may provide pain relief when medical interventions have failed. Osteotomy, arthrodesis or arthroplasties may be beneficial in later stages of disease.

JUVENILE IDIOPATHIC ARTHRITIS

Systemic juvenile idiopathic arthritis (JIA; formerly known as Still's disease) is a systemic disorder of children characterised by fever, rash, arthritis, hepatosplenomegaly and serositis with a raised ESR and CRP. Autoantibody tests are negative.

The principles of management are similar to those in adult inflammatory disease, starting with corticosteroids and methotrexate for systemic JIA. TNF blockers and other biological agents may be effective in resistant cases.

Oligoarthritis frequently resolves at puberty, but those with polyarticular or systemic manifestations have a poorer prognosis; ~50% of cases persist into adulthood, requiring transition to adult rheumatology services.

Adult-onset Still's disease

This is a rare idiopathic systemic inflammatory disorder, similar to JIA, which presents with intermittent fever, rash and arthralgia. Splenomegaly, hepatomegaly and lymphadenopathy may be present. Tests for RF and antinuclear antibody (ANA) are negative.

Most patients respond to corticosteroids, but DMARDs may also be required as steroid-sparing agents.

This term is applied to a group of inflammatory joint diseases distinct from RA that share a number of clinical features (Box 15.12):
• Ankylosing spondylitis. • Reactive arthritis, including Reiter's disease. • Psoriatic arthropathy. • Arthritis associated with inflammatory bowel disease (Crohn's disease, ulcerative colitis).

An association with HLA-B27 occurs in all seronegative spondarthritides but is particularly strong for ankylosing spondylitis and Reiter's disease (>90%). The suggested pathogenesis is an aberrant response to infection in genetically predisposed individuals. In some situations a triggering organism can be identified, as in Reiter's disease following bacterial dysentery or chlamydial urethritis, but in others the environmental trigger remains obscure.

Ankylosing spondylitis

Ankylosing spondylitis is a chronic inflammatory arthritis predominantly affecting the sacroiliac joints and spine. The onset is typically between the ages of 20 and 30, with a male:female ratio of 3:1.

Clinical features

The cardinal feature is low back pain radiating to the buttocks or posterior thighs and early morning stiffness. Symptoms are exacerbated by inactivity and relieved by movement. The disease tends to ascend slowly, ultimately involving the whole spine. Examination reveals a reduced range of lumbar spine movements and pain on sacroiliac stressing. As the disease progresses, the spine and chest become rigid as ankylosis occurs. Secondary vertebral osteoporosis frequently occurs, causing an increased fracture risk.

15.12 Clinical features common to seronegative spondarthritis

• Asymmetrical inflammatory oligoarthritis (lower >upper limb)
• Sacroiliitis and inflammatory spondylitis
• Inflammatory enthesitis (e.g. tendons, ligaments)
• Tendency for familial aggregation
• RF and ACPA negative
• Absence of nodules and other extra-articular features of RA
• Extra-articular features:
    Mucosal: conjunctivitis, buccal ulceration, urethritis, prostatitis, bowel ulceration
    Pustular skin lesions, nail dystrophy
    Anterior uveitis
    Aortic root fibrosis (aortic incompetence, conduction defects)
    Erythema nodosum

Spinal fusion is usually mild, but a few patients develop incapacitating kyphosis of the thoracic and cervical spine with fixed flexion contractures of hips or knees. Pleuritic chest pain is common and results from costovertebral joint involvement. Plantar fasciitis, Achilles tendinitis and tenderness over bony prominences such as the iliac crest and greater trochanter may occur, reflecting inflammation at tendon insertions (enthesitis).

Up to 40% of patients also have asymmetrical peripheral arthritis, affecting large joints such as the hips, knees, ankles and shoulders. In ~10%, involvement of a peripheral joint antedates spinal symptoms, and in a further 10%, symptoms begin in childhood.

Fatigue is common and reflects both chronic sleep disturbance by pain, and systemic inflammation with direct effects of inflammatory cytokines on the brain. Anterior uveitis is the most common extra-articular feature, which occasionally precedes joint disease.

Investigations

In established ankylosing spondylitis, X-rays of the sacroiliac joint show irregularity and loss of cortical margins, sclerosis, joint space narrowing and fusion. Lateral thoracolumbar spine X-rays may show anterior 'squaring' of vertebrae, bridging syndesmophytes, ossification of the anterior longitudinal ligament and facet joint fusion ('bamboo' spine). Erosive changes may be seen in the symphysis pubis, ischial tuberosities and peripheral joints. Osteoporosis and atlanto-axial dislocation can occur. MRI is valuable for detecting spinal or sacroiliac inflammation in early disease.

The ESR and CRP are usually raised in active disease but may be normal. HLA-B27 is usually present. Autoantibodies such as RF, ACPA and ANA are negative.

Management and prognosis

Education and regular back exercises are essential to maintain mobility and avoid deformity. NSAIDs are effective in relieving symptoms and may alter the course of the disease. Long-acting NSAIDs at night are particularly helpful for morning stiffness. Sulfasalazine, methotrexate or azathioprine may control peripheral arthritis but these drugs have no effect on axial disease. Anti-TNF therapy may improve symptoms in active disease resistant to standard therapy but does not alter disease course.

Local corticosteroid injections may help persistent plantar fasciitis, other enthesitis and peripheral arthritis. Severe hip, knee, ankle or shoulder symptoms may require surgery.

Reactive arthritis

Reactive arthritis classically affects young men. It follows an episode of bacterial dysentery (due to *Salmonella*, *Shigella*, *Campylobacter* or *Yersinia*) or non-specific urethritis (due to *Chlamydia*). The triad of urethritis, conjunctivitis and reactive arthritis constitutes classical Reiter's disease but incomplete forms are common.

Clinical features

Patients present with acute-onset, inflammatory oligoarthritis affecting the large and small joints of the lower limbs 1–3 wks following sexual exposure or an attack of dysentery. Symptoms of urethritis and conjunctivitis may be present. It occasionally presents with insidious onset of single joint involvement, minimal features of urethritis and conjunctivitis, and no clear history of 'trigger' illness. Achilles tendinitis or plantar fasciitis may occur.

Additional extra-articular features include:

• Circinate balanitis: causes vesicles (often painless) on the prepuce and glans. • Buccal erosions. • Keratoderma blennorrhagica: waxy yellow–brown skin lesions, particularly affecting the palms and soles. • Nail dystrophy identical to psoriatic nail dystrophy.

The first attack of reactive arthritis is usually self-limiting, with spontaneous remission within 2–4 mths. Recurrent arthritis develops in >60% of patients. Uveitis is rare with the first attack but occurs in 30% of patients with recurring arthritis.

Investigations

• Raised ESR and CRP. • Aspirated synovial fluid: leucocyte-rich with multinucleated macrophages. • High vaginal swab: may reveal *Chlamydia*. • Stool cultures: usually negative by the time the arthritis presents. • Serum RF, ACPA and ANA: negative. • X-ray changes: usually absent during the acute attack, other than soft tissue swelling. Joint space narrowing and marginal erosions may develop with recurrent disease.

Management

Rest and NSAIDs provide symptomatic relief during the acute phase. Intra-articular corticosteroid injections may help severe synovitis. Non-specific chlamydial urethritis is treated with a short course of doxycycline. DMARDs are occasionally used for severe progressive arthritis and keratoderma blennorrhagica. Anterior uveitis is a medical emergency requiring topical or systemic corticosteroids.

Psoriatic arthropathy

Psoriatic arthritis affects 7–20% of patients with psoriasis. It typically presents between the ages of 25 and 40 yrs. The seronegative arthritis usually occurs in individuals with pre-existing cutaneous psoriasis but can predate the skin disease.

Clinical features

Five major presentations of joint disease are recognised:

Asymmetrical inflammatory oligoarthritis (40%): May affect lower and upper limb joints. Involvement of a finger or toe by synovitis, together with enthesitis and inflammation of intervening tissue, can give rise to a 'sausage digit' or dactylitis. Usually only one or two large joints are involved, mainly knees.

Symmetrical polyarthritis (25%): May strongly resemble RA, with symmetrical involvement of small and large joints in both upper and lower limbs. However, nodules and other extra-articular features of RA are absent.

Distal interphalangeal joint (DIPJ) arthritis (15%): Predominantly affects men, almost invariably with accompanying nail dystrophy.

Psoriatic spondylitis (15%): Presents a similar clinical picture to ankylosing spondylitis but tends to be less severe.

Arthritis mutilans (5%): This deforming erosive arthritis targets fingers and toes. Marked cartilage and bone attrition results in loss of the joint and instability.

The general pattern of psoriatic arthritis is one of intermittent exacerbation followed by periods of remission. Residual damage and disability are relatively mild, except in arthritis mutilans.

Extra-articular features include:

• Skin lesions. • Nail changes: pitting, onycholysis (separation of the nail from the nail bed) and subungual hyperkeratosis. • Uveitis (in HLA-B27–positive cases with spondylitis).

Investigations

• ESR and CRP: may be raised but are often normal. • Serum RF and ANA: negative. • X-rays: may be normal or show erosive change with joint space narrowing.

Management and prognosis

Simple analgesics and NSAIDs provide symptomatic relief. Intra-articular corticosteroids may help control florid synovitis. Regular exercise is important in preventing ankylosis. DMARDs may be required for persistent unresponsive synovitis. Methotrexate is the treatment of choice, as it may also help severe skin psoriasis. Anti-TNF therapy should be considered in those unresponsive to DMARDs. The retinoid acitretin is effective in treating both the arthritis and the skin lesions but is teratogenic.

Enteropathic arthritis

This inflammatory arthritis is associated with ulcerative colitis and Crohn's disease, predominantly affecting large lower limb joints. The arthritis coincides with exacerbations of the underlying bowel disease and improves with effective treatment of the bowel disease. Sacroiliitis and ankylosing spondylitis indistinguishable from classic ankylosing spondylitis also occur with bowel disease but are not correlated with the activity of the bowel disease.

CONNECTIVE TISSUE DISEASE

These diseases share overlapping clinical features, characterised by dysregulation of immune responses, autoantibody production often directed at components of the cell nucleus, and widespread tissue damage.

Systemic lupus erythematosus

Systemic lupus erythematosus (SLE) is a rare multisystem connective tissue disease, mainly occurring in women (90%), with a peak onset in the second and third decades. Prevalence is 0.2% in Afro-Caribbeans and 0.03% in Caucasians.

Several autoantibodies are associated with SLE. Many of the target autoantigens are intracellular and intranuclear components. It is likely that the wide spectrum of autoantibody production results from polyclonal B- and T-cell activation. Although the triggers that lead to autoantibody production in SLE are unknown, one mechanism may be exposure of intracellular antigens on the cell surface during apoptosis.

Clinical features

Fever, weight loss and mild lymphadenopathy occur during flares of disease activity; fatigue, malaise and fibromyalgia-like symptoms are not particularly associated with active disease.

Arthritis: This is a common symptom, occurring in 90% of patients and often associated with early morning stiffness. Tenosynovitis may also be a feature but clinically apparent synovitis with joint swelling is rare.

Raynaud's phenomenon: Arthralgia or arthritis in combination with Raynaud's phenomenon is the most common presentation of SLE. Raynaud's phenomenon in a teenage girl with no other associated symptoms is likely to be idiopathic 'primary' Raynaud's. By contrast, onset in a male, or in a woman over the age of 30 yrs, suggests underlying connective tissue disease.

Skin: Three types of rash are characteristic:
• The classic butterfly (malar) facial rash: raised and painful or pruritic, and spares the nasolabial folds (Fig. 15.7). • The subacute cutaneous lupus erythematosus (SCLE) rash: migratory, non-scarring and either annular or psoriaform. • The discoid lupus rash: characterised by hyperkeratosis and follicular plugging, with scarring alopecia if it occurs on the scalp.

Other skin manifestations include periungual erythema, vasculitis and livedo reticularis, which is also a common feature of the antiphospholipid syndrome.

Kidney: The typical renal lesion is a proliferative glomerulonephritis, characterised by haematuria, proteinuria and casts on urine microscopy.

Cardiovascular: Pericarditis is the most common feature. Myocarditis and Libman–Sacks endocarditis (sterile fibrin containing vegetations) also occur. Atherosclerosis, stroke and myocardial infarction are increased due to the adverse effects of inflammation on the endothelium, chronic steroid therapy and the procoagulant effects of antiphospholipid antibodies.

Lung: Pleurisy can cause pleuritic chest pain, a rub or a pleural effusion. Alveolitis, lung fibrosis and diaphragmatic paralysis can also occur.

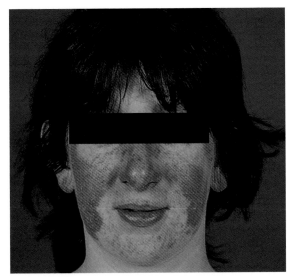

Fig. 15.7 Butterfly (malar) rash of systemic lupus erythematosus.

Neurological: Cerebral lupus causes visual hallucinations, chorea, organic psychosis, transverse myelitis and lymphocytic meningitis.

Haematological: Neutropenia, lymphopenia, thrombocytopenia and haemolytic anaemia occur.

GI: Oral ulcers are common. Mesenteric vasculitis can cause bowel infarction.

Investigations

The criteria for diagnosis of SLE are given in Box 15.13. Blood should be sent for haematology, biochemistry, ANA, antibodies to extractable nuclear antigens, and complement levels. Patients with active SLE almost always test positive for ANA, but ANA-negative SLE occurs very rarely with antibodies to the Ro antigen. Anti-dsDNA antibodies are characteristic of severe active SLE but only occur in ~30% of cases. Patients with active disease tend to have low C3 and C4, but this may reflect inherited complement deficiency that predisposes to SLE. Studies of other family members help to differentiate inherited deficiency from complement consumption. A raised ESR, leucopenia and lymphopenia are typical of active SLE, as are anaemia, haemolytic anaemia and thrombocytopenia. CRP is often normal in active SLE, except in the presence of serositis; elevated CRP suggests coexisting infection.

Management

Patients should avoid sun exposure and should apply high-factor sun blocks.

15.13 American Rheumatism Association criteria for SLE

Features	Characteristics
Malar rash	Fixed erythema, flat or raised, sparing nasolabial folds
Discoid rash	Erythematous raised patches, keratotic scarring, follicular plugging
Photosensitivity	Rash on sunlight exposure
Oral ulcers	Oral or nasopharyngeal; may be painless
Arthritis	Non-erosive, ≥2 peripheral joints
Serositis	Pleuritis *or* pericarditis
Renal disorder	Persistent proteinuria >0.5 g/day *or* cellular casts
Neurological	Seizures or psychosis, without provoking drugs/metabolic derangement
Haematological disorder	Haemolytic anaemia *or* leucopenia* (<4 × 10^9/L) *or* lymphopenia* (<1 × 10^9/L) *or* thrombocytopenia* (<100 × 10^9/L) not due to drugs
Immunological	Raised anti-DNA antibodies *or* antibody to Sm antigen *or* positive antiphospholipid antibodies
ANA disorder	Abnormal ANA titre by immunofluorescence

SLE is diagnosed if any 4 of these 11 features are present serially or simultaneously.

*On two separate occasions.

Mild disease: Disease restricted to skin and joints may require only analgesics, NSAIDs and hydroxychloroquine. Short courses of oral prednisolone may be needed for flares of disease (e.g. synovitis, pleuro-pericarditis).

Life-threatening disease (e.g. renal, cerebral, cardiac): This requires high-dose corticosteroids (IV methylprednisolone) in combination with IV cyclophosphamide, repeated at intervals of 2–3 wks. Haemorrhagic cystitis and *Pneumocystis* pneumonia are important complications of this treatment. Mycophenolate mofetil (MMF) is a less toxic alternative to cyclophosphamide.

Maintenance therapy: Azathioprine, methotrexate and MMF are used for maintenance. Patients with thrombosis and the antiphospholipid syndrome require lifelong warfarin.

Systemic sclerosis

Systemic sclerosis (scleroderma) is a generalised multisystem connective tissue disorder. The peak age of onset is in the fourth and fifth decades, and it has a 4:1 female:male ratio. It is subdivided into diffuse cutaneous systemic sclerosis (DCSS) and limited cutaneous systemic sclerosis (LCSS). Many patients with LCSS have features that are grouped into the 'CREST' syndrome (calcinosis, Raynaud's, oesophageal involvement, sclerodactyly, telangiectasia).

The aetiology of systemic sclerosis is unknown. Early in the disease, there is skin infiltration by T lymphocytes and abnormal fibroblast activation, leading to increased production of collagen in

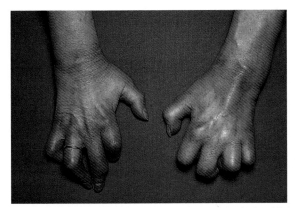

Fig. 15.8 Systemic sclerosis. Hands showing tight shiny skin, sclerodactyly and flexion contractures of the fingers.

the dermis. This results in symmetrical thickening, tightening and induration of the skin, and then sclerodactyly in the fingers. In addition to skin changes, there is arterial and arteriolar narrowing due to intimal proliferation and vessel wall inflammation. Endothelial injury causes release of vasoconstrictors and platelet activation, resulting in further ischaemia.

Clinical features

Skin: The skin of the fingers becomes tight, shiny and thickened (sclerodactyly, Fig. 15.8). Raynaud's phenomenon occurs early in the disease. In the distal extremities, the combination of intimal fibrosis and vasculitis may cause tissue ischaemia, skin ulceration and localised infarcts. Subcutaneous calcium deposition can cause nodules on the fingers (calcinosis). Involvement of the face causes thinning and radial furrowing of the lips. Telangiectasia may be present. Skin involvement restricted to sites distal to the elbow or knee (apart from the face) is classified as LCSS or CREST syndrome; more proximal involvement is classified as DCSS.

Musculoskeletal features: Arthralgia, morning stiffness and flexor tenosynovitis are common. Restricted hand function is usually due to skin rather than joint disease.

GI features: Smooth muscle atrophy and fibrosis in the lower oesophagus lead to acid reflux with erosive oesophagitis; this may in turn progress to further fibrosis. Dysphagia may also occur. Involvement of the stomach causes early satiety and occasionally outlet obstruction. Small intestine involvement may lead to malabsorption due to bacterial overgrowth and intermittent bloating or pain. Dilatation of the large or small bowel due to autonomic neuropathy may cause pseudo-obstruction.

Cardiorespiratory features: Pulmonary involvement is a major cause of morbidity and mortality. Pulmonary fibrosis mainly affects patients with diffuse disease. Pulmonary hypertension is a complication of long-standing limited disease, characterised by rapidly progressive dyspnoea and right heart failure.

Renal features: One of the main causes of death is hypertensive renal crisis characterised by rapidly developing malignant hypertension and renal failure. It is much more common in patients with diffuse disease.

Investigations

The diagnosis is primarily a clinical one. ANA is positive in 70%. Anti-topoisomerase I (anti-Scl-70) antibodies occur in 30% of those with diffuse systemic sclerosis, and anti-centromere antibodies occur in 60% of those with CREST syndrome.

Management and prognosis

Raynaud's and digital ulcers: Patients should avoid cold exposure; conventional or heated mittens can be effective. Calcium antagonists (e.g. nifedipine, amlodipine) and angiotensin II receptor antagonists (e.g. valsartan) promote vasodilatation, and epoprostenol infusions may be helpful for severe digital ischaemia. Prompt antibiotics are required for infected skin ulcers.

Oesophageal reflux: This should be treated with proton pump inhibitors (PPIs) and prokinetic agents such as metoclopramide.

Hypertension: This should be treated aggressively with ACE inhibitors.

Pulmonary hypertension: This is managed with the oral endothelin 1 antagonist bosentan, but if severe may require heart–lung transplantation.

Mixed connective tissue disease

This is an overlap connective tissue disease with features of SLE, systemic sclerosis and myositis. Most patients have anti-ribonucleoprotein (anti-RNP) antibodies, although these can also occur in SLE without overlap features.

Sjögren's syndrome

This idiopathic autoimmune disorder is characterised by lymphocytic infiltration of salivary and lachrymal glands, leading to glandular fibrosis and exocrine failure. It predominantly affects women and has a peak onset between the ages of 40 and 60 yrs. There is an association with HLA-B8 and DR3. The disease may be primary or secondary in association with other autoimmune diseases such as RA, SLE or primary biliary cirrhosis.

Clinical features

• Dry eyes (keratoconjunctivitis sicca) due to a lack of tears. • Dry mouth (xerostomia). • Vaginal dryness. • Other features: fatigue, non-erosive arthritis and Raynaud's phenomenon. • There is a 40-fold increase in lifetime risk of lymphoma.

Investigations

The diagnosis can be established by the Schirmer test, which measures the flow of tears using an absorbent paper strip placed in the lower eyelid; a normal result is >6 mm of wetting over 5 mins. If the diagnosis is in doubt, lip biopsy may identify lymphocytic infiltration of the minor salivary glands.

• ESR: usually elevated. • Autoantibodies: RF, ANA, anti-Ro (SS-A) and anti-La (SS-B).

Management

Treatment is largely symptomatic:

• Artificial tears and lubricants for dry eyes. • Artificial saliva for xerostomia. • Lubricants such as K-Y jelly for vaginal dryness. • Corticosteroids for extraglandular and musculoskeletal manifestations.

Polymyositis and dermatomyositis

These rare connective tissue disorders are characterised by muscle weakness and inflammation. The onset is usually between 40 and 60 yrs of age. There is a threefold increased risk of malignancy in patients with dermatomyositis and polymyositis.

Clinical features

Polymyositis: Presents with symmetrical proximal muscle weakness, usually affecting the lower limbs first. Patients report difficulty rising from a chair, climbing stairs and lifting, sometimes in combination with muscle pain. The onset is typically gradual, over a few weeks. Systemic features of fever, weight loss and fatigue are common. Respiratory or pharyngeal muscle involvement leading to ventilatory failure/aspiration is ominous and requires urgent treatment. Interstitial lung disease occurs in up to 30%, most of whom have antisynthetase (Jo-1) antibodies.

Dermatomyositis: Presents similarly but in combination with characteristic cutaneous manifestations. Gottron's papules are scaly erythematous/violaceous plaques or papules occurring over the extensor surfaces of the fingers (see Fig. 17.14, p. 721). A characteristic heliotrope rash may develop – a violaceous discoloration of the eyelid associated with periorbital oedema.

Investigations

Muscle biopsy shows typical features of fibre necrosis and inflammatory cell infiltration. MRI can help identify areas of abnormal muscle. CK is usually raised and tracks disease activity. ANA and anti-Jo1 antibodies may be positive. EMG may confirm the presence of myopathy and exclude neuropathy.

Management

Oral corticosteroids (e.g. prednisolone) are the mainstay of initial treatment. Patients with severe weakness or respiratory or pharyngeal involvement may require IV methylprednisolone. Additional immunosuppressive therapy (e.g. azathioprine or methotrexate) is often required.

VASCULITIS

This heterogeneous group of diseases is characterised by inflammation and necrosis of blood vessel walls. Vasculitis may also occur in many types of inflammatory or infectious diseases, such as SLE, RA and endocarditis. Clinical features (Box 15.14) involve many systems and are due to a combination of local tissue ischaemia and systemic effects of widespread inflammation.

Takayasu's disease

This is a granulomatous large-vessel vasculitis affecting the aorta and its major branches, and occasionally the pulmonary arteries. The typical age at onset is between 25 and 30 yrs, with an 8:1 female preponderance. The usual presentation is with claudication, fever, arthralgia and weight loss. Examination may reveal loss of pulses, bruits and aortic incompetence. Diagnosis is based on angiographic findings of coarctation, occlusion and aneurysmal dilatation. Treatment is with high-dose steroids and immunosuppressants, as for SLE.

Kawasaki disease

This rare vasculitis causes coronary arteritis in children aged under 5. It presents with fever, rash and pericarditis, myocarditis or infarction.

Polyarteritis nodosa

Polyarteritis nodosa (PAN) is a rare necrotising vasculitis involving medium-sized and small arteries; it predominantly affects middle-aged men. Hepatitis B is a risk factor for PAN.

Presentation is with myalgia, arthralgia, fever and weight loss, together with manifestations of multisystem disease. Skin involvement can cause a palpable purpuric rash, ulceration, infarction and livedo reticularis. Arteritis of the vasa nervorum leads to a symmetrical sensory and motor neuropathy. Severe hypertension and renal impairment may occur due to multiple renal infarctions.

15.14 Clinical features of systemic vasculitis	
Systemic	Malaise, fever, night sweats, weight loss, arthralgia, myalgia
Rashes	Palpable purpura, pulp infarcts, ulceration, livedo reticularis
ENT	Epistaxis, sinusitis, deafness
Respiratory	Haemoptysis, cough, poorly controlled asthma
GI	Abdominal pain (mucosal inflammation or enteric ischaemia), mouth ulcers, diarrhoea
Neurological	Sensory or motor neuropathy

Diagnosis is confirmed by finding multiple aneurysms and narrowing of the mesenteric, hepatic or renal vessels on angiography. Muscle or sural nerve biopsy may also be diagnostic. Treatment is with high-dose steroids and immunosuppressants, as for SLE.

Giant cell arteritis and polymyalgia rheumatica

Giant cell arteritis (GCA) is a granulomatous arteritis mainly affecting medium-sized arteries in the head and neck. It is commonly associated with polymyalgia rheumatica (PMR), which causes pain and stiffness in the shoulders and hips. Since many patients with GCA have symptoms of PMR, and many patients with PMR go on to develop GCA if untreated, they may be different manifestations of one underlying disorder. Both are rare under the age of 60 yrs. The average age at onset is 70, with a female preponderance of ~3:1. The overall prevalence is ~20/100 000 in those over the age of 50 yrs.

Clinical features

The cardinal symptom of GCA is temporal or occipital headache, which may be accompanied by scalp tenderness. Jaw pain develops in some patients, brought on by chewing or talking, due to ischaemia of the masseter muscles. Visual disturbance can occur and GCA may present with blindness in one eye due to occlusion of the posterior ciliary artery. On fundoscopy, the optic disc may appear pale and swollen with haemorrhages, but these changes take 24–36 hrs to develop and the fundi may initially appear normal. Other visual symptoms include loss of visual acuity, reduced colour perception and papillary defects. Rarely, transient ischaemic attacks, brainstem infarcts and hemiparesis may occur.

PMR presents with symmetrical muscle pain and stiffness affecting the shoulder and pelvic girdles. Weight loss, fatigue, malaise and night sweats are systemic features. Symptoms usually appear over a few days but onset may be more insidious. Examination reveals stiffness and painful restriction of active shoulder movement but passive movements are preserved. Muscles may be tender to palpation but weakness and muscle-wasting are absent.

Investigations

• Raised ESR and CRP. • Normochromic, normocytic anaemia.

Diagnosis is based on a combination of the typical clinical features, raised ESR and prompt response to steroid. If doubt persists, however, a temporal artery biopsy may reveal characteristic inflammatory changes. Whilst a positive biopsy is helpful, a negative biopsy does not exclude the diagnosis because the lesions are focal. USS or arteriography may be used to help guide the biopsy.

Management

Corticosteroids are the treatment of choice and should be commenced urgently in suspected GCA to prevent visual loss. Symptoms will completely resolve within 48–72 hrs of starting corticosteroids in virtually all patients. The prednisolone dose should be reduced progressively, guided by symptoms and ESR, until an acceptable dose is achieved (5–7.5 mg daily). If symptoms recur, the dose should be temporarily increased again. Most patients need steroids for an average of 12–24 mths. Prophylaxis against osteoporosis should be given in patients with low bone mineral density.

ANCA-associated vasculitis and other small-vessel vasculitis

Antineutrophil cytoplasmic antibodies (ANCA) occur in two patterns of immunofluorescence: cytoplasmic (c-ANCA, directed against proteinase 3) and perinuclear (p-ANCA, directed against myeloperoxidase). They are associated with two types of vasculitis:

Microscopic polyangiitis (MPA): A necrotising small-vessel vasculitis associated with rapidly progressive glomerulonephritis, alveolar haemorrhage, neuropathy and pleural effusions. Patients are usually p-ANCA–positive.

Granulomatosis with polyangiitis (formerly Wegener's granulomatosis): Characterised by granuloma formation in the nasopharynx, airways and kidney (glomerulonephritis). It presents with epistaxis, nasal crusting and sinusitis, but haemoptysis, mucosal ulceration and deafness are also seen. Proptosis occurs due to retro-orbital inflammation, causing diplopia or visual loss. Untreated nasal disease may erode bone and cartilage. Pulmonary infiltrates and cavitating nodules occur in 50% of patients. Patients are usually c-ANCA–positive, with elevated CRP and ESR. MRI is useful in localising abnormalities but the diagnosis should be confirmed by biopsy of the kidney or upper airway lesions.

Management is with high-dose steroids and cyclophosphamide, followed by maintenance with lower-dose steroids and azathioprine, methotrexate or mycophenolate. A chronic relapsing course is usual.

Churg–Strauss syndrome

This is a small-vessel vasculitis presenting with skin lesions (purpura or nodules), mononeuritis multiplex and eosinophilia on a background of resistant asthma. Pulmonary infiltrates may be present. Mesenteric vasculitis can cause abdominal symptoms. Either c-ANCA or p-ANCA is present in up to 60% of cases.

Henoch–Schönlein purpura

This small-vessel vasculitis is caused by immune complex deposition and usually affects children and young adults. Typical presentation is with purpura over the buttocks and lower legs, abdominal symptoms (pain and bleeding) and arthritis (knee or ankle) following an upper respiratory tract infection. Nephritis may occur and can result in renal impairment. The diagnosis is confirmed by demonstrating IgA within blood vessel walls. Henoch–Schönlein purpura usually settles without treatment but corticosteroids and immunosuppressants may be used for severe disease, e.g. nephritis.

Behçet's syndrome

This is a rare vasculitis that characteristically targets venules. The diagnosis is clinical, and is based on the presence of recurrent oral ulceration together with two of the following:

• Recurrent genital ulceration. • Eye lesions: anterior or posterior uveitis, retinal vasculitis. • Skin lesions: erythema nodosum, papulopustular lesions, acneiform nodules. • Positive pathergy test: skin pricking with a needle results in pustule development within 48 hrs.

Other features include meningitis, encephalitis and recurrent thromboses.

Oral ulceration is treated with topical corticosteroids. Thalidomide is effective for resistant oral and genital ulceration but is teratogenic. Systemic disease requires oral corticosteroids in combination with other immunosuppressive drugs.

DISEASES OF BONE

Osteoporosis

Osteoporosis is the most common bone disease. It is characterised by reduced bone mineral density (BMD) with an increased risk of fracture, and increases markedly with age. Osteoporotic fractures affect up to 30% of women and 12% of men at some time during their life.

In normal individuals, bone mass increases to reach a peak between the ages of 20 and 40 yrs but falls thereafter. Bone turnover throughout life depends on the balance between bone formation by osteoblasts and bone resorption by osteoclasts. There is an accelerated phase of bone loss in women after the menopause as a result of oestrogen deficiency, which alters this balance in favour of increased bone resorption. This leads to an increased risk of osteoporosis and fractures, particularly in women who have attained a low peak bone mass. Conditions increasing the risk of osteoporosis are shown in Box 15.15.

15.15 Risk factors for osteoporosis	
Endocrine disease	Early menopause, hypogonadism, hyperthyroidism, hyperparathyroidism, Cushing's syndrome
Inflammatory disease	Inflammatory bowel disease, RA, ankylosing spondylitis
Drugs	Corticosteroids, anticonvulsants, heparin, alcohol excess
GI disease	Malabsorption, chronic liver disease
Respiratory disease	Chronic obstructive pulmonary disease (COPD), cystic fibrosis
Miscellaneous	Myeloma, anorexia nervosa, lack of exercise, immobilisation, poor diet/low body weight, smoking, HIV

Corticosteroid therapy is an important cause of osteoporosis. Although there is no 'safe' dose of corticosteroid, the risk increases when the dose of prednisolone exceeds 7.5 mg daily for >3 mths. Corticosteroids reduce bone formation by inhibiting osteoblast function and promoting apoptosis in osteoblasts and osteocytes. Corticosteroids also inhibit intestinal calcium absorption and cause renal calcium leak, reducing serum calcium and leading to secondary hyperparathyroidism with increased osteoclastic bone resorption. Hypogonadism may also occur with high-dose steroids.

Clinical features

Osteoporosis is asymptomatic until a fracture occurs. The most common sites are the forearm (Colles fracture), spine (vertebral fractures causing back pain, height loss and kyphosis) and femur (hip fracture).

Investigations

BMD is measured using dual energy X-ray absorptiometry (DEXA) of the lumbar spine and hip. DEXA should be performed in patients sustaining low trauma fractures or other features of osteoporosis, and individuals with an elevated 10-yr fracture risk as judged by a risk-assessment tool (e.g. www.shef.ac.uk/FRAX/).

The T-score measures by how many standard deviations the patient's BMD value differs from that of a young healthy control. The Z-score measures by how many standard deviations the BMD deviates from that of an age-matched control. Osteoporosis is diagnosed when the T-score value falls to −2.5 or below. T-scores between −1.0 and −2.5 indicate osteopenia, and values above −1.0 are regarded as normal.

If osteoporosis is confirmed by bone densitometry, any predisposing factors should be sought (see Box 15.15). Relevant blood tests include:

• U&Es, calcium, phosphate. • TFTs. • Immunoglobulins. • ESR. • Anti-tissue transglutaminase (for coeliac disease). • 25(OH) vitamin D. • Parathyroid hormone (PTH). • Sex hormone and gonadotrophin levels.

Management

Patients with osteopenia should be given lifestyle advice:

• Cessation of smoking. • Limitation of alcohol intake. • Adequate dietary calcium intake (1500 mg daily). • Regular exercise.

Referral to a falls prevention team should be made if the patient is unsteady on examination. Osteopenic patients should be offered a repeat BMD measurement in 2–3 yrs.

Pharmacological treatment is indicated in those with T-scores below −2.5, steroid-treated patients with T-scores between −2.5 and −1.5, and patients with non-traumatic vertebral fractures.

Bisphosphonates: Bisphosphonates are first-line drugs in the treatment of osteoporosis (p. 787).

Calcium and vitamin D supplements: Calcium (500 mg daily) and vitamin D supplements (800 U daily) are used as an adjunct to other treatments. They do not reduce fracture risk in osteoporosis when given as monotherapy.

Strontium ranelate: Strontium ranelate inhibits bone resorption and increases BMD. It is effective in secondary prevention of vertebral and non-vertebral fractures in post-menopausal women but can cause diarrhoea and thrombosis.

Hormone replacement therapy (HRT) and raloxifene: HRT with oestrogen and progestogens prevents post-menopausal bone loss and reduces vertebral and non-vertebral osteoporotic fractures. It is mainly used to prevent osteoporosis in women with an early menopause and to treat women in their early fifties with osteoporosis and troublesome menopausal symptoms. HRT should be avoided in older women with osteoporosis because it increases the risk of breast cancer and cardiovascular disease. Raloxifene is a selective oestrogen receptor modulator, which is useful in post-menopausal patients with vertebral osteoporosis who are intolerant of bisphosphonates.

To monitor response, DEXA may be repeated not less than 2 yrs into treatment or if recurrent fracture occurs.

Osteomalacia and rickets

These conditions result from defective bone mineralisation due to vitamin D deficiency, resistance to vitamin D or hypophosphataemia. In adults, osteomalacia describes a syndrome of bone pain, bone fragility and fractures. Rickets is the equivalent in children and features enlargement of the growth plate and bone deformity. The disease remains prevalent in frail older people with a poor diet and limited sunlight exposure, and in some Muslim women who live in northern latitudes. Causes of osteomalacia and rickets include:

• Deficiency of vitamin D or defects in vitamin D metabolism.
• Hypophosphataemia. • Drug-induced inhibition of bone mineralisation.

Vitamin D deficiency can result from lack of sunlight exposure, dietary deficiency or malabsorption in patients with GI disease. In normal individuals, ~70% is made in the skin from 7-dehydrocholesterol under the influence of ultraviolet light, whereas the remaining 30% is derived from the diet. Lack of vitamin D is accompanied by a reduction in $25(OH)D_3$ synthesis in the liver. This causes reduced production of the active metabolite $1,25(OH)_2D_3$ in the kidneys, reduced intestinal calcium absorption and low serum calcium. The low serum calcium level stimulates PTH secretion, resulting in secondary hyperparathyroidism and subsequent increased osteoclastic bone resorption, reduced renal calcium excretion and increased renal phosphate excretion. This sequence represents an attempt by the parathyroid glands to restore serum calcium levels to normal; however, this cannot be achieved with continuing vitamin D deficiency so there is progressive loss of both calcium and phosphate from bone and defective mineralisation.

Osteomalacia also occurs in association with defects of vitamin D metabolism and function:

Chronic renal failure: Renal synthesis of the active metabolite of vitamin D $(1,25(OH)_2D_3)$ fails.

Mutations in the renal α-hydroxylase enzyme: These mutations render the enzyme unable to convert $25(OH)D_3$ to $1,25(OH)_2D_3$ and cause vitamin D-resistant rickets type I.

Mutations in the vitamin D receptor: These mutations render the receptor resistant to activation by $1,25(OH)_2D_3$ and cause vitamin D-resistant rickets type II.

Clinical features

In children, rickets causes enlargement of epiphyses at the lower end of the radius and swelling of the costochondral junctions ('rickety rosary').

Osteomalacia in adults presents more insidiously and may be asymptomatic. When symptomatic, it causes bone pain, pathological fractures and proximal muscle weakness, causing a waddling gait and difficulty climbing stairs or rising from a chair.

Investigations

Renal function, serum calcium, phosphate, albumin, alkaline phosphatase, serum $25(OH)D_3$ and PTH levels should be measured. Vitamin D-deficient osteomalacia is suggested by low or low–normal calcium and phosphate, raised alkaline phosphatase, low $25(OH)D_3$ and raised PTH. X-rays are of limited value in diagnosis, but may show focal radiolucent areas (Looser's zones) in advanced cases. Osteopenia is a common finding. Bone biopsy can be used to confirm the diagnosis.

Management

Rickets and osteomalacia caused by vitamin D deficiency respond rapidly to oral vitamin D and calcium supplementation. Higher doses may be required in patients with malabsorption. Osteomalacia due to renal failure and vitamin D-resistant rickets type I requires treatment with active vitamin D metabolites (1-α-$(OH)D_3$ or $1,25(OH)_2D_3$) since these bypass the defect in 1-α-hydroxylation of $25(OH)D_3$. Serum calcium and alkaline phosphatase should be monitored to assess response to treatment.

Paget's disease

Paget's disease of bone (PDB) is a common condition characterised by focal areas of increased and disorganised bone remodelling. It increases in frequency with age, affecting 8% of the UK population by the age of 85. Genetic factors are implicated in the aetiology of PDB; mutations in the *SQSTM1* gene are a common cause of classical PDB. The presence of inclusion bodies within osteoclasts has led to speculation that a slow virus infection may also play a role. The primary abnormality in PDB is increased osteoclastic bone resorption accompanied by increased osteoblast activity. The resultant bone is architecturally abnormal and has reduced mechanical strength. Other features of PDB are marrow fibrosis and increased bone vascularity.

Clinical features

PDB most commonly affects the pelvis, femur, tibia, lumbar spine and skull. Patients classically present with bone pain, deformity and pathological fractures, although many cases are asymptomatic. Clinical signs include bone deformity and expansion with increased warmth over affected bones. Bone deformity is most evident in the femur, tibia and skull. Neurological complications include deafness and spinal cord compression. The deafness is often conductive in nature due to osteosclerosis of the temporal bone. Other rare complications include high-output cardiac failure (due to increased bone vascularity) and osteosarcoma.

Investigations

Alkaline phosphatase is raised with normal calcium and phosphate levels. X-rays show areas of osteosclerosis alternating with areas of radiolucency, together with bone expansion and deformity. Radionuclide bone scanning is useful in confirming PDB and documenting its extent. Bone biopsy is not usually required to make the diagnosis, but can occasionally be helpful in differentiating PDB from sclerotic bony metastases.

Management

Treatment of PDB is primarily indicated for control of bone pain.

If paracetamol and NSAIDs are ineffective, then bisphosphonates (e.g. oral risedronate, IV pamidronate, IV zoledronic acid) are helpful in suppressing bone turnover, reducing serum alkaline phosphatase and controlling pain. SC calcitonin is an alternative to bisphosphonates but is less convenient and more expensive. The long-term effects of therapy with bisphosphonates and calcitonin on complications such as deafness, bone deformity and fracture are unknown. Currently, there is no evidence to show that prophylactic therapy with bisphosphonates in asymptomatic patients is effective in preventing complications.

Scheuermann's osteochondritis

This predominantly affects adolescent boys, who develop a dorsal kyphosis with irregular radiographic ossification of the vertebral end plates. It has a strong genetic component and may be inherited as an autosomal dominant trait. Most patients are asymptomatic, but back pain, aggravated by exercise and relieved by rest, may occur. Management consists of avoidance of excessive activity and performance of protective postural exercises. Rarely, corrective surgery may be required for severe deformity.

Osteogenesis imperfecta

This rare disease is characterised by bone fragility presenting with multiple fractures in infancy and childhood. It is caused by genetic defects of collagen production. Other common features include blue sclerae and abnormal dentition. Treatment is multidisciplinary in nature, involving orthopaedic surgery for the management of fractures and limb deformities, physiotherapy and occupational therapy.

Primary bone tumours

Primary bone tumours are less common than secondary bone metastases. They have a peak incidence in childhood and adolescence, although osteosarcoma secondary to PDB develops in later adulthood.

Primary bone tumours present with local pain and swelling. Plain X-rays show expansion of the bone, CT and MRI are used for staging, and diagnosis is confirmed by biopsy. Treatment usually involves surgical removal followed by chemotherapy and radiotherapy. The prognosis is generally good in cases presenting in childhood and adolescence, but poor in elderly patients with osteosarcoma related to PDB.

Neurological disease

16

The brain, spinal cord and peripheral nerves constitute an organ responsible for perception of the environment, a person's behaviour within it, and the maintenance of the body's internal milieu in readiness for this behaviour. In the UK some 10% of the population consult their GP each year with a neurological symptom, and neurological disorders account for about one-fifth of acute medical admissions and a large proportion of chronic physical disability.

PRESENTING PROBLEMS IN NEUROLOGICAL DISEASE

Headache and facial pain

Headache is common and causes considerable worry, but rarely represents sinister disease. The causes may be divided into:
• Primary (benign): e.g. migraine, tension headache, cluster headache, thunderclap headache (p. 639). • Secondary: e.g. medication overuse, intracerebral bleed, infection, temporal arteritis, referred pain.

Most patients have primary syndromes. Sudden-onset headache, maximal immediately, is always a 'red flag' and should prompt rapid hospital assessment for possible subarachnoid haemorrhage or other sinister causes, although only 10–25% will have serious pathology. Clues to other possible causes (e.g. rash in meningitis) should be sought. Headache evolving over hours to days is much less likely to be sinister.

It is important to establish whether the headache is intermittent (usually migraine) or constant. Associated visual symptoms, nausea/vomiting or photophobia/phonophobia may suggest migraine, but progressive focal symptoms, weight loss or fever may suggest a more sinister cause (e.g. cancer or meningitis). Migraine patients typically retire to bed to sleep in a dark room, whereas cluster headache often induces agitated and restless behaviour.

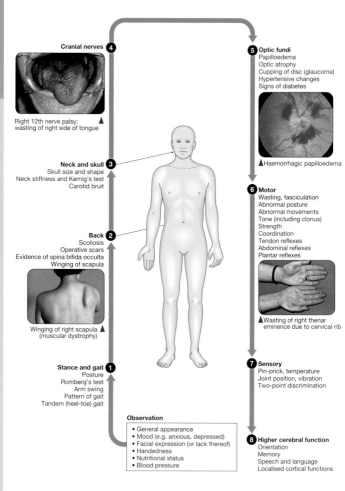

Cranial nerves ❹

Right 12th nerve palsy: ▲
wasting of right side of tongue

Neck and skull ❸
Skull size and shape
Neck stiffness and Kernig's test
Carotid bruit

Back ❷
Scoliosis
Operative scars
Evidence of spina bifida occulta
Winging of scapula

Winging of right scapula ▲
(muscular dystrophy)

Stance and gait ❶
Posture
Romberg's test
Arm swing
Pattern of gait
Tandem (heel-toe) gait

Observation
• General appearance
• Mood (e.g. anxious, depressed)
• Facial expression (or lack thereof)
• Handedness
• Nutritional status
• Blood pressure

❺ **Optic fundi**
Papilloedema
Optic atrophy
Cupping of disc (glaucoma)
Hypertensive changes
Signs of diabetes

▲Haemorrhagic papilloedema

❻ **Motor**
Wasting, fasciculation
Abnormal posture
Abnormal movements
Tone (including clonus)
Strength
Coordination
Tendon reflexes
Abdominal reflexes
Plantar reflexes

▲Wasting of right thenar
eminence due to cervical rib

❼ **Sensory**
Pin-prick, temperature
Joint position, vibration
Two-point discrimination

❽ **Higher cerebral function**
Orientation
Memory
Speech and language
Localised cortical functions

Headaches that have been present for months or years worry patients yet are almost never sinister, whereas new-onset headache, especially in the elderly, is more of a concern. In patients >60 yrs with pain localised to one or both temples, temporal arteritis (p. 597) should be considered, especially if temporal pulses are absent and/or the arteries are enlarged and tender. Most outpatients with headache have migraine (intermittent, lasting a few hours, associated with migrainous symptoms) or chronic daily headache syndrome (often present for months to years, without associated symptoms and refractory to analgesia). Sinusitis, 'eye strain', food allergies and uncomplicated hypertension are almost never the explanation for persistent headache.

Ocular pain

Assuming ocular disease (such as acute glaucoma) has been excluded, ocular pain may be due to trigeminal autonomic cephalalgias (TACs) or, rarely, inflammatory or infiltrative lesions at the apex of the orbit or the cavernous sinus, when 3rd, 4th, 5th or 6th cranial nerve involvement is usually evident.

Facial pain

Pain in the face can be due to dental, temporomandibular joint or sinus problems but this is usually apparent from other features. Facial pain is common in migraine but some syndromes can present solely with facial pain. The most common neurological causes are trigeminal neuralgia, herpes zoster (shingles) and post-herpetic neuralgia, all characterised by their extreme severity. In trigeminal neuralgia, the patient describes brief bouts of lancinating pain ('electric shocks'), most frequently in the second and third divisions of the nerve, triggered by talking or chewing. Facial shingles most commonly affects the ophthalmic division of the trigeminal nerve, and pain usually precedes the rash. Post-herpetic neuralgia may follow, typically a continuous burning pain throughout the affected territory, with marked sensitivity to light touch (allodynia) and resistance to treatment. Destructive lesions of the trigeminal nerve usually cause numbness rather than pain.

Dizziness, blackouts and 'funny turns'

Episodes of lost or altered consciousness are frequent. After a careful history from the patient, supplemented by a witness account, it should be clear whether the patient is describing loss of consciousness, altered consciousness, vertigo, transient amnesia or something else. The diagnostic approach is shown in Figure 16.1.

Loss of consciousness

Transient loss of consciousness occurs because of a recoverable loss of adequate blood supply to the brain (syncope), or from sudden electrical dysfunction of the brain during a seizure (epileptic fit). Many patients have psychogenic blackouts or non-epileptic seizures, which may confuse this distinction. No amount of

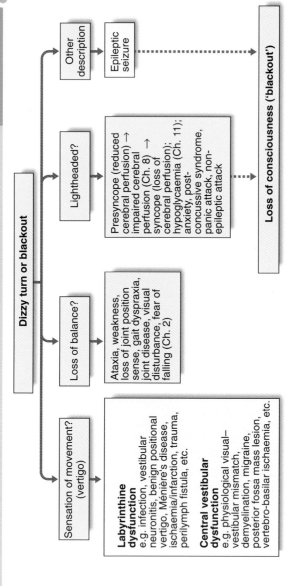

Dizzy turn or blackout

Sensation of movement? (vertigo)

Labyrinthine dysfunction
e.g. infection, vestibular neuronitis, benign positional vertigo, Ménière's disease, ischaemia/infarction, trauma, perilymph fistula, etc.

Central vestibular dysfunction
e.g. physiological visual–vestibular mismatch, demyelination, migraine, posterior fossa mass lesion, vertebro-basilar ischaemia, etc.

Loss of balance?

Ataxia, weakness, loss of joint position sense, gait dyspraxia, joint disturbance, fear of falling (Ch. 2)

Lightheaded?

Presyncope (reduced cerebral perfusion) → impaired cerebral perfusion (Ch. 8) → syncope (loss of cerebral perfusion); hypoglycaemia (Ch. 11); anxiety, post-concussive syndrome, panic attack, non-epileptic attack

Other description

Epileptic seizure

Loss of consciousness ('blackout')

Fig. 16.1 A diagnostic approach to the patient with dizziness, funny turns or blackouts.

16.1 How to distinguish seizures from faints		
	Seizure	**Faint**
Aura (e.g. olfactory)	+	−
Cyanosis	+	−
Tongue-biting	+	−/+
Post-ictal confusion	+	−
Post-ictal amnesia	+	−
Post-ictal headache	+	−
Rapid recovery	−	+

investigation can replace a clear history in these circumstances. Features in the history useful in distinguishing a seizure from a faint are shown in Box 16.1.

Syncope

A brief feeling of 'lightheadedness' often precedes syncope; vision then darkens and there may be a ringing in the ears. Neurocardiogenic syncope (p. 212) may be provoked by emotion or pain and usually occurs while standing. During a syncopal attack, incontinence of urine can occur and there is often stiffening and brief twitching of the limbs, but tongue-biting never occurs. Cardiac syncope, caused by a sudden decline in cardiac output and hence cerebral perfusion, may be exertional (e.g. with severe aortic stenosis) or may occur completely 'out of the blue' (as in heart block). Recovery is rapid and without confusion.

Seizures

The diagnosis of generalised tonic–clonic seizures, in which there is loss of consciousness, falling to the ground and clonic movements (p. 643), is easy, but unobserved episodes can leave uncertainty. Less dramatic episodes, such as absences (p. 643) or some focal seizures (p. 643), which cause alteration of consciousness without falling, may merely be experienced as 'lost time'. Since epileptic seizures are the result of specific processes that vary between individuals, they tend to be intermittent and stereotyped with clusters in time, for reasons incompletely understood.

Non-epileptic attack disorder, psychogenic seizures, pseudoseizures, psychogenic non-epileptic seizures

Around 10% of patients referred to a first seizure clinic have loss of consciousness resulting from psychological reactions to circumstances or traumatic events. Clues include specific emotional triggers, partially retained awareness, dramatic movements or vocalisation, very prolonged duration (hours), rapid recovery or subsequent emotional distress. Diagnosis is important, as such patients are at risk of harm from inappropriate anti-epileptic treatment. Conversely, a hasty diagnosis may lead to treatment being withheld in atypical or prolonged seizures.

16.2 Management of status epilepticus

Initial

* Check airway, pulse, BP, blood glucose stick, respiratory rate
* Secure IV access
* Send blood for glucose, U&Es, Ca, Mg, LFTs, drug levels
* Give diazepam 10 mg IV (or rectally); repeat *once only* after 15 mins; *or* lorazepam 4 mg IV
* Correct any metabolic trigger, e.g. hypoglycaemia

Ongoing

If seizures continue >30 mins
* IV infusion (with cardiac monitoring) with one of:
   Phenytoin: 15 mg/kg at 50 mg/min
   Fosphenytoin: 15 mg/kg at 100 mg/min
   Phenobarbital: 10 mg/kg at 100 mg/min

If seizures still continue after 30–60 mins
* Transfer to ICU for intubation and ventilation, and general anaesthesia using propofol or thiopental, EEG monitor

Once status controlled
* Commence longer-term anticonvulsant medication with one of:
   Sodium valproate 10 mg/kg IV over 3–5 mins, then 800–2000 mg/day
   Phenytoin: give loading dose (if not already used) of 15 mg/kg, infuse at <50 mg/min, then 300 mg/day
   Carbamazepine 400 mg by nasogastric tube, then 400–1200 mg/day
* Investigate cause

Status epilepticus

Status epilepticus is seizure activity not resolving spontaneously, or recurrent seizure without recovery of consciousness in between. It is an emergency with a recognised mortality.

Diagnosis is clinical, based on the description of prolonged rigidity and/or clonic movements with loss of awareness. Cyanosis, pyrexia, acidosis and sweating may occur, and complications include aspiration, hypotension, arrhythmias and renal or hepatic failure.

In patients with pre-existing epilepsy, the commonest cause is a subtherapeutic anti-epileptic drug level. In de novo status epilepticus, precipitants such as infection (meningitis, encephalitis), neoplasia and metabolic derangement (hypoglycaemia, hyponatraemia, hypocalcaemia) should be excluded. Management is outlined in Box 16.2.

Coma

Conscious level should be measured using the Glasgow Coma Scale (GCS, Box 16.3). Although developed for head injury, GCS is widely used in medical coma, but disorders affecting language or limb function may reduce its usefulness. Nevertheless, serial recordings provide useful prognostic information. Persistent coma indicates

16.3 Glasgow Coma Scale	
Eye-opening (E)	
Spontaneous	4
To speech	3
To pain	2
Nil	1
Best motor response (M)	
Obeys commands	6
Localises	5
Withdraws	4
Abnormal flexion	3
Extensor response	2
Nil	1
Verbal response (V)	
Orientated	5
Confused conversation	4
Inappropriate words	3
Incomprehensible sounds	2
Nil	1
Coma score = E + M + V	
Minimum	3
Maximum	15

disorder of the arousal mechanisms in the brainstem and diencephalon. There are many causes of coma (Box 16.4). A history from any witnesses is crucial to establishing the cause. Neurological examination may reveal evidence of head injury, papilloedema, meningism or eye movement disorder.

Brain death

Brain death is a state in which cortical and brainstem function is irreversibly lost. If diagnostic criteria for brain death are met, this allows support to be withdrawn and natural death to occur. Diagnosing brain death is complex and should only be done by a clinician with appropriate expertise, as clinical differentiation of brain death from conditions causing complete paralysis can be challenging.

Delirium and acute confusion

In delirium, unlike in dementia, there is a disturbance of arousal that accompanies the global impairment of mental function. There is drowsiness with disorientation, perceptual disturbances and muddled thinking. Patients typically fluctuate, confusion being worse at night, and there may be associated emotional disturbance or psychomotor changes.

16.4 Causes of coma	
Metabolic disturbance	Drug overdose, diabetes mellitus (hypoglycaemia, ketoacidosis, hyperosmolar coma), hyponatraemia, uraemia, liver failure, respiratory failure, hypothermia, hypothyroidism, thiamine deficiency
Trauma	Cerebral contusion, extradural/subdural haematoma, deceleration injury
Vascular disease	Subarachnoid haemorrhage, intracerebral haemorrhage, brainstem infarction/haemorrhage, cerebral venous sinus thrombosis
Infections	Meningitis, encephalitis, cerebral abscess, systemic sepsis
Others	Epilepsy, brain tumour, functional

Diagnosis

There are many possible causes (Box 16.5). A history from a witness is vital, and examination may yield other clues. It is important to distinguish confusion from a fluent aphasia. Often, however, the cause is not obvious and a wide screen of tests must be performed (Box 16.6).

Management

Identify the cause and correct it where possible. Nurse in a well-lit room and avoid sedative drugs that may exacerbate confusion. Occasionally, haloperidol may be required. In delirium tremens (alcohol withdrawal), the treatment is a tapered course of diazepam with IV thiamine.

Amnesia

Memory disturbance is common. In the absence of significant functional impairment, many patients prove to have benign memory dysfunction related to age, mood or psychiatric disorders. Investigation and treatment of the dementias are discussed elsewhere (pages 652–4).

Temporary memory loss may be due to a toxic confusional state, a post-ictal state or transient global amnesia. These are distinguished from the history.

Transient global amnesia

This predominantly affects middle-aged patients with an abrupt, discrete and reversible loss of anterograde memory function, leading to repetitive questioning. Consciousness is preserved, and after 4–6 hrs, memory and behaviour return to normal. There are none of the phenomena associated with seizures, and transient global amnesia recurs in only 10–20%. There are no physical signs and further investigation may not be needed if epilepsy can be excluded.

16.5 Causes of acute confusional state

Type	Common	Unusual
Infective	Chest infection Urinary infection Septicaemia Viral illness Meningitis, encephalitis	Cerebral abscess Subdural empyema
Metabolic/ endocrine	Hypoxia (cardiac/respiratory failure) Acute haemorrhage Hyper-/hypoglycaemia Hyper-/hypocalcaemia Hyponatraemia Liver failure, renal failure	Hypo-/hyperthyroidism Adrenal disease Porphyria
Vascular	Acute cerebral haemorrhage/infarction Subarachnoid haemorrhage	Vasculitis (e.g. systemic lupus erythematosus) Cerebral venous thrombosis
Toxic	Alcohol intoxication/withdrawal Drugs (therapeutic/illicit)	Carbon monoxide poisoning Industrial exposure (e.g. heavy metals)
Neoplastic	Secondary deposits	Primary cerebral tumour Paraneoplastic syndrome
Trauma	Cerebral contusion, subdural haematoma	
Other	Post-ictal state Peri-operative Acute decompensation of dementia	Acute hydrocephalus Complex partial status epilepticus Hashimoto's encephalopathy

16.6 Investigation of acute confusional state

	First-line	Other useful tests
Blood tests	FBC, ESR U&Es, Ca, Mg Glucose LFTs TFTs	Cardiac enzymes Protein electrophoresis, tumour markers Vitamin B_{12}, copper studies Syphilis serology Autoantibodies
CNS tests	Head imaging (CT and/or MRI)	Lumbar puncture, EEG
Other	ABGs, ECG Infection screen (blood cultures, CXR, urine culture)	Viral screen, as appropriate (e.g. HIV) Urinary porphyrins

Permanent amnesia

This more commonly signifies serious disease. When short-term memory is affected, Korsakoff's syndrome (often secondary to alcohol) is likely. Progressive loss should lead to testing for underlying dementia.

Weakness

Lesions in various parts of the motor system produce distinctive patterns of motor deficit. These can be 'negative' symptoms (weakness, lack of coordination, lack of stability and stiffness) or 'positive' symptoms (tremor, dystonia, chorea, athetosis, hemiballismus, tics and myoclonus). When the lower limbs are affected, characteristic patterns of gait disorder may result.

The motor system

A programme of movement formulated by the pre-motor cortex is converted into a series of muscle movements in the motor cortex and then transmitted to the spinal cord in the pyramidal tract. The anatomy of the motor system is summarised in Figure 16.2.

Lower motor neuron lesions: These cause loss of contraction in their units' muscle fibres and the muscle will be weak and flaccid. Denervated muscle fibres atrophy, causing wasting. Re-innervation from neighbouring motor neurons occurs but the neuromuscular junctions are unstable, causing fasciculations (visible to the naked eye because the motor units are larger than normal).

Upper motor neuron (pyramidal) lesions: Upper motor neurons have both excitatory and inhibitory influences on anterior horn cells. Upper motor neuron lesions cause increased tone, most evident in the strongest muscle groups (i.e. leg extensors and arm flexors); weakness is conversely more pronounced in the opposing muscle groups. Loss of inhibition leads to brisk reflexes and enhanced reflex patterns of movement, such as flexion withdrawal to noxious stimuli and spasms of extension.

Extrapyramidal lesions: There is an increase in tone, which is continuous throughout the range of movement at any speed of stretch ('lead-pipe' rigidity). Involuntary movements are present, and a tremor combined with rigidity produces typical 'cogwheel' rigidity. Rapid movements are slowed (bradykinesia). Extrapyramidal lesions also cause postural instability, precipitating falls.

Cerebellar lesions: These cause lack of coordination on the same side of the body. The initial movement is normal but accuracy deteriorates as the target is approached, producing an 'intention tremor'. The distances of targets are misjudged (dysmetria), resulting in 'past-pointing'. The ability to produce rapid, regularly alternating movements is impaired (dysdiadochokinesis). Disorders of the central vermis of the cerebellum produce a characteristic ataxic gait.

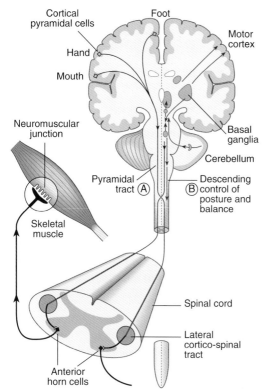

Fig. 16.2 The motor system. Neurons from the motor cortex descend as the pyramidal tract in the internal capsule and cerebral peduncle to the ventral brainstem, where most cross low in the medulla (A). In the spinal cord, the upper motor neurons form the cortico-spinal tract in the lateral column before synapsing with the lower motor neurons in the anterior horns. The activity in the motor cortex is modulated by influences from the basal ganglia and cerebellum. Pathways descending from these structures control posture and balance (B).

Labels in figure:
Cortical pyramidal cells
Foot
Motor cortex
Hand
Mouth
Neuromuscular junction
Basal ganglia
Cerebellum
Skeletal muscle
Pyramidal tract (A)
(B) Descending control of posture and balance
Spinal cord
Lateral cortico-spinal tract
Anterior horn cells

Clinical assessment of weakness

The pattern of symptoms and signs usually indicates the nature of the lesion (Box 16.7, Fig. 16.3). It is important to establish whether the patient has loss of power, altered sensation or generalised fatigue. Pain may restrict movement, mimicking weakness, while sensory neglect (p. 632) may leave patients unaware of severe weakness.

Patients with parkinsonism may complain of weakness; examination reveals rigidity (cogwheel or lead pipe), bradykinesia should be evident, and there is a resting tremor, usually asymmetrical (p. 621). Movement restricted by pain should be apparent to

16.7 How to assess weakness	
Clinical finding	**Likely level of lesion/diagnosis**
Pattern and distribution	
Isolated muscles	Radiculopathy or mononeuropathy
Both limbs on one side (hemiparesis)	Cerebral hemisphere, less likely cord or brainstem
One limb	Neuronopathy, plexopathy, cord/brain
Both lower limbs (paraparesis)	Spinal cord; look for a sensory level
Fatigability	Myasthenia gravis
Bizarre, fluctuating, not following anatomical rules	Functional
Signs	
Upper motor neuron	Brain/spinal cord
Lower motor neuron	Peripheral nervous system
Evolution of the weakness	
Sudden and improving	Stroke/mononeuropathy
Evolving over months or years	Meningioma, cervical spondylotic myelopathy
Gradually worsening over days or weeks	Cerebral mass, demyelination
Associated symptoms	
Absence of sensory involvement	Motor neuron disease, myopathy, myasthenia

observation, as should contractures, wasting, fasciculations and abnormal movements/postures.

Functional weakness is common. On examination, the signs are often variable (e.g. the patient can walk but appears to have no leg movement when assessed on the couch), and strength may appear to 'give way', with the patient able to achieve full power for brief bursts. This does not occur in disease. In functional weakness, one may see hip extension weakness (rarely organic), which then returns to full strength on testing contralateral hip flexion. This sign may be demonstrated to the patient in a non-confrontational manner, to show that the potential limb power is intact.

Facial nerve palsy (Bell's palsy)

One of the most common causes of facial weakness is Bell's palsy, a lower motor neuron lesion of the 7th (facial) nerve within the facial canal, affecting all ages and both sexes.

Symptoms develop subacutely over a few hours, with pain around the ear preceding unilateral facial weakness. Patients often describe numbness but there is no objective sensory loss (except to taste, if the chorda tympani is involved). Hyperacusis may occur if the nerve to stapedius is involved, and there may be diminished salivation and tear secretion. Vesicles in the ear or on the palate may indicate primary herpes zoster infection (p. 66).

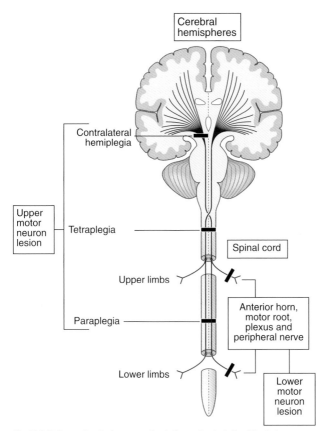

Fig. 16.3 Patterns of motor loss according to the anatomical site of the lesion.

About 80% of patients recover spontaneously within 12 wks. Steroids improve recovery if started within 72 hrs of onset but antiviral drugs are ineffective. Unlike Bell's palsy, lesions with an upper motor neuron origin partly spare the upper face.

Sensory disturbance

Sensory symptoms are common and are frequently benign, but sensory examination is difficult for both doctor and patient. While neurological disease can cause sensory symptoms, systemic disorders can also be responsible. Perioral and digital tingling occurs with hyperventilation (p. 267) or hypocalcaemia (p. 356). When there is dysfunction of the relevant cerebral cortex, the patient's perception of the relevant part of the body may be distorted.

A diagnostic approach to sensory symptoms

In the history, the most useful features are:
• Anatomical distribution. • Mode of onset of numbness.
• Paraesthesia or pain.

Certain patterns can be recognised. For example, in migraine the aura may consist of a front of paraesthesia followed by numbness that takes 20–30 mins to spread over one half of the body. Sensory loss due to a vascular lesion, on the other hand, will occur more or less instantaneously. The numbness and paraesthesia of spinal cord lesions often ascend one or both lower limbs to a level on the trunk over hours or days.

Patterns of sensory disturbance

See Figure 16.4.

Sensory loss in peripheral nerve lesions

In peripheral nerve lesions, the symptoms are usually of sensory loss and simple paraesthesia. Single peripheral nerve lesions will cause disturbance in the sensory distribution of that nerve. In diffuse neuropathies the longest neurons are affected first, giving the characteristic 'glove and stocking' distribution. Diabetes typically affects small fibres, preferentially impairing temperature and pin-prick, while demyelination may particularly affect large fibres subserving vibration and proprioception.

Sensory loss in nerve root lesions

Pain is more often a feature of lesions of nerve roots within the spine or in the limb plexuses. It is often felt in the muscles innervated by a root. The site of nerve root lesions may be deduced from the dermatomal pattern of sensory loss.

Sensory loss in spinal cord lesions

Sensory information ascends the nervous system in two anatomically discrete systems, differential involvement of which is often of diagnostic assistance (Fig. 16.5).

Transverse spinal cord lesions: There is loss of all modalities below that segmental level. Often a band of paraesthesia or hyperaesthesia is found at the top of the area of loss. If vascular in origin (e.g. due to anterior spinal artery thrombosis), the posterior one-third of the spinal cord (dorsal column modalities) may be spared.

Unilateral spinal cord lesions: There is loss for spinothalamic modalities (pain and temperature) on the opposite side of the lesion. There is also loss for dorsal column modalities (joint position and vibration) on the same side as the lesion (e.g. Brown–Séquard syndrome).

Central spinal cord lesions (e.g. syringomyelia): These spare the dorsal columns but affect spinothalamic fibres from both sides over the length of the lesion. The sensory loss is therefore dissociated (in terms of the modalities affected) and suspended (segments above and below the lesion are spared).

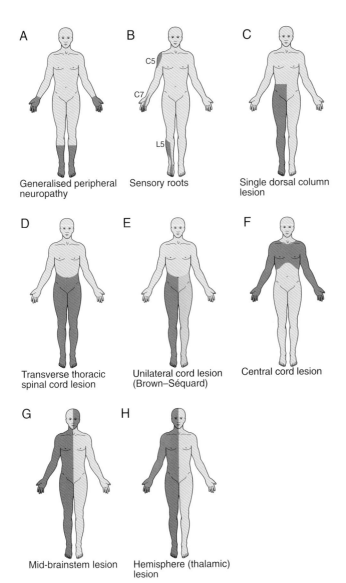

Fig. 16.4 Patterns of sensory loss. A Generalised peripheral neuropathy. **B** Sensory roots. **C** Single dorsal column lesion (proprioception and some touch loss). **D** Transverse thoracic spinal cord lesion. **E** Unilateral cord lesion (Brown–Séquard): ipsilateral dorsal column (and motor) deficit and contralateral spinothalamic deficit. **F** Central cord lesion: 'cape' distribution of spinothalamic loss. **G** Mid-brainstem lesion: ipsilateral facial sensory loss and contralateral loss on body. **H** Hemisphere (thalamic) lesion: contralateral loss on one side of face and body.

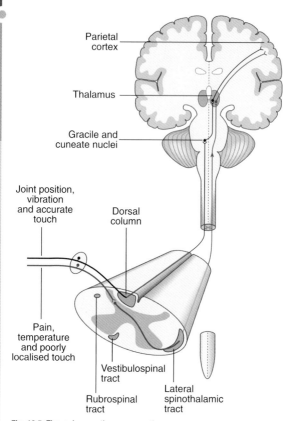

Fig. 16.5 The main somatic sensory pathways.

Single dorsal column lesion (e.g. multiple sclerosis): The patient experiences an unpleasant tight feeling over the limb involved. There is loss of proprioception without any loss of pin-prick or temperature sensation.

Sensory loss in brainstem lesions

Brainstem lesions produce complex patterns of sensory loss, depending on the anatomy of the lesion and its influence on the trigeminal nuclei.

Sensory loss in hemispheric lesions

These may affect all modalities of sensation. In the thalamus, discrete lesions (e.g. small lacunar strokes) can cause loss of sensation over the whole contralateral half of the body. With substantial lesions of the parietal cortex (as with large strokes) there is severe loss of proprioception and even loss of conscious awareness of the existence of the affected limb(s).

Neuropathic pain

Pain is of two main types:

• Nociceptive pain, arising from a pathological process in a body part. • Neuropathic pain, caused by dysfunction of the pain perception apparatus itself.

Neuropathic pain is a very unpleasant persistent burning sensation, often with increased sensitivity to touch. The most common syndromes include partial damage to peripheral nerves ('causalgia'), the trigeminal nerve (post-herpetic neuralgia) or the thalamus. Drugs (carbamazepine, tricyclics or phenothiazines) may help but usually only partially. Neurosurgical attempts to interrupt pain pathways sometimes succeed. Implantation of electrical stimulators has occasionally proved successful.

Abnormal movements

Abnormal movements usually imply a disorder in the basal ganglia, in which there is disinhibition of intrinsic rhythm generators or a disorder of postural control.

Tremor

The many causes of tremor have different characteristics:

Parkinsonian: 'Pill-rolling', asymmetrical and present at rest.

Physiological: Exaggerated by anxiety, emotion, thyrotoxicosis, drugs and toxins.

Essential: Slower than physiological tremor; often familial and responsive to propranolol.

Dystonic: Affects head, arms and legs; jerky, associated with dystonias.

Functional: Variable pattern; disappears on distraction.

Other hyperkinetic syndromes

Chorea: Jerky, brief, purposeless involuntary movements, appearing as fidgety; they suggest disease in the caudate nucleus. Causes include:

• Hereditary (Huntington's disease, Wilson's disease). • Drugs (levodopa, antipsychotics, anticonvulsants, oral contraceptives). • Autoimmune disease (e.g. Sydenham's chorea, antiphospholipid syndrome, systemic lupus erythematosus). • Endocrine factors (pregnancy, thyrotoxicosis, hypoparathyroidism, hypoglycaemia). • Other: vascular causes, demyelination, brain tumour.

Athetosis: Slower writhing movements of the limbs. These are often combined with chorea and have similar causes.

Ballism: More dramatic than chorea. These flinging movements of the limbs usually occur unilaterally (hemiballismus) in vascular lesions of the subthalamic nucleus.

Dystonia: A movement disorder in which a limb (or the head) involuntarily takes up an abnormal posture. This may be generalised in basal ganglia disease, or may be focal or segmental, as in spasmodic torticollis when the head involuntarily turns to one side. Other segmental dystonias may cause abnormal disabling postures during specific actions (e.g. writer's cramp) and can be treated with botulinum toxin to the responsible muscles.

Myoclonus: Brief, isolated, random, non-purposeful jerks of muscle groups in the limbs. They occur normally at the onset of sleep (hypnic jerks). Myoclonus can occur in epilepsy, from subcortical structures or from segments of the spinal cord.

Tics: Repetitive semi-purposeful movements, such as blinking, winking, grinning or screwing up of the eyes. Unlike with other involuntary movements, patients can suppress tics, at least for a short time.

Abnormal perception

The parietal lobes are involved in the higher processing and integration of sensory information. This takes place in areas of 'association' cortex, damage to which causes sensory (including visual) inattention, disorders of spatial perception, and disruption of spatially orientated behaviour, leading to apraxia. Apraxia is the inability to perform complex, organised activity in the presence of normal basic motor, sensory and cerebellar function (after weakness, numbness and ataxia have been excluded). Examples of complex motor activities include dressing, using cutlery and geographical orientation. Other abnormalities that can result from damage to the association cortex involve difficulty reading (dyslexia) or writing (dysgraphia), or the inability to recognise familiar objects (agnosia).

Altered balance and vertigo

Disorders of balance can arise from abnormalities affecting:
• Input: loss of vision, vestibular disorders or lack of joint position sense. • Processing: damage to vestibular nuclei or cerebellum. • Motor function: spinal cord lesions, leg weakness of any cause.

Disturbance of cerebellar function may also cause nystagmus, dysarthria or ataxia.

Disordered balance due to failure of proprioception or cerebellar function causes unsteadiness, while failure of the vestibular and labyrinthine apparatus causes vertigo, an illusory sensation of movement of the environment or self.

Vertigo occurs as a result of a mismatch between the information about a person's position reaching the brain from the eyes, limb proprioception and the vestibular system. Vertigo arising from inappropriate labyrinthine input is usually short-lived, though it may recur, whilst vertigo arising from central (brainstem) disorders is often persistent and accompanied by other signs of brainstem dysfunction.

Gait disorders

Patterns of weakness, loss of coordination and proprioceptive sensory loss produce a range of abnormal gaits. Neurogenic disorders need to be distinguished from skeletal abnormalities, usually characterised by pain producing an antalgic gait, or limp.

Pyramidal gait: Upper motor neuron lesions cause extension of the leg. The tendency for the toes to strike the ground on walking requires the leg to swing outwards at the hip (circumduction). In a hemiplegia, the asymmetry between affected and normal sides is obvious. In a paraparesis, both lower limbs move slowly, swung from the hips and dragged on the ground in extension.

Foot drop: Weakness of ankle dorsiflexion disrupts normal gait. Descent of the foot is less controlled, making a slapping noise, and the foot may be lifted higher, producing a high-stepping gait.

Myopathic gait: In proximal muscle weakness, usually caused by muscle disease, the hips are not properly fixed and trunk movements are exaggerated, producing a rolling or waddling gait.

Ataxic gait: Patients with lesions of the central parts of the cerebellum (the vermis) walk with a characteristic broad-based gait, 'as if drunk'.

Apraxic gait: There is normal power in the legs and no abnormal cerebellar signs or proprioception loss, yet the patient cannot formulate the motor act of walking. This higher cerebral dysfunction occurs in bilateral hemisphere disease, such as normal pressure hydrocephalus and diffuse frontal lobe disease.

Marche à petits pas: This gait is characterised by small, slow steps and marked instability. The usual cause is small-vessel cerebrovascular disease, and there are accompanying bilateral upper motor neuron signs.

Extrapyramidal gait: Patients have difficulty initiating walking and controlling the pace of their gait. This produces the festinant gait: initial stuttering steps that quickly increase in frequency while decreasing in length.

Abnormal speech and language

Speech disturbance may be isolated to disruption of sound output (dysarthria) or may involve language disturbance (dysphasia). Dysphonia (reduction in the sound/volume) is usually due to mechanical laryngeal disruption, whereas dysarthria is more typically neurological in origin. Dysphasia is always neurological and localises to the dominant cerebral hemisphere (usually left, regardless of handedness).

Dysphonia and dysarthria

The vocal cords may fail to generate sounds properly in speech, resulting in hoarse or whispered speech (dysphonia). This may be due to a local problem affecting the cords or a higher-level problem (dystonia) of vocal cord operation. If the muscles or nerves controlling the mouth, tongue, pharynx and lips are not functioning correctly, poorly articulated speech will result (dysarthria). Cerebellar or brainstem disease, lower cranial nerve lesions, myasthenia and muscle disease may all result in dysarthria.

Dysphasia

Dysphasia (or aphasia) is a disorder of the language content of speech that causes an inability to produce the correct word. It can occur with lesions over a wide area of the dominant hemisphere. It is categorised as fluent or non-fluent. In non-fluent (expressive) aphasias, such as Broca's aphasia, verbal comprehension may be preserved. If a patient has difficulty with speech comprehension, there is likely to be a lesion in Wernicke's area. Patients with large lesions over much of the speech area have no language production and have 'global aphasia'.

Disturbance of smell

Symptomatic olfactory loss almost always is due to local causes (nasal obstruction), follows head injury or is idiopathic. Hyposmia may occur early in Parkinson's disease. Frontal lobe lesions are a rare cause. Positive olfactory symptoms may arise from Alzheimer's disease or epilepsy.

Visual disturbance and ocular abnormalities

Visual loss

The visual pathway from the retina to the occipital cortex is topographically organised, so the pattern of visual field loss allows localisation of the site of the lesion (Fig. 16.6, Box 16.8). Patients often present with transient visual loss.

Visual loss lasting less than 15 mins is likely to have a vascular cause. This can affect one eye (amaurosis fugax) or one visual field. The field loss may be monocular (carotid circulation) or a homonymous hemianopia (vertebro-basilar circulation). Transient visual disturbance lasting 10–60 mins suggests migraine, especially if accompanied by headache and/or positive visual phenomena (e.g. zigzag lines, flashing coloured lights).

Visual hallucinations may be due to drugs or epilepsy.

Eye movement disorders

The control of eye movements begins in the cerebral hemispheres, and the pathway then descends to the brainstem with input from the visual cortex and cerebellum. Horizontal and vertical gaze centres in the pons and mid-brain coordinate output to the ocular motor nerve nuclei (3, 4 and 6). These are connected to each other by the medial longitudinal fasciculus. The extraocular muscles are then supplied by the oculomotor (3rd), trochlear (4th) and abducens (6th) nerves.

Diplopia ('double vision')

The pattern of double vision and associated features allow localisation of the lesion, whilst the mode of onset and subsequent behaviour suggest the aetiology (e.g. fatigability in myasthenia). The trochlear (4th) nerve innervates the superior oblique muscle, and the abducens (6th) nerve innervates the lateral rectus. The oculomotor

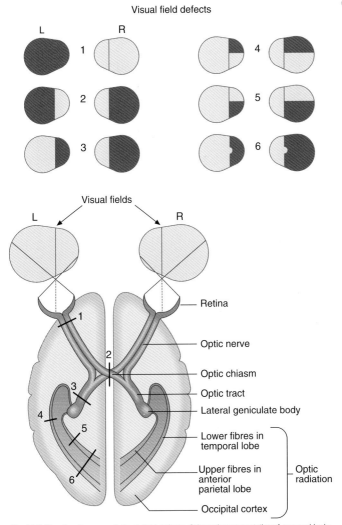

Fig. 16.6 **Visual pathways and visual field defects.** Schematic representation of eyes and brain in transverse section.

16.8 Clinical manifestations of visual field loss

Site	Common causes	Complaint	Visual field loss	Associated physical signs
Retina/optic disc	Vascular disease (including vasculitis) Glaucoma Inflammation	Partial/complete visual loss depending on site	Altitudinal field defect Arcuate scotoma	Reduced acuity Visual distortion (macula) Abnormal retinal appearance
Optic nerve	Optic neuritis Sarcoidosis Tumour Leber's hereditary optic neuropathy	Partial/complete loss of vision in one eye Often painful Central vision particularly affected	Central scotoma Paracentral scotoma Monocular blindness	Reduced acuity Reduced colour vision Relative afferent pupillary defect
Optic chiasm	Pituitary tumours Craniopharyngioma Sarcoidosis	May be none Rarely diplopia ('hemifield slide')	Bitemporal hemianopia	Pituitary function abnormalities
Optic tract	Tumour Inflammatory disease	Disturbed vision to one side of midline	Incongruous contralateral homonymous hemianopia	
Temporal lobe	Stroke Tumour Inflammatory disease	Disturbed vision to one side of midline	Contralateral homonymous upper quadrantanopia	Memory/language disorders
Parietal lobe	Stroke Tumour Inflammatory disease	Disturbed vision to one side of midline Bumping into things	Contralateral homonymous lower quadrantanopia	Contralateral sensory disturbance Asymmetry of optokinetic nystagmus
Occipital lobe	Stroke Tumour Inflammatory disease	Disturbed vision to one side of midline Difficulty reading Bumping into things	Homonymous hemianopia (may be macula-sparing)	Damage to other structures supplied by posterior cerebral circulation

(3rd) nerve innervates the remainder of the extraocular muscles, along with the levator palpebrae superioris and the ciliary body (pupil constriction and accommodation). Causes of ocular motor nerve palsies are given in Box 16.9.

Nystagmus

If the eye movement control systems are defective, the eyes may drift off target, resulting in a repetitive to-and-fro movement (drift–correction–drift) known as nystagmus. The direction of the fast phase is designated as the direction of the nystagmus because it is easier to see, although the abnormality is the slower drift of the eyes off target.

Vestibular lesions: Damage to the horizontal canal allows output from the healthy, contralateral side to cause the eyes to drift towards the side of the lesion. Recurrent compensatory fast movements away from the lesion cause unidirectional horizontal nystagmus to the opposite side. Nystagmus of peripheral labyrinthine lesions fatigues quickly and is always accompanied by vertigo and/or nausea and vomiting. Central vestibular nystagmus is more persistent.

Brainstem/cerebellar lesions: Lesions allow the eyes to drift back in towards primary position, producing nystagmus with fast component that beats in the direction of gaze. They are bi-directional and not accompanied by vertigo. Brainstem disease may also cause vertical nystagmus. Unilateral cerebellar lesions may cause nystagmus in the direction of the lesion (fast phases are directed towards the side of the lesion).

Other causes: These include physiological (in response to vestibular stimulation), toxicity (especially drugs), nutritional (thiamine) deficiency and congenital ('pendular' rather than 'jerking') causes.

Ptosis

Ptosis may result from a 3rd nerve palsy (see Box 16.9), sympathetic nerve damage (Horner's syndrome) or muscle disorders (e.g. myasthenia gravis or myotonic dystrophy).

Abnormal pupillary responses

Pupillary response to light is due to a combination of parasympathetic and sympathetic activity.

• Third nerve lesions: pupillary dilatation, complete ptosis and extraocular muscle palsy. • Sympathetic lesions (e.g. Horner's syndrome): partial ptosis and pupillary constriction. • Holmes–Adie pupils: dilation and constriction to accommodation but not to light. • Afferent pupillary disorders: impairment of the direct light reflex because of optic nerve damage (consensual response from stimulation of the normal eye remains intact).

Optic disc disorders

Optic disc swelling: This occurs with:
• Raised intracranial pressure ('papilloedema'). • Venous obstruction (cavernous sinus or retinal). • Systemic disorders affecting retinal

16.9 Common causes of damage to cranial nerves 3, 4 and 6

Site	Common pathology	Nerve(s) involved	Associated features
Brainstem	Infarction	3 (mid-brain)	Contralateral pyramidal signs
	Haemorrhage	6 (ponto-medullary junction)	Ipsilateral lower motor neuron 7 palsy
	Demyelination		Other brainstem/cerebellar signs
	Intrinsic tumour		
Intrameningeal	Meningitis	3 and/or 6	Meningism
	Raised intracranial pressure	6	Papilloedema
		3 (uncal herniation)	Features of space-occupying lesion
	Aneurysms	3 (posterior communicating artery)	Pain
		6 (basilar artery)	Features of subarachnoid haemorrhage
			8, 7, 5 lesions
	Cerebello-pontine angle tumour		Ipsilateral cerebellar signs
Cavernous sinus	Trauma	3, 4 and/or 6	Other features of trauma
	Infection/thrombosis	3, 4 and/or 6	May be 5th nerve involvement also
	Carotid artery aneurysm		Pupil may be fixed, mid-position
	Carotico-cavernous fistula		
Superior orbital fissure	Tumour (e.g. sphenoid wing meningioma)	3, 4 and/or 6	May be proptosis, chemosis
	Granuloma		
Orbit	Vascular, infections, tumour, granuloma, trauma	3, 4 and/or 6	Pain
			Pupil often spared in vascular 3 palsy

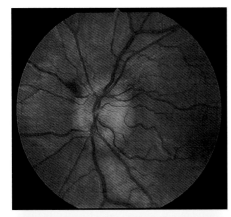

Fig. 16.7 Optic disc oedema (papilloedema). Fundus photograph of the left eye showing optic disc oedema with a small haemorrhage on the nasal side of the disc.

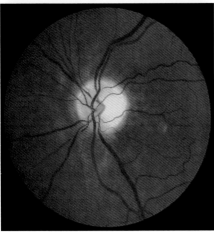

Fig. 16.8 Fundus photograph of the left eye of a patient with familial optic atrophy. Note marked pallor of optic disc.

vessels (hypertension, hypercapnia, vasculitis). • Optic nerve damage (e.g. demyelination, ischaemia, sarcoid, glioma).

There is the cessation of normal venous pulsation at the disc, and the disc margins then become red and indistinct; the whole disc is raised up, often with haemorrhages in the retina (Fig. 16.7).

Optic atrophy: Optic nerve damage makes the optic disc appear pale (Fig. 16.8). Causes include:
• Previous optic neuritis. • Ischaemic damage. • Chronic papilloedema. • Optic nerve compression. • Trauma. • Degenerative conditions.

Hearing disturbance

Each cochlear organ has bilateral cortical representation, so unilateral hearing loss indicates peripheral organ damage. Bilateral hearing dysfunction is usual, and is usually due to age-related degeneration or noise damage, although infection and drugs (particularly diuretics and aminoglycoside antibiotics) can cause deafness.

Bulbar symptoms – dysphagia and dysarthria

Swallowing is a complex activity involving the lips, tongue, soft palate, pharynx, larynx and cranial nerves 7, 9, 10, 11 and 12. Structural causes of dysphagia are considered on page 413. Neurological mechanisms usually cause dysphagia accompanied by dysarthria. Acute onset suggests a brainstem stroke or a rapidly developing neuropathy, such as Guillain–Barré syndrome or diphtheria. Intermittent fatigable muscle weakness (including dysphagia) suggests myasthenia gravis. Dysphagia developing over weeks or months occurs in motor neuron disease, polymyositis, basal meningitis and inflammatory brainstem disease. More slowly developing dysphagia suggests a myopathy or possibly a brainstem or skull-base tumour.

Pathologies affecting lower cranial nerves (9–12) frequently manifest bilaterally, producing dysphagia and dysarthria. 'Bulbar palsy' is the term for lower motor neuron lesions either within or outside the brainstem. The tongue is wasted and fasciculating, and palatal movement reduced.

Upper motor neuron innervation of swallowing is bilateral, so persistent dysphagia is unusual with a unilateral upper motor lesion (except in the acute stages of a hemispheric stroke). Widespread lesions above the medulla will cause upper motor neuron bulbar paralysis, known as 'pseudobulbar palsy'. Here the tongue is small and contracted, and moves slowly; the jaw jerk is brisk.

Bladder, bowel and sexual disturbance
Bladder

The bladder is analogous to skeletal muscle in that neural control can be divided into upper and lower motor neuron components.

Atonic (lower motor neuron) bladder: Distended with overflow, and loss of perineal sensation. It occurs in disease affecting the sacral cord or roots.

Hypertonic (upper motor neuron) bladder: Occurs in cortical, spinal cord or brainstem disease, and presents with a loss of awareness of bladder fullness and reflex micturition. Parasympathetic over-activity causes incontinence and loss of coordination between detrusor contraction and sphincter relaxation.

Rectum

The rectum has an excitatory cholinergic input from the parasympathetic sacral outflow, and inhibitory sympathetic supply similar to that of the bladder. Continence depends on skeletal muscle contraction in the pelvic floor muscles supplied by the pudendal nerves, as well as the internal and external anal sphincters.

Damage to the autonomic components usually causes constipation. Lesions affecting the conus medullaris, the somatic S2–4 roots and the pudendal nerves cause faecal incontinence.

Erectile failure and ejaculation failure

These related functions are under autonomic control via the pelvic (parasympathetic, S2–4) and hypogastric nerves (sympathetic, L1–2). Erection is largely parasympathetic and is impaired by several anticholinergic, antihypertensive and antidepressant drugs. Sympathetic activity is important for ejaculation and may be inhibited by α-adrenoceptor antagonists.

Changes in personality and behaviour

Organic conditions can result in altered personality and behaviour. This particularly applies to disorders affecting the frontal lobes, which control executive function, movement and behaviour. The frontal lobes may be damaged structurally (e.g. trauma, strokes, hydrocephalus or tumour) or functionally (e.g. metabolic disturbances). Three main patterns are seen:

Mesial frontal lesions: Cause patients to become withdrawn, unresponsive and mute, often with urinary incontinence, gait apraxia and increased tone.

Dorsolateral pre-frontal cortical lesions: Cause difficulties with speech, motor planning and organisation.

Orbitofrontal lesions: Cause disinhibited or irresponsible behaviour. Memory is substantially intact, and there may be focal physical signs such as a grasp reflex, palmo-mental response or pout.

STROKE DISEASE

Stroke is a common medical emergency with an annual incidence of between 180 and 300 per 100 000. The incidence rises with age. One-fifth of patients with an acute stroke will die within a month of the event, and at least half of those who survive will be left with physical disability.

Acute stroke

Acute stroke is characterised by the rapid appearance (over minutes) of a focal deficit of brain function, which can take several forms:

Weakness: Unilateral weakness is the classical presentation of stroke. The weakness starts suddenly, and progresses rapidly in a hemiplegic pattern. Reflexes are initially reduced but later tone and reflexes are increased. Upper motor neuron facial weakness is often present.

Speech disturbance: Dysphasia and dysarthria are the usual speech manifestations in stroke (p. 623). Dysphasia indicates dominant frontal or parietal lobe damage, while dysarthria is caused by weakness or incoordination of the face and pharyngeal muscles.

Visual deficit: Monocular blindness in stroke can be caused by reduced blood flow in the internal carotid or ophthalmic arteries. If transient, this is called amaurosis fugax. Ischaemic damage to the occipital cortex or optic tracts causes contralateral hemianopia (p. 624).

Visuo-spatial dysfunction: Damage to the non-dominant cortex often results in contralateral sensory or visual neglect and apraxia (p. 622). This is sometimes mistaken for confusion.

Ataxia: Stroke causing damage to the cerebellum and its connections can present as acute ataxia (p. 657), sometimes with brainstem features, e.g. diplopia (p. 624) and vertigo (p. 622). The differential diagnosis includes vestibular disorders (p. 622).

Headache: Sudden severe headache is the cardinal symptom of subarachnoid haemorrhage but also occurs in intracerebral haemorrhage. Headache is also a feature of cerebral venous disease.

Seizure: Seizure is unusual in acute stroke but may occur in cerebral venous disease.

Coma: Coma is an uncommon feature of stroke, though it may occur with a brainstem event. In the first 24 hrs, coma usually indicates a subarachnoid or intracerebral haemorrhage.

Cerebral infarction

Cerebral infarction (85%) is mostly due to thromboembolic disease secondary to atherosclerosis in the major extracranial arteries (carotid artery and aortic arch). About 20% are due to embolism from the heart, and 20% are due to intrinsic disease of small perforating vessels, producing so-called 'lacunar' infarctions. Perhaps 5% have rare causes, including vasculitis, endocarditis and cerebral venous disease. Risk factors for ischaemic stroke are similar to those for coronary artery disease (p. 230).

In the affected territory, as blood flow falls below the threshold for the maintenance of electrical activity, neurological deficit develops. At this point, the neurons are still viable; if the blood flow increases again, function returns and the patient will have had a transient ischaemic attack (TIA). If the blood flow falls further, however, a level is reached at which irreversible cell death (infarction) occurs.

Intracerebral haemorrhage

Intracerebral haemorrhage (10%) usually results from rupture of a blood vessel within the brain parenchyma: a primary intracerebral haemorrhage. It may also occur with subarachnoid haemorrhage (5%) if the artery ruptures into the brain substance, as well as the subarachnoid space. Haemorrhage frequently occurs into an area of brain infarction; if large, it may be difficult to distinguish from primary intracerebral haemorrhage. Risk factors for intracerebral haemorrhage include:

• Age. • Hypertension. • Anticoagulant therapy. • Intracranial vascular malformations. • Substance abuse.

Clinical features

The common clinical stroke syndromes depend on which vascular territories are affected (Fig. 16.9). Stroke can also be classified by the time course of the deficit:

16.10 Differential diagnosis of stroke and TIA

'Structural' stroke mimics

- Primary cerebral tumours
- Metastatic cerebral tumours
- Subdural haematoma
- Cerebral abscess
- Peripheral nerve lesions (vascular or compressive)
- Demyelination

'Functional' stroke mimics

- Todd's paresis (after epileptic seizure)
- Hypoglycaemia
- Migrainous aura (with or without headache)
- Focal seizures
- Ménière's disease or other vestibular disorder
- Conversion disorder
- Encephalitis

Transient ischaemic attack (TIA): Symptoms resolve completely within 24 hrs. This includes amaurosis fugax (see above).

Stroke: Symptoms last >24 hrs. With a clear history of rapid-onset transient or sustained focal deficit, the alternative diagnoses (Box 16.10) account for only 5% of cases.

Progressing stroke ('stroke in evolution'): Focal neurological deficit worsens after the patient first presents. It may be due to increasing volume of infarction, haemorrhage or related oedema.

Completed stroke: Focal deficit persists but is not progressing.

Investigations

Investigation aims to:

• Confirm the vascular nature of the lesion. • Distinguish cerebral infarction from haemorrhage. • Identify the underlying vascular disease and risk factors (Box 16.11).

Further investigations are indicated if the nature of the stroke is uncertain, especially for younger patients who are less likely to have atherosclerotic disease.

Neuroimaging

CT or MRI should be performed in all patients. CT (Figs 16.9 and 16.10) can exclude non-stroke lesions (e.g. subdural haematomas, tumours) and demonstrate intracerebral haemorrhage. CT changes in cerebral infarction may be absent in the first few hours after symptom onset. Usually, CT scan within the first day or so is adequate. However, an immediate CT scan is essential if the patient has abnormal coagulation, a progressing deficit or suspected cerebellar haematoma, or if thrombolysis is planned. MRI detects infarction earlier than CT and is more sensitive for strokes affecting the brainstem and cerebellum.

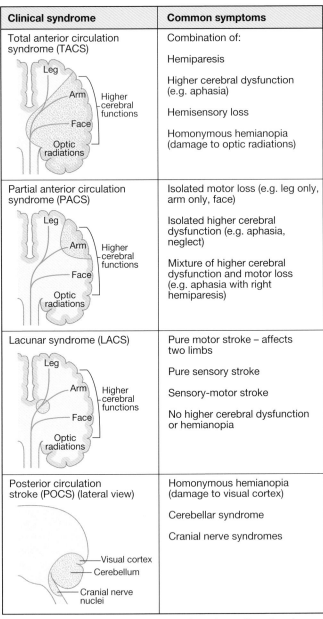

Clinical syndrome	Common symptoms
Total anterior circulation syndrome (TACS)	Combination of: Hemiparesis Higher cerebral dysfunction (e.g. aphasia) Hemisensory loss Homonymous hemianopia (damage to optic radiations)
Partial anterior circulation syndrome (PACS)	Isolated motor loss (e.g. leg only, arm only, face) Isolated higher cerebral dysfunction (e.g. aphasia, neglect) Mixture of higher cerebral dysfunction and motor loss (e.g. aphasia with right hemiparesis)
Lacunar syndrome (LACS)	Pure motor stroke – affects two limbs Pure sensory stroke Sensory-motor stroke No higher cerebral dysfunction or hemianopia
Posterior circulation stroke (POCS) (lateral view)	Homonymous hemianopia (damage to visual cortex) Cerebellar syndrome Cranial nerve syndromes

Fig. 16.9 Clinical and radiological features of the stroke syndromes. The top three diagrams show coronal brain sections, the bottom one a sagittal section. Infarcted areas (shown in red) can cause damage to the relevant cortex (PACS), nerve tracts (LACS) or both (TACS). In corresponding CT scans, the lesion is highlighted by arrows.

Common cause	CT scan features
Middle cerebral artery occlusion (Embolism from heart or major vessels)	
Occlusion of a branch of the middle cerebral artery or anterior cerebral artery (Embolism from heart or major vessels)	
Thrombotic occlusion of small perforating arteries (Thrombosis in situ)	
Occlusion in vertebral, basilar or posterior cerebral artery territory (Cardiac embolism or thrombosis in situ)	

Fig. 16.9 cont'd

Is it a vascular lesion?	CT/MRI
Is it ischaemic or haemorrhagic?	CT/MRI
Is it a subarachnoid haemorrhage?	CT, LP
Is there any cardiac source of embolism?	ECG, 24-hr ECG, echocardiogram
What is the underlying vascular disease?	Duplex USS of carotids
	Magnetic resonance angiography (MRA)
	CT angiography (CTA)
	Contrast angiography
What are the risk factors?	FBC, cholesterol, glucose
Is there an unusual cause?	ESR, protein electrophoresis, clotting and thrombophilia screen

Vascular imaging

Detection of extracranial vascular disease can help establish why the patient has had an ischaemic stroke and may lead on to specific treatments, including carotid endarterectomy, to reduce the risk of further stroke. A carotid bruit is not a reliable indicator of the degree of carotid stenosis. Extracranial arterial disease can be non-invasively identified with duplex USS, MR angiography or CT angiography.

Cardiac investigations

The most common causes of cardiac embolism are atrial fibrillation, prosthetic heart valves, other valvular abnormalities and recent myocardial infarction. A transthoracic or transoesophageal echocardiogram can identify an unsuspected source such as endocarditis, atrial myxoma, intracardiac thrombus or patent foramen ovale.

Management

Management is aimed at:
• Minimising the volume of brain that is irreversibly damaged. • Preventing complications. • Reducing disability and handicap through rehabilitation. • Reducing the risk of recurrent episodes.

Early admission to a specialised stroke unit facilitates coordinated care from a multidisciplinary team and reduces mortality and residual disability amongst survivors. In the acute phase it may be useful to refer to a checklist (Box 16.12) to ensure that all the factors that might influence outcome have been addressed.

The deteriorating stroke patient

Neurological deficits may worsen during the hours or days after their onset. This is most common with lacunar infarction but may occur in other patients, due to extension of the area of infarction, haemorrhage into it or the development of oedema with consequent mass effect. It is important to distinguish this from

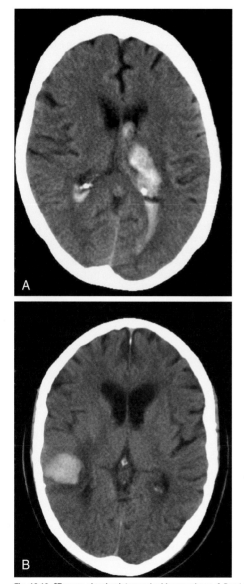

Fig. 16.10 CT scans showing intracerebral haemorrhage. A Basal ganglia haemorrhage with intraventricular extension. **B** Small cortical haemorrhage.

16.12 Acute stroke management: admission checklist	
Airway	Perform a swallow screen and keep patient nil by mouth if swallowing unsafe
Breathing	Check respiratory rate, O_2 saturation; give oxygen if SaO_2 <95%
Circulation	Check peripheral perfusion, pulse and BP are adequate
Hydration	If dehydrated, give IV or NG fluids if swallow is unsafe
Nutrition	Consider nutritional supplements. If persistent dysphagia, feed via NG tube
Medication	If dysphagic, consider alternative routes for essential medications
BP	Unless there is heart failure/renal failure/hypertensive encephalopathy/aortic dissection, do not lower BP in 1st wk, as it compromises cerebral perfusion. BP usually normalises within a few days
Blood glucose	If blood glucose ≥11.1 mmol/L, use insulin (via infusion or glucose/potassium/insulin (GKI)) to normalise levels
Temperature	If pyrexial, investigate and treat cause but give antipyretics early
Pressure areas	Anticipate and manage risk: treat infection, maintain nutrition, provide a pressure-relieving mattress and turn immobile patients regularly
Incontinence	Ensure patient is not constipated or in urinary retention. Avoid catheterisation unless retention or incontinence is threatening pressure areas
Mobilisation	Avoid bed rest

deterioration caused by complications (hypoxia, sepsis, seizures, metabolic abnormalities), which may be more easily reversed. Patients with cerebellar haematomas or infarcts with mass effect may develop obstructive hydrocephalus and might benefit from insertion of a ventricular drain and/or decompressive surgery. Patients with massive cerebral oedema may benefit from anti-oedema agents (mannitol), artificial ventilation and/or surgical decompression to reduce intracranial pressure, although evidence for these interventions is still incomplete.

Thrombolysis

IV thrombolysis with recombinant tissue plasminogen activator (rt-PA) increases the risk of haemorrhagic transformation of the cerebral infarct with potentially fatal results. However, if given within 4.5 hrs of symptom onset to highly selected patients, the haemorrhagic risk may be offset by an improvement in overall outcome. Earlier treatment maximises benefit.

Aspirin

Aspirin (300 mg daily) should be started immediately after an ischaemic stroke unless rt-PA has been given, in which case it should be withheld for at least 24 hrs. Aspirin reduces the risk of early recurrence and improves long-term outcome. Heparin does not improve outcomes and should not be used in acute stroke.

Coagulation abnormalities

In intracerebral haemorrhage, coagulation abnormalities (most commonly due to oral anticoagulants), should be reversed immediately to reduce the likelihood of the haematoma enlarging.

Management of risk factors

The average risk of a further stroke is 5–10% within the first week of a stroke or TIA, 15% in the first year and 5%/yr thereafter. Patients with ischaemic events should be put on long-term antiplatelet drugs and statins to lower cholesterol. For patients in atrial fibrillation, the risk can be reduced by ~60% by oral anticoagulation to achieve an INR of 2–3. The risk of recurrence after both ischaemic and haemorrhagic strokes can be reduced by lowering BP.

Carotid endarterectomy and angioplasty

Patients with a carotid territory ischaemic event and >70% carotid artery stenosis on the side of the brain lesion have a higher risk of stroke recurrence. For those without major residual disability, removal of the stenosis reduces the overall risk of recurrence, although the operation itself carries a 5% risk of stroke. Carotid angioplasty and stenting are technically feasible but the long-term effects are unclear.

Subarachnoid haemorrhage

About 85% of cases of spontaneous arterial bleeding into the subarachnoid space are caused by rupture of saccular ('berry') aneurysms at bifurcations of the cerebral arteries; 10% are non-aneurysmal haemorrhages; and 5% are due to rarities (arteriovenous malformations, vertebral artery dissection). Subarachnoid haemorrhage is rare (incidence 6/100000); women are more frequently affected and most present <65 yrs. The immediate mortality is ~30%. Survivors have a rebleed rate of 40% in the first 4 wks and 3% annually thereafter.

Clinical features

There is typically a sudden, severe 'thunderclap' headache (often occipital), which lasts for hours or even days, often accompanied by vomiting. Physical exertion, straining and sexual excitement are common antecedents. Usually the patient is distressed and irritable, with photophobia, but there may be loss of consciousness. Neck stiffness, focal hemisphere signs and subhyaloid haemorrhage on fundoscopy may be found.

Investigations

About 1 patient in 8 with a sudden severe headache has subarachnoid haemorrhage; therefore, all should be investigated to exclude it, starting with a CT scan. If the CT scan is negative (small amounts of blood may not be visible), then CSF should be obtained by LP at least 12 hrs after symptom onset, in order to detect blood and xanthochromia. If the CT scan and CSF at 12 hrs are negative, then subarachnoid haemorrhage can be excluded. If either is positive, cerebral angiography is indicated.

Management

Nimodipine (30–60 mg IV) is given to prevent vasospasm in the acute phase. Endovascular insertion of coils into an aneurysm or surgical clipping of the aneurysm neck reduces recurrence.

Cerebral venous disease

Thrombosis of cerebral veins and venous sinuses is relatively uncommon.

Predisposing systemic causes include:

• Dehydration. • Pregnancy. • Thrombophilia. • Oral contraceptives.
• Hypotension. • Behçet's disease.

Local causes include:

• Paranasal sinusitis. • Meningitis. • Facial skin infection. • Otitis media, mastoiditis. • Penetrating head/eye wounds. • Skull fracture.

Anticoagulation is usually given, and management of underlying causes and complications is important.

Cortical vein thrombosis

This may present with focal cortical deficits (aphasia, hemiparesis) or epilepsy, according to the area involved.

Cerebral venous sinus thrombosis

Cavernous sinus thrombosis causes proptosis, ptosis, headache, ophthalmoplegias, papilloedema and numbness in the trigeminal first division dermatome. Superior sagittal sinus thrombosis causes headache, papilloedema and seizures. Transverse sinus thrombosis causes hemiparesis, seizures and papilloedema.

About 10% of cases are associated with infection and require antibiotics; otherwise, treatment is by anticoagulation.

HEADACHE SYNDROMES

The general approach to headache is described on page 605. The primary headache syndromes are described here.

Tension-type headache

This is the most common type of headache.

Clinical features

The pain is constant and generalised but often radiates forward from the occipital region. It is described as 'dull', 'tight' or like a 'pressure'. The pain may continue for weeks without interruption, although the severity may vary. There is no vomiting or photophobia. The pain characteristically becomes more troublesome as the day goes on.

Management

Discussion of likely precipitants and explanation that the symptoms are not due to sinister pathology are more likely to help than analgesics. Excessive use of analgesics, particularly codeine, may worsen the headache (analgesic headache). Physiotherapy (with muscle relaxation and stress management) may be useful, as may low-dose amitriptyline. Patients benefit most from reassurance and rigorous assessment.

Migraine

Migraine affects 20% of women and 6% of men at some point. The aetiology is largely unknown. The headache phase is associated with vasodilatation of extracranial vessels. There is often a family history, suggesting a genetic predisposition. The female preponderance hints at hormonal influences. The contraceptive pill appears to exacerbate migraine in many patients. Doctors and patients often overestimate the role of dietary precipitants such as cheese, chocolate or red wine. When psychological stress is involved, the migraine attack often occurs after the period of stress.

Clinical features

A prodrome of malaise, irritability or behavioural change may occur. In ~20% of patients, migraine starts with aura (previously called 'classical' migraine). Shimmering, silvery zigzag lines (fortification spectra) march across the visual fields for up to 40 mins, sometimes leaving a trail of temporary field loss (scotoma). Patients may feel tingling followed by numbness, spreading over 20–30 mins, from one part of the body to another. Dominant hemisphere involvement may cause transient speech disturbance. Some 80% of patients have migraine without aura (previously 'common' migraine).

Migraine headache is usually severe and throbbing, with photophobia, phonophobia and vomiting lasting 4–72 hrs. Movement exacerbates pain and patients seek a quiet, dark room.

Before ascribing limb weakness or isolated aura without headache to migraine, other structural brain disorders, or focal epilepsy, should be considered.

Rarely, the aura does not resolve, leaving permanent neurological disturbance. This persistent migrainous aura may occur with or without evidence of brain infarction.

Management

Acute attack: Simple analgesia with aspirin or paracetamol, often with an antiemetic. Severe attacks can be treated with one of the 'triptans' (e.g. sumatriptan), 5-HT agonists that are potent vasoconstrictors of the extracranial arteries.

Prevention: Avoidance of identified triggers or exacerbating factors. If frequent, try calcium channel blockers, propranolol, amitriptyline or anti-epileptic drugs (e.g. sodium valproate). Women with aura should avoid oestrogen treatment for contraception or HRT, although the risk of ischaemic stroke is minimal.

Medication overuse headache

Headache syndromes perpetuated by analgesia intake (particularly codeine and other opiate-containing preparations) are becoming more common. Medication overuse headache is usually associated with use on more than 10–15 days/mth.

Management is by withdrawal of the responsible analgesics; patients should be warned that the initial effect will be to exacerbate the headache.

Cluster headache (migrainous neuralgia)
Clinical features

This is much less common than migraine. Males predominate 5:1, and onset is usually in the third decade. The syndrome comprises runs of severe, unilateral periorbital pain accompanied by unilateral lacrimation, nasal congestion and conjunctival injection, lasting 30–90 mins. The headache may occur repeatedly for a number of weeks, followed by months of respite before another cluster occurs.

Management

Acute attacks are usually halted by SC injections of sumatriptan or inhalation of 100% oxygen. Attacks can sometimes be prevented by sodium valproate, verapamil, methysergide or short courses of corticosteroids. Severe, debilitating clusters can be helped with lithium therapy.

Trigeminal neuralgia
Clinical features

Trigeminal neuralgia causes unilateral lancinating facial pains in the second and third divisions of the trigeminal nerve territory. The pain is severe and very brief but repetitive, causing the patient to flinch as if with a motor tic. It may be precipitated by touching trigger zones within the trigeminal territory or by eating. There is a tendency for the condition to remit and relapse over years.

Management

The pain usually responds at least partially to carbamazepine. If patients cannot tolerate carbamazepine, gabapentin, pregabalin, amitriptyline or steroids may help.

Surgical treatment should be considered, especially where response is incomplete in younger patients. Decompression of the vascular loop encroaching on the trigeminal root is said to have a 90% success rate. Otherwise, localised injection of alcohol or phenol into a peripheral branch of the nerve may be effective.

EPILEPSY

A seizure is any clinical event caused by an abnormal electrical discharge in the brain, whilst epilepsy is the tendency to have recurrent seizures. A single seizure is not epilepsy but is an indication for investigation. The recurrence rate after a first seizure approaches 70% in the first year. The lifetime risk of a single seizure is ~5%, whilst the prevalence of epilepsy is ~0.5%.

The division of seizure types on physiological grounds is between focal seizures in which paroxysmal neuronal activity is limited to one part of the cortex, and generalised seizures in which the electrophysiological abnormality involves both hemispheres simultaneously.

Clinical features

To classify seizure type, establish first whether there is a focal onset, and second whether the seizures conform to one of the recognised patterns (Box 16.13). Epilepsy that starts over the age of 35 almost invariably reflects a focal cerebral event. Where activity remains focal, signs may indicate the site. Even when generalised tonic–clonic seizures occur, seizures beginning in one cortical area will cause neurological symptoms and signs corresponding to the function of that area.

• Occipital onset: causes visual changes (lights/blobs of colour). • Temporal lobe onset: false recognition (déjà vu). • Sensory strip involvement: sensory alteration (burning, tingling). • Motor strip involvement: jerking.

Focal seizures

These may be idiopathic or may reflect focal structural lesions. The latter may be:

• Genetic (e.g. tuberous sclerosis). • Developmental. • Cerebrovascular (e.g. arteriovenous malformation). • Neoplastic. • Traumatic. • Infective. • Inflammatory (e.g. vasculitis).

Focal neurological signs may localise the source, but the signs may spread, causing impairment of awareness or bizarre behaviour.

Generalised seizures

Tonic–clonic seizures: May be preceded by an initial 'aura'. The patient then goes rigid, stops breathing, becomes unconscious and cyanosed, and may fall heavily. After a few moments, the rigidity is periodically relaxed, producing clonic jerks. Urinary incontinence or tongue-biting may occur. After a period of flaccid coma, the patient then regains consciousness, but is drowsy or confused for some hours.

Absence seizures: Generalised seizures, which always start in childhood. The child goes blank and stares for a few seconds only. The attacks are brief but may be frequent, and are not associated with post-ictal confusion. They may be mistaken for daydreaming.

16.13 Classification of seizures (2010 International League Against Epilepsy classification)

Generalised seizures

- Tonic–clonic (in any combination)
- Absence:
    Typical
    Atypical
    Absence with special features
- Myoclonic absence
- Eyelid myoclonia
- Myoclonic:
    Myoclonic
    Myoclonic atonic
    Myoclonic tonic
- Clonic
- Tonic
- Atonic

Focal seizures

- Without impairment of consciousness or awareness (was 'simple partial'):
    Focal motor
    Focal sensory
- With impairment of consciousness or awareness (was 'complex partial')
- Evolving to a bilateral, convulsive seizure (was 'secondarily generalised seizure'):
    Tonic
    Clonic
    Tonic–clonic

Unknown

- Epileptic spasms

Myoclonic seizures: Brief, jerking movements, predominating in the arms. They occur in the morning or on waking, or may be provoked by fatigue, alcohol or sleep deprivation.

Atonic seizures: Seizures involving brief loss of muscle tone, usually resulting in heavy falls with or without loss of consciousness.

Tonic seizures: Associated with a generalised increase in tone and an associated loss of awareness. Atonic and tonic seizures are usually seen as part of an epilepsy syndrome.

Clonic seizures: Similar to tonic–clonic seizures, but without a preceding tonic phase.

Many patients with epilepsy follow specific patterns of seizure type(s), age of onset and treatment responsiveness: the so-called electroclinical syndromes. Genetic testing may ultimately demonstrate similarities in molecular pathophysiology.

Investigations

No cause is found in most patients. However, investigations are necessary to confirm the diagnosis, characterise the type of epilepsy, and identify any underlying cause.

Cerebral imaging: After a single seizure, head CT or MRI is advisable, although the yield of structural lesions is low unless there are focal features.

EEG: May be more helpful in showing focal features if performed very soon after a seizure than after an interval. It can also help establish the type of epilepsy and guide therapy; however, an interictal EEG is normal in 50% so it cannot exclude epilepsy.

Other investigations: These should identify any metabolic, infective, inflammatory or toxic causes. They include FBC, ESR, CRP, U&Es, glucose, LFTs, CXR, syphilis serology, HIV, tests for collagen disease and CSF examination.

Management

Explain the nature and cause of seizures to patients and their relatives. Instruct relatives in the first aid management of major seizures. Emphasise that epilepsy is common and that full control can be expected in ~70% of patients.

The recognised mortality of epilepsy should be discussed sensitively with patients to encourage a serious approach to lifestyle modification and adherence to medication.

Immediate care: Little can or need be done for a person whilst a major seizure is occurring, except for first aid and common-sense manœuvres (Box 16.14).

Lifestyle advice: Patients should be made aware of the riskiness of activities in which loss of awareness would be dangerous, until good control of seizures has been established. This includes work or recreational activities involving exposure to heights, dangerous machinery, open fires or water. In the UK and many other countries,

16.14 Immediate care of seizures

First aid (by relatives and witnesses)

- Move person away from danger (fire, water, machinery, furniture)
- After convulsions cease, turn into 'recovery' position (semi-prone)
- Ensure airway is clear but do **not** insert anything in mouth (tongue-biting occurs at onset and cannot be prevented)
- If convulsions continue for >5 mins or recur without person regaining consciousness, summon urgent medical attention
- Person may be drowsy/confused for 30–60 mins and should not be left alone until recovered

Immediate medical attention

- See Box 16.2

16.15 Guidelines for choice of anti-epileptic drugs

Epilepsy type	First-line	Second-line
Focal onset and/or secondary GTCS	Lamotrigine	Carbamazepine Levetiracetam Sodium valproate Topiramate Zonisamide
GTCS	Sodium valproate Levetiracetam	Lamotrigine Topiramate Zonisamide
Absence	Ethosuximide	Sodium valproate
Myoclonic	Sodium valproate	Levetiracetam Clonazepam

N.B. Use as few drugs as possible. (GTCS = generalised tonic–clonic seizure.)

legal restrictions regarding vehicle driving apply to patients with epilepsy.

Anticonvulsant drug therapy (see also p. 761): Drug treatment should be considered after more than one unprovoked seizure. In most patients, full control is achieved with a single drug. Dose regimens should be kept as simple as possible to promote compliance. Guidelines are listed in Box 16.15. For seizures of focal onset, lamotrigine is the best-tolerated monotherapy and has few side-effects. Unclassified or specific syndromes respond best to valproate. Sodium valproate should not be used in women of reproductive age unless the benefits outweigh the risks. The first choice should be an established first-line drug, with more recently introduced drugs as second choice. Newer drugs have predictable pharmacokinetics, so drug levels are mainly used to monitor adherence. Gradual medication withdrawal may be considered after 2 seizure-free yrs.

Surgery: Some patients with drug-resistant epilepsy respond to resection of epileptogenic foci or nerve stimulation.

Prognosis

Generalised seizures are more readily controlled than partial seizures. A structural lesion makes complete control less likely. After 20 yrs:

• 50% have been seizure-free for the last 5 yrs without medication. • 20% are seizure-free with medication. • 30% continue to have seizures despite medication.

Withdrawal of anticonvulsant therapy: After complete control of seizures for 2–4 yrs, withdrawal of medication may be considered. Childhood-onset epilepsy carries the best prognosis for successful drug withdrawal. Overall, the recurrence rate of seizures after drug withdrawal is ~40%. Withdrawal should be undertaken slowly, reducing the drug dose gradually over 6–12 mths.

VESTIBULAR DISORDERS

Vertigo is the typical symptom of vestibular dysfunction, and most patients with vertigo have acute vestibular failure, benign paroxysmal positional vertigo or Ménière's disease. Central (brain) causes of vertigo are rare by comparison, with the exception of migraine.

Acute vestibular failure (labyrinthitis, vestibular neuronitis): Usually presents in the 3rd or 4th decade as severe vertigo, with vomiting and ataxia. The vertigo is most severe at onset and settles down over the next few days but may be provoked by head movement for longer. Nystagmus is present for a few days during the attack. Symptomatic relief can be achieved with short-term use of vestibular sedatives (e.g. cinnarizine, prochlorperazine, betahistine). A few patients have persisting symptoms requiring vestibular rehabilitation by a physiotherapist.

Benign paroxysmal positional vertigo: Paroxysms of vertigo occurring with certain head movements may be due to otolithic debris affecting endolymph flow in the labyrinth. Each attack lasts seconds but patients may become reluctant to move their head, producing a muscle tension-type headache. The diagnosis can be confirmed by using the 'Hallpike manœuvre', in which the head is swung briskly back to demonstrate positional nystagmus. The vertigo fatigues with repetitive positioning of the head and can be treated with vestibular exercises.

Ménière's disease: Patients usually present with tinnitus and deafness, and then develop episodic vertigo accompanied by a sense of fullness in the ear. Examination shows sensorineural hearing loss on the affected side. Vestibular sedatives may be helpful for acute attacks.

SLEEP DISORDERS

Sleep disturbances include too much sleep (hypersomnolence or excessive daytime sleepiness), insufficient or poor-quality sleep (insomnia) and abnormal behaviour during sleep (parasomnias). Insomnia is usually caused by psychological or psychiatric disorders, shift work, other environmental causes, pain, and so on, and will not be discussed further.

Hypersomnolence

The most common cause is obstructive sleep apnoea (p. 319). The history in narcolepsy is strikingly different.

Narcolepsy

In this disorder, sudden, irresistible sleep 'attacks' are experienced, often interrupting normal activities. Patients will report at least one other of the classical symptoms:

• Cataplexy (sudden loss of muscle tone, triggered by surprise, laughter or emotion). • Frightening ('hypnagogic') hallucinations at sleep onset. • Sleep paralysis.

Narcoleptic attacks can be treated with sodium oxybate or modafinil. Cataplexy responds to sodium oxybate, clomipramine or venlafaxine.

Parasomnias

Parasomnias are abnormal motor behaviours occurring in either REM or non-REM sleep.

Non-REM parasomnias: These manifest as night terrors, sleep walking and confusional arousals. Patients have little or no recollection of episodes, even though they appear 'awake'. Treatment is usually not required but clonazepam can be used.

REM sleep behaviour disorder: Patients 'act out' their dreams during REM sleep due to failure of the usual muscle atonia. Sleep partners describe patients 'fighting' or 'struggling' in their sleep, sometimes injuring themselves or their partner. Polysomnography confirms the diagnosis, and clonazepam is the most successful treatment.

Restless leg syndrome: This is a common disorder, also known as Ekbom's syndrome. Unpleasant sensations in the legs that are eased by moving the legs occur when the patient is tired and at sleep onset. Restless legs can also be symptomatic of a peripheral neuropathy, iron deficiency or uraemia. Treatment, if required, is with clonazepam or dopaminergic drugs.

NEURO-INFLAMMATORY DISEASES

Multiple sclerosis

Multiple sclerosis (MS) is an important cause of chronic disability in adults. In the UK the prevalence is 120/100000, with an annual incidence of 7/100000. Although the exact cause is uncertain, an interplay of genetic and environmental factors is probably responsible. The incidence is higher at temperate than equatorial latitudes, and the disease is twice as common in women as men. The risk of familial recurrence is 15%. Pathogenesis involves recurrent cell-mediated autoimmune attack on the myelin-producing oligodendrocytes of the CNS. Histologically, the characteristic lesion is a plaque of demyelination in the periventricular regions of the brain, the optic nerves or the subpial regions of the spinal cord.

Clinical features

A diagnosis of MS requires the demonstration of otherwise unexplained CNS lesions separated in time and space. There are several recognisable clinical courses:

• Relapsing and remitting clinical course (80%) with variable recovery. • Primary progressive clinical course (10–20%). • Secondary progressive disease (supersedes relapse and remission phase). • Fulminant disease (<10%), leading to early death.

There are a number of clinical syndromes suggestive of multiple sclerosis (Box 16.16). Demyelinating lesions cause symptoms and signs that come on over days or weeks and resolve over weeks or

> ## 16.16 Clinical features of MS
>
> **Common presentations of MS**
>
> - Optic neuritis
> - Relapsing and remitting sensory symptoms
> - Subacute painless spinal cord lesion
> - Acute brainstem syndrome
> - Subacute loss of function of upper limb (dorsal column deficit)
> - 6th cranial nerve palsy
>
> **Other symptoms and syndromes suggestive of CNS demyelination**
>
> - Afferent pupillary defect and optic atrophy (previous optic neuritis)
> - Lhermitte's symptom (tingling in spine or limbs on neck flexion)
> - Progressive non-compressive paraparesis
> - Partial Brown–Séquard syndrome
> - Internuclear ophthalmoplegia with ataxia
> - Postural ('rubral', 'Holmes') tremor
> - Trigeminal neuralgia <50 yrs of age
> - Recurrent facial palsy

months. Frequent relapses with incomplete recovery indicate a poor prognosis. In a minority, there is an interval of years between attacks, and in some there is no recurrence. The physical signs depend on the anatomical site of demyelination. Combinations of spinal cord and brainstem signs are common, maybe with evidence of previous optic neuritis. Significant intellectual impairment is unusual until late in the disease.

Investigations

There is no specific test for MS, and the clinical diagnosis should be supported by investigations to:

• Exclude other conditions. • Provide evidence of an inflammatory disorder. • Identify multiple sites of neurological involvement.

MRI: The most sensitive test for demyelinating lesions in the brain and spinal cord (Fig. 16.11), which excludes other causes of the neurological deficit. However, appearances may be confused with small-vessel disease or cerebral vasculitis.

Visual evoked potentials: Detect clinically silent lesions in up to 70% of patients.

CSF: Lymphocytic pleocytosis in the acute phase and oligoclonal bands of IgG in 70–90% of patients between attacks. Oligoclonal bands denote intrathecal inflammation and occur in a range of other disorders.

Management

This involves treatment of the acute relapse, prevention of future relapses, treatment of complications and management of disability.

Acute relapse: Pulses of high-dose methylprednisolone, either IV or orally, shorten the duration of relapse but do not affect long-term

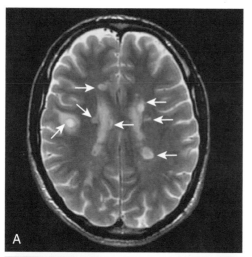

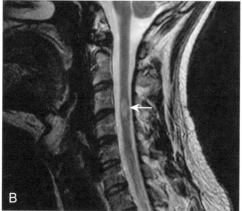

Fig. 16.11 Multiple sclerosis. A Brain MRI in MS: multiple high-signal lesions (arrows) are seen particularly in the paraventricular region on T2 image. **B** Demyelinating lesion in cervical spinal cord: high-signal T2 image (sagittal plane).

outcome. Pulsed steroids can be given up to 3 times/yr but should be restricted to significant function-threatening deficits. Prophylaxis against osteoporosis should be considered.

Disease-modifying treatment: Steroids, immunoglobulins and standard chemotherapies are neither practical nor helpful in established MS. In relapsing and remitting MS, SC or IM interferon beta reduces relapses by ~30%, with a small effect on long-term disability. Glatiramer acetate and mitoxantrone also reduce relapse rates.

16.17 Treatment of complications of MS	
Spasticity	Physiotherapy
	Baclofen, dantrolene, gabapentin, tizanidine
	Local injection of botulinum toxin, chemical neuronectomy
Ataxia	Isoniazid, clonazepam
Dysaesthesia	Carbamazepine, gabapentin, phenytoin, amitriptyline
Bladder symptoms	Anticholinergics for hypertonic bladder, intermittent catheterisation
Fatigue	Amantadine, modafinil, amitriptyline
Impotence	Sildenafil, tadalafil

Newer immunomodulatory treatments include natalizumab and fingolimod; trial outcomes are awaited to direct use.

Complications: Treatment of complications is summarised in Box 16.17. Specialist nurses are of great value in managing the chronic phase of the disease. Physiotherapy and occupational therapy may improve functional capacity in patients who become disabled. Bladder care is particularly important. Urgency and frequency may be treated pharmacologically, but this may lead to retention and infection. Retention can be managed initially by intermittent self-catheterisation but an in-dwelling catheter may become necessary.

Prognosis

This is difficult to predict, especially early in the disease:
• ~15% of those having one attack of demyelination do not suffer further events. • Those with relapsing and remitting symptoms have ~1–2 relapses every 2 yrs. • After 10 yrs ~one-third of patients are sufficiently disabled to need help with walking.

Acute disseminated encephalomyelitis

This is an acute monophasic condition with areas of perivenous demyelination throughout the brain and spinal cord. The illness often occurs a week or so after a viral infection (e.g. measles, chickenpox, recent vaccination), suggesting that it is immunologically mediated.

Clinical features

• Headache, vomiting, pyrexia, confusion and meningism, often with focal brain and spinal cord signs. • Occasionally, seizures or coma.

Investigations

MRI shows multiple high-signal areas in a pattern similar to that of MS. CSF may be normal or show an increase in protein and lymphocytes; oligoclonal bands may be found acutely but do not persist on recovery (unlike in MS).

Management

The disease may be fatal in the acute stages but is otherwise self-limiting. Treatment is with high-dose IV methylprednisolone.

Transverse myelitis

Transverse myelitis is an acute, monophasic, inflammatory demyelinating disorder affecting the spinal cord. Patients present with a subacute paraparesis with a sensory level, often with severe neck or back pain at onset. MRI is needed to distinguish this from a compressive spinal cord lesion. CSF examination shows cellular pleocytosis, and oligoclonal bands are usually absent. Treatment is with high-dose IV methylprednisolone. The outcome is variable; in some cases, near-complete recovery occurs despite a severe initial deficit. Some patients go on to develop MS.

PARANEOPLASTIC NEUROLOGICAL DISEASE

Neurological disease may occur with systemic malignant tumours in the absence of metastases. In most cases, tumour antigens lead to the development of autoantibodies to parts of the CNS.

Clinical features

These are summarised in Box 16.18. The neurological disease often precedes clinical presentation of the primary neoplasm.

Investigations

Characteristic autoantibodies are present in many cases (e.g. anti Jo-1 in dermatomyositis). CT of the chest or abdomen or PET scanning is often necessary to find the causative tumour. CSF often shows increased protein and lymphocytes with oligoclonal bands.

Management

This is directed at the primary tumour. Some improvement may occur following administration of IV immunoglobulin.

NEURODEGENERATIVE DISEASES

Whilst MS is the most common cause of disability in young people in the UK, vascular and neurodegenerative diseases are increasingly important in later life. These diseases lead to specific neuronal death, causing relentlessly progressive symptoms that increase with age. Degeneration of the cerebral cortex causes dementia. Degeneration of the basal ganglia results in movement disorder. Cerebellar degeneration usually causes ataxia. Degeneration can also occur in the spinal cord or peripheral nerves, giving rise to motor, sensory or autonomic disturbance.

Degenerative causes of dementia

Dementia is characterised by a loss of previously acquired intellectual function in the absence of impairment of arousal, and affects 5%

	16.18 Paraneoplastic syndromes	
Syndrome	**Clinical features**	**Associated tumours**
CNS		
Limbic encephalitis	Memory loss, progressive dementia Seizures	SCLC, testicular, breast, thymoma, ovarian/ testicular teratoma
Myelopathy	Progressive spinal cord lesion (usually cervical)	SCLC, thymoma
Cerebellar degeneration	Progressive ataxia, nystagmus, vertigo	SCLC, breast, ovarian, lymphoma
Motor neuron disease	Subacute, patchy progressive, usually lower limb, weakness and wasting	SCLC, others
Peripheral		
Sensory neuropathy	Limb pain, paraesthesia, distal numbness	Lymphoma, SCLC, others
Sensorimotor peripheral neuropathy	Mild, non-disabling peripheral limb numbness and paraesthesia	Lymphoma, SCLC, others
Lambert–Eaton syndrome	Weakness of proximal limb muscles, fatigue with exertion after initial improvement, areflexia	SCLC
Dermatomyositis/ polymyositis	Proximal limb weakness and pain, heliotrope skin rash, Gottron's papules on knuckles	Lung, breast
Myasthenia gravis	Muscle fatigue reversible with anticholinesterase	Thymoma

(SCLC = small cell lung cancer.)

of those over 65 and 20% of those over 85. It is defined as a global impairment of cognitive function, and is typically progressive and non-reversible. Although memory is most affected initially, deficits in visuo-spatial function, language ability, concentration and attention gradually become apparent. Alzheimer's disease and diffuse vascular disease are the most common causes, but rarer causes include:

• MS. • Chronic head trauma. • Creutzfeldt–Jakob disease.
• Alcohol. • HIV. • Syphilis. • Vitamin B_{12} deficiency. • Hydrocephalus.

Rarer causes of dementia should be actively sought in younger patients and those with short histories.

Alzheimer's disease

This is the most common cause of dementia. About 15% of cases are familial. The brain is atrophic, with senile plaques and neurofibrillary tangles in the cerebral cortex. Many different neurotransmitter abnormalities have been described, in particular impairment of cholinergic transmission.

Clinical features

The key feature is impairment of the ability to remember new information. Memory impairment is gradual and usually associated with disorders of other cortical functions. Both short-term memory and long-term memory are affected. Later in the disease, patients commonly deny their disabilities, and additional features are apraxia, visuo-spatial impairment, depression and aphasia.

Investigations and management

Investigation is aimed at excluding the less common treatable causes of dementia (see above). Anticholinesterases (donepezil, rivastigmine, galantamine) and the NMDA receptor antagonist memantine have been shown to be of some benefit. Depression should be treated with antidepressants. Support for carers is crucial.

Fronto-temporal dementia

This term encompasses a number of different syndromes, including Pick's diseases and primary progressive aphasia; all are much rarer than Alzheimer's disease. Patients may present with personality change due to frontal lobe involvement or with language disturbance due to temporal lobe involvement. Memory is relatively preserved in the early stages. There is no specific treatment.

Lewy body dementia

This is a neurodegenerative disorder clinically characterised by dementia and signs of Parkinson's disease. The cognitive state often fluctuates and there is a high incidence of visual hallucinations. Affected individuals are particularly sensitive to the side-effects of anti-Parkinsonian medication and also to antipsychotic drugs. There is no specific treatment but anticholinesterase agents may well be helpful.

Wernicke–Korsakoff disease

A rare but important effect of chronic alcohol misuse is the Wernicke–Korsakoff syndrome. This organic brain disorder results from damage to the mamillary bodies, dorsomedial nuclei of the thalamus and adjacent areas of periventricular grey matter; it is caused by a deficiency of thiamine (vitamin B_1), most commonly from long-standing heavy drinking and an inadequate diet. It can also arise from malabsorption or even protracted vomiting. Without prompt treatment, the acute presentation of Wernicke's encephalopathy (nystagmus, ophthalmoplegia, ataxia and confusion) can progress to the irreversible deficits of Korsakoff's syndrome (severe short-term memory deficits and confabulation, and also reduced red blood cell transketolase).

It must be considered in any confused patient; if in doubt, treat anyway. Prevention of the Wernicke–Korsakoff syndrome requires the immediate use of high doses of thiamine, which is initially given parenterally in the form of Pabrinex (two vials 3 times daily for 48 hrs) and then orally (100 mg 3 times daily). There is no treatment for Korsakoff's syndrome once it has arisen.

Movement disorders

Movement disorders present with a wide range of symptoms. They may be genetic or acquired, and the most important is Parkinson's disease. Most movement disorders are categorised clinically, with few confirmatory investigations available other than for those with a known gene abnormality.

Idiopathic Parkinson's disease

Parkinsonism is a clinical syndrome characterised by bradykinesia, increased tone (rigidity), tremor and loss of postural reflexes. Although it may be caused by drugs, degenerative disease (e.g. Alzheimer's), anoxic or other injury, or genetic conditions (e.g. Huntington's disease), >80% of cases are due to Parkinson's disease (PD). PD has an annual incidence of 18/100000 in the UK and a prevalence of 180/100000. Average age of onset is ~60 yrs; <5% present under 40.

Single genes causing parkinsonism have been identified, although only in a small proportion of cases. Having a first-degree relative with PD confers a 2–3 times increased risk of PD. It is a progressive and incurable condition, with a variable prognosis. Whilst motor symptoms are the usual presenting features, cognitive impairment, depression and anxiety become increasingly common as the disease progresses, and significantly reduce quality of life.

Clinical features

The presentation is usually asymmetrical, e.g. a resting tremor in an upper limb. Typical features of an established case include:

Bradykinesia: Slowness in initiating or repeating movements, impaired fine movements (causing small handwriting) and expressionless face. The patient is slow to start walking, with reduced arm swing, rapid small steps and a tendency to run (festination).

Tremor: Present at rest (4–6 Hz), diminished on action; it starts in the fingers/thumb and may affect arms, legs, feet, jaw and tongue.

Rigidity: Cogwheel type mostly affects upper limbs; plastic (lead-pipe) type mostly affects legs.

Non-motor symptoms may precede typical motor symptoms and include:

• Depression. • Anxiety. • Cognitive impairment: develops in one-third of patients as the disease progresses.

Investigations

Diagnosis is clinical. CT may be needed if any features suggest pyramidal, cerebellar or autonomic involvement, or if the diagnosis is in doubt, but is usually normal for age. Patients <50 yrs should be tested for Wilson's disease and Huntington's disease.

Management: drug therapy

Levodopa: This remains the mainstay of treatment, together with a peripheral-acting dopa-decarboxylase inhibitor. Therapy should be started when symptoms are impacting on daily life. Decarboxylase inhibitors (carbidopa and benserazide) reduce peripheral side-effects and are available as combination preparations with levodopa (Sinemet and Madopar). Levodopa is particularly effective at improving bradykinesia and rigidity. Side-effects are:

• Postural hypotension. • Nausea and vomiting. • Involuntary movements (orofacial dyskinesias, limb and axial dystonias). • Occasionally, depression, hallucinations and delusions.

Late deterioration despite levodopa occurs after 3–5 yrs in up to 50% of patients. The simplest form is end-of-dose deterioration; this may be improved by using smaller, more frequent doses or a slow-release preparation. More complex fluctuations present as periods of severe parkinsonism alternating with dyskinesia and agitation (the 'on–off' phenomenon).

Dopamine receptor agonists: These drugs are less powerful than levodopa but cause fewer dose fluctuations or dyskinesia. Oral options include bromocriptine, pergolide, cabergoline and lisuride. Apomorphine causes marked vomiting and has to be administered parenterally with concomitant antiemetic medication (e.g. domperidone). Side-effects include:

• Nausea. • Vomiting. • Confusion. • Hallucinations.

MAOI-B inhibitors: Monoamine oxidase type B facilitates breakdown of excess dopamine in the synapse. Two inhibitors are used in PD: selegiline and rasagiline. The effects of both are modest, although usually well tolerated. Neither is neuroprotective, despite initial hopes.

COMT (catechol-O-methyl-transferase) inhibitors: When used with levodopa, entacapone prolongs the effects of each dose and reduces motor fluctuations. This allows the levodopa dose to be reduced.

Amantadine: This has a mild, short-lived effect on bradykinesia but may be useful early in the disease. It can help control the dyskinesias produced by dopaminergic treatment later on. Side-effects are:

• Livedo reticularis. • Peripheral oedema. • Confusion and seizures.

Anticholinergic agents: These were the main treatment for PD prior to the introduction of levodopa. Their role is now limited by lack of efficacy (apart from an effect on tremor sometimes) and adverse effects, including dry mouth, blurred vision, constipation, urinary retention, confusion and hallucinosis.

Management: non-pharmacological

Surgery: Stereotactic surgery most commonly involves deep brain stimulation (DBS), rather than the destructive approach of previous eras. Various targets have been identified, including the thalamus (only effective for tremor), globus pallidus and subthalamic nucleus. DBS is usually reserved for patients with medically refractory tremor or motor fluctuations.

Physiotherapy and speech therapy: Physiotherapy reduces rigidity and corrects abnormal posture. Speech therapy may help dysarthria and dysphonia.

Other parkinsonian syndromes

Cerebrovascular disease and drug-induced parkinsonism are the most common alternative causes of parkinsonism. There are several degenerative conditions that cause parkinsonism, including multiple systems atrophy, progressive supranuclear palsy and corticobasal degeneration. They typically have a more rapid progression than PD and tend to be resistant to treatment with levodopa.

Multiple systems atrophy

Features of parkinsonism are combined with degrees of autonomic failure, cerebellar involvement and pyramidal tract dysfunction. Diagnosis is assisted by autonomic function tests. Falls are more common than in idiopathic Parkinson's disease, and life expectancy is reduced.

Progressive supranuclear palsy

Clinical features include parkinsonism (rigidity in extension rather than flexion) with supranuclear paralysis of eye movements. Other features are pyramidal signs and cognitive impairment.

Huntington's disease

This is an autosomal dominant inherited disorder, usually presenting in adult life. It is due to expansion of a trinucleotide repeat on chromosome 4 and frequently demonstrates anticipation (younger age of onset in subsequent generations).

Clinical features: Gradually progressive chorea and behavioural disturbance are the earliest symptoms. There is cognitive impairment, which later becomes frank dementia. Seizures may occur late in the disease.

Investigations: The diagnosis is confirmed by genetic testing; presymptomatic testing for other family members is available but must be preceded by appropriate counselling. Brain imaging may show caudate atrophy but is not reliable.

Management: Chorea may respond to risperidone or tetrabenazine. Depression is common and may be helped by antidepressant medication. Long-term psychological support and eventually institutional care are often needed.

Ataxias

This is a group of inherited disorders in which degenerative changes occur to varying extents in the cerebellum, brainstem, pyramidal tracts, spinocerebellar tracts, and optic and peripheral nerves. They usually present in childhood with ataxia, and sometimes with other neurological deficits, e.g. spasticity and impaired cognitive function. Genetic testing facilitates diagnosis and counselling in some.

Motor neuron disease

In this disease there is progressive degeneration of upper and lower motor neurons in the spinal cord, cranial nerve nuclei, and motor cortex. Annual incidence is $2/100\,000$ and prevalence is $7/100\,000$. Most cases are sporadic but 5–10% are familial. Average age at onset is 65 yrs and <10% present before the age of 45. Males are more commonly affected.

Clinical features

Patients present with a combination of lower and upper motor neuron signs without sensory involvement. Symptoms often begin focally, and then spread gradually but relentlessly. The presence of brisk reflexes in wasted fasciculating limb muscles is typical. There may also be dysarthria or dysphagia. Up to 50% have some cognitive impairment on formal testing and ~10% develop fronto-temporal dementia. Three common clinical patterns are described in Box 16.19.

Investigations

The diagnosis is clinical. Exclude potentially treatable disorders (e.g. cervical myeloradiculopathy, immune-mediated multifocal motor neuropathy). EMG confirms fasciculation and denervation. Nerve conduction studies may show low-amplitude motor action potentials.

16.19 Patterns of involvement in motor neuron disease

Progressive muscular atrophy

- Predominantly spinal motor neurons affected
- Weakness and wasting of distal limb muscles at first
- Fasciculation in muscles; tendon reflexes may be absent

Progressive bulbar palsy

- Early involvement of tongue, palate and pharyngeal muscles (dysarthria/dysphagia)
- Wasting and fasciculation of tongue
- Pyramidal signs

Amyotrophic lateral sclerosis

- Combination of distal and proximal muscle-wasting and weakness, fasciculation
- Spasticity, ↑ reflexes, extensor plantars; bulbar/pseudobulbar palsy follow eventually
- Pyramidal tract features may predominate

Management and prognosis

Multidisciplinary team management is required, including physiotherapists, occupational therapists, speech therapists, dietitians and palliative care specialists. Riluzole has a modest effect in amyotrophic lateral sclerosis. Feeding by percutaneous gastrostomy may be necessary if bulbar palsy is marked. Non-invasive ventilatory support may ease distress from weak respiratory muscles. MND is relentlessly progressive and up to 50% die within 2 yrs of diagnosis.

INFECTIONS OF THE NERVOUS SYSTEM

Meningitis

Acute infection of the meninges presents with pyrexia, headache and meningism. Meningism, which can occur in other situations (e.g. subarachnoid haemorrhage), consists of stiffness of the neck. Abnormalities in the CSF (Box 16.20) are helpful in distinguishing the cause of meningitis. Causes are listed in Box 16.21.

Viral meningitis

Viral infection is the most common cause of meningitis.

Clinical features

The condition occurs mainly in children or young adults, with acute headache, irritability and meningism. In viral meningitis, the headache is usually the most severe feature.

Investigations

CSF contains an excess of lymphocytes, but glucose and protein are commonly normal or the protein may be raised. This picture can also be found in partially treated bacterial meningitis.

Management

There is no specific treatment. Disease is usually benign and self-limiting. Treat the patient symptomatically in a quiet environment. Recovery usually occurs within days.

Meningitis may also occur as a complication of viral infection in other organs (e.g. mumps, measles, infectious mononucleosis, herpes zoster and hepatitis). Complete recovery without specific therapy is the rule.

Bacterial meningitis

Many bacteria can cause meningitis and certain organisms are particularly common at different ages (see Box 16.21). Bacterial meningitis is usually secondary to a bacteraemic illness. Several of the organisms are normal upper respiratory tract commensals and infection may complicate otitis media, skull fracture or sinusitis. Bacterial meningitis has become less common but mortality and morbidity remain significant. *Streptococcus pneumoniae* and *Neisseria meningitidis* (meningococcus) are the most frequent causes in Western

16.20 CSF findings in meningitis and subarachnoid haemorrhage

	Normal	Subarachnoid haemorrhage	Acute bacterial meningitis	Viral meningitis	Tuberculous meningitis
Pressure	50–250 mmH$_2$O	Increased	Normal/increased	Normal	Normal/increased
Colour	Clear	Blood-stained Xanthochromic	Cloudy	Clear	Clear/cloudy
Red cell count ×10^6/L	0–4	Raised	Normal	Normal	Normal
White cell count ×10^6/L	0–4	Normal/slightly raised	1000–5000 polymorphs	10–2000 lymphocytes	50–5000 lymphocytes
Glucose	>50–60% of blood level	Normal	Decreased	Normal	Decreased
Protein	<0.45 g/L	Increased	Increased	Normal/increased	Increased
Microbiology	Sterile	Sterile	Organisms on Gram stain and/or culture	Sterile/virus detected	Ziehl–Nielsen/auramine stain or TB culture positive
Oligoclonal bands	Negative	Negative	Can be positive	Can be positive	Can be positive

16.21 Causes of meningitis

Infective

Bacteria	Adults: *Neisseria meningitidis*, *Strep. pneumoniae*, *Listeria*, *Mycobacterium tuberculosis*, *Staph. aureus* Young children: *Haemophilus influenzae*, *Strep. pneumoniae*, *N. meningitidis* Neonates: Gram −ve bacilli, group B streptococci, *Listeria*
Viruses	Enteroviruses (echo, Coxsackie, polio), mumps, influenza, Herpes simplex, varicella zoster, Epstein–Barr, HIV
Protozoa and parasites	*Cysticercus*, *Amoeba*, *Toxoplasma*, *Coccidioides*
Fungi	*Cryptococcus*, *Candida*, *Histoplasma*

Non-infective ('sterile')

Malignant disease	Breast cancer, bronchial cancer, leukaemia, lymphoma
Inflammatory disease (may be recurrent)	Sarcoidosis, systemic lupus erythematosus, Behçet's disease

Europe, while *Haemophilus influenzae* and *Strep. pneumoniae* are most common in India. Epidemics of meningococcal meningitis occur, particularly in cramped living conditions or where the climate is hot and dry.

Clinical features

Headache, drowsiness, fever and neck stiffness are the usual presenting features. Around 90% of patients with meningococcal meningitis have two of the following:

• Fever. • Neck stiffness. • Altered consciousness. • Purpuric rash.

When accompanied by septicaemia, it may present very rapidly, with abrupt obtundation due to cerebral oedema and circulatory collapse. Pneumococcal meningitis may be associated with pneumonia and occurs especially in older patients, alcoholics and patients with no spleen. *Listeria monocytogenes* is seen increasingly as a cause of meningitis and brainstem encephalitis in the immunosuppressed, people with diabetes, alcoholics and pregnant women.

Investigations

CT head: If there is drowsiness, focal neurological signs or seizures, CT is required prior to LP to exclude a mass lesion (there is a risk of coning if LP is performed with raised intracranial pressure).

LP: CSF is cloudy due to neutrophils. Protein is significantly elevated and glucose is reduced. A Gram film and culture may identify the organism.

Other: Blood cultures may be positive. PCR of blood and CSF can identify bacterial DNA.

16.22 Chemotherapy of bacterial meningitis when cause is known

Pathogen	Regimen of choice	Alternative agent(s)
N. meningitidis	Benzylpenicillin 2.4 g IV 6 times daily for 5–7 days	Cefuroxime, ampicillin Chloramphenicol*
Strep. pneumoniae or Strep. suis (sensitive to β-lactams)	Cefotaxime 2 g IV 4 times daily or ceftriaxone 2 g IV twice daily for 10–14 days	Chloramphenicol*
Strep. pneumoniae (resistant to β-lactams)	Add vancomycin 1 g IV twice daily or rifampicin 600 mg IV twice daily	Vancomycin + rifampicin*
H. influenzae	Cefotaxime 2 g IV 4 times daily or ceftriaxone 2 g IV twice daily for 10–14 days	Chloramphenicol*
L. monocytogenes	Ampicillin 2 g IV 6 daily plus gentamicin 5 mg/kg IV daily	Ampicillin + co-trimoxazole 50 mg/kg daily

*For patients with a history of anaphylaxis to β-lactam antibiotics.

Management

If bacterial meningitis is suspected, the patient should be given parenteral antibiotics immediately and admitted to hospital. Before the cause of meningitis is known, patients should receive cefotaxime (2 g IV 4 times daily) or ceftriaxone (2 g IV twice daily). The antibiotic regimen may be modified after CSF examination, depending on the infecting organism (Box 16.22). Adjunctive corticosteroid therapy is useful in both children and adults.

Prevention of meningococcal infection: Close contacts of patients with meningococcal infections should be given 2 days of oral rifampicin. In adults, a single dose of ciprofloxacin is an alternative. If not treated with ceftriaxone, meningitis patients should be given similar treatment to clear nasopharyngeal carriage. Vaccines against meningococcus are available but not for the most common subgroup (B).

Tuberculous meningitis

Tuberculous meningitis is uncommon in healthy people in developed countries but remains common in developing countries, where it is seen more frequently as a secondary infection in AIDS. It may occur as part of a primary infection in childhood or as part of miliary TB. The usual source is a caseous focus in the meninges or brain.

Clinical features

There is a slow onset of headache, low-grade fever, vomiting, lassitude, depression, confusion and behavioural changes. Signs include meningism, oculomotor palsies, papilloedema, reduced conscious level and focal hemisphere signs.

Investigations

CSF is clear and under increased pressure, and contains up to 500 $\times 10^6$ cells/L, predominantly lymphocytes. There is elevated protein and markedly reduced glucose. CSF culture takes up to 6 wks and so treatment must be started empirically. Brain imaging may show hydrocephalus, brisk meningeal enhancement on enhanced CT, and/or an intracranial tuberculoma.

Management and prognosis

Chemotherapy should be started with a regimen including pyrazinamide (p. 295). Corticosteroids may improve mortality but not focal neurological damage. Surgical ventricular drainage may be needed if obstructive hydrocephalus develops.

Untreated tuberculous meningitis is fatal. Complete recovery is the rule if treatment is started before focal signs or stupor. When treatment is started later, the risk of death or serious neurological deficit is 30%.

Parenchymal viral infections
Viral encephalitis

Infection of nervous tissues will produce both focal dysfunction (deficits and/or seizures) and general signs of infection. Only a minority of patients have a history of recent viral infection. In Europe, the most serious cause is herpes simplex. In some parts of the world, viruses transmitted by mosquitoes and ticks (arboviruses) are an important cause. Acute encephalitis may occur in HIV infection.

Clinical features

Viral encephalitis presents with acute onset of headache, fever, focal neurological signs (aphasia and/or hemiplegia) and seizures. Disturbance of consciousness, ranging from drowsiness to deep coma, supervenes early. Meningism is common.

Investigations

CT (which should precede LP) may show low-density lesions in the temporal lobes but MRI is more sensitive to early abnormalities. CSF usually contains excess lymphocytes but is occasionally normal. The protein may be elevated but the glucose is normal. The EEG is usually abnormal in the early stages, especially in herpes simplex encephalitis. Virological investigations of the CSF may reveal the causative organism but treatment should not await this.

Management

Herpes simplex encephalitis responds to aciclovir (10 mg/kg IV 3 times daily for 2–3 wks). This has reduced mortality from 70% to 10%, and should be given early to all patients with suspected viral encephalitis. Raised intracranial pressure is treated with dexamethasone, and seizures controlled with anticonvulsants.

Brainstem encephalitis

This presents with ataxia, dysarthria, diplopia or other cranial nerve palsies. The CSF is lymphocytic, with a normal glucose. The causative agent is presumed to be viral. However, *L. monocytogenes* may cause a similar syndrome and requires specific treatment with ampicillin (500 mg 4 times daily).

Rabies

Rabies is caused by a rhabdovirus, which infects the central nervous tissue and salivary glands of mammals, and is usually conveyed by saliva through bites. Humans are most frequently infected from dogs. The incubation period varies, but is usually between 4 and 8 wks.

Clinical features

A prodromal period of 1–10 days leads to 'hydrophobia'; although the patient is thirsty, drinking provokes violent contractions of the diaphragm and inspiratory muscles. Delusions and hallucinations may develop, with lucid intervals. Cranial nerve lesions and terminal hyperpyrexia are common. Death ensues, usually within a week of symptoms.

Investigations

The diagnosis is made on clinical grounds. Rapid immunofluorescent techniques can detect antigen in corneal smears or skin biopsies.

Management

A few patients have survived; all received post-exposure prophylaxis and needed ICU facilities. Only palliative treatment is possible once symptoms have appeared. The patient should be heavily sedated with diazepam, supplemented by chlorpromazine if necessary.

Prevention

Pre-exposure prophylaxis: This is required by those who professionally handle potentially infected animals, work with rabies virus in laboratories or live at special risk in rabies-endemic areas. Protection is afforded by two injections of human diploid cell strain vaccine given 4 wks apart, followed by yearly boosters.

Post-exposure prophylaxis: The wounds should be cleaned, damaged tissues excised and the wound left unsutured. Rabies can usually be prevented if treatment is started within a day or two of biting. For maximum protection, hyperimmune serum (human rabies immunoglobulin) and vaccine (human diploid cell strain vaccine) are required.

Poliomyelitis

The disease is caused by one of three polioviruses. It is much less common in developed countries following the use of oral vaccines. Infection occurs through the nasopharynx, causing a lymphocytic meningitis and infecting the grey matter of the nervous system. There is a propensity to damage anterior horn cells.

Clinical features

The incubation period is 7–14 days. Many patients recover fully after a few days of mild fever and headache. In others, there is recurrence of pyrexia, headache and meningism. Weakness may start later and can progress to widespread paresis. Respiratory failure may supervene if intercostal muscles or the medullary motor nuclei are involved.

Investigations

CSF shows a lymphocytic pleocytosis, raised protein and normal glucose. Poliomyelitis virus may be cultured from CSF and stool.

Management and prognosis

Bed rest is imperative, as exercise appears to worsen or precipitate the paralysis. A tracheostomy and ventilation are required for respiratory difficulties. Subsequent treatment is by physiotherapy and orthopaedic measures. Epidemics vary widely in mortality rate. Death occurs from respiratory paralysis. Gradual recovery may take place over several months. Muscles showing no signs of recovery after 1 mth will probably not regain function. Prevention is by immunisation with live (Sabin) vaccine. Killed vaccine is used increasingly in countries where polio is rare.

Subacute sclerosing panencephalitis

This is a rare, chronic, progressive and eventually fatal complication of measles. It occurs in children and adolescents, usually many years after the primary virus infection. The onset is insidious, with intellectual deterioration, apathy and clumsiness, followed by myoclonic jerks, rigidity and dementia. The EEG is distinctive, with periodic bursts of triphasic waves. Antiviral therapy is ineffective and death ensues within years.

Progressive multifocal leucoencephalopathy

This is an infection of oligodendrocytes by human polyomavirus JC, which causes widespread demyelination of the white matter of the cerebral hemispheres. It is found most frequently as a feature of AIDS but also occurs in lymphoma and leukaemia. Clinical signs include dementia, hemiparesis and aphasia, which progress rapidly, leading to death within weeks or months. MRI reveals diffuse high signal in the cerebral white matter. Restoring the immune system may be beneficial.

Parenchymal bacterial infections
Cerebral abscess

Bacteria can enter the cerebral substance in many ways. The site of abscess formation and the causative organism are both related to the source of infection (Box 16.23).

	16.23 Aetiology and treatment of bacterial cerebral abscess		
Site of abscess	**Source of infection**	**Likely organisms**	**Recommended treatment**
Frontal lobe	Paranasal sinuses Teeth	Streptococci Anaerobes	Cefotaxime 2–3 g IV 4 times daily *plus* metronidazole 500 mg IV 3 times daily
Temporal lobe	Middle ear	Streptococci Enterobacteriaceae	Ampicillin 2–3 g IV 3 times daily *plus* metronidazole 500 mg IV 3 times daily *plus either* ceftazidime 2 g IV 3 times daily *or* gentamicin* 5 mg/kg IV daily
Cerebellum	Sphenoid sinus Mastoid/middle ear	*Pseudomonas* spp. Anaerobes	As for temporal lobe
Any site	Penetrating trauma	Staphylococci	Flucloxacillin 2–3 g IV 4 times daily *or* cefuroxime 1.5 g IV 3 times daily
Multiple	Metastatic and cryptogenic	Streptococci Anaerobes	Benzylpenicillin 1.8–2.4 g IV 4 times daily if endocarditis or cyanotic heart disease Otherwise cefotaxime 2–3 g IV 4 times daily *plus* metronidazole 500 mg IV 3 times daily

*Monitor gentamicin levels.

Clinical features

A cerebral abscess may present acutely with fever, headache, meningism and drowsiness, but more commonly presents over days or weeks as a cerebral mass lesion with little or no evidence of infection, making distinction from tumour difficult. Seizures, raised intracranial pressure and focal hemisphere signs occur alone or in combination.

Investigations

LP is potentially hazardous in the presence of raised intracranial pressure and CT should always precede it. CT reveals single or multiple low-density areas, which show ring enhancement and surrounding cerebral oedema. There may be an elevated WBC and ESR with active infection. Cerebral toxoplasmosis or tuberculous disease secondary to HIV infection should always be considered.

Management and prognosis

Antimicrobial therapy is indicated once the diagnosis is made (see Box 16.23). Surgical treatment by burr-hole aspiration or excision may be necessary. Anticonvulsants are often required, as epilepsy frequently develops. The mortality rate remains high at 10–20%.

Spinal epidural abscess

The characteristic clinical features are pain in a root distribution and progressive transverse spinal cord syndrome with paraparesis, sensory impairment and sphincter dysfunction. Infection is usually haematogenous. Staphylococcal infection, often linked to IV drug misuse, has contributed to a marked rise in incidence. MRI or myelography should precede urgent neurosurgical intervention. Decompressive laminectomy with draining of the abscess relieves the pressure on the dura. This, together with appropriate antibiotics, may prevent complete and irreversible paraplegia.

Neurosyphilis

Neurosyphilis may involve the meninges, blood vessels and/or the brain and spinal cord. In developed countries, syphilis is now most commonly seen in AIDS. Although it is rare, early diagnosis and treatment remain important.

Clinical features

The three most common presentations are summarised in Box 16.24. The 'Argyll Robertson' pupillary abnormality may accompany any neurosyphilitic syndrome; the pupils are small and react to convergence but not directly to light.

Investigations

Routine screening is warranted in many neurological patients. Serological tests are positive in most patients but CSF examination

16.24 Clinical and pathological features of neurosyphilis		
Type (interval from primary)	**Pathology**	**Clinical features**
Meningovascular (5 yrs)	Endarteritis obliterans Meningeal exudates Granuloma (gumma)	Stroke Cranial nerve palsies Seizures/mass lesion
General paralysis of the insane (5–15 yrs)	Degeneration in cerebral cortex/cerebral atrophy Thickened meninges	Dementia Tremor Bilateral upper motor signs
Tabes dorsalis (5–20 yrs)	Degeneration of sensory neurons Wasting of dorsal columns Optic atrophy	Lightning pains Sensory ataxia Visual failure Abdominal crises Incontinence Trophic changes
Any of the above		Argyll Robertson pupils

is essential; active disease is suggested by an elevated lymphocyte count, and protein may be elevated.

Management

Procaine benzylpenicillin and probenecid are given for 17 days. Further courses must be given if symptoms persist/recur or if the CSF continues to show signs of active disease.

Tetanus

This results from infection with *Clostridium tetani*, a commensal in the gut of humans and domestic animals, which is found in soil. Infection enters the body through wounds. It is rare in the UK but is a major killer in developing countries. Spores germinate and bacilli multiply in areas of tissue necrosis. The bacilli remain localised but produce an exotoxin with an affinity for motor nerve endings and cells. The anterior horn cells are affected, resulting in rigidity and convulsions. Symptoms appear from 2 days to several weeks after injury – the shorter the incubation period, the worse the prognosis.

Clinical features

The most important early symptom is trismus – painless spasm of the masseter muscles ('lockjaw'). The tonic rigidity spreads to the muscles of the face, neck and trunk. Contraction of facial muscles leads to the so-called 'risus sardonicus'. The back is usually slightly arched ('opisthotonus') and there is a board-like abdominal wall. In more severe cases, painful violent spasms or convulsions can occur, which may lead to exhaustion, asphyxia or aspiration pneumonia. Autonomic involvement may cause cardiovascular complications such as hypertension.

Investigations and management

The diagnosis is made on clinical grounds. Treatment of an established case involves:
• Human tetanus antitoxin (3000 U IV) to neutralise absorbed toxin. • Débridement of wounds. • IV benzylpenicillin (or metronidazole if allergic). • Nursing in a quiet room and avoidance of unnecessary stimuli. • Diazepam IV to control spasms; if ineffective, paralyse and ventilate. • Fluid and nutritional support.

Prevention

• Débridement of contaminated injuries. • Penicillin (1.2 g injection followed by a 7-day oral course). • IM injection of 250 U of human tetanus antitoxin, along with toxoid (repeated at 1 and 6 mths). • If already immunised: only a booster of toxoid is required.

Botulism

Botulism means paralysis and neurological dysfunction produced by the neurotoxins of *Clostridium botulinum*. Common contaminated sources include sealed and preserved foods, and honey. Wound botulism is a growing problem in injection drug-users. Ingestion of even picogram amounts of this potent neurotoxin causes bulbar and ocular palsies (dysphagia, blurred or double vision, ptosis), progressing to limb weakness and respiratory paralysis. Management includes ventilation and supportive measures until the toxin dissociates from nerve endings at 6–8 wks following ingestion. Antitoxin is available against some toxin types.

Transmissible spongiform encephalopathies

Transmissible spongiform encephalopathies (TSEs) are characterised by the histopathological triad of cortical spongiform change, neuronal cell loss and gliosis. There is also deposition of an abnormal prion protein. These diseases can be transmitted by inoculation; they may also occur spontaneously or as an inherited disorder. Diseases affecting animals include bovine spongiform encephalopathies (BSE). These diseases achieved media prominence in the 1990s, when a form of Creutzfeldt–Jakob disease emerged that was associated with prion protein ingestion.

Creutzfeldt–Jakob disease

Creutzfeldt–Jakob disease (CJD) is the best-characterised human TSE. Some 10% of cases arise from a mutation in the gene coding for the prion protein. The sporadic form is the most common, presenting in middle-aged to elderly patients with rapidly progressive dementia, myoclonus and a characteristic EEG pattern (repetitive slow wave complexes). Death occurs after a mean of 4–6 mths. There is no known treatment.

Variant CJD

A variant of CJD has been described in a few patients, mostly in the UK. The causative agent appears identical to that causing BSE in cows, and the disease may have appeared as a result of the BSE epidemic in the UK in the 1980s. Affected patients are typically younger than those with sporadic CJD and present with neuropsychiatric changes and sensory symptoms in the limbs, followed by ataxia, dementia and death (mean time to death is over a year). Characteristic EEG changes are not present but MRI scans show typical changes.

INTRACRANIAL MASS LESIONS AND RAISED INTRACRANIAL PRESSURE

Intracranial mass lesions may be:
• Traumatic: subdural or extradural haematoma. • Vascular: intracranial haemorrhage. • Infective: e.g. abscess, tuberculoma, cysticercosis. • Neoplastic: benign or malignant.

   Symptoms and signs are produced by direct effects on adjacent tissue, raised intracranial pressure and false localising signs.

Raised intracranial pressure

Raised intracranial pressure (RIP) may be caused by mass lesions, cerebral oedema, obstruction to CSF circulation causing hydrocephalus, impaired CSF absorption and cerebral venous obstruction.

Clinical features

In adults, intracranial pressure is <10–15 mmHg. If pressure increases slowly, compensatory alteration in the volume of fluid in CSF spaces and venous sinuses may minimise symptoms. Rapid pressure increase overwhelms this compensation, causing early symptoms, including sudden death. Papilloedema may be absent.

False localising signs (i.e. signs distant from the primary pathology) occur in RIP. Cerebral swelling may stretch or compress the 6th cranial nerve against the petrous temporal bone ridge. Transtentorial herniation of the uncus may compress the ipsilateral 3rd nerve, causing a dilated pupil; however, a contralateral 3rd nerve palsy may also occur, due to compression by the tentorial margin. Vomiting, coma, bradycardia and arterial hypertension are later features of RIP.

Downward displacement of the medial temporal lobe (uncus) through the tentorium due to a cortical mass may cause 'temporal coning'. This may stretch the 3rd and/or 6th cranial nerves, or compress the contralateral cerebral peduncle (causing ipsilateral upper motor neuron signs), usually with progressive coma. Downward movement of the cerebellar tonsils through the foramen magnum may compress the medulla – 'tonsillar coning', causing brainstem haemorrhage and/or acute obstruction of the CSF pathways. Unless the condition is treated rapidly, coma and death occur.

Management is that of the causative lesion.

Intracranial neoplasms
Primary and secondary brain tumours

Common sources of metastases from extracranial primary tumours are bronchus, breast and GI tract. Primary intracerebral tumours are classified by their cell of origin and degree of malignancy (Box 16.25). Even when malignant, they do not metastasise outside the nervous system.

Clinical features

Rapidly growing tumours present with a short history of mass effects (headache, nausea), while indolent tumours present with slowly progressive focal deficits, reflecting their location; generalised or focal seizures are common. Headache, if present, is accompanied by focal deficits or seizures; isolated stable headache is almost never due to intracranial tumour.

The size of a brain tumour is of far less prognostic significance than its location. Brainstem tumours cause early neurological deficits, while frontal tumours may be large before symptoms occur.

Investigations

Diagnosis is by neuroimaging and pathological grading following biopsy, or resection where this is possible. The more malignant

16.25 Primary intracranial tumours		
Histological type	**Common site**	**Age**
Malignant		
Glioma	Cerebral hemisphere	Adulthood
(astrocytoma)	Cerebellum	Childhood/adulthood
	Brainstem	Childhood/young adulthood
Oligodendroglioma	Cerebral hemisphere	Adulthood
Medulloblastoma	Posterior fossa	Childhood
Ependymoma	Posterior fossa	Childhood/adolescence
Cerebral lymphoma	Cerebral hemisphere	Adulthood
Benign		
Meningioma	Cortical dura, parasagittal, sphenoid ridge, suprasellar, olfactory groove	Adulthood
Neurofibroma	Acoustic neuroma	Adulthood
Craniopharyngioma	Suprasellar	Childhood/adolescence
Pituitary adenoma	Pituitary fossa	Adulthood
Colloid cyst	Third ventricle	Any age
Pineal tumours	Quadrigeminal cistern	Childhood (teratomas) Young adult (germ cell)

tumours are more likely to demonstrate contrast enhancement on imaging. If the tumour appears to be metastatic, further investigation to find the primary will be required.

Management

Medical: Dexamethasone (orally or IV in acute RIP) lowers intracranial pressure by resolving the reactive oedema. Seizures should be treated with anticonvulsants. Prolactin or growth hormone-secreting pituitary tumours may respond to dopamine agonists.

Surgical: Surgery is the mainstay of treatment. Only partial excision may be possible if tumour is inaccessible or if removal will cause unacceptable brain damage. Biopsy should be considered even if tumour cannot be removed (histology has implications for management). Meningiomas and acoustic neuromas offer the best prospects for complete removal. Pituitary adenomas may be removed by a trans-sphenoidal route, avoiding craniotomy.

Radiotherapy and chemotherapy: These have only a marginal effect on cerebral metastases and malignant gliomas in adults, although temozolomide may slightly extend survival in grade IV glioblastomas. Radiotherapy reduces recurrence of pituitary adenoma after surgery. Radiotherapy may be an adjunct to surgery for meningiomas that cannot be completely excised or whose histology suggests an increased tendency to recurrence.

Prognosis

Gliomas are rarely completely excised and recurrence is therefore common. Prognosis is related to histological grade; patients with better grades may survive many years, whilst those with high-grade stage IV gliomas have a median survival of just over a year. The prognosis for benign tumours is good, provided complete surgical excision can be achieved.

Neurofibromatosis

Neurofibromatosis encompasses two clinically and genetically separate conditions, with an autosomal dominant pattern of inheritance. Multiple fibromatous tumours develop from the neurilemmal sheaths of peripheral and cranial nerves.

Type 1 (NF1, von Recklinghausen's disease): Caused by a mutation on chromosome 17. Clinical features include multiple cutaneous neurofibromas, café au lait spots in the skin, plexiform and spinal neurofibroma, scoliosis and endocrine tumours. Investigation and treatment are only indicated if there are new symptoms or if malignant change is suspected.

Type 2 (NF2): Caused by a mutation on chromosome 22. Characterised by schwannomas (benign nerve sheath Schwann cell tumours), with little skin involvement. Clinical manifestations include acoustic and/or spinal schwannomas, meningiomas, ependymomas and ocular hamartomas or meningiomas.

Acoustic neuroma

This is a benign tumour of Schwann cells of the 8th cranial nerve, which may arise in isolation or as part of NF2. As an isolated finding, it occurs after the third decade and is more frequent in females.

Clinical features

There is unilateral hearing loss, often with tinnitus. Vertigo is an unusual symptom, as slow growth allows compensatory brainstem mechanisms to develop. Distortion of the brainstem or cerebellum may cause ataxia and/or cerebellar signs. Distortion of the fourth ventricle and cerebral aqueduct may cause hydrocephalus.

Investigations and management

MRI is the investigation of choice. Management involves surgical removal. If this is complete, the prognosis is excellent. Deafness and facial weakness may result from the operation.

Von Hippel–Lindau disease

This is a dominantly inherited disease characterised by the combination of retinal and intracranial (typically cerebellar) haemangiomas and haemangioblastomas. There may be associated extracranial hamartomatous lesions.

Hydrocephalus

Hydrocephalus (dilatation of the ventricular system) may be due to increased CSF production, reduced absorption or obstruction of CSF

16.26 Causes of hydrocephalus

Congenital malformations

- Aqueduct stenosis
- Chiari malformations
- Dandy–Walker syndrome
- Benign intracranial cysts
- Vein of Galen aneurysms
- Congenital CNS infections
- Craniofacial anomalies

Acquired causes

- Mass lesions (esp. posterior fossa):
  Tumour
  Colloid cyst of third ventricle
  Abscess
  Haematoma
- Absorption blockages:
  Inflammation (e.g. meningitis, sarcoidosis)
  Intracranial haemorrhage

circulation. Causes are given in Box 16.26. In obstructive hydrocephalus, diversion of the CSF by a shunt placed between the ventricular system and peritoneal cavity or right atrium may relieve symptoms.

Normal pressure hydrocephalus

Dilatation of the ventricular system is caused by intermittent rises in CSF pressure. It occurs in old age and is suggested by gait apraxia and dementia, often with urinary incontinence. The result of shunting procedures is unpredictable.

Idiopathic intracranial hypertension

This usually occurs in obese young women. Raised intracranial pressure develops without a space-occupying lesion, ventricular dilatation or impairment of consciousness. The aetiology is uncertain. It can be precipitated by drugs (tetracycline, vitamin A, retinoids).

Clinical features

Headache is present, sometimes with transient diplopia and visual obscurations. There are usually no signs other than papilloedema.

Investigations

CT or MR angiography is performed to exclude cerebral venous sinus thrombosis or stenosis of other cause. LP (after CT) confirms a CSF pressure >30 cm CSF with normal content.

Management

Avoid precipitants; reduce weight if obese. Acetazolamide may lower intracranial pressure. Repeated LP helps headache but is often unacceptable to the patient. Patients failing to respond, in whom chronic papilloedema threatens vision, may require optic nerve sheath fenestration or a lumbo-peritoneal shunt.

DISORDERS OF THE SPINE AND SPINAL CORD

Cervical spondylosis

Degeneration of the intervertebral discs and secondary osteoar-throsis (cervical spondylosis) is often asymptomatic but may cause neurological dysfunction. The C5/6, C6/7 and C4/5 vertebral levels affecting C6, C7 and C5 roots, respectively, are most commonly affected.

Cervical spondylotic radiculopathy

Compression of a nerve root occurs when a disc prolapses laterally, which may develop acutely or more gradually due to osteophytic encroachment of the intervertebral foramina.

Clinical features

Neck pain may radiate in the distribution of the affected nerve root. Neck movements may exacerbate pain. Paraesthesia and sensory loss may be found in the affected segment and there may be lower motor neuron signs (Box 16.27).

Investigations

X-rays are unhelpful except for trauma or destructive lesions. MRI is the investigation of choice for radicular symptoms. Electro-physiological studies rarely add to clinical examination.

Management

Analgesia and physiotherapy usually suffice. A minority require surgery (discectomy or radicular decompression).

Cervical myelopathy

Dorsomedial herniation of a disc or dorsal osteophytes may com-press the spinal cord or the anterior spinal artery (which supplies the anterior two-thirds of the cord).

Clinical features

The onset is usually insidious and painless, but acute deterioration may occur after trauma. Spasticity in the legs, together with

16.27 Physical signs in cervical root compression			
Root	Muscle weakness	Sensory loss	Reflex loss
C5	Biceps, deltoid, spinati	Upper lateral arm	Biceps
C6	Brachioradialis	Lower lateral arm, thumb, index finger	Supinator
C7	Triceps, finger and wrist extensors	Middle finger	Triceps

numbness, tingling and proprioceptive loss in the hands, is a common pattern. Disturbance of micturition is a very late feature.

Investigations

MRI or myelography is used to direct surgical intervention.

Management and prognosis

Surgery, including laminectomy and anterior discectomy, may arrest progression but neurological improvement is not the rule. The decision whether to operate may be difficult. Manual manipulation of the cervical spine is of no benefit and may cause acute deterioration.

Lumbar spondylosis

This term covers degenerative disc disease and osteoarthritic change in the lumbar spine. Pain in the distribution of the lumbar or sacral roots ('sciatica') is usually due to disc protrusion but can rarely be a feature of spinal tumour, pelvic malignancy or vertebral TB.

Lumbar disc herniation

Acute lumbar disc herniation is often precipitated by lifting heavy weights while the spine is flexed.

Clinical features

The onset may be sudden or gradual. Constant aching pain in the lumbar region may radiate to the buttock, thigh, calf and foot. Pain is exacerbated by straining but may be relieved by lying flat. Root pressure is suggested by limited hip flexion on the affected side if the straight leg is raised (Lasègue's sign). If the L3 or L4 is involved, back pain may be induced by hyperextension of the hip (femoral nerve stretch test). The roots most frequently affected are L4, L5 and S1 (Box 16.28).

Investigations

MRI is the investigation of choice; plain X-rays of the lumbar spine are of little value.

Management

Some 90% of patients recover with analgesia and early mobilisation. Physical manœuvres likely to strain the lumbar spine should be avoided. Local anaesthetic or corticosteroid injections may help in

16.28 Physical signs in lumbar root compression				
Disc level	**Root**	**Sensory loss**	**Weakness**	**Reflex loss**
L3/L4	L4	Inner calf	Inversion of foot	Knee
L4/L5	L5	Outer calf and dorsum of foot	Dorsiflexion of hallux/toes	Hamstring
L5/S1	S1	Sole and lateral foot	Plantar flexion	Ankle

ligamentous injury or joint dysfunction. Consider surgery if there is no response to conservative treatment or if there is a progressive neurological deficit. Central disc prolapse with bilateral symptoms and sphincter dysfunction requires urgent surgical decompression.

Lumbar canal stenosis

This is congenital narrowing of the lumbar spinal canal, exacerbated by age-related degenerative change. Patients are usually elderly. There is exercise-induced weakness and paraesthesia in the legs, which is quickly relieved by rest ('spinal claudication'). Peripheral pulses are preserved and ankle reflexes are absent. MRI will demonstrate narrowing of the lumbar canal. Lumbar laminectomy often results in complete relief of symptoms.

Spinal cord compression

Acute spinal cord compression is a common neurological emergency and is most commonly caused by trauma or metastatic tumours. Rarer causes include intervertebral disc prolapse, epidural abscess, tuberculoma, and tumours of the meninges or spinal cord. The early stages of damage are reversible but severely damaged neurons do not recover; patients with a short history should therefore be investigated urgently.

Clinical features

• Pain: localised over the spine or in a root distribution, which may be aggravated by coughing, sneezing or straining. • Sensory: paraesthesia, numbness or cold sensations, especially in the lower limbs, which spread proximally, often to a level on the trunk. • Motor: weakness, heaviness or stiffness of the limbs, most commonly the legs. • Sphincters: urgency or hesitancy of micturition, leading eventually to urinary retention

The Brown–Séquard syndrome (p. 619) results if damage is confined to one side of the cord.

Box 16.29 lists the expected signs, according to the level of cord damage.

16.29 **Signs of spinal cord compression**	
Cervical, above C5	Upper motor neuron signs and sensory loss in all four limbs Diaphragm weakness (phrenic nerve)
Cervical, C5–T1	Lower motor neuron signs and segmental sensory loss in the arms; upper motor neuron signs in the legs Respiratory (intercostal) muscle weakness
Thoracic cord	Spastic paraplegia with a sensory level on the trunk. Sacral loss of sensation and extensor plantar responses
Cauda equina	Spinal cord ends at approximately the T12/L1 spinal level; lesions below this can only cause lower motor neuron signs by affecting the cauda equina

Investigations

• Urgent MRI of the spine: the investigation of choice. • Plain X-rays: may show bony destruction and soft-tissue abnormalities. • Routine investigations, including CXR: may reveal systemic disease. • Needle biopsy: required prior to radiotherapy to establish tumour histology.

Management

Benign tumours: These should be surgically excised. Recovery is good unless there is a marked neurological deficit before diagnosis.

Extradural compression due to malignancy: Prognosis is poor; useful function may be regained if treatment is initiated within 24 hrs of severe weakness or sphincter dysfunction. Surgical decompression may be appropriate in some; outcome is similar to that of radiotherapy.

Spinal cord compression due to TB: Surgical treatment is performed if the patient is seen early. Appropriate anti-tuberculous chemotherapy should be given.

Traumatic lesions of the vertebral column: These require specialised neurosurgical treatment.

Intrinsic diseases of the spinal cord

There are many disorders that interfere with spinal cord function due to non-compressive involvement of the spinal cord itself (Box 16.30). The symptoms and signs are similar to those of extrinsic compression, although a suspended sensory loss can only occur with intrinsic disease such as syringomyelia. Investigation starts with imaging, which is important for excluding a compressive lesion. MRI provides the most information about structural lesions (e.g. diastematomyelia, syringomyelia or intrinsic tumours, Fig. 16.12). Non-specific signal change may be seen in inflammatory or infective conditions. Other investigations, such as LP or blood tests, are required to make a specific diagnosis.

DISEASES OF PERIPHERAL NERVES

Pathological processes may affect the nerve roots (radiculopathy), the nerve plexuses (plexopathy) and/or the individual nerves (neuropathy). Nerve fibres of different types (motor, sensory or autonomic) may be involved. Disorders may be primarily directed at the axon, the myelin sheath (Schwann cells) or both. An acute or chronic peripheral nerve disorder may be focal (affecting a single nerve: mononeuropathy), multifocal (several nerves: mononeuritis multiplex) or generalised (polyneuropathy). Neurophysiological tests, and sometimes nerve biopsy, will help determine whether the pathology is primarily affecting the nerve axon (axonal neuropathy) or the myelin sheath (demyelinating neuropathy).

16.30 Intrinsic diseases of the spinal cord

Type of disorder	Condition	Clinical features
Congenital	Diastematomyelia (spina bifida)	LMN features, deformity and sensory loss of legs, sphincter dysfunction Hairy patch or pit over low back Incidence ↓ by maternal intake of folic acid during pregnancy
	Hereditary spastic paraplegia	Autosomal dominant; onset usually in adult life. Slowly progressive UMN features (legs >arms), little sensory loss
Infective/ inflammatory	Transverse myelitis (viruses, e.g. HZV, HIV), schistosomiasis, MS, sarcoidosis	Weakness, sensory loss pain, developing over hours to days UMN features below lesion, impaired sphincter function
Vascular	Anterior spinal artery infarct	Abrupt onset LMN signs at level of lesion, UMN features below it
	Intervertebral disc embolus	Spinothalamic sensory loss below lesion (spared dorsal column sensation)
	Spinal AVM/dural fistula	Onset variable (acute to slowly progressive) Variable LMN, UMN, sensory and sphincter disturbance
Neoplastic	Glioma, ependymoma	Weakness, sensory loss, pain, developing over months/years UMN features below lesion; LMN features in conus; sphincter dysfunction
Metabolic	Vitamin B_{12} deficiency (subacute combined degeneration)	Progressive spastic paraparesis with proprioception loss, absent reflexes due to peripheral neuropathy, optic nerve and cerebral involvement
Degenerative	Motor neuron disease	Progressive LMN and UMN features, bulbar weakness, no sensory loss
	Syringomyelia	Gradual onset over months or years, pain in cervical segments LMN signs at level of lesion, UMN features below it Suspended spinothalamic sensory loss at lesion, dorsal columns preserved

(AVM = arteriovenous malformation; HZV = herpes zoster virus; LMN/UMN = lower/upper motor neuron)

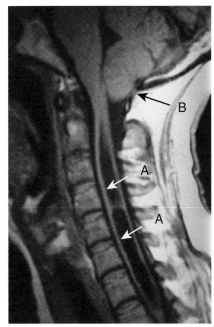

Fig. 16.12 MRI scan showing syrinx (arrows A), with herniation of cerebellar tonsils (arrow B).

Causes of polyneuropathy include:

• Genetic: e.g. Charcot–Marie–Tooth disease. • Toxins: alcohol, lead, thallium, many drugs. • Metabolic disease: diabetes, chronic kidney disease. • Inflammatory: e.g. Guillain–Barré syndrome, polyarteritis nodosa, systemic lupus erythematosus, rheumatoid arthritis. • Infections: e.g. HIV, brucella, leprosy. • Neoplasms: lymphoma, carcinoma, myeloma. • Vitamin deficiencies: especially B_{12}, thiamine, folic acid, E.

Investigations required in peripheral neuropathy reflect this spectrum of causes (Box 16.31).

Entrapment neuropathy

Focal compression is the usual cause of a mononeuropathy (Box 16.32). Certain conditions increase the risk of entrapment neuropathies, including acromegaly, hypothyroidism, diabetes and bone damage near the nerve. Unless axonal loss has occurred, entrapment neuropathies will recover, provided the pressure on the nerve is relieved, either by avoidance of precipitating activities or by surgical decompression.

Multifocal neuropathy (mononeuritis multiplex)

When multiple nerve root, peripheral nerve or cranial nerve lesions occur serially or concurrently, the pathology is due either

16.31 Investigation of peripheral neuropathy

Initial tests

- Glucose (fasting)
- ESR, CRP
- FBC
- U&Es
- LFTs
- Serum protein electrophoresis
- Vitamin B$_{12}$, folate
- ANA, ANCA
- CXR
- HIV testing

If initial tests are negative

- Nerve conduction studies
- Vitamins E and A
- Genetic testing
- Lyme serology (p. 79)
- Serum ACE
- Serum amyloid

(ANCA = antineutrophil cytoplasmic antibody; ANA = antineutrophil antibody)

to involvement of the vasa nervorum or to malignant infiltration of the nerves. Investigation should be urgent since vasculitis is a common cause.

Polyneuropathy

The clinical effects of a generalised pathological process occur in the longest peripheral nerves first, affecting the distal lower limbs before the upper limbs, with sensory symptoms and signs of an ascending 'glove and stocking' distribution. In inflammatory demyelinating neuropathies, the pathology may be patchier and variations from this ascending pattern occur.

Guillain–Barré syndrome

Guillain–Barré syndrome (GBS) is a heterogeneous group of immune-mediated conditions with an incidence of 1–2/100000/yr. In Europe and North America, the most common variant is an acute inflammatory demyelinating polyneuropathy (AIDP). Axonal or sensorimotor variants are more common in China and Japan (often associated with *Campylobacter jejuni*). The hallmark is an acute paralysis evolving over days or weeks with loss of reflexes. About two-thirds of those with AIDP have a prior history of infection, and an autoimmune response triggered by the preceding infection causes demyelination.

Clinical features

Distal paraesthesia and pain precede weakness that ascends rapidly from lower to upper limbs, and is more marked proximally than

	16.32 Symptoms and signs in common entrapment neuropathies			
Nerve	**Symptoms**	**Muscle weakness/ muscle-wasting**	**Area of sensory loss**
Median (at wrist; carpal tunnel syndrome)	Pain and paraesthesia on palmar aspect of hands. Pain may extend to arm and shoulder	Abductor pollicis brevis	Lateral palm and thumb, index, middle and lateral half 4th finger
Ulnar (at elbow)	Paraesthesia on medial border of hand, wasting and weakness of hand muscles	All small hand muscles, excluding abductor pollicis brevis	Medial palm and little finger, and medial half 4th finger
Radial	Weakness of extension of wrist and fingers, often precipitated by sleeping in abnormal posture, e.g. arm over back of chair	Wrist and finger extensors, supinator	Dorsum of thumb
Common peroneal	Foot drop, trauma to head of fibula	Dorsiflexion and eversion of foot	Nil or dorsum of foot
Lateral cutaneous nerve of the thigh	Tingling and dysaesthesia on lateral border of the thigh	Nil	Lateral border of thigh

distally. Facial and bulbar weakness is common, and respiratory weakness requiring ventilation occurs in 20% of cases. Weakness progresses for up to 4 wks. Rapid deterioration to respiratory failure can develop within hours. Examination shows diffuse weakness with loss of reflexes. A rare variant, Miller Fisher syndrome, presents with internal and external ophthalmoplegia, ataxia and areflexia.

Investigations

CSF protein is elevated (or may initially be normal) but there is no rise in CSF cell number. Electrophysiology shows conduction block and motor slowing after a week. Other causes of neuromuscular paralysis should be excluded (e.g. poliomyelitis, botulism, diphtheria, spinal cord syndromes or myasthenia).

Management and prognosis

• Regular monitoring of vital capacity to detect respiratory failure.
• Supportive measures to protect the airway, and prevent pressure sores and venous thrombosis. • Plasma exchange or IV immunoglobulin therapy: shorten the illness and improve prognosis if started within 14 days.

Overall, 80% of patients recover completely within 3–6 mths, 4% die and the remainder suffer residual neurological disability. Adverse prognostic features include older age, rapid deterioration to ventilation and evidence of axonal loss on EMG.

Chronic polyneuropathy

A chronic symmetrical axonal polyneuropathy, evolving over months or years, is the most common form of chronic neuropathy. Diabetes mellitus is the most common cause but in ~25–50% no cause can be found.

Hereditary neuropathy

Charcot–Marie–Tooth disease (CMT) is an umbrella term for the inherited neuropathies. This group of syndromes has different clinical and genetic features. The most common CMT is the autosomal dominantly inherited CMT type 1, which causes distal wasting ('inverted champagne bottle' legs), often with pes cavus, and predominantly motor involvement. X-linked and recessive forms of CMT also occur.

Chronic demyelinating polyneuropathy

The acquired chronic demyelinating neuropathies include chronic inflammatory demyelinating peripheral neuropathy (which responds to steroids, plasma exchange or IV immunoglobulin), multifocal motor neuropathy and paraprotein-associated demyelinating neuropathy (sometimes associated with a lymphoproliferative malignancy). They may also demonstrate positive antibodies to myelin-associated glycoprotein.

Plexus lesions

Brachial plexopathy

Trauma usually damages either the upper or the lower parts of the brachial plexus, according to the mechanics of the injury. The clinical features depend upon the site of damage (Box 16.33). The lower brachial plexus is vulnerable to breast or apical lung tumours, therapeutic irradiation, birth trauma or compression by thoracic outlet anomalies such as a cervical rib.

16.33 Physical signs in brachial plexus lesions			
Site	**Root**	**Affected muscles**	**Sensory loss**
Upper plexus (Erb–Duchenne)	C5/6	Biceps, deltoid, spinati, rhomboids, brachioradialis	Patch over deltoid
Lower plexus (Déjerine–Klumpke)	C8/T1	Small hand muscles, lumbricals (claw hand), ulnar wrist flexors	Ulnar border hand/ forearm
Thoracic outlet syndrome	C8/T1	Small hand muscles, lumbricals (claw hand), long finger flexors	Ulnar border hand/ forearm/upper arm

Lumbosacral plexopathy

This may be caused by neoplastic infiltration or compression by retroperitoneal haematomas. A small-vessel vasculopathy can produce a lumbar plexopathy, especially in elderly patients with type 2 diabetes mellitus ('diabetic amyotrophy') or a vasculitis. This presents with painful wasting of the quadriceps and an absent knee reflex.

Spinal root lesions

These are caused by compression at or near spinal exit foramina by prolapsed intervertebral discs or degenerative spinal disease. Clinical features include muscle weakness and wasting and dermatomal sensory loss with reflex changes reflecting the roots involved (see Boxes 16.27 and 16.28). Pain in the muscles innervated by the affected roots is common.

DISORDERS OF THE NEUROMUSCULAR JUNCTION

Myasthenia gravis

This is characterised by progressive fatigable weakness, particularly of the ocular, neck, facial and bulbar muscles. In 80% of cases it is caused by autoantibodies to acetylcholine receptors in the neuromuscular junction. About 15% of patients have a thymoma, and a majority of the remainder have thymic follicular hyperplasia. Penicillamine can trigger an antibody-mediated myasthenic syndrome and some drugs (e.g. aminoglycosides) may exacerbate the neuromuscular blockade.

Clinical features

The disease usually presents between 15 and 50 yrs, with women affected more often than men in the younger age groups and the reverse at older ages. The cardinal symptom is abnormal fatigable weakness of the muscles; movement is initially strong but rapidly weakens. Worsening towards the end of the day or following exercise is characteristic. Intermittent ptosis or diplopia is common but weakness of chewing, swallowing, speaking or limb movement also occurs. Respiratory muscle weakness is an avoidable cause of death. Aspiration may occur and cough may be ineffectual. Ventilatory support is required where weakness is severe or of abrupt onset.

Investigations

Tensilon test: IV injection of an anticholinesterase, edrophonium, causes improved muscle power within 30 secs, which persists for 2–3 mins.

EMG: Repetitive stimulation may show a characteristic decremental response.

Autoantibodies: Anti-acetylcholine receptor antibody is found in >80% of cases, and anti-muscle-specific kinase antibodies in others. Screen for associated autoimmune disorders.

Thoracic CT: This is required to exclude thymoma (may not be visible on plain X-ray).

Management

Anticholinesterases: These maximise activity of acetylcholine at receptors in the neuromuscular junction using anticholinesterases, e.g. pyridostigmine. Muscarinic side-effects may be controlled by propantheline. Anticholinesterase over-dosage may cause a cholinergic crisis (muscle fasciculation, paralysis, pallor, sweating, salivation and small pupils); this may be distinguished from a myasthenic crisis clinically and, if necessary, by a dose of edrophonium.

Immunological treatment: Acutely, plasma exchange or IV immunoglobulin reduces antibody levels and causes marked, though brief improvement. This is mainly used for severe myasthenia or preoperative preparation. For long-term treatment, corticosteroids (which may initially exacerbate symptoms) may be used, with azathioprine to minimise dose and side-effects. Thymectomy should be considered in young female patients with generalised disease but is less likely to cause remission in older patients. Rapid progression of the disease more than 5 yrs after onset is uncommon.

Other myasthenic syndromes

In the Lambert–Eaton myasthenic syndrome, transmitter release is impaired, often with antibodies to prejunctional calcium channels. The cardinal sign is absent tendon reflexes, which return immediately after sustained contraction of the relevant muscle. The syndrome is often associated with underlying malignancy. It is diagnosed electrophysiologically and treatment is with 3,4-diaminopyridine, or pyridostigmine with immunosuppression.

DISEASES OF MUSCLE

Disease of voluntary muscle most commonly presents as symmetrical weakness of the large proximal muscles (proximal myopathy). Other presenting symptoms include myotonia (an abnormality of muscle relaxation) and muscle pain. Diagnosis depends on the clinical picture, along with EMG studies, muscle biopsy and sometimes genetic studies.

Muscular dystrophies

These inherited disorders are characterised by progressive degeneration of muscle groups, sometimes with cardiac or respiratory involvement or non-myopathic features (Box 16.34).

Clinical features

Onset is often in childhood, with symmetrical wasting and weakness. There is no fasciculation and no sensory loss. Tendon reflexes are preserved until a late stage, except in myotonic dystrophy.

16.34 The muscular dystrophies

Type	Genetics	Age of onset (yrs)	Muscles affected	Other features
Myotonic dystrophy	AD: expanded triplet repeat chromosome 19q	Any	Face (incl. ptosis), sternomastoids, distal limb, generalised later	Myotonia, cognitive impairment, cardiac conduction abnormalities, lens opacities, frontal balding, hypogonadism
Proximal myotonic myopathy	AD: quadruplet repeat in chromosome 3q	8–50	Proximal, especially thigh, muscle hypertrophy	As above but cognition not affected Muscle pain
Duchenne	X-linked; deletions in *dystrophin* gene	<5	Proximal and limb girdle	Cardiomyopathy and respiratory failure
Becker	X-linked; deletions in *dystrophin* gene	Childhood/ early adult	Proximal and limb girdle	Cardiomyopathy; respiratory failure uncommon
Limb girdle	Many mutations on different chromosomes	Childhood/ early adult	Limb girdle	Variable with mutation. Some have cardiorespiratory involvement
Facioscapulohumeral	AD: repeat deletion chromosome 4q	7–30	Face and upper limb girdle; distal leg	Pain in shoulder girdle common, deafness
Oculopharyngeal	AD or AR	30–60	Ptosis, ophthalmoplegia, dysphagia, tongue	Mild leg weakness

(AD = autosomal dominant; AR = autosomal recessive)

16.35	Causes of acquired proximal myopathy
Inflammatory	Polymyositis, dermatomyositis
Endocrine and metabolic	Hypothyroidism, hyperthyroidism, acromegaly, Cushing's syndrome, Addison's disease, Conn's syndrome, osteomalacia, hypokalaemia (liquorice, diuretic and purgative abuse), hypercalcaemia (disseminated bony metastases)
Toxic	Alcohol, amphetamines, cocaine, heroin, vitamin E, organophosphates, snake venoms
Drugs	Corticosteroids, chloroquine, amiodarone, β-blockers, statins, clofibrate, ciclosporin, vincristine, zidovudine, opiates
Paraneoplastic	Carcinomatous neuromyopathy, dermatomyositis

Investigations

• Specific genetic testing, with EMG and muscle biopsy if necessary.
• Creatine kinase: markedly elevated in Duchenne and Becker muscular dystrophies but normal or moderately elevated in other dystrophies. • Screening for cardiomyopathy or dysrhythmia: important.

Management

There is no specific therapy, but physiotherapy and occupational therapy help with managing disability. Treatment of associated cardiac failure or arrhythmia (with pacemaker insertion, if necessary) may be required; similarly, management of respiratory complications (including nocturnal hypoventilation) can improve quality of life. Improvements in non-invasive ventilation have led to significant improvements in survival for patients with Duchenne muscular dystrophy. Genetic counselling is important.

Acquired myopathies

Muscle weakness may be caused by a range of metabolic, endocrine, toxic or inflammatory disorders (Box 16.35). Disorders affecting the muscles' structural integrity can be distinguished by EMG from those caused by metabolic derangement. In metabolic disorders, weakness is often acute and generalised, while a proximal myopathy predominantly affecting the pelvic girdle is a feature of some endocrine disorders.

Skin disease is common, and is important because impaired skin function not only can be life-threatening but also can severely impair quality of life. People with skin disease may suffer the effects of stigma, stemming from others' belief that skin changes represent contagious disease. Assessment of the skin is valuable in the management of any medical problem and, conversely, assessment of other body systems is important when managing skin disease. This chapter covers common skin diseases and those that are important as components of general medical conditions. Skin infections are also discussed in Chapter 5.

A glossary of dermatological words is shown in Box 17.1.

PRESENTING PROBLEMS IN SKIN DISEASE

Lumps – new or changing lesions

This is one of the key dermatology presentations. The challenge is distinguishing benign from malignant disease. Detailed history and examination are essential:

Lesion: Is this new or has a pre-existing lesion changed – in size, colour, shape or surface? Has change been rapid or slow? Is there pain, itch, inflammation, bleeding or ulceration?

Patient: Age? Fair-skinned and freckled? Sun exposure (sunbeds/ lived in sunny climates, photoprotection)?

Site: Sun-exposed or covered? The scalp, face, upper limbs and back in men, and face, hands and lower legs in women are the most sun-exposed sites.

Are there other similar lesions? These might include actinic keratoses or basal cell papillomas.

Morphology of lesion: Tenderness, size, symmetry, regularity of border, colour, surface characteristics and the presence of crust, scale and ulceration must be assessed. Stretching the skin and using a magnifying lens can be helpful.

Dermatoscopy: This can be used to detect the presence of abnormal vessels, such as in basal cell carcinoma or the characteristic

CLINICAL EXAMINATION IN SKIN DISEASE

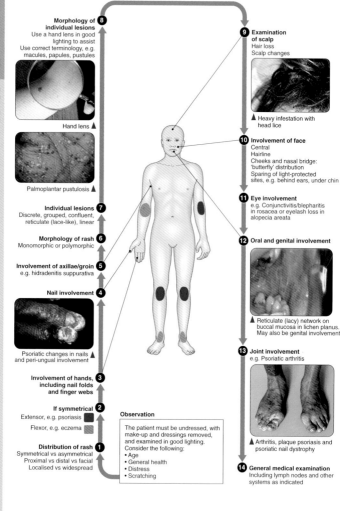

8 Morphology of individual lesions
Use a hand lens in good lighting to assist
Use correct terminology, e.g. macules, papules, pustules

Hand lens ▲

Palmoplantar pustulosis ▲

7 Individual lesions
Discrete, grouped, confluent, reticulate (lace-like), linear

6 Morphology of rash
Monomorphic or polymorphic

5 Involvement of axillae/groin
e.g. hidradenitis suppurativa

4 Nail involvement

Psoriatic changes in nails and peri-ungual involvement ▲

3 Involvement of hands, including nail folds and finger webs

2 If symmetrical
Extensor, e.g. psoriasis
Flexor, e.g. eczema

1 Distribution of rash
Symmetrical vs asymmetrical
Proximal vs distal vs facial
Localised vs widespread

9 Examination of scalp
Hair loss
Scalp changes

▲ Heavy infestation with head lice

10 Involvement of face
Central
Hairline
Cheeks and nasal bridge: 'butterfly' distribution
Sparing of light-protected sites, e.g. behind ears, under chin

11 Eye involvement
e.g. Conjunctivitis/blepharitis in rosacea or eyelash loss in alopecia areata

12 Oral and genital involvement

▲ Reticulate (lacy) network on buccal mucosa in lichen planus. May also be genital involvement

13 Joint involvement
e.g. Psoriatic arthritis

▲ Arthritis, plaque psoriasis and psoriatic nail dystrophy

14 General medical examination
Including lymph nodes and other systems as indicated

Observation

The patient must be undressed, with make-up and dressings removed, and examined in good lighting.
Consider the following:
• Age
• General health
• Distress
• Scratching

17.1 Terms used to describe skin lesions	
Macule	A circumscribed flat area of altered colour, ≤1 cm diameter
Patch	As for macule, but larger
Papule	A discrete elevation of skin
Nodule	As for papule, but >1 cm diameter and involving dermis
Plaque	A raised area of skin with a flat top, >1 cm across
Vesicle/bulla	A small (≤1 cm)/larger (>1 cm) blister, respectively
Pustule	A visible accumulation of pus in a blister
Abscess	A localised collection of pus in a cavity
Weal	An evanescent discrete area of dermal oedema
Scale	A flake arising from the stratum corneum
Petechiae, purpura, ecchymosis	Petechiae are flat, pinhead-sized macules of extravascular blood in the dermis; larger ones (purpura) may be palpable; deeper bleeding causes ecchymosis
Burrow	A linear or curvilinear papule, caused by a burrowing scabies mite
Comedone	A plug of keratin and sebum in a dilated pilosebaceous orifice
Telangiectasia	Visible dilatation of small cutaneous blood vessels
Crust	Dried exudate of blood or serous fluid
Ulcer	An area from which the epidermis and the upper dermis have been lost
Excoriation	A linear ulcer or erosion resulting from scratching
Erosion	An area of skin denuded by complete or partial loss of the epidermis
Fissure	A deep, slit-shaped ulcer, e.g. irritant dermatitis of the hands
Sinus	A cavity or channel that permits the escape of pus or fluid
Scar	Permanent fibrous tissue resulting from healing
Atrophy	Loss of substance due to diminution of the epidermis, dermis or subcutaneous fat
Stria	A linear, atrophic, pink/purple/white lesion in the connective tissue

keratin cysts in basal cell papillomas. It is invaluable for pigmented and vascular lesions.

Melanocytic naevus or malignant melanoma?

The precise nature of the change should be determined (as above). Does the patient have other pigmented lesions? If the presenting lesion looks different from the others, then suspicion is needed; conversely, if the patient has multiple basal cell papillomas, this may be reassuring. Is there a positive family history of melanoma? A suspicious naevus in a patient with a first-degree relative with melanoma probably warrants excision.

The ABCDE 'rule' is a guide to the characteristic features of melanoma:

• Asymmetry. • Border irregularity or bleeding. • Colour (moles developing pigment variegation). • Diameter (increase in size over

<table>
<tr><td colspan="4">i 17.2 Clinical features of common scaly rashes</td></tr>
<tr><td>Type of rash</td><td>Distribution</td><td>Morphology</td><td>Associated clinical signs</td></tr>
<tr><td>Atopic eczema</td><td>Face/flexures</td><td>Poorly defined erythema and scaling; lichenification</td><td>Shiny nails, infra-orbital crease, 'dirty neck'</td></tr>
<tr><td>Psoriasis</td><td>Extensor surfaces</td><td>Well-defined plaques with a silvery scale</td><td>Nail pitting and onycholysis; scalp involvement, axillae and genital areas often affected</td></tr>
<tr><td>Pityriasis rosea</td><td>'Fir tree' pattern on torso</td><td>Well-defined Small, erythematous plaques Collarette of scale</td><td>Herald patch</td></tr>
<tr><td>Pityriasis versicolor</td><td>Upper trunk and shoulders</td><td>Hypo- and hyperpigmented scaly patches</td><td></td></tr>
<tr><td>Drug eruption</td><td>Widespread</td><td>Macules and papules Erythema and scale Exfoliation</td><td>Mucosal involvement, erythroderma</td></tr>
<tr><td>Lichen planus</td><td>Distal limbs Flexor aspect of wrists; lower back</td><td>Shiny, flat-topped violaceous papules with Wickham's striae</td><td>White lacy network on buccal mucosa; nail changes, alopecia</td></tr>
<tr><td>Tinea corporis</td><td>Asymmetrical, often isolated lesions</td><td>Scaly plaques that expand with central healing</td><td>Nail involvement</td></tr>
<tr><td>Secondary syphilis</td><td>Trunk, proximal limbs, palms and soles</td><td>Red macules and papules</td><td>History of chancre Malaise, fever</td></tr>
</table>

time). • Evolution (any change noted by the patient in a pigmented lesion).

Rashes – papulosquamous eruptions

A common presenting complaint in general practice is an eruptive scaly rash, sometimes associated with itching. Causes are summarised in Box 17.2.

History

Age at onset and duration? Atopic eczema often starts in infancy or early childhood, pityriasis rosea and psoriasis between the ages of 15 and 40. Drug eruptions are acute in onset with a clear temporal relationship between starting the medicine and the onset of the rash.

Site of onset? For example, flexural sites are involved in atopic eczema and extensor surfaces and scalp in psoriasis. Symmetry suggests endogenous disease, such as psoriasis, whereas asymmetry is more common with exogenous causes, such as contact dermatitis or herpes zoster.

17.3 Causes of acquired blisters		
	Localised	**Generalised**
Vesicular	Herpes (simplex or zoster), impetigo, pompholyx	Eczema herpeticum*, dermatitis herpetiformis, acute eczema
Bullous	Impetigo, cellulitis, stasis oedema, acute eczema, insect bites, fixed drug eruptions	Toxic epidermal necrolysis*, erythema multiforme/Stevens–Johnson syndrome*, bullous pemphigoid, pemphigus*, epidermolysis bullosa acquisita, bullous lupus erythematosus, porphyria cutanea tarda, pseudoporphyria, drug eruptions

*Usually also mucosal involvement.

Is it itchy? Atopic eczema is extremely itchy, psoriasis and pityriasis rosea less so.

Was there a preceding illness or systemic symptoms? Guttate psoriasis is often preceded by a β-haemolytic streptococcal sore throat. Almost all patients with infectious mononucleosis (p. 69) treated with amoxicillin develop an erythematous maculopapular eruption.

The morphology of the rash and the characteristics of the lesions are important (see Box 17.2).

Blisters

There are a limited number of conditions that present with blisters (Box 17.3). Blistering occurs due to loss of cell adhesion within the epidermis or subepidermal region, and the presentation depends on the site or level of blistering within the skin. This in turn reflects the underlying pathogenesis:

Split high in the epidermis (below the stratum corneum): Intact blisters are uncommon, as the blister roof is so fragile that it ruptures easily, leaving erosions (e.g. pemphigus foliaceus, staphylococcal scalded skin syndrome and bullous impetigo).

Split lower in the epidermis: Intact flaccid blisters and erosions may be seen (e.g. pemphigus vulgaris and toxic epidermal necrolysis).

Subepidermal split: Tense-roofed blisters occur (e.g. bullous pemphigoid, Fig. 17.1), epidermolysis bullosa acquisita and porphyria cutanea tarda.

Foci of separation at different levels of the epidermis: Multilocular bullae (made up of coalescing vesicles) occur, as in a dermatitis.

A history of onset, progression, mucosal involvement, drugs and systemic symptoms should be taken. Clinical assessment of the distribution, extent and morphology of the rash should then be made. The Nikolsky sign is useful: sliding pressure from a finger on normal-looking epidermis can dislodge the epidermis in conditions

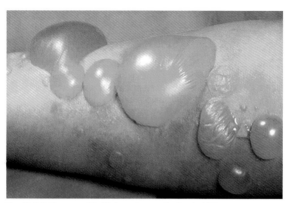

Fig. 17.1 Bullous pemphigoid. Large tense and unilocular blisters.

with intra-epidermal defects, such as pemphigus and toxic epidermal necrolysis.

A systematic approach should be taken to diagnosis:

Exclude infection: e.g. herpes simplex, varicella zoster, *Staphylococcus aureus*.

Consider common skin disorders in which blistering **uncommonly** *occurs:* e.g. severe peripheral oedema, cellulitis, allergic contact dermatitis, eczema.

Remember bullae may develop in drug eruptions: e.g. fixed drug eruption, erythema multiforme and vasculitis. Toxic epidermal necrolysis (p. 715) is a medical emergency.

Consider immunobullous disease: The age of the patient may be informative (p. 716).

Investigations and management are guided by the clinical presentation and differential diagnosis, and are described in this chapter under the specific diseases.

Itch (pruritus)

Diagnosis is important and a full history, examination and, sometimes, investigations, are necessary. When a patient presents with generalised itch, it is important to determine whether skin changes are primary (a process in the skin causing itch) or secondary (skin changes caused by rubbing and scratching because of itch). Many common primary skin disorders are associated with itch:

Generalised pruritus:
• Scabies. • Eczemas. • Pre-bullous pemphigoid. • Urticarias.
• Xeroderma of old age. • Psoriasis.

Localised pruritus:
• Eczemas. • Lichen planus. • Dermatitis herpetiformis. • Pediculosis.
• Tinea infections.

If itch is not connected with primary skin disease, many causes should be considered, including:

• Liver diseases (mainly cholestatic diseases, e.g. primary biliary cirrhosis). • Malignancies (e.g. generalised itch in lymphoma). • Haematological conditions (e.g. generalised itch in chronic iron deficiency or itch provoked by water contact (aquagenic) in polycythaemia). • Endocrine diseases (including hypo- and hyperthyroidism). • Chronic kidney disease (severity of itch not always clearly associated with plasma creatinine). • Psychogenic causes (such as in 'delusions of infestation').

Pruritus is common in pregnancy and may be due to one of the pregnancy-specific dermatoses. Diagnosis is particularly important in pregnancy, as some disorders can be associated with increased fetal risk.

Management

Management of the underlying primary skin condition or medical condition may alleviate the itch. For those with persisting symptoms despite specific management, symptomatic relief includes sedation (H_1 antagonist antihistamines), emollients and counter-irritants (e.g. topical menthol-containing preparations). Ultraviolet B (UVB) phototherapy is useful in itch from a variety of causes, although the only robust evidence of efficacy in generalised itch (not due to skin disease) is in chronic kidney disease. Other treatments include tricyclic antidepressants and opiate antagonists.

Photosensitivity

Photosensitivity is an abnormal response of the skin to ultraviolet (UVR) or visible radiation, either from sunlight, sunbeds or phototherapy. The UVB band of sunlight (wavelength 300–320 nm) accounts for its 'sunburning' effects. Chronic UVR exposure increases skin cancer risk and photoageing. Erythema on acute exposure is a normal response. Abnormal photosensitivity occurs when a patient reacts to lower doses than would normally cause a response. Photoaggravated skin diseases (e.g. lupus erythematosus, erythema multiforme and rosacea) are exacerbated by sunlight but not caused by it.

Clinical assessment

Key sites are the face, top of ears, neck, bald scalp, back of hands and forearms. Shaded sites, e.g. under the chin, are spared. Some conditions (e.g. solar urticaria) develop rapidly after sunlight exposure, while others, such as cutaneous lupus, can take several days to evolve.

Investigations and management

The patient should be referred to a specialist centre for phototesting, provocation, patch or photopatch testing, and screening for lupus and porphyrias.

Management depends on diagnosis. Phototoxic drugs should be stopped, and associated diseases treated. Counselling regarding sun avoidance, protective clothing and sunscreens is essential.

17.4 Causes of leg ulceration	
Venous hypertension	Sometimes following DVT
Arterial disease	Atherosclerosis, vasculitis, Buerger's disease
Small-vessel disease	Diabetes mellitus, vasculitis
Haematological disorders	Sickle-cell disease, cryoglobulinaemia, spherocytosis, immune complex disease, polycythaemia
Neuropathy	Diabetes mellitus, leprosy, syphilis
Tumour	Squamous cell carcinoma, basal cell carcinoma, malignant melanoma, Kaposi's sarcoma
Trauma	Injury, artefact

Sunscreens: Modern sunscreens offer protection against UVB and most UVA wavelengths. The sun protection factor (SPF) describes the ratio of the dose of UVR required to produce erythema with, as opposed to without, the sunscreen. In practice, people use 25–33% of the amount of sunscreen required for the stated SPF; thus, an SPF30 sunscreen will usually offer SPF10 in practice. All sunscreens offer only partial protection, at best, and are no substitute for avoiding exposure and covering up.

Leg ulcers

Ulceration of the skin is the complete loss of the epidermis and part of the dermis. There are numerous aetiologies, summarised in Box 17.4, but when present on the lower limb, ulceration is usually due to arterial or venous insufficiency. The site of the ulceration gives clues as to its aetiology (Fig. 17.2).

Clinical assessment
• Urinalysis to detect glycosuria ± fasting blood glucose to rule out diabetes. • Bacterial swab to exclude infection. • Blood count to exclude anaemia and dyscrasias. • Doppler USS to assess arterial sufficiency.

Leg ulceration due to venous disease
Clinical assessment
This is a common clinical problem in middle to old age. Clinical signs include:
• Varicose veins. • Haemosiderin deposition. • Oedema. • Lipo-dermatosclerosis: firm induration of the skin of the leg, with a shiny appearance, producing the 'inverted champagne bottle' sign. • Ulceration: typically on the medial lower leg. • Malignant transformation of a chronic ulcer into squamous cell carcinoma: termed 'Marjolin's ulcer'.

Leg ulceration due to arterial disease
Deep, painful and punched-out ulcers on the lower leg, especially if they occur on the shin and foot and in the context of intermittent

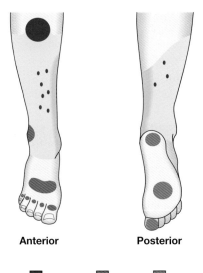

Anterior   Posterior

☐ Venous ■ Vasculitis ▨ Arterial ▨ Neuropathic

Fig. 17.2 Causes of lower leg ulceration.

claudication, are likely to be due to arterial disease. Risk factors include smoking, hypertension, diabetes mellitus and hyperlipidaemia. The foot is cyanotic and cold, and the skin surrounding the ulcer is atrophic and hairless. The peripheral arterial pulses are absent or reduced. Doppler studies are required, and if arterial insufficiency is confirmed, compression bandaging should be prohibited and advice sought from a vascular surgeon.

Leg ulceration due to vasculitis

Vasculitis can cause leg ulceration directly through epidermal necrosis due to damage to the underlying vasculature, or indirectly due to neuropathy (e.g. in systemic polyarteritis nodosa, p. 596).

Leg ulceration due to neuropathy

The most common cause of a neuropathic ulcer is diabetes. The ulcers occur over weight-bearing areas such as the heel. Microangiopathy also contributes to ulceration in diabetes. This is discussed in detail on page 410.

Management

Advise weight loss (if obese), smoking cessation and gentle exercise. Oedema should be reduced with the use of compression bandages (once arterial sufficiency is excluded, ratio of ankle:brachial systolic pressure >0.8), elevation of the legs when sitting and the judicious use of diuretics. If purulent, use weak potassium permanganate soaks. Non-adherent absorbent dressings (alginates, hydrogels or hydrocolloids) should be changed daily for highly exudative ulcers. Surrounding venous eczema should be treated with topical steroid. Skin grafts may hasten healing of clean ulcers.

Abnormal skin colour

Depigmentation, hypopigmentation and hyperpigmentation are covered on pages 717–719.

Hair and nail abnormalities

These may be a marker for systemic disease or a feature of skin conditions (e.g. psoriasis). Specific disorders are covered on pages 719–722.

Acute skin failure

Erythroderma, defined as erythema with or without scaling involving >90% of the body surface, is associated with systemic symptoms due to excessive cutaneous heat loss, and haemodynamic upset characterised by hypotension and tachycardia as a response to a large increase in insensible losses. Causes include:
• Eczema. • Psoriasis. • Pityriasis rubra pilaris (a variant of psoriasis).
• Cutaneous T-cell lymphoma (Sézary's syndrome).

Skin failure without erythroderma can occur with autoimmune blistering disease and Stevens–Johnson syndrome.

SKIN TUMOURS

Skin cancer is categorised as non-melanoma skin cancer (NMSC) and melanoma. NMSC comprises basal cell carcinoma (BCC) and squamous cell carcinoma (SCC). The latter has precursor non-invasive states of intra-epithelial carcinoma (Bowen's disease; BD) and dysplasia (actinic keratosis; AK). Melanoma is much rarer than NMSC, but because of its metastatic risk it causes most skin cancer deaths.

UVR is the main risk factor for skin cancer; it is strongly linked to risk of SCC and AK, and modestly to BCC risk. Melanoma usually arises on intermittently exposed sites, and episodes of sunburn are an additional risk factor. Other factors include genetic predisposition (e.g. in xeroderma pigmentosum) and immunosuppression; organ transplant recipients have an increased risk of skin cancer, particularly SCC. Chronic inflammation is also a risk factor for SCC (e.g. chronic skin ulcers, lupus), as is scarring skin disease, e.g. epidermolysis bullosa.

Malignant tumours
Basal cell carcinoma

This is a common, slow-growing malignant tumour that rarely metastasises but which can invade locally ('rodent ulcer'). Early BCCs usually present as pale, translucent papules or nodules, with

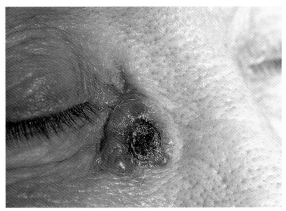

Fig. 17.3 Basal cell carcinoma. A slowly growing, pearly nodule just below the inner canthus. The central crust overlies an ulcerated area.

overlying superficial telangiectatic vessels (nodular BCC). If untreated, they increase in size and ulcerate, forming a crater with a rolled, pearled edge and ectatic vessels (Fig. 17.3). A superficial multifocal type of BCC presents as a red/brown plaque or patch with a raised, thread-like edge, often on the trunk, and may be up to 10 cm in diameter. Less commonly, a morphoeic, infiltrative BCC presents as an ill-defined, slowly enlarging, sclerotic yellow/grey plaque.

Management
The choice of treatment modality depends on local expertise and interest, and includes surgery, cryotherapy, radiotherapy, photodynamic therapy or the topical immunomodulator imiquimod. All treatments used optimally can produce excellent cure rates.

Squamous cell carcinoma
SCC usually arises on sun-exposed areas with diverse clinical appearances, including keratotic nodules, exophytic erythematous nodules, infiltrating firm tumours and ulcers. Histological grade varies from well differentiated to anaplastic, and lymph node metastasis may occur.

Management
Complete surgical excision is the treatment of choice. Other options include curettage and cautery for small, low-risk lesions and radiotherapy if surgery is not feasible. Wide excision has a cure rate of ~90–95%. In patients who are at high risk for further SCC, systemic retinoids may reduce the rate of occurrence, but rapid appearance of tumours occurs on drug cessation.

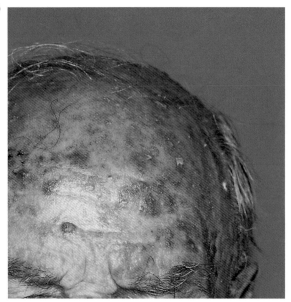

Fig. 17.4 Numerous actinic keratoses in a white patient who had lived for years in the tropics.

Actinic keratosis

Actinic keratoses are hyperkeratotic erythematous lesions arising on chronically sun-exposed sites (Fig. 17.4). Histology shows dysplasia, although the diagnosis is usually clinical. They are treated easily and effectively with liquid nitrogen. If there is a large number of lesions, then the topical cytotoxic 5-fluorouracil may be required; alternatively, topical imiquimod or photodynamic therapy may be used. Progression to SCC is rare, but should be suspected if there is ulceration, bleeding or pain.

Intra-epidermal carcinoma (Bowen's disease)

Intra-epidermal carcinoma (IEC) usually presents as a slow-growing, erythematous, scaly plaque, on the lower legs of fair-skinned elderly women. Histology demonstrates intra-epithelial carcinoma not penetrating the basement membrane. IEC may develop into SCC and should always be treated. A biopsy may be required to make the diagnosis but non-surgical photodynamic or immunomodulatory therapies are commonly preferred on the legs, as they are associated with improved healing.

Keratoacanthoma

Although benign, this squamous tumour can be hard to distinguish from SCC and therefore is included here. It presents as a rapidly growing, isolated nodule often ≥5 cm in diameter, with a central keratin plug. It is associated with chronic sun exposure and usually occurs on the face. Clinically and histologically, it resembles SCC. Most are treated by curettage or excision to rule out SCC and to avoid the scar resulting from spontaneous resolution.

Cutaneous lymphoma

Cutaneous T-cell lymphoma (mycosis fungoides, MF) develops slowly over many years from polymorphic patches and plaques through to nodules and then a systemic stage. As it can resemble other common conditions, such as persistent eczema and psoriasis, a high index of suspicion is required for diagnosis.

Treatment is symptomatic and does not alter prognosis. In early disease, systemic or local corticosteroids may be indicated; alternatively, psoralen (photosensitiser) + UVA (PUVA; for plaque stage MF) or UVB (for patch stage MF) may be used. In advanced disease, localised radiotherapy, electron beam radiation or anti-lymphoma chemotherapy may be needed.

Melanoma

Melanoma is a malignant tumour of epidermal melanocytes and has metastatic potential. Incidence has increased over recent decades. Early detection and treatment are essential because of the lack of effective therapies for metastatic disease. The main risk factors for melanoma are:

• Prolonged UVR exposure. • Pale skin. • Large numbers of naevi. • Positive family history (several associated genes now identified).

Clinical features

Melanoma can occur at any age and site, but is rare before puberty and typically affects the leg in females and back in males.

Five subtypes occur:

Superficial spreading malignant melanoma (Fig. 17.5): Most common in Caucasians and characterised by a superficial radial growth pattern, which over time may progress to vertical spread.

Nodular melanoma: A rapidly growing nodule, typically found on the trunk in men. It may bleed, ulcerate and metastasise.

Lentigo maligna melanoma: Occurs most often on exposed skin of the elderly as a pigmented macular area. It is preceded by a prolonged pre-invasive phase (lentigo maligna).

Acral lentiginous melanoma: Occurs on the palms and soles, particularly in dark-skinned people.

Subungual melanoma: Rare. It presents with a painless streak of pigmentation under a nail.

Diagnosis

Any new or changed naevi should be assessed using the ABCDE rule (p. 689), and excised if doubt remains.

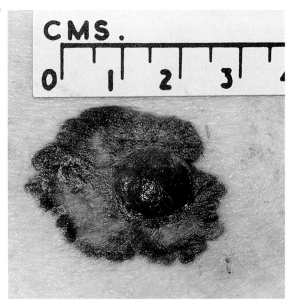

Fig. 17.5 Superficial spreading melanoma. The radial growth phase was present for ~3 yrs before the invasive amelanotic nodule developed within it. Note the irregular outline, asymmetrical shape and different hues, including depigmented areas signifying spontaneous regression.

Management

The lesion should be excised with a wide margin. The Breslow thickness of tumour (i.e. the maximal depth from granular cell layer to deepest tumour cells) is critical for management and prognosis. Clinical staging is essential, to establish whether disease is localised or metastatic. Treatment may involve wider local excision, sentinel lymph node mapping and biopsy. Prognosis for metastatic disease is poor and chemotherapy is palliative, but tumour-targeted genetic treatments are under development.

Benign skin lesions mimicking tumours
Freckles

These are most common in sun-exposed sites in fair-skinned individuals and represent focal over-production of melanin with normal melanocyte number. They become darker with sun exposure and are associated with a familial sun-sensitive phenotype.

Lentigines

These are dark brown macules 1 mm–1 cm across. They are associated with chronic sun exposure and become more common with age. Biopsy may be needed to distinguish them from melanoma.

Basal cell papilloma (seborrhoeic wart)

Seborrhoeic warts are common benign epidermal tumours, which appear over the age of 35. They vary in colour from yellow to dark brown, and have a greasy, 'stuck-on' appearance. Although they may be a cosmetic problem, their principal significance lies in the differential diagnosis of melanoma or other skin tumours, which may require biopsy.

Melanocytic naevi

Melanocytic naevi (moles) are localised benign clonal proliferations of melanocytes. Moles are a usual feature of most human beings and it is quite normal to have 20–50. Individuals with high sun exposure also show more moles, i.e. there is clear evidence for both genetic and environmental factors. Most melanocytic naevi appear in early childhood, at adolescence, and during pregnancy or oestrogen therapy. The appearance of a new mole is less common after the age of 25.

Clinical features

Acquired melanocytic naevi are classified according to the microscopic location of the melanocyte nests:
• Junctional naevi are usually circular and macular, and mid- to dark brown. • Compound and intradermal naevi are nodules, because of the dermal component, and may be hair-bearing. • Intradermal naevi are usually less pigmented than compound naevi. Their surface may be smooth, cerebriform, hyperkeratotic or papillomatous.

Management

Melanocytic naevi are normal and do not require excision, except when malignancy is suspected (p. 689) or when they repeatedly become inflamed or traumatised. Some individuals wish to have them removed for cosmetic reasons.

COMMON SKIN INFECTIONS AND INFESTATIONS

Bacterial infections
Impetigo

Impetigo is a common, highly contagious, superficial bacterial skin infection. There are two main presentations: bullous impetigo, caused by a staphylococcal epidermolytic toxin, and non-bullous impetigo (Fig. 17.6), which can be caused by either *Staph. aureus* or streptococcus, or both. *Staphylococcus* is the most common agent in temperate climates; streptococcal impetigo is seen in hot, humid areas. Non-bullous disease particularly affects young children, often in late summer. It can be sporadic, although outbreaks can arise with overcrowding or poor hygiene, or in institutions. Coexisting skin conditions, such as abrasions, infestations or eczema, predispose to impetigo.

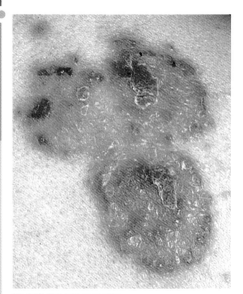

Fig. 17.6 Non-bullous impetigo.

In non-bullous impetigo, a thin-walled vesicle develops, ruptures rapidly and is rarely seen intact. Dried exudate, forming golden crusting, arises on an erythematous base. In bullous disease, the toxins cleave the superficial epidermis, causing intact blisters containing clear to cloudy fluid; these last 2–3 days. The face, scalp and limbs are commonly affected but sites of eczema can also be involved. Constitutional symptoms are uncommon. A bacterial swab should be taken from blister fluid or active lesions before treatment. Around one-third of the population are nasal carriers of *Staphylococcus*, so nasal swabs should also be obtained.

In mild, localised disease, topical treatment with mupirocin or fusidic acid usually suffices and limits spread. Staphylococcal nasal carriage should be treated with topical mupirocin. In severe cases, oral flucloxacillin or erythromycin is indicated. If a nephritogenic streptococcus is suspected, systemic antibiotics should be given, as post-streptococcal glomerulonephritis can occur (p. 185).

Staphylococcal scalded skin syndrome

This is a serious exfoliating condition predominantly affecting children, particularly neonates. Systemic circulation of epidermolytic toxins from a *Staph. aureus* infection cause a split in the superficial epidermis and peeling of the skin.

The child presents with fever, irritability, skin tenderness and erythema, often starting in the groin, in the axilla and around the mouth. Blisters and superficial erosions develop over 1–2 days.

Bacterial swabs should be taken from possible sites of primary infection (throat, nose, etc.). Diagnosis is made on the clinical appearance and histological examination of a skin snip taken from the edge of one of the peeling areas, to determine the plane of cleavage and thus exclude the differential diagnosis of toxic epidermal necrolysis, which involves the full thickness of the epidermis. Management consists of immediate systemic antibiotics (e.g. flucloxacillin) and supportive measures in an HDU. Family members should be screened and treated for staphylococcal carriage.

Folliculitis, furuncles and carbuncles

Folliculitis can be superficial, involving just the ostium of the hair follicle (folliculitis), or deep (furuncles and carbuncles).

Superficial folliculitis: This is very common, usually minor, and subacute or chronic. It is often infective, caused by *Staph. aureus*, but can also be due to physical (e.g. traumatic epilation) or chemical (e.g. mineral oils) injury. In these cases, the folliculitis is usually sterile. Staphylococcal folliculitis is most common in children and often occurs on the scalp or limbs. The pustules usually heal in 7–10 days but can become more chronic, and in older children and adults can progress to a deeper form of folliculitis.

Deep folliculitis (furuncles and carbuncles): A furuncle (boil) is an acute *Staph. aureus* infection of the hair follicle, which becomes pustular and fluctuant, and is often exquisitely tender. The lesions eventually rupture to discharge pus and, because they are deep, leave a scar. They can progress to form a carbuncle, which is an exquisitely tender nodule, often on the neck, shoulders or hips, and is associated with severe constitutional symptoms. It implies the involvement of several contiguous hair follicles. Treatment, as for furuncles, is with an appropriate antistaphylococcal antibiotic.

Cellulitis and erysipelas

Cellulitis is inflammation of subcutaneous tissue, due to bacterial infection. In contrast, erysipelas is bacterial infection of the dermis and upper subcutaneous tissue, although in practice it may be difficult to distinguish between them. The most common organism causing both conditions is group A streptococcus.

Diagnosis is based on clinical findings of erythema, heat, swelling, pain and sometimes fever, with a leucocytosis, raised inflammatory markers and a swab isolating a causative organism. Erysipelas (Fig. 17.7) typically has well-defined edge, indicating involvement of the dermis. It usually affects the face. Cellulitis most commonly involves the legs. Blistering and regional lymphadenopathy may occur in both conditions. There is often a predisposing cause, such as a portal of entry for infection, e.g. tinea pedis, or an underlying predisposition to infection such as varicose leg ulcer or diabetes. Treatment is usually with an IV antistreptococcal agent such as benzylpenicillin, or in cases of penicillin sensitivity, erythromycin or ciprofloxacin. In mild cases, oral antibiotics are indicated.

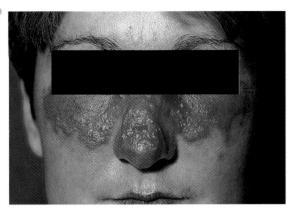

Fig. 17.7 Erysipelas. Note the blistering and crusted rash with raised erythematous edge.

Erythrasma

Erythrasma is a mild localised infection of the skin caused by *Corynebacterium minutissimum*, which often is part of the normal skin flora.

C. minutissimum can provoke an asymptomatic or mildly itchy eruption between the toes and in the flexures. Lesions are well defined and reddish-brown, with some scale. The bacterium is identified by coral pink fluorescence with Wood's light. Treatments include a topical azole cream such as miconazole or a topical antibiotic.

Viral infections

Herpes virus infections

These are described on pages 71–73.

Papillomaviruses and viral warts

Viral warts are caused by the DNA human papillomavirus (HPV) and are extremely common, being transmitted by direct contact with the virus in either living skin or shed skin fragments. Most people suffer from one or more warts at some point during their life. There are >90 different subtypes. HPV subtypes 16 and 18 are spread by sexual contact and are strongly associated with subsequent development of cervical carcinoma. Vaccinations are now available against HPV-16 and 18 and are recommended for adolescent females before they become sexually active. Immunosuppressed patients are at greater risk of infection with HPV.

Clinical features

Common warts appear initially as smooth, skin-coloured papules. As they enlarge, their surface becomes irregular and hyperkeratotic, producing the typical warty appearance. One method of classifying warts is based on their clinical appearance:

Plantar warts (verrucae): Found on the sole of the foot. These are characterised by a horny collar surrounding a roughened surface. Paring reveals capillary loops that distinguish plantar warts from corns.

Mosaic warts: Mosaic-like sheets of warts.

Plane warts: Smooth, flat-topped papules, usually on the face and the dorsum of the hands.

Filiform warts: Often found on the face.

Genital warts: Papillomatous and protuberant.

Management

Most viral warts resolve spontaneously but often very slowly. Therapeutic options to speed resolution include:

• Topical salicylic acid (first-line). • Cryotherapy. • Imiquimod or podophyllin for genital warts. • Intralesional bleomycin (for recalcitrant warts).

Molluscum contagiosum

Molluscum contagiosum is caused by a DNA poxvirus infection. It can affect any age group but usually targets children over the age of 1 and the immunosuppressed. The classic lesion is a dome-shaped, 'umbilicated', skin-coloured papule with a central punctum. Lesions tend to be multiple and are often in sites of apposition, such as the side of the chest and the inner arm. No treatment is required, as these lesions resolve spontaneously but can take several months to do so. If active resolution is sought, curettage or cryotherapy may be tried, or topical agents such as salicylic acid, podophyllin or imiquimod.

Orf

Orf is an occupational hazard for those who work with sheep and goats. It is a cutaneous infection with a parapoxvirus carried by these animals. Inoculation of the virus, usually into the skin of a finger, causes significant inflammation and necrosis, which resolve in 2–6 wks. No specific treatment is available unless there is evidence of secondary infection. Erythema multiforme can be triggered by orf virus infection.

Fungal infections

Dermatophytes are fungi capable of causing superficial skin infections known as ringworm or dermatophytosis. The causative fungi (*Microsporum, Trichophyton, Epidermophyton*) can originate from the soil (geophilic) or animals (zoophilic), or be confined to human skin (anthropophilic).

Clinical forms of cutaneous infection include:

• Tinea corporis (involvement of the body). • Tinea capitis (scalp involvement). • Tinea cruris (groin involvement). • Tinea pedis (involvement of the feet). • Onychomycosis (fungal infection of the nail).

Tinea corporis: This condition should be considered in the differential diagnosis of the red scaly rash (p. 690). Lesions are erythematous, annular and scaly, with a well-defined edge and central clearing. They may be single or multiple and are usually asymmetrical. *Microsporum canis* and *Trichophyton verrucosum* are common culprits and are zoophilic (from dogs and cats, respectively). Inadvertent topical corticosteroid application leads to disguising and worsening of the signs (tinea incognito).

Tinea cruris: This is common worldwide and is usually caused by *T. rubrum.* Itchy erythematous plaques extend from the groin flexures on to the thighs.

Tinea pedis (athlete's foot): This is the most common fungal skin infection in the UK and USA, and is usually caused by anthropophilic fungi such as *T. rubrum*, *T. interdigitale* and *Epidermophyton floccosum.* Clinical features include an itchy rash between the toes, with peeling, fissuring and maceration.

Tinea capitis: This dermatophyte scalp infection is most common in children. It presents with inflammation and scaling, pustules and partial hair loss. Infection may be within the shaft (endothrix), causing broken hairs at the surface ('black dot'), or outside the hair shaft (ectothrix) with minimal inflammation. Kerion is a boggy, inflammatory area of tinea capitis, usually caused by zoophilic fungi and treated with systemic antifungals.

Onychomycosis: This causes yellow–brown discoloration and crumbling of the nail plate, which usually starts distally and spreads proximally.

Diagnosis and management

In all cases of suspected dermatophyte infection, the diagnosis should be confirmed by skin scraping or nail clippings. Treatment can be topical (terbinafine or miconazole cream) or systemic (terbinafine, griseofulvin or itraconazole).

Scabies

Scabies is caused by the *Acarus* mite, *Sarcoptes scabiei*. The infestation causes intense itch and can lead to secondary infection and complications such as post-streptococcal glomerulonephritis. Scabies spreads in households and environments where there is a high frequency of intimate personal contact.

Diagnosis is made by identifying the scabietic burrow, usually found on the edges of the fingers, toes or sides of the hands and feet. The clinical features include secondary eczematisation elsewhere on the body; the face and scalp are rarely involved, except in infants. Even after successful treatment, the itch can continue and occasionally nodular lesions persist. Treatment involves two applications, 1 wk apart, of an aqueous solution of either permethrin or malathion to the whole body, excluding the head. Household contacts should also be treated. In some clinical situations, such as poor compliance, immunocompromised individuals and heavy infestations

(Norwegian scabies), systemic treatment with a single dose of ivermectin is appropriate.

Lice

Infestation with the head louse, *Pediculus humanus capitis*, is common and highly contagious. Head lice are spread by direct head-to-head contact.

Scalp itching leads to scratching, secondary infection and cervical lymphadenopathy. The diagnosis is confirmed by identifying the living louse or nymph on the scalp or on a black sheet of paper after careful fine-toothed combing of wet hair following conditioner application. The empty egg cases ('nits') are easily seen adhering strongly to the hair shaft.

Treatment with malathion, permethrin and carbaryl in lotion or aqueous form is recommended for the infected individual and any infected household/school contacts. Treatment is applied on two separate occasions at 7–10 days' interval. Body lice and pubic (crab) lice are similar, the latter being predominantly sexually transmitted. They also respond to malathion.

ACNE AND ROSACEA

Acne vulgaris

Acne is a common chronic inflammation of the pilosebaceous units affecting >90% of adolescents. The key components are increased sebum production; colonisation of pilosebaceous ducts by *Propionibacterium acnes*, which in turn causes inflammation; and occlusion of pilosebaceous ducts. Family history may be positive, suggesting that genetic factors are important.

Acne usually affects the face and trunk. Greasiness of the skin (seborrhoea) accompanies open comedones (blackheads – dilated keratin-filled follicles) and closed comedones (whiteheads – caused by accumulation of sebum and keratin deeper in the pilosebaceous ducts). Inflammatory papules, nodules and cysts occur and may arise from comedones.

Management

Mild disease is managed with topical antibiotics such as erythromycin, dessicants such as benzoyl peroxide, or topical retinoids.

Moderate inflammatory acne is treated with prolonged courses of oral tetracyclines. Oestrogen-containing oral contraceptives may help in women.

In severe cases, oral retinoid therapy with isotretinoin has revolutionised the management of acne. The side-effect profile includes drying of the skin and mucous membranes but this is generally manageable. Isotretinoin may elevate serum triglycerides and derange liver function; both should be checked prior to commencing the drug. Isotretinoin is highly teratogenic, and female patients must be counselled about this prior to commencing treatment.

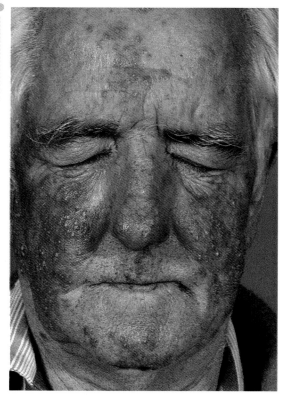

Fig. 17.8 Rosacea. The colour is distinctive and the typical papulo-pustular rash involves the cheeks, centre of the forehead and chin.

Rosacea

Rosacea is a persistent facial eruption of unknown cause, largely occurring in middle age (Fig. 17.8). It is characterised by erythema, telangiectasia, papules and pustules. A bulbous appearance to the nose, known as rhinophyma, may be seen as part of the disease and is caused by sebaceous gland hypertrophy. The papulo-pustular element of disease usually responds well to tetracyclines, but the erythema and telangiectasia do not; these may require laser therapy.

ECZEMA

The terms 'eczema' and 'dermatitis' are synonymous. There are a number of clinical variants, which are all characterised by acute or chronic inflammation and spongiosis (oedema) of the dermis and epidermis on histology.

Atopic eczema

Generalised, prolonged hypersensitivity to common environmental antigens, including pollen and house dust mites, is the hallmark of atopy, in which there is a genetic predisposition to over-production of IgE. Atopic individuals manifest one or more of a group of diseases that includes asthma, hay fever, food and other allergies, and atopic eczema. The identification of null alleles in the filaggrin gene predisposing to atopic eczema (and asthma in association with atopic eczema) has dramatically increased our understanding of the pathogenesis of atopic eczema. Filaggrin is an important component of the skin barrier and it is the combination of this defect with exposure to environmental allergens that is likely to cause the clinical signs of atopic eczema.

Clinical features

Acute atopic eczema presents with severe itch, redness and swelling. Papules and vesicles may be evident, along with scaling and cracking of the skin, which is excessively dry. In patients with chronic eczema, lichenification may be found (dry, leathery thickening of the skin with increased skin markings, secondary to constant rubbing/scratching). The distribution of atopic eczema varies with the age of the patient: in infancy and adulthood the eczema tends to affect the face and trunk, while in childhood it affects the limb flexures, wrists and the ankles (Fig. 17.9).

Seborrhoeic eczema

This condition, which is characterised by a red scaly rash, classically affects the scalp (dandruff), central face, nasolabial folds, eyebrows and central chest. It is thought to be a reaction to *Pityrosporum* yeast infection of the skin. Management includes the use of ketoconazole or selenium-containing shampoo, in combination with a weak- to moderate-potency topical steroid.

Discoid eczema

This is common and characteristically consists of discrete coin-shaped eczematous lesions, which may become infected, most commonly on the limbs of men.

Irritant eczema and allergic contact eczema

These terms refer to eczematous eruptions of the skin in response to exogenous agents. Detergents, alkalis, acids, solvents and abrasive dusts are common causes of irritant eczema. Allergic contact eczema represents a type IV hypersensitivity reaction to an exogenous agent. Nickel, parabens (a preservative in cosmetics and creams), colophony (in sticking plasters) and balsam of Peru (in perfumes) are common causes of allergic contact eczema. Both types of eczema account for a large amount of work loss. Patch testing may be helpful in diagnosis.

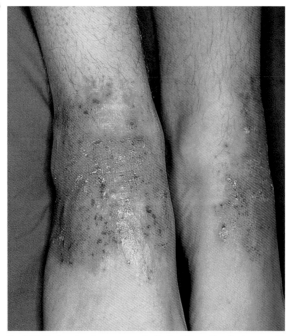

Fig. 17.9 Atopic subacute eczema on the fronts of the ankles of a teenager. These are sites of predilection, along with the cubital and popliteal fossae, in atopic eczema.

Asteatotic eczema

This occurs in dry skin, most often on the lower legs of the elderly, as a rippled or 'crazy paving' pattern of fine fissuring on an erythematous background. Low humidity caused by central heating, over-washing and diuretics are contributory factors.

Gravitational (stasis) eczema

This occurs on the lower legs and is often associated with signs of venous insufficiency (oedema, red or bluish discoloration, loss of hair, induration, haemosiderin pigmentation and ulceration).

Lichen simplex

This describes a localised plaque of lichenified eczema caused by repeated rubbing or scratching. Common sites include the neck, lower legs and anogenital area.

Pompholyx

Intensely itchy vesicles and bullae occur on the palms, palmar surface and sides of the fingers and soles. Pompholyx may have several causes, which include atopic eczema, irritant and contact allergic dermatitis and fungal infection.

Investigation and management of eczema

Patch tests are performed if contact allergic dermatitis is suspected. Bacterial and viral swabs should be taken where supra-infection is suspected. Herpes simplex virus (HSV) may cause a widespread infection, eczema herpeticum; small, punched-out lesions within worsening eczema suggest secondary HSV infection. Skin scrapings to rule out secondary fungal infection should be considered.

Regular emollients (e.g. emulsifying ointment): Applied as bath additives, soap substitutes or directly to the skin. These are the mainstay of treatment in eczema, as they limit water loss and reduce the amount of topical corticosteroid required. Sedative antihistamines are useful if sleep is interrupted.

Topical steroids: Available in a range of potencies from highly potent (clobetasol propionate), potent (betamethasone valerate) and moderately potent (clobetasone butyrate) to weakly potent (hydrocortisone, used on the face). The side-effects of topical corticosteroid therapy (thinning, striae, fragility, purpura and systemic effects) need to be considered when patients are using them for a long period of time, although 'steroid phobia' and under-treatment are often more of a problem. The least potent corticosteroid that is effective should be used for the shortest possible time. Topical calcineurin inhibitors (tacrolimus, pimecrolimus) may be useful steroid-sparing agents, particularly on the face.

PSORIASIS AND OTHER ERYTHEMATOUS ERUPTIONS

Psoriasis

Psoriasis is a chronic inflammatory hyperproliferative skin disease, characterised by well-defined erythematous scaly plaques, particularly affecting the extensor surfaces and scalp. It follows a relapsing and remitting course. The prevalence is 1.5–3% in European populations but less in African and Asian populations. Pathology reveals keratinocyte proliferation and an inflammatory infiltrate. The cause is unknown but there is a large familial component, and several linked genes have been identified. Precipitating factors include:

• Trauma. • Intercurrent infection. • Certain drugs (β-blockers, antimalarials, lithium). • Stress/anxiety.

There are five main clinical presentations:

Plaque psoriasis: This the most common type, consisting of the well-recognised salmon-pink plaques with silvery scale arising on the elbows, knees and back (Fig. 17.10). The scalp is involved in ~60% of patients. Nail disease is common, with pitting of the nail plate, onycholysis or subungual hyperkeratosis (Fig. 17.11). Psoriasis of the flexures (e.g. natal cleft, axillae, submammary folds) looks red, shiny and symmetrical, but not scaly.

Guttate psoriasis: This is most common in children and adolescents, and often follows a streptococcal sore throat. The onset is rapid, and the lesions consist of small, raindrop-sized, scaly plaques.

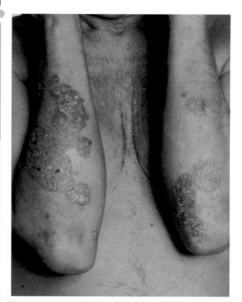

Fig. 17.10 Chronic plaque psoriasis affecting the extensor surfaces.

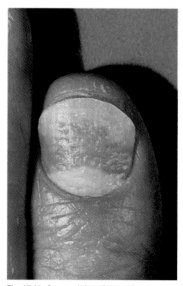

Fig. 17.11 Coarse pitting of the nail and separation of the nail from the nail bed (onycholysis). These are both classic features of psoriasis.

Guttate psoriasis responds well to phototherapy. The majority of these patients later develop plaque psoriasis.

Erythrodermic psoriasis: Generalised erythrodermic psoriasis is a medical emergency that may cause acute skin failure (p. 696).

Pustular psoriasis: This may be generalised or localised. The rare generalised form is a dermatological emergency, presenting with large numbers of sterile pustules on an erythematous base. The patient is unwell with swinging pyrexia, and requires hospital admission. The localised form is less serious, though extremely uncomfortable, and generally affects the palms and the soles (palmoplantar pustulosis). This condition is closely linked to smoking.

Psoriatic arthropathy: See page 588.

Diagnosis and management

The diagnosis is clinical, but should include swabs to exclude infection and liaison with Rheumatology if joints are affected. Disease impact scores (e.g. Dermatology Life Quality Index, DLQI) are also valuable.

The psychosocial impact of psoriasis is considerable, and reassurance and counselling are vital to management. Treatment should be individualised according to disease impact and after full discussion of side-effects. Limited chronic plaque psoriasis should be manageable with topical agents only, whereas more extensive disease may require phototherapy or systemic agents.

Topical agents: Dithranol, tar and vitamin D analogues (calcitriol, calcipotriol) all reduce plaques. Corticosteroids are used sparingly, mainly for flexures.

Phototherapy: UVB or PUVA is effective in moderate to severe psoriasis but extensive PUVA carries a long-term risk of skin cancer.

Systemic agents: Retinoids, methotrexate and ciclosporin are effective but may cause significant side-effects. Infliximab, etanercept and adalimumab may be considered when other treatments have failed.

Lichen planus

Lichen planus is an idiopathic rash characterised by intensely itchy polygonal papules with a violaceous hue, most commonly involving the volar aspects of the wrists, and the lower back (Fig. 17.12). Between 30 and 70% of patients have oral mucosal involvement: an asymptomatic fine, white, lacy network of papules known as Wickham's striae (p. 690).

The diagnosis is clinical but biopsy for histopathology may be required in atypical cases. Potent topical steroids may ease the itch; ciclosporin, retinoids and phototherapy have all been tried for more recalcitrant cases. Resolution usually occurs after ~1 yr, leaving post-inflammatory staining of the skin.

Urticaria (nettle rash, hives)

Urticaria refers to an area of focal dermal oedema secondary to a transient increase in capillary permeability, largely mediated by

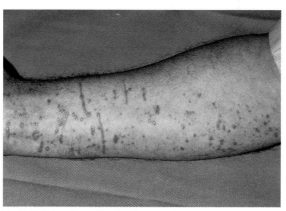

Fig. 17.12 Lichen planus. Glistening discrete papules involving the volar aspects of the forearm and wrist. Note the lesions along scratch marks (Köbner phenomenon).

17.5 Causes of urticaria

Acute and chronic urticaria

- Autoimmune due to production of antibodies that cross-link the IgE receptor on mast cells
- Allergens in foods, inhalants and injections
- Drugs (see Box 17.9)
- Physical, e.g. heat, cold, pressure, sun, water
- Contact, e.g. animal saliva, latex
- Infection, e.g. intestinal parasites
- Other conditions, e.g. systemic lupus erythematosus, pregnancy
- Idiopathic

Urticarial vasculitis

- Hepatitis B
- Systemic lupus erythematosus
- Idiopathic

mast cell degranulation releasing histamine and other mediators. If oedema involves subcutaneous or submucosal layers, the term angioedema is used. Acute urticaria may be associated with angioedema of the lips, face, tongue and throat, and even with anaphylaxis (p. 27).

Clinical features

By definition the swelling lasts <24 hrs. Urticarial vasculitis has a similar clinical presentation but lesions last >24 hrs. Most cases are idiopathic but physical, drug-induced, infection-related and autoimmune forms exist (Box 17.5). A record of possible allergens, including drugs (see Box 17.9 below), should be determined. A family history must be sought in cases of angioedema, in order to determine the likelihood of underlying C1 esterase inhibitor deficiency. Dermographism (urticaria appearing after firm pressure on the skin) may be elicited on examination.

Investigations

These should be guided by the history. Some or all of the following may be appropriate:
- FBC: eosinophils suggest parasitic infection or drug reaction. • ESR: elevated in vasculitis. • U&Es, LFTs and TFTs: to detect underlying disorders. • Total and specific IgE to possible allergens, e.g. shellfish and peanuts. • Antinuclear factor: positive in systemic lupus erythematosus (SLE) and urticarial vasculitis. • C_3 and C_4 complement levels: if low (complement consumption), check for C1 esterase inhibitor deficiency. • Skin biopsy: if urticarial vasculitis suspected.

Management

Avoid potential triggers, such as NSAIDs and codeine-containing preparations. Non-sedating antihistamines (e.g. loratadine) are the mainstay of management. H_2-blockers (e.g. ranitidine) may be added in cases refractory to H_1-blockers alone. Montelukast, UVB therapy or short-course steroids may be tried in resistant cases. Those with features of angioedema should carry a kit for self-administration of adrenaline (epinephrine) (p. 28).

BULLOUS DISEASES

Toxic epidermal necrolysis

Toxic epidermal necrolysis (TEN) is a severe mucocutaneous blistering disease that is usually caused by a drug reaction (see Box 17.9 below). Some 1–4 wks after drug commencement, pyrexia, erythema and blistering develop, rapidly involving all skin and mucous membranes. Blisters coalesce and denude, leaving painful erythematous skin. Skin snip allows early diagnosis.

The causative drug is stopped. Treatment is supportive in an intensive care environment, with sterile dressings and emollients, scrupulous fluid balance and monitoring for infection. Sepsis and multi-organ failure are major risks. Corticosteroids increase mortality and are contraindicated.

Immunobullous diseases

Box 17.6 summarises the clinical features of the immunobullous disorders.

Bullous pemphigoid

Bullous pemphigoid (BP) is the most common immunobullous disease, with an average age of onset of 65 yrs.

17.6 Clinical and investigational findings in the immunobullous disorders

Disease	Age	Site of blisters	Nature of blisters	Involves mucous membranes	Treatment
Pemphigus vulgaris	40–60 yrs	Trunk, head	Flaccid and fragile, many erosions	100%	Systemic steroids, cyclophosphamide
Bullous pemphigoid	≥60 yrs	Trunk (esp. flexures) and limbs	Tense (see Fig. 17.1)	Occasionally	Systemic steroids, azathioprine
Dermatitis herpetiformis	Young, associated with coeliac disease	Elbows, lower back, buttocks	Excoriated and often ruptured	No	Dapsone, gluten-free diet
Pemphigoid gestationis	Young pregnant female	Periumbilical and limbs	Tense	Rare	
Epidermolysis bullosa acquisita	All ages	Widespread	Tense, scarring	Common (50%)	Immunosuppressants, but poor response
Linear IgA disease	All ages	Widespread	Tense, annular ('string of beads')	Frequent	Dapsone, prednisolone

Clinical features and diagnosis

After a prodrome of itchy erythematous rash, tense bullae develop (see Fig. 17.1). Mucosal involvement is uncommon. Biopsy reveals subepidermal blistering, an eosinophil-rich infiltrate, and IgG and C3 at the basement membrane on immunofluorescence.

Management

Very potent topical steroids may be sufficient in frail elderly patients. Tetracyclines have a role; however, most require systemic corticosteroids, often with azathioprine. The condition often burns out over a few years.

Pemphigus

Pemphigus is less common than BP and affects patients aged 40–60. It may occur secondary to drugs or malignancy ('paraneoplastic pemphigus').

Clinical features and diagnosis

Skin and mucosae are usually involved, although the skin may be spared. The blisters are flaccid, easily ruptured and often not seen intact. Biopsy shows intra-epidermal blistering, acantholysis and positive direct immunofluorescence. Circulating epidermal autoantibodies can be used to monitor activity. Investigations should screen for underlying autoimmune disease and malignancy.

Management

High-dose systemic corticosteroids are usually required. Azathioprine, cyclophosphamide and IV immunoglobulins may be used as steroid-sparing agents.

Dermatitis herpetiformis

Dermatitis herpetiformis (DH) is an autoimmune blistering disorder that occurs in up to 10% of individuals with coeliac disease. Almost all patients with DH have evidence of partial villous atrophy, even if asymptomatic.

Intact vesicles or blisters are uncommon, as the condition is so pruritic that excoriations on extensor surfaces of arms, knees, buttocks, shoulders and scalp may be the only signs.

Direct immunofluorescence shows granular IgA in the papillary dermis. A gluten-free diet may suffice but, if not, the condition is usually highly responsive to dapsone.

PIGMENTATION DISORDERS

Decreased pigmentation
Vitiligo

Vitiligo is an acquired condition affecting 1% of the population worldwide. It may be familial and is associated with other autoimmune diseases.

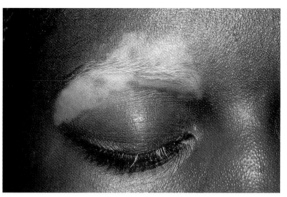

Fig. 17.13 Vitiligo. Localised patches of depigmented skin, including some white hairs. *(From White GM, Cox NH. Diseases of the skin. London: Mosby; 2000; copyright Elsevier)*

Clinical features

Focal loss of melanocytes causes patches of sharply defined depigmentation. Generalised vitiligo is often symmetrical and frequently involves the hands, wrists, knees and neck, as well as the area around the body orifices. Associated hair may also depigment (Fig. 17.13). Segmental vitiligo is restricted to one part of the body but not necessarily a dermatome. Some spotty perifollicular pigment may be seen within the depigmented patches and is sometimes the first sign of repigmentation. Sensation in the depigmented patches is normal (in contrast to tuberculoid leprosy). The course is unpredictable but most patches remain static or enlarge; a few repigment spontaneously.

Management

Protecting the patches from excessive sun exposure with clothing or sunscreen may be helpful to avoid sunburn. Camouflage cosmetics may help those with dark skin, as can potent topical corticosteroids. Narrowband UVB is the most effective repigmentary treatment available for generalised vitiligo but even very prolonged courses often do not produce a satisfactory outcome. Autologous melanocyte transfer, using split-skin or blister roof grafts, is sometimes employed on dermabraded recipient skin.

Oculocutaneous albinism

Albinism results from genetic abnormalities of melanin biosynthesis in skin and eyes but the number of melanocytes is normal (in contrast to vitiligo). It is usually inherited as an autosomal recessive trait; several types can be distinguished by genetic analysis. From birth, patients have complete absence of pigment, resulting in pale skin and white hair, and also failure of melanin production in the retina and iris. This causes photophobia, poor vision not correctable with refraction, rotatory nystagmus and alternating strabismus.

17.7 Drug-induced pigmentation	
Drug	**Appearance**
Amiodarone	Slate-grey, exposed sites
Arsenic	Diffuse bronze pigmentation with raindrop depigmentation
Bleomycin	Often flexural, brown
Busulfan	Diffuse brown
Chloroquine	Blue–grey, exposed sites
Clofazimine	Brown–grey, exposed sites
Mepacrine	Yellow
Minocycline	Slate-grey, scars, temples, shins and sclera
Phenothiazines	Slate-grey, exposed sites
Psoralens	Brown, exposed sites

These patients are at greatly increased risk of sunburn and skin cancer, and assiduous protection from sun damage is essential.

Increased pigmentation

This is mostly due to hypermelanosis but other pigments may occasionally be deposited in the skin, e.g. an orange tint in carotenaemia or a bronze hue in haemochromatosis.

Endocrine pigmentation

Chloasma describes discrete patches of facial pigmentation that occur in pregnancy and in some women taking oral contraceptives. Diffuse pigmentary change may also occur in Addison's disease, Cushing's syndrome, Nelson's syndrome and chronic renal failure.

Drugs causing hyperpigmentation

These are shown in Box 17.7.

HAIR DISORDERS

Alopecia

The term means nothing more than loss of hair and is a sign rather than a diagnosis. It is subdivided into localised or diffuse types and also into scarring or non-scarring alopecia. The causes of alopecia are summarised in Box 17.8.

Alopecia areata: This common, non-scarring autoimmune condition appears as well-defined, non-inflamed bald patches, usually on the scalp. Pathognomonic 'exclamation mark' hairs are seen (broken-off hairs 3–4 mm long, tapering towards the scalp) during active hair loss. The condition may affect the eyebrows, eyelashes and beard. The hair usually regrows spontaneously in small bald patches, but the outlook is less good with larger patches and when the alopecia appears early in life or is associated with atopy. Alopecia totalis describes complete loss of scalp hair and alopecia universalis

17.8 Classification of alopecia

Localised	Diffuse
Non-scarring	
Tinea capitis, alopecia areata, androgenetic alopecia, traumatic (trichotillomania, traction, cosmetic), syphilis	Androgenetic alopecia, telogen effluvium, hypo- or hyperthyroidism, hypopituitarism, diabetes mellitus, HIV disease, nutritional deficiency, liver disease, post-partum, alopecia areata, syphilis, drug-induced (chemotherapy)
Scarring	
Developmental defects, discoid lupus erythematosus, herpes zoster, pseudopelade, tinea capitis/kerion, morphoea, idiopathic	Discoid lupus erythematosus, radiotherapy, folliculitis decalvans, lichen planopilaris

complete loss of all hair. There is an association of alopecia areata with autoimmune disorders, atopy and Down's syndrome.

Androgenetic alopecia: Male-pattern baldness is physiological in men >20 yrs old, although rarely it may be extensive and develop at an alarming pace in the late teens. It also occurs in females, most obviously after the menopause. The distribution is of bitemporal recession and then crown involvement.

Investigations

These should include FBC, U&Es, LFTs, TFTs, iron studies, an autoantibody profile and, in cases where lupus or lichen planus is suspected, a scalp biopsy.

Management of alopecia

Specific causes, such as fungal infection, should be treated. Alopecia areata sometimes responds to topical or intralesional corticosteroids. Some males with androgenetic alopecia may be helped by systemic finasteride or topical minoxidil solution. In females, anti-androgen therapy, such as cyproterone acetate, is sometimes useful. A wig may be the most appropriate treatment for extensive alopecia.

Hypertrichosis

A generalised increase in hair, hypertrichosis is commonly a side-effect of drugs, e.g. ciclosporin, minoxidil or diazoxide. Eflornithine inhibits hair growth and may be useful if the cause cannot be removed.

Hirsutism

Hirsutism is the growth of terminal hair in a male pattern in a female. The cause of most cases is unknown and, while it may occur in hyperandrogenism, Cushing's syndrome and polycystic ovary syndrome, only a small minority of patients have a demonstrable hormonal abnormality. Psychological distress is often significant and oral contraceptives containing an anti-androgen (e.g. cyproterone acetate), laser therapy or topical eflornithine may be beneficial.

NAIL DISORDERS

The nails can be affected by both local and systemic disease. The nail apparatus consists of the nail matrix and the nail plate, which arises from the matrix and lies on the nail bed. The cells of the matrix and, to a lesser extent, the bed produce the keratinous plate.

Nail-fold examination may reveal dilated capillaries and ragged cuticles in connective tissue disease (Fig. 17.14) or the boggy inflammation of paronychia, which occurs in individuals undertaking wet work, those with diabetes or poor peripheral circulation, and subsequent to vigorous manicuring.

Common nail changes and disorders
Normal variants

Longitudinal ridging and beading of the nail plate occur with age. White transverse patches (striate leuconychia) are often caused by airspaces within the plate.

Effects of trauma

Nail biting/picking: These are very common. Repetitive proximal nail-fold trauma results in transverse ridging and central furrowing of the nail.

Chronic trauma: Trauma from poorly fitting shoes and sport can cause thickening, disordered nail growth (onychogryphosis) and subsequent ingrowing toenails.

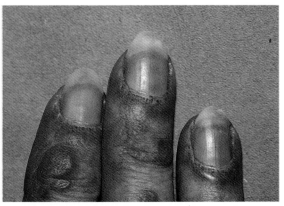

Fig. 17.14 Dermatomyositis. Erythema, dilated and tortuous capillaries in the proximal nail fold, and Gottron's papules on the digits are important diagnostic features (p. 595).

Splinter haemorrhages: Fine, linear, dark brown longitudinal streaks in the plate (p. 202) are usually caused by trauma, especially if distal. Uncommonly, they can occur in nail psoriasis and are a hallmark of infective endocarditis (p. 255).

Subungual haematoma: Red, purple or grey–brown discoloration of the nail plate, usually of the big toe, is usually due to trauma, although a history of trauma may not be clear. The main differential is subungual melanoma, although rapid onset, lack of nail-fold involvement and proximal clearing as the nail grows are clues to the diagnosis of haematoma. If there is diagnostic doubt, a biopsy may be needed.

The nail in systemic disease

Beau's lines: These transverse grooves appear at the same time on all nails, a few weeks after an acute illness, moving out to the free margins as the nails grow.

Koilonychia: This concave or spoon-shaped deformity of the plate is a sign of iron deficiency.

Clubbing: In its most gross form, this is seen as a bulbous swelling of the tip of the finger or toe. The normal angle between the proximal part of the nail and the skin is lost. Causes include:

• Respiratory: bronchogenic carcinoma, asbestosis, suppurative lung disease (empyema, bronchiectasis, cystic fibrosis), idiopathic pulmonary fibrosis. • Cardiac: cyanotic congenital heart disease, subacute bacterial endocarditis. • Other: inflammatory bowel disease, biliary cirrhosis, thyrotoxicosis, familial causes.

Discoloration of the nails: Whitening is a rare sign of hypoalbuminaemia. 'Half and half' nails (white proximally and red-brown distally) occur occasionally in patients with renal failure. Rarely, drugs (e.g. antimalarials) may discolour nails.

SKIN DISEASE IN GENERAL MEDICINE

Conditions involving cutaneous vasculature
Vasculitis

Vasculitis usually presents as palpable purpura. Causes include drugs, infection, connective tissue disease, malignancy and Henoch–Schönlein purpura. The diagnosis is confirmed by biopsy.

Pyoderma gangrenosum

Pyoderma gangrenosum (PG) presents initially as a painful, tender, inflamed nodule or pustule, which breaks down centrally and rapidly progresses to an ulcer with an indurated, undermined purplish or pustular edge (Fig. 17.15). Lesions may be single or multiple and may be ulcerative, pustular, bullous or vegetative. PG usually occurs in adults in association with underlying inflammatory bowel disease, inflammatory arthritis, blood dyscrasias, immunodeficiencies and HIV. The diagnosis is largely clinical, as histology is not specific. Analgesia, treatment of secondary bacterial infection and

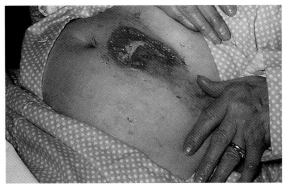

Fig. 17.15 **Pyoderma gangrenosum.** A large indolent ulcer in a patient with rheumatoid arthritis. Note healing in one part.

supportive dressings are important. Very potent topical corticosteroids or calcineurin inhibitors may be beneficial. Systemic treatment with tetracyclines, systemic steroids, dapsone, ciclosporin or other immunosuppressants is often required.

Pressure sores

Localised, prolonged, pressure-induced ischaemia can cause pressure sores, which occur in up to 30% of the hospitalised elderly, with considerable morbidity, mortality and expense. The main risk factors are immobility, poor nutrition and tissue hypoxia – e.g. with anaemia, peripheral vascular disease, diabetes, sepsis and skin atrophy.

Prevention is key and involves identification of at-risk patients and regular repositioning and use of pressure-relieving mattresses.

Connective tissue disease

Lupus erythematosus

The autoimmune disorder lupus erythematosus can be subdivided into systemic lupus erythematosus (SLE) and cutaneous lupus, which includes discoid lupus (DLE) and subacute cutaneous lupus erythematosus (SCLE).

DLE: This presents as scaly red plaques, with follicular plugging, on photo-exposed areas of the face, head and neck, which resolve with scarring and pigmentary change. Scalp involvement causes scarring alopecia. Most patients with DLE do not develop SLE.

SCLE: Patients may have extensive cutaneous involvement, usually aggravated by sun exposure, with an annular, polycyclic or papulosquamous eruption. Systemic involvement is uncommon and the prognosis usually good.

A diagnosis of cutaneous lupus is confirmed by histopathology and immunofluorescence. SLE is a described on page 590. Drug-induced lupus should always be considered (Box 17.9).

17.9 Clinical patterns of drug eruptions

Reaction pattern	Appearance	Examples of causative drugs
Exanthematous	Erythema, maculopapular	Antibiotics, anticonvulsants, gold, penicillamine, NSAIDs, carbimazole, biological therapies
Urticaria and angioedema	Itchy weals, sometimes with angioedema	Salicylates, opiates, NSAIDs, antibiotics, dextran, ACEI
Lichenoid	See Fig. 17.12	Gold, penicillamine, antimalarials, anti-TB drugs, thiazides, NSAIDs, β-blockers, ACEI, PPIs, quinine, sulphonamides, lithium, sulphonylureas, dyes
Purpura and vasculitis	Palpable purpura/ necrosis	Allopurinol, antibiotics, ACEI, NSAIDs, aspirin, anticonvulsants, diuretics, OCP
Erythema multiforme	See Fig. 17.17	See p. 727
Erythema nodosum	See p. 728	See p. 728
Exfoliative dermatitis	May be erythroderma	Allopurinol, carbamazepine, penicillins, isoniazid, gold, lithium, penicillamine, ACEI
Toxic epidermal necrolysis	See p. 715	Anticonvulsants, sulphonamides, sulphonylureas, NSAIDs, terbinafine, antiretrovirals, allopurinol
Photosensitivity	See p. 693	Thiazides, amiodarone, quinine, fluoroquinolones, sulphonamides, phenothiazines, tetracyclines, NSAIDs, retinoids, psoralens
Drug-induced lupus	Discoid or urticarial	Allopurinol, thiazides, ACEI, hydralazine anticonvulsants, β-blockers, gold, minocycline, penicillamine, lithium
Psoriasiform rash	See Fig. 17.10	Antimalarials, β-blockers, NSAIDs, lithium, anti-TNF
Acneiform eruptions	Rash resembles acne	Lithium, anticonvulsants, OCP, anti-TB drugs, androgenic/glucocorticoid steroids, EGFR antagonists, e.g. cetuximab
Pigmentation	–	See Box 17.7 (p. 719)
Pseudoporphyria	Blisters, hypertrichosis on hands	NSAIDs, tetracyclines, retinoids, furosemide, nalidixic acid
Drug-induced immunobullous disease	See Fig. 17.1	Penicillamine, ACEI, vancomycin
Fixed drug eruptions	Round erythema, oedema ± bullae	Tetracyclines, sulphonamides, penicillins, quinine, NSAIDs, barbiturates, anticonvulsants
Hair loss	Diffuse	Cytotoxics, retinoids, anticoagulants, lithium, anticonvulsants, antithyroid drugs, OCP, infliximab
Hypertrichosis	See p. 720	Diazoxide, minoxidil, ciclosporin

(ACEI = angiotensin-converting enzyme inhibitor; EGFR = epidermal growth factor receptor; OCP = oral contraceptive; PPI = proton pump inhibitor)

17 · **SKIN DISEASE**

724

Cutaneous lupus may respond to topical corticosteroids or immunosuppressants. Antimalarials and photoprotection are also important, and systemic immunosuppression or low-dose UVA1 phototherapy may be required for resistant disease.

Systemic sclerosis

This autoimmune multisystem disease is described on page 592. Skin features start with Raynaud's phenomenon, followed by progressive skin tightening and oedema. Constricted mouth opening, perioral radial furrows, matted telangiectasiae and pigmentary change are common. Fixed flexion deformities of the hands, ulceration, dilated nail-fold capillaries, calcification, scarring and digital gangrene may develop.

Morphoea

Morphoea is a localised cutaneous form of scleroderma that can affect any site at any age. It presents as a thickened violaceous plaque, which may become hyper- or hypopigmented. Topical corticosteroids, immunosuppressants or phototherapy can be effective.

Dermatomyositis

This rare multisystem disease is described on page 595. Cutaneous features include a violaceous 'heliotrope' rash periorbitally, involving the upper eyelids. A more extensive, photoaggravated rash may involve the trunk, limbs and hands, with papules over the knuckles (Gottron's papules, see Fig. 17.14).

Granulomatous disease

Granuloma annulare

This is a common cutaneous condition of uncertain aetiology; any association with diabetes is now thought to be spurious. Dermal nodules occur singly or in an annular configuration. They are asymptomatic and commonly occur on highly visible sites, such as the hands and feet. Intralesional corticosteroids can be helpful but most nodules spontaneously resolve over years.

Necrobiosis lipoidica

This condition is important to recognise because of its association with diabetes mellitus. Typically, the lesions appear as shiny, atrophic and slightly yellow plaques on the shins (Fig. 17.16). Underlying telangiectasia is easily seen. Minor knocks may precipitate slow-healing ulcers. Fewer than 1% of people with diabetes have necrobiosis, but more than 85% of patients with necrobiosis will have or will develop diabetes.

No treatment is very effective. Topical and intralesional corticosteroids are used, as is PUVA.

Sarcoidosis

Cutaneous manifestations of sarcoid are seen in about one-third of patients with systemic disease. Variants include:

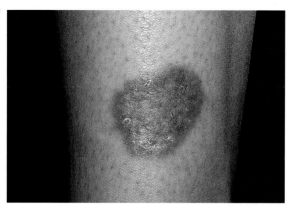

Fig. 17.16 Necrobiosis lipoidica. An atrophic yellowish plaque on the skin of a person with diabetes.

• Erythema nodosum. • Dusky infiltrated plaques on the nose and fingers (lupus pernio). • Scattered brownish-red, violaceous or hypo-pigmented papules or nodules that vary in number, size and distribution.

Metabolic disease
Porphyria

The porphyrias are a group of rare disorders of the haem biosynthe-sis pathway (p. 156). Some have cutaneous manifestations.

Photoexposed site blistering and fragility

Acquired porphyria cutanea tarda (PCT) is the most common por-phyria to cause these symptoms. PCT is due to a chronic liver disease (e.g. alcohol, hepatitis C), in combination with liver iron overload. The underlying liver disease is usually only diagnosed on investigation of the skin presentation. Typical features are increased skin fragility, blistering erosions, hypertrichosis and milia occurring on light-exposed areas, such as the backs of the hands. Other por-phyrias that can cause similar skin features include variegate por-phyria and hereditary coproporphyria.

Pain on daylight exposure

Erythropoietic protoporphyria is a rare inherited porphyria but is important to consider. The presentation is usually in early child-hood, although the diagnosis is often delayed, in part because physi-cal signs are often minimal despite the prominence of symptoms on sunlight exposure.

Abnormal deposition disorders
Xanthomas
Deposits of fatty material in the skin, subcutaneous fat and tendons may be the first clue to primary or secondary hyperlipidaemia (see page 202).

Amyloidosis
Cutaneous amyloid may present as periocular plaques in primary systemic amyloidosis (p. 155) and amyloid associated with multiple myeloma, but is uncommon in amyloidosis secondary to chronic inflammatory diseases. Amyloid infiltration of blood vessels may manifest as 'pinch purpura' following skin trauma. Macular amyloid, pruritic grey–brown macules or patches, usually on the back, is more common in darker skin types.

Genetic disorders
Neurofibromatosis
This is described on page 672.

Tuberous sclerosis
This is an autosomal dominant condition with hamartomas affecting many systems. Diagnosis is made on the basis of the classical triad of mental retardation, epilepsy and skin lesions:
• Pale oval patches on the skin (ash leaf macules). • Yellowish-pink papules on the face (adenoma sebaceum). • Peri-/subungual fibromas. • Connective tissue naevi (shagreen patches, often on the lower back).

Gum hyperplasia, retinal phakomas (fibrous overgrowth), renal, lung and heart tumours, cerebral gliomas and calcification of the basal ganglia may also occur.

Reactive disorders
Erythema multiforme
Erythema multiforme has characteristic clinical and histological features, and is thought to be an immunological reaction triggered by infections (e.g. herpes simplex, orf, *Mycoplasma*), drugs (especially sulphonamides, penicillins and barbiturates) and occasionally by sarcoidosis, malignancy or SLE. A cause is not always identified. Lesions are multiple, erythematous, annular, targetoid 'bull's eyes' and may blister (Fig. 17.17). Stevens–Johnson syndrome is a severe variant with marked blistering, mucosal involvement (mouth, eyes and genitals) and systemic upset.

Identification and removal/treatment of triggers are essential. Analgesia and topical steroids may provide symptomatic relief. Supportive care is required in Stevens–Johnson syndrome, including ophthalmology input. Systemic corticosteroids may increase the risk of infection, and the role for IV immunoglobulins is controversial.

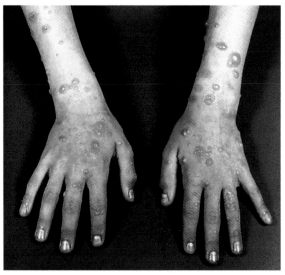

Fig. 17.17 Erythema multiforme with blistering lesions in a young woman.

Erythema nodosum

This septal panniculitis of subcutaneous fat causes painful, indurated violaceous nodules on the shins and lower legs. Malaise, fever and joint pains are common. The lesions resolve slowly over a month, leaving bruise-like marks.

Causes include:

• Infections: bacteria (streptococcus, mycobacteria, *Brucella*, *Rickettsia*, *Chlamydia*, *Mycoplasma*), viruses (hepatitis B, infectious mononucleosis) and fungi. • Drugs: e.g. sulphonamides, sulphonylureas, oral contraceptive pill. • Systemic diseases, especially sarcoidosis, inflammatory bowel disease, malignancy.

The underlying cause should be determined and treated. Bed rest and oral NSAIDs may hasten resolution. Tapering systemic corticosteroid courses may be required in stubborn cases.

Acanthosis nigricans

This is a velvety hyperkeratosis and pigmentation of the major flexures, particularly the axillae. Causes include obesity, insulin resistance syndromes and malignancy, usually adenocarcinoma, particularly gastric. Pruritus is a feature of malignancy-associated acanthosis, and the mucous membranes may be involved.

Drug eruptions

Cutaneous drug reactions are common and almost any drug can cause them. Drug reactions may reasonably be included in the differential diagnosis of most skin diseases. Presentations are summarised in Box 17.9. Common to most drug eruption is symmetry, and a temporal relationship to the commencement of the suspected drug. Eosinophilia or abnormal LFTs may occur but there are no specific investigations that help.

Management

• Withdrawal of the offending drug. • Oral antihistamines for itch. • Short course of oral prednisolone or potent topical steroid for symptomatic relief. • Emollient.

Therapeutics and prescribing

Simon Maxwell

18

Prescribing medicines is the major tool used by most doctors to cure or ameliorate disease, alleviate symptoms and prevent future illness. However, the beneficial effects of the drugs these medicines contain must be weighed against the risks of adverse drug reactions (ADRs) and interactions, often caused by injudicious prescribing decisions and by prescribing errors. Good prescribers take into account the diagnosis and disease pathophysiology, the realistic goals of treatment for the patient, the pharmacology of the proposed medication, and the impact of individual patient-related factors (e.g. age, sex, comorbidities such as hepatic or renal failure, and interacting drugs) when selecting a treatment regimen, and only prescribe when the balance of benefit to harm is favourable. They will then counsel the patient about the prescription and monitor the outcome, both beneficial and harmful, before deciding to amend or change the prescription.

Prescribing is probably the greatest challenge facing newly qualified doctors. They are required to prescribe a wide variety of drugs, many unfamiliar, for patients with diverse clinical problems who are often elderly and vulnerable, have several established conditions, and take several other drugs. These encounters often happen in busy, time-pressured clinical environments with minimal supervision. In these circumstances, the new doctor should ideally be able to draw on a good understanding of the principles of therapeutics and prescribing, a reasonable knowledge of commonly prescribed drugs and the ability to find additional information when it is required.

This chapter provides some basic advice on writing prescriptions and on the specific factors that should be taken into account when prescribing for patients with special requirements. It also provides concise summaries of some important drug classes, including the mode of action, important adverse effects, contraindications and interactions, and a guide to their use in clinical practice. The list is not comprehensive and is intended to be a brief introduction. Readers should refer to the *British National Formulary* or other equivalent resources for more detailed and regularly updated guidance.

WRITING A DRUG PRESCRIPTION

A prescription is the means by which a prescriber communicates the intended plan of treatment to the pharmacist who dispenses a medicine and to a nurse or patient who administers it. It should be precise, accurate, clear and legible. This is easy to achieve when using the electronic prescribing systems that are now common in primary care but the majority of hospital prescriptions are still hand-written. Simple guidance on writing a prescription is given in Box 18.1.

In the UK, the Misuse of Drugs Act (1971), and subsequent updates such as the Controlled Drugs (Supervision of Management and Use) Regulations (2006) regulate the possession and supply of 'controlled drugs' that are at risk of misuse. The requirements for the prescription of controlled drugs are listed in Box 18.1. Doctors in other countries should make themselves familiar with local regulations.

ALTERING DOSAGES IN RENAL IMPAIRMENT

If a drug (or an active metabolite) is predominantly eliminated from the body by the kidneys, there is a risk of accumulation and adverse effects in patients with renal impairment. This can be avoided by reducing the regular maintenance dosage or choosing an alternative drug. It is not usually necessary to reduce the dosage of drugs given as a single dose. Patients with renal impairment are readily identified by having a low estimated glomerular filtration rate (eGFR <60 mL/min) based on their serum creatinine, age, sex and ethnic group (p. 159), and this can be used as a guide to reducing maintenance dosages.

The pharmacodynamic response to some drugs is significantly enhanced in renal impairment, even if elimination is unimpaired, and these require careful monitoring or should be avoided. In contrast, the response to diuretics is reduced because of the poor access to their site of action in the renal tubules and reduced filtration of sodium and water. Box 18.2 gives a brief list of drugs that require dosage reduction or additional monitoring, or which should be avoided altogether in renal impairment.

ALTERING DOSAGES IN HEPATIC FAILURE

The liver has a large functional capacity for drug metabolism, and hepatic insufficiency has to be advanced before it significantly alters

18.1 How to write a prescription

General

- Write in block capitals, legibly, with black ballpoint pen
- Do not amend what is already written; if you make a mistake, start again

Patient identity

- Write this clearly and unambiguously, including surname, one forename, initials, date of birth (with age if <12 or >60 yrs), health-care number and address
- For hospital charts, use the correct 'addressograph' label on the front of the chart and write the identity on subsequent pages
- Give the patient's weight and height when this required in order to calculate safe doses for many drugs with narrow therapeutic indices

Drug sensitivities/allergies

- Fill in this box on hospital charts and check it before writing new prescriptions
- Obtain further details of the drug history if in doubt

Drug names

- Use the generic International Non-proprietary Name (INN) rather than brand name (e.g. 'SIMVASTATIN' not 'ZOCOR®'). The only exceptions are when variation occurs in the properties of alternative branded formulations (e.g. modified-release preparations of drugs such as lithium, theophylline, phenytoin and nifedipine) or when the drug is a combination product with no generic name (e.g. 'Kliovance®')
- Do not use abbreviations (e.g. write 'ISOSORBIDE MONONITRATE' not 'ISMN')
- If outside hospital, identify the formulation, its strength and the quantity to be supplied

Drug dosage

- Remember that the only acceptable abbreviations are 'g' and 'mg'. 'Units' (e.g. of insulin or heparin), 'micrograms' and 'nanograms' must always be written in full, never as 'U', 'μg' (nor 'mcg', nor 'ug') or 'ng'
- Avoid decimal points (e.g. 500 mg not 0·5 g) or, if unavoidable, put a '0' in front of it (e.g. '0·5 micrograms' not '·5 micrograms')
- Do not use a decimal point for round numbers (e.g. '7 mg' not '7.0 mg')
- For liquid preparations write the dose in mg; 'mL' can only be written for a combination product (e.g. Gaviscon® liquid) or if the strength is not expressed in weight (e.g. adrenaline (epinephrine) 1 in 1000)
- Use numbers/figures (e.g. 1 or 'one') to denote use of a sachet/enema but avoid prescribing numbers of tablets without specifying their strength
- Always include the dose of inhaled drugs in addition to stating numbers of 'puffs', as strengths can vary
- State a maximum dose as necessary for some drugs (e.g. colchicine in gout)

Route and method of administration

- If you wish to abbreviate, use these widely accepted abbreviations: intravenous – 'IV'; intramuscular – 'IM'; subcutaneous – 'SC'; sublingual

Continued

– 'SL'; per rectum – 'PR'; per vaginam – 'PV'; nasogastric – 'NG'; inhaled – 'INH'; topical – 'TOP'. Prefer 'ORAL' to per oram – 'PO'
* Never abbreviate 'INTRATHECAL'
* Take care when specifying 'RIGHT' or 'LEFT' for eye and ear drops. It may be necessary to specify the method of giving a medicine intravenously (e.g. as a single undiluted bolus injection, or as an infusion in a specified volume of saline over a specified time)

Frequency and timing of administration

* Write as: e.g. furosemide 40 mg orally once daily; amoxicillin 250 mg orally three times daily
* If you wish to abbreviate, use these widely accepted Latin abbreviations for dose frequency: once daily – 'OD'; twice daily – 'BD'; three times daily – 'TDS'; four times daily – 'QDS'; as required – 'PRN'; in the morning – 'OM' (omni mane); at night – 'ON' (omni nocte); immediately – 'STAT'
* On hospital charts identify specific times for regular medicines that coincide with nursing 'drug rounds'
* If treatment is for a known time period, cross off subsequent days when the medicine is not required. If a drug is not to be given every day, cross off the days when it is not required
* For 'as required' (PRN) medicines describe the indication, frequency, minimal time interval between doses, and maximum dose in any 24-hr period

Additional information

* Add any important information, e.g. whether a medicine should be taken with food, type of inhaler device to be used, and anything else that the drug dispenser or patient should know
* In hospital, indicate the times for peak/trough plasma levels for drugs requiring therapeutic monitoring

Controlled drugs

* Remember the need for clarity concerning the form and strength of all preparations; for liquids, the total volume in millilitres (in both words and figures) of the preparation to be supplied; for dosage units, the number (in both words and figures) of dosage units to be supplied; in any other case, the total quantity (in both words and figures) of the controlled drug to be supplied (e.g. 'diamorphine 30 (thirty) mg injection, 60 (sixty) mg daily by subcutaneous infusion, supply 6 (six) ampoules')

Prescriber identity

* Sign and print your name clearly (with your address if outside hospital) so that you can be identified by professional colleagues
* Date the prescription

18.2 Drugs to be used with caution in renal impairment*

GI diseases	H_2-receptor antagonists (e.g. ranitidine, cimetidine) Aminoglycosides (e.g. sulfasalazine, mesalazine) Metoclopramide
Cardiovascular diseases	Digoxin Potassium-sparing diuretics (e.g. spironolactone) ACE inhibitors (e.g. lisinopril) Angiotensin-receptor antagonists (e.g. losartan) Some β-blockers (e.g. atenolol, bisoprolol, sotalol) Fibrates Low molecular weight heparins (e.g. enoxaparin)
Neurological diseases	Opioid analgesics (e.g. morphine, codeine, fentanyl, oxycodone) Other analgesics (e.g. gabapentin, pregabalin) Anti-epileptics (e.g. levetiracetam, topiramate, vigabatrin)
Psychiatric diseases	Lithium – *monitor plasma concentration* Some tricyclic antidepressants (e.g. trazodone, lofepramine) Some selective serotonin re-uptake inhibitors (e.g. sertraline, citalopram) Some second-generation antipsychotics (e.g. amisulpride, risperidone, clozapine)
Infectious diseases	Penicillins (e.g. amoxicillin, co-amoxiclav) Cephalosporins (e.g. ceftazidime) Piperacillin Tetracyclines – *avoid (except doxycycline and minocycline)* Carbapenems (e.g. meropenem) Nitrofurantoin Chloramphenicol Aminoglycosides (e.g. gentamicin) – *monitor plasma concentration* Vancomycin – *monitor plasma concentration* Fluconazole Isoniazid Antiviral drugs (e.g. famciclovir, aciclovir, ganciclovir, zidovudine, lamivudine)
Endocrine diseases	Insulin Metformin – *avoid if eGFR <30 mL/min* Sulphonylureas (e.g. gliclazide, chlorpropamide) Dipeptidyl peptidase-IV inhibitors (e.g. sitagliptin)
Musculoskeletal diseases	Methotrexate NSAIDs (e.g. ibuprofen, diclofenac) – *avoid* Allopurinol Colchicine Penicillamine Azathioprine

*More detailed guidance is available in the *British National Formulary* and comparable national guidelines. Renal replacement therapy will improve the clearance of some of these drugs.

THERAPEUTICS AND PRESCRIBING · **18**

the pharmacokinetic handling of most drugs. Patient features that should alert prescribers to this situation are:

• Jaundice. • Ascites. • Prolonged prothrombin time. • Hypo-albuminaemia. • Malnutrition. • Encephalopathy.

Any of these features makes clinically relevant impairment of drug metabolism more likely. This may mean that orally administered drugs with extensive 'first-pass' metabolism after absorption from the gut are more readily bioavailable and achieve higher peak concentrations after oral administration. They will then tend to accumulate after regular doses because of the reduced rate of clearance.

In contrast to renal impairment, there is no easy way of predicting the appropriate reduction in dosage in patients with impaired hepatic function. Dosages of drugs that are metabolised by the liver should therefore be altered according to the therapeutic response, and with careful clinical monitoring for signs of known adverse effects. Box 18.3 gives a brief list of drugs that require dosage reduction or additional monitoring, or which should be avoided altogether in hepatic failure.

ALTERING DOSAGES IN OLDER PEOPLE

Both the pharmacokinetic handling and pharmacodynamic responses to drugs change with age, increasing the inter-individual variability and vulnerability to ADRs. The major underlying causes are:

Altered pharmacokinetic handling: Renal function declines and drugs are more likely to accumulate in the frail elderly, even when given in standard dosage (e.g. digoxin). Drug distribution is sometimes altered because of reduced body weight and a greater proportion of fat, favouring accumulation of lipid-soluble drugs.

Reduced physiological reserve: Organs such as the CNS, cardiovascular system and kidneys are less able to compensate for any adverse pharmacological effects than in younger patients (e.g. antihypertensive drugs causing falls, drugs acting on the brain causing sedation or delirium).

Comorbidities: Coexisting conditions are more likely and may be adversely affected by drug therapy (e.g. calcium channel blockers exacerbating left ventricular (LV) dysfunction, NSAIDs exacerbating renal impairment).

Polypharmacy: Elderly patients are increasingly prescribed drugs to treat or prevent the diseases of old age, and many of these have the potential for pharmacokinetic or pharmacodynamic interactions (Box 18.4).

Adherence: Adherence to the treatment regimen may be compromised because of cognitive impairment, reduced manual dexterity, difficulty swallowing (e.g. dry mouth) and complex therapeutic regimens.

For all of these reasons prescribers should generally begin treatment with lower doses, titrate more cautiously and monitor the

i 18.3 Drugs to be used with caution in liver disease

High-clearance drugs*

- Antipsychotics
- β-blockers (e.g. propranolol, labetolol)
- Calcium channel blockers
- Lidocaine
- Nitrates (e.g. glyceryl trinitrate)
- Opioids (e.g. morphine)
- Selective serotonin re-uptake inhibitors
- Statins (e.g. simvastatin)
- Tricyclic antidepressants

Low-clearance drugs

- Amiodarone
- Anticonvulsants (most)
- Antimalarials
- Antiparkinsonian drug
- Antithyroids
- Benzodiazepines
- Corticosteroids
- NSAIDs
- Paracetamol
- Proton pump inhibitors
- Quinidine
- Retinoids
- Rifampicin
- Spironolactone
- Sulphonylureas
- Theophylline
- Warfarin

Drugs that have increased risks of adverse effects

- Metformin – *lactic acidosis*
- Sulphonylureas – *hypoglycaemia*
- NSAIDs – *GI bleeding*
- Warfarin – *over-anticoagulation*

*Drugs with high hepatic clearance (i.e. extraction ratio) are particularly sensitive to the effects of liver disease, which reduces their first-pass metabolism and significantly increases oral bioavailability. They require greater dose reductions than those with a lower clearance, which are less sensitive to the effects of liver disease.

effects of new drugs or dosages with even more care in elderly patients, especially when using drugs with a low therapeutic index. Adherence may be improved by:

• Supplying medicines in pill organisers (e.g. dosette boxes or calendar blister packs). • Providing automatic reminders. • Choosing formulations that are easily swallowed. • Regularly reviewing and simplifying the drug regimen (e.g. once-daily drugs if possible).

18.4 Common drug interactions

Mechanism	Interacting drugs		Result
	Object	Precipitant	
Pharmacokinetic interactions			
Absorption			
Reduced absorption	Tetracyclines	Calcium, aluminium, magnesium salts	Reduced tetracycline absorption
Distribution			
Reduced protein binding	Phenytoin	Aspirin	Reduced phenytoin plasma concentration with same therapeutic effect
Metabolism			
Reduced metabolism (CYP3A4)	Terfenadine	Grapefruit juice	Cardiac arrhythmias because of prolonged QT interval
	Warfarin	Clarithromycin	Enhanced anticoagulation
Reduced metabolism (CYP2C19)	Phenytoin	Ticlopidine	Phenytoin toxicity
Reduced metabolism (CYP2D6)	Clozapine	Paroxetine	Clozapine toxicity
Reduced metabolism (other enzymes)	Azathioprine (xanthine oxidase)	Allopurinol	Azathioprine toxicity
Increased metabolism (induction)	Ciclosporin	St John's wort	Loss of immunosuppression
Excretion			
Reduced renal elimination	Lithium	Diuretics	Lithium toxicity
	Methotrexate	NSAIDs	Methotrexate toxicity
Pharmacodynamic interactions			
Direct antagonism at same receptor	Opioid analgesics	Naloxone	Reversal of opiate effects used therapeutically
	Salbutamol	Atenolol	Inhibits bronchodilator effect
Direct potentiation at same organ system	Benzodiazepines	Alcohol	Increased sedation
	ACE inhibitors	NSAIDs	Increased risk of renal impairment
Indirect potentiation	Digoxin	Diuretics	Digoxin toxicity enhanced because of hypokalaemia
	Warfarin	Aspirin/NSAIDs	Increased risk of bleeding because of gastrotoxicity and antiplatelet effects

The following sections contain a list of drugs that are commonly prescribed by junior hospital doctors and GPs. Where possible, these are gathered together into drug classes, for which examples are provided.

Class	Drug class
Drugs	Important examples in common use
Action	Mode of action
Indications	Major clinical indications for prescribing (and any contraindications)
Usage	How the drug is used, including route and dosage
ADRs	Important side-effects, other adverse effects or interactions
Advice	Any other important advice for patients or prescribers

GI diseases
Drugs used for dyspepsia and peptic ulcer disease

The management of peptic ulcer disease is described on page 437. Important drugs used to treat symptoms of dyspepsia related to gastro-oesophageal reflux disease (GORD) and peptic ulcers include antacids, H_2-receptor antagonists and proton pump inhibitors. Other drugs, such as bismuth chelates, mucosal protectants (e.g. sucralfate) and prostaglandin analogues (e.g. misoprostol), are rarely used.

Class	Antacids
Drugs	aluminium hydroxide, magnesium carbonate, magnesium trisilicate
Action	Neutralise gastric acid
Indications	Dyspepsia
Usage	Antacids are given when symptoms occur, typically between meals and at bedtime. They may be given several times a day. They relieve symptoms but do not generally lead to ulcer healing. Liquid preparations are more effective than tablet preparations. Simeticone is added to some antacid preparations as an antifoaming agent to reduce flatulence. Alginates are added to others used in GORD to aid symptomatic relief by forming a protective mucosal raft on the surface of the stomach contents that reduces reflux
ADRs	Aluminium salts inhibit absorption of some drugs (e.g. digoxin) and are constipating, while magnesium salts can cause diarrhoea. Some antacid preparations have high sodium content and can exacerbate cardiac failure

THERAPEUTICS AND PRESCRIBING • 18

Class	Histamine₂-receptor antagonists
Drugs	ranitidine, cimetidine, famotidine
Action	Competitively inhibit H_2-receptors on parietal and enterochromaffin-like cells, thereby reducing secretion of hydrogen ions
Indications	Benign gastric or duodenal ulceration, GORD, prophylaxis of acid aspiration in obstetrics and surgery, prophylaxis of stress ulceration in critically ill patients
Usage	H_2-antagonists (e.g. ranitidine 150 mg orally twice daily) have a good safety profile and are effective in the symptomatic relief of GORD and healing of peptic ulceration (4–8-wk course). However, they provide less potent acid suppression than proton pump inhibitors and their use is therefore declining
ADRs	Diarrhoea and other GI upset, altered LFTs, headache, dizziness. Cimetidine binds to microsomal cytochrome P450 and retards oxidative hepatic drug metabolism of some other drugs (e.g. warfarin, phenytoin, theophylline)

Class	Proton pump inhibitors (PPIs)
Drugs	omeprazole, lansoprazole, pantoprazole
Action	Irreversibly inhibit H^+/K^+ ATPase (the 'proton pump') on the surface of parietal cells, thereby reducing hydrogen ion secretion
Indications	GORD, benign gastric and duodenal ulceration, eradication of *H. pylori*, prophylaxis of NSAID-associated ulcer, prophylaxis of acid aspiration due to general anaesthesia, Zollinger–Ellison syndrome, acid-related dyspepsia
Usage	PPIs (e.g. omeprazole 10–40 mg orally daily, lansoprazole 15–30 mg orally daily) cause potent acid suppression and rapid ulcer healing, and have become the treatment of choice for many of the above conditions. They are combined with two antibacterial drugs (e.g. amoxicillin, clarithromycin, metronidazole) in standard *H. pylori* eradication regimens (p. 437) and are effective in both the prevention and treatment of NSAID-associated ulcer. They are superior to H_2-antagonists for healing ulcers and oesophagitis. IV PPI treatment reduces the rate of rebleeding and need for surgery following endoscopic therapy for major peptic ulcer haemorrhage but has not been shown to influence mortality
ADRs	PPIs are well tolerated, but more common effects are GI upset (e.g. nausea, diarrhoea, flatulence), headache and dizziness. Reduced gastric acidity may increase the risk of GI infections

Drugs used for irritable bowel syndrome

Irritable bowel syndrome (IBS, p. 464) is associated with discomfort related to smooth muscle spasm, constipation or diarrhoea. Painful spasms may be relieved by antispasmodic drugs (e.g. antimuscarinic drugs, direct smooth muscle relaxants). Opioid analgesics (e.g.

codeine) should be avoided because of the risk of dependence. An osmotic laxative (e.g. macrogols) can be used to treat constipation. Loperamide may relieve diarrhoea. Many patients benefit from an increase in soluble fibre (e.g. ispaghula husk). For some patients there are important psychological factors that may be tackled with reassurance or antidepressant medication (e.g. low doses of a tricyclic antidepressant or a selective serotonin re-uptake inhibitor).

Class	Antimuscarinic antispasmodics
Drugs	atropine sulfate, hyoscine butylbromide, propantheline bromide
Action	Antagonism of the stimulatory effects of acetylcholine at muscarinic cholinergic receptors on GI smooth muscle
Indications	Management of spasm in IBS and diverticular disease. Arrhythmias, COPD, motion sickness, parkinsonism, urinary incontinence, mydriasis and cycloplegia. Used as a pre-medication and as an antidote to organophosphorus poisoning
Usage	Dicycloverine 10–20 mg orally 3 times daily, propantheline 15 mg orally 3 times daily
ADRs	Predictable adverse effects include dry mouth, blurred vision (loss of accommodation), tachycardia (palpitation and arrhythmias), urinary retention, constipation and confusion. General contraindications to antimuscarinics are myasthenia gravis, toxic megacolon, obstructive prostatic disease and angle-closure glaucoma

Class	Direct smooth muscle relaxants
Drugs	mebeverine hydrochloride, peppermint oil
Action	Direct relaxation of intestinal smooth muscle
Indications	Relieve pain in IBS and diverticular disease
Usage	Mebeverine 135–150 mg orally 3 times daily before meals
ADRs	Well tolerated but should be avoided in paralytic ileus. Peppermint oil can cause heartburn

Drugs used for diarrhoea

The most important therapeutic approach for diarrhoea is prompt fluid and electrolyte replacement (e.g. oral rehydration preparations or IV fluids) to prevent dehydration, especially in vulnerable patients such as infants and the elderly. However, there are some drugs that may be useful in reducing stool frequency in acute diarrhoea. These include antimotility drugs such as co-phenotrope, loperamide hydrochloride and opioids (e.g. codeine phosphate, morphine). Rarely, infective diarrhoeas can be treated with specific antibacterial drugs (e.g. ciprofloxacin), and diarrhoea secondary to malabsorption of bile salts in the ileum can be managed with sequestrants (e.g. colestyramine).

Drugs used for constipation

Before treating constipation it is important to establish that the patient is not being unrealistic in their expectation regarding bowel frequency and to consider the potential underlying causes. Important classes of laxative include bulk-forming laxatives, stimulant laxatives, faecal softeners and osmotic laxatives.

Class	Bulk-forming laxatives
Drugs	wheat bran, ispaghula husk, methylcellulose, sterculia
Action	Increase faecal mass, which stimulates peristalsis
Indications	Constipation, especially when secondary to inadequate dietary intake of fibre and fluid. Other indications include patients with a colostomy, ileostomy, haemorrhoids, anal fissure, IBS, and chronic diarrhoea associated with diverticular disease
Usage	Ispaghula husk is typically taken as 1 sachet in water twice daily after meals. Methylcellulose is taken as tablets twice daily with plenty of fluid
ADRs	Bulk-forming laxatives may cause flatulence and abdominal distension, and may rarely promote GI obstruction in vulnerable patients
Advice	Patients should be advised to maintain an adequate fluid intake

Class	Stimulant laxatives
Drugs	bisacodyl, sodium picosulfate, senna, glycerol, docusate sodium (also a softening agent)
Action	Stimulate intestinal motility
Indications	Constipation
Usage	Senna (15 mg orally) and bisacodyl (15 mg orally) are given as tablets at night. Glycerol is given as a suppository. Co-danthramer is a combination laxative (stimulant/softener) usually reserved for use in patients with terminal disease due to concern over potential carcinogenicity in animal studies
ADRs	Commonly cause abdominal cramp. Excessive use causes diarrhoea and associated hypokalaemia. Prolonged use may lead to an atonic, poorly functioning colon (degeneration of the myenteric plexus). Contraindicated in intestinal obstruction

Class	Faecal softeners
Drugs	arachis oil, liquid paraffin
Action	Soften and lubricate the faeces
Indications	Constipation with faecal impaction
Usage	Arachis oil (contains peanut oil) is given as an enema. Liquid paraffin is given orally
ADRs	Liquid paraffin can leak from the anus to cause local irritation

Class	Osmotic laxatives
Drugs	lactulose, macrogols, phosphates, magnesium salts, sodium citrate
Action	Increase the amount of fluid in the large bowel either by drawing fluid in or retaining the fluid they were given with. Lactulose is a semi-synthetic disaccharide. Macrogols are inert polymers of ethylene glycol
Indications	Constipation, bowel preparation for radiological investigations, hepatic encephalopathy (lactulose).
Usage	Lactulose (15 mL orally twice daily) and macrogols (Movicol® 1–2 sachets orally daily) are given as sachets dissolved in liquid. Phosphate and sodium citrate are given as enemas, especially before radiological or surgical procedures. Lactulose (30–50 mL orally 3 times daily) is given in high dose for hepatic encephalopathy, where it reduces the pH of colonic contents, thereby inhibiting ammonia-producing bacteria. Phosphate enemas are used in severe constipation (after a faecal softener such as an arachis oil enema if the stool is very hard) and for bowel evacuation prior to endoscopic and surgical procedures
ADRs	Abdominal distension, nausea, flatulence, diarrhoea

Drugs used in inflammatory bowel disease

Ulcerative colitis and Crohn's disease are chronic inflammatory diseases of the bowel that are managed with a combination of aminosalicylates (e.g. sulfasalazine), corticosteroids (e.g. prednisolone, p. 785) and drugs that affect the immune response (e.g. azathioprine, infliximab) (see p. 463 and p. 790).

Class	Aminosalicylates
Drugs	sulfasalazine (a combination of 5-aminosalicylic acid and sulfapyridine), mesalazine (5-aminosalicylic acid), balsalazide (a 5-aminosalicylic acid prodrug), olsalazine (a 5-aminosalicylic acid dimer)
Action	Exact mechanism unknown but seems to be a local anti-inflammatory effect at the colonic mucosa
Indications	Ulcerative colitis and Crohn's disease; rheumatoid arthritis (sulfasalazine)
Usage	Given either orally (e.g. sulfasalazine 1–2 g 4 times daily, mesalazine 2–4 g daily) or rectally (sulfasalazine suppository 0.5–1 g twice daily, mesalazine foam enema 1–2 g daily)
ADRs	Many potential adverse effects include GI upset, hypersensitivity reactions (e.g. rash, urticaria, Stevens–Johnson syndrome), blood disorders (e.g. anaemia, neutropenia, thrombocytopenia) and renal dysfunction
Advice	Patients should report any unexplained bleeding, bruising, sore throat or fever and an FBC should be performed. Renal function should be monitored

Drugs used in diverticular disease

Diverticular disease is treated with a diet high in fibre, including bran supplements if necessary, bulk-forming drugs (e.g. ispaghula husk), antispasmodics (e.g. mebeverine hydrochloride) for colic, and antibacterials if diverticula become infected. Antimotility drugs (e.g. codeine, loperamide) that slow intestinal motility are contraindicated.

Other drugs

For antiemetic drugs, see page 763.

Bile acid sequestrants (e.g. colestyramine) are anion-exchange resins, which form an insoluble complex with bile acids that are not absorbed from the GI tract and relieve diarrhoea in patients with ileal resections or disease. This action also promotes a reduction in serum cholesterol and is used in the treatment of hypercholesterolaemia. Colestyramine can interfere with the absorption of a number of drugs.

Supplements of pancreatin are given orally to replace the exocrine pancreatic secretions and promote the digestion of starch, fat and protein in patients with cystic fibrosis, and following pancreatectomy, gastrectomy or chronic pancreatitis.

Obesity is predominantly managed by encouraging a healthy lifestyle and restricting energy intake. For those patients with a BMI $>30 \text{ kg/m}^2$ or more, the intestinal lipase inhibitor orlistat reduces fat absorption but produces steatorrhoea as a predictable adverse effect.

Cardiovascular diseases
Drugs for hypertension

The most important drug classes used to treat hypertension, usually in combination, are the thiazide diuretics, calcium channel blockers, angiotensin-converting enzyme (ACE) inhibitors and angiotensin receptor antagonists. Guidelines for treatment of hypertension are given on page 247. Other antihypertensive drugs used in patients who are resistant to (or intolerant of) first-line drugs include alpha-adrenoceptor blocking drugs ('α-blockers'), beta-adrenoceptor blocking drugs ('β-blockers'), aldosterone antagonists (e.g. spironolactone) and vasodilator drugs (e.g. hydralazine, minoxidil). Methyldopa is a centrally acting drug that is still commonly used to treat hypertension in pregnancy.

Class	Thiazide diuretics
Drugs	bendroflumethiazide, metolazone, indapamide, chlortalidone
Action	Inhibit sodium reabsorption at the beginning of the distal convoluted tubule, causing increased loss of sodium and water
Indications	Hypertension, oedema

Class	Thiazide diuretics *(Continued)*
Usage	Low-dose thiazides (e.g. bendroflumethiazide 2.5–5 mg orally daily, chlortalidone 25–50 mg orally daily, indapamide 2.5 mg orally daily) are used to treat hypertension. The newer thiazide-like drugs chlortalidone and indapamide are increasingly prescribed because of evidence suggesting that they are more effective in preventing cardiovascular events than bendroflumethiazide. They are less effective than loop diuretics in relieving oedema, but the combination of a loop diuretic (p. 748) and a thiazide (e.g. bendroflumethiazide 5–10 mg daily) or thiazide-like diuretic (e.g. metolazone 5–10 mg daily) may produce an intense diuresis and can be helpful in resistant oedema
ADRs	Common predictable effects are dehydration and postural hypotension, and various electrolyte disturbances including hypokalaemia, hyponatraemia, hypomagnesaemia, hypercalcaemia and hypochloraemic alkalosis. Thiazides also cause metabolic disturbances, including hyperlipidaemia, hyperglycaemia, hyperuricaemia and gout

Class	Beta-adrenoceptor-blocking drugs
Drugs	propranolol, atenolol, bisoprolol, labetalol
Action	Block cardiac β_1-adrenoceptors, thereby reducing heart rate and myocardial contractility. Individual drugs vary in their relative selectivity for β_1- and β_2-adrenoceptors. Propranolol is relatively unselective, while atenolol, metoprolol and bisoprolol are relatively β_1-selective. Labetalol and carvedilol tend to cause some vasodilatation and reduce peripheral vascular resistance
Indications	Prophylaxis of angina, unstable angina, hypertension, treatment and prevention of supraventricular tachycardia and atrial fibrillation, stable heart failure, prophylaxis after myocardial infarction (MI), symptomatic relief in anxiety and thyrotoxicosis
Usage	β-blockers are effective antihypertensives but are no longer first-line treatment (p. 248), unless there is another specific indication (e.g. angina), because of uncertainty about their ability to reduce cardiovascular endpoints and an increased risk of type 2 diabetes associated with their use. Cardioselective agents (atenolol 25–100 mg orally daily, bisoprolol 2.5–10 mg orally daily) are first-line therapy for stable angina and are also used in acute coronary syndromes and as secondary prevention post-MI. β-blockers (e.g. bisoprolol 1.25 mg orally daily, increased gradually over 12 wks to a target dose of 10 mg daily) are now an important therapeutic approach in chronic heart failure. Labetalol blocks both β- and α-receptors; it is used in pregnancy and can be given as an IV infusion in accelerated phase hypertension. Propranolol (40–120 mg orally twice daily) is non-selective and has more adverse effects; it is now used mainly to relieve adrenergic symptoms (e.g. palpitation, tremor, anxiety) in thyrotoxicosis. β-blockers are also class II anti-arrhythmic drugs (p. 218)

Class	Beta-adrenoceptor-blocking drugs *(Continued)*
ADRs	Predictable effects include fatigue, reduced exercise capacity, peripheral vasoconstriction (cold peripheries, worsening of intermittent claudication and Raynaud's phenomenon), bronchospasm (even cardioselective drugs are contraindicated in asthma but may be tolerated in COPD), bradycardia and conduction disorders (contraindicated in sick sinus syndrome and heart block). Sleep disturbance and nightmares occur more frequently with lipid-soluble (e.g. propranolol) than water-soluble (e.g. atenolol) agents. Other effects include reduced awareness of hypoglycaemia in diabetes and sexual dysfunction. Abrupt withdrawal may worsen angina

Class	Calcium channel blockers (CCBs)
Drugs	amlodipine, nifedipine, diltiazem, verapamil
Action	Inhibit the slow inward calcium current in cardiac and arteriolar muscle cells, reducing contractility, sinus node activity, atrioventricular (AV) node conduction and vascular tone. Dihydropyridine CCBs (e.g. nifedipine, amlodipine) bind more selectively to vascular cells and principally cause arteriolar vasodilatation. Non-dihydropyridine CCBs (verapamil, diltiazem) bind equally to cardiac and vascular cells and possess powerful negative inotropic and chronotropic properties
Indications	Prophylaxis and treatment of angina, hypertension, supraventricular arrhythmias
Usage	Dihydropyridine CCBs (e.g. amlodipine 5–10 mg orally daily, nifedipine 20–60 mg orally daily) cause arteriolar and coronary vasodilatation, and are used in the treatment of hypertension and angina. They have no anti-arrhythmic activity and often cause a reflex tachycardia, which may be counterproductive in angina (consider combining with β-blockers). They are particularly helpful in disorders caused by vasospasm (e.g. Raynaud's phenomenon). Verapamil (40–120 mg orally 3 times daily) and diltiazem (60–120 mg orally 3 times daily) slow heart rate and inhibit conduction through the AV node. CCBs are also class IV anti-arrhythmic drugs that are used in the treatment of supraventricular arrhythmias (p. 248) and are often employed for their rate-limiting properties (e.g. in angina, permanent atrial fibrillation) in patients unable to take β-blockers. Verapamil can be given IV (5–10 mg) in emergencies
ADRs	Dihydropyridine CCBs cause predictable vasodilator effects such as peripheral oedema, flushing, headache and postural lightheadedness. The most common adverse effect of verapamil is constipation. It is also highly negatively inotropic (more so than diltiazem) and chronotropic, and may cause profound bradycardia and hypotension (IV verapamil must be avoided in patients taking β-blockers). CCBs are contraindicated in heart failure, significantly impaired LV function, sick sinus syndrome, and second- or third-degree AV block

Class	Angiotensin-converting enzyme (ACE) inhibitors
Drugs	enalapril, ramipril, lisinopril
Action	Inhibit the conversion of angiotensin I to angiotensin II, and also inhibit the breakdown of the vasodilating hormone, bradykinin. The major haemodynamic effect is a reduction in peripheral vascular resistance
Indications	Hypertension, heart failure, asymptomatic LV systolic dysfunction, diabetic nephropathy, secondary prevention in coronary artery and cerebrovascular disease
Usage	For hypertension, ACE inhibitors (e.g. enalapril 20 mg orally daily, ramipril 2.5–5 mg orally daily, lisinopril 10–40 mg orally daily) are first-line therapy for younger patients (<55 yrs) but are less effective in Afro-Caribbean patients. BP reduction is potentiated by diuretics, which activate the renin–angiotensin system. For diabetic nephropathy, ACE inhibitors retard the progression of renal failure and reduce proteinuria independently of BP reduction. For heart failure (p. 205), ACE inhibitors relieve symptoms, improve exercise capacity and reduce hospital admissions and mortality. They also reduce cardiovascular events and can delay the development of overt heart failure in patients with asymptomatic LV systolic dysfunction. For patients with established CAD or cerebrovascular disease, ACE inhibitors reduce the risk of recurrent events, irrespective of the presence of hypertension or LV dysfunction
ADRs	The most common effect is dry cough (due to increased bradykinin), which leads to discontinuation in 10–20% of patients. Other predictable effects are hypotension (including severe first-dose hypotension), rash, angioedema, hyperkalaemia and renal impairment. Particular care is required for patients taking concomitant thiazide or loop diuretics (risk of severe hypotension), potassium-sparing diuretics (risk of hyperkalaemia) or NSAIDs (risk of nephrotoxicity) and those with impaired renal function (reduction in glomerular filtration pressure may exacerbate renal failure). ACE inhibitors are contraindicated in pregnancy, bilateral renal artery stenosis and critical aortic stenosis
Advice	All patients should have their renal function checked before and during treatment. More frequent monitoring is required for certain groups (e.g. patients with renal impairment, elderly patients)

Class	Angiotensin receptor antagonists (ARAs)
Drugs	candesartan, losartan, valsartan, irbesartan
Action	Block the angiotensin II receptor, reducing the vasoconstrictor, volume regulation and other actions of angiotensin II
Indications	Hypertension, heart failure, and diabetic nephropathy in patients intolerant of ACE inhibitors

Class	Angiotensin receptor antagonists (ARAs) *(Continued)*
Usage	ARAs (e.g. losartan 25–100 mg orally daily, candesartan 4–32 mg orally daily) have similar effects to ACE inhibitors and are generally better tolerated. They are the logical alternative for patients intolerant of ACE inhibitors because of a dry cough
ADRs	Similar adverse effect profile to ACE inhibitors but generally better tolerated because they do not potentiate the effects of kinins
Advice	All patients should have their renal function monitored during treatment

Class	Alpha-adrenoceptor-blocking drugs
Drugs	doxazosin, prazosin, indoramin
Action	Post-synaptic α-blockers lead to vasodilatation and reduced peripheral vascular resistance. Relaxation of prostatic smooth muscle
Indications	Resistant hypertension, benign prostatic hypertrophy (p. 194)
Usage	α-blockers (e.g. doxazosin 1–16 mg orally daily) are reserved as additional treatment in patients resistant to (or intolerant of) the treatments above
ADRs	Hypotension and dizziness, drowsiness, weakness, reflex tachycardia
Advice	May reduce BP rapidly after the first dose and should be introduced with caution and warnings in the elderly

Drugs for heart failure

The pathophysiology of heart failure is described on page 206. A key feature is the compensatory neurohumoral responses involving the sympathetic nervous and renin–angiotensin systems that promote vasoconstriction and sodium retention. The therapeutic approach is to mitigate these responses and associated symptoms (dyspnoea and oedema) with the use of loop diuretics (e.g. furosemide), ACE inhibitors (e.g. ramipril), angiotensin receptor antagonists (e.g. candesartan), β-blockers (e.g. bisoprolol) and aldosterone antagonists (e.g. spironolactone). Cardiac glycosides (e.g. digoxin) (p. 751) are now rarely used unless heart failure is accompanied by atrial fibrillation. Patients who cannot tolerate ACE inhibitors or angiotensin receptor antagonists are sometimes given alternative vasodilators (e.g. isosorbide dinitrate, hydralazine). Acute LV failure is normally treated with a combination of oxygen, IV loop diuretics, IV opioids and IV nitrates.

Class	Loop diuretics
Drugs	furosemide, bumetanide
Action	Inhibit sodium reabsorption in the thick ascending limb of the loop of Henle in the renal tubule and have a powerful natriuretic and diuretic effect

Class	Loop diuretics *(Continued)*
Indications	Oedema, resistant hypertension
Usage	For chronic heart failure, oedema is usually controlled with furosemide 40–160 mg or bumetanide 1–4 mg orally daily. For resistant oedema caused by heart failure or other conditions, very high oral doses (e.g. 250 mg daily), an IV infusion (e.g. 10 mg/hr) or combination with a thiazide diuretic can sometimes initiate a diuresis. For acute pulmonary oedema, furosemide 50–100 mg IV normally achieves a diuresis with 30 mins when a small but significant degree of arterial and venous dilatation may also be of therapeutic benefit. For resistant hypertension associated with renal impairment, furosemide 20–80 mg orally daily may be used instead of a thiazide diuretic
ADRs	Predictable effects include dehydration, acute urinary retention, and electrolyte disturbances including hyponatraemia, hypokalaemia, hypocalcaemia, hypochloraemia, hypomagnesaemia and metabolic alkalosis. Metabolic disturbances include hyperlipidaemia, hyperglycaemia (less common than with thiazides), hyperuricaemia and gout. Ototoxicity with tinnitus and deafness (usually with high IV doses and rapid administration, and in renal impairment) is a rare but important adverse effect
Advice	Patients should have their serum electrolytes and renal function reviewed

Class	Aldosterone antagonists
Drugs	spironolactone, eplerenone
Action	Inhibit the sodium-retaining (and potassium-excreting) effects of aldosterone at the distal convoluted tubule and collecting duct
Indications	Oedema and ascites in cirrhosis of the liver, nephrotic syndrome and heart failure. Resistant hypertension. Primary hyperaldosteronism
Usage	For oedema, spironolactone 100–200 mg orally daily is normally given in combination with loop diuretics. For heart failure and resistant hypertension, lower doses (e.g. 25–50 mg daily) are given to selected patients
ADRs	Common effects include potassium retention and hyperkalaemia, particularly in patients with renal impairment or those taking interacting drugs (e.g. ACE inhibitors, ARAs). Spironolactone causes gynaecomastia but this is less likely with eplerenone, which has weaker pharmacological effects
Advice	Patients should have their serum electrolytes and renal function reviewed

Drugs for angina

Angina therapy includes the use of drugs that reduce ventricular workload by slowing the heart rate, reducing venous return, reducing arterial BP and promoting coronary vasodilatation. Standard treatment is with organic nitrates (e.g. glyceryl trinitrate), β-blockers (e.g. atenolol) and calcium channel blockers (e.g. verapamil). Nicorandil is a potassium channel activator with a nitrate component that has both arterial and venous vasodilating properties. Ivabradine reduces heart rate by a direct action on the sinus node.

Class	Organic nitrates
Drugs	glyceryl trinitrate (GTN), isosorbide dinitrate, isosorbide mononitrate
Action	Potent vasodilators with most clinical benefit resulting from venodilatation and a reduction in venous return, which reduces LV work. Long-term administration of nitrates leads to tolerance due to reduced tissue responsiveness and neurohumoral activation
Indications	Angina pectoris (prophylaxis and treatment), heart failure
Usage	GTN is given sublingually by spray or tablet (300 micrograms) to provide rapid symptomatic relief of angina, although the effects are short-lasting (20–30 mins). Isosorbide dinitrate and mononitrate are given orally as angina prophylaxis but require a daily 'nitrate-free' interval to avoid tolerance. GTN can be given IV (10–200 micrograms/min) in the emergency treatment of acute myocardial ischaemia and heart failure
ADRs	Common predictable effects are flushing, headache, and postural hypotension shortly after administration
Advice	Patients should be counselled about sublingual administration, warned about the vasodilator effects and advised when to seek help if their chest pain does not settle

Anti-arrhythmic drugs

Effective treatment of cardiac arrhythmias depends on making the correct diagnosis. AF is the most common arrhythmia and not only compromises cardiac function but significantly increases the risk of thromboembolic stroke, meaning that anticoagulation is indicated for some patients (p. 221). The main therapeutic approach is to reduce the ventricular response rate using β-blockers (e.g. atenolol), calcium channel blockers (e.g. verapamil) or cardiac glycosides (e.g. digoxin). Patients uncontrolled on standard therapy may respond to amiodarone, which has more serious adverse effects.

Paroxysmal supraventricular tachycardia frequently terminates spontaneously or with reflex vagal stimulation (e.g. a Valsalva manœuvre, carotid sinus massage) but sometimes requires IV doses of adenosine, which temporarily blocks AV node conduction. IV verapamil is an alternative but is contraindicated in patients treated with β-blockers because of the risk of complete heart block.

Ventricular tachycardia is a serious arrhythmia that usually requires urgent treatment with DC cardioversion and/or IV administration of membrane-stabilising class I (e.g. flecainide, propafenone, lidocaine) or class III (e.g. amiodarone) anti-arrhythmic drugs. Patients who remain at risk of recurrence require an implantable defibrillator and/or maintenance drug therapy with β-blockers (e.g. sotalol) or amiodarone.

Class	Cardiac glycosides
Drugs	digoxin
Action	Inhibits the Na$^+$/K$^+$ ATPase pump on cardiac myocytes, leading indirectly to an increase in intracellular calcium and causing a positive inotropic effect. Also increases vagal activity via a central effect, thereby slowing conduction through the AV node
Indications	Rate control in AF. Heart failure
Usage	For AF, digoxin 62.5–250 micrograms orally daily is effective in limiting the ventricular response rate. Its long half-life means that more urgent treatment must be initiated with a loading dose (e.g. 0.75–1.5 mg orally over 24 hrs in divided doses). It has the advantage over alternative drugs in having a positive rather than negative inotropic effect. When used as maintenance therapy, it may provide inadequate control of heart rate during exercise and is often combined with a β-blocker. For chronic heart failure, digoxin is helpful in patients with coexistent AF but of uncertain benefit in those who remain in sinus rhythm (no effect on overall survival but may reduce the need for hospitalisation). Digoxin is largely excreted by the kidneys, and the maintenance dose should be reduced in the elderly and those with renal impairment
ADRs	Common effects include anorexia, nausea, vomiting, altered colour vision, drowsiness and confusion. Cardiac manifestations include bradycardia, increased ectopy, and atrial and ventricular tachyarrhythmias. The adverse effects of digoxin are all more common in the presence of hypokalaemia or renal impairment (digoxin is renally excreted). Measurement of plasma digoxin concentration (at least 6 hrs post-dose) helps to confirm toxicity; if confirmed, treatment entails discontinuation of the drug, correction of hypokalaemia and, in severe cases, administration of digoxin-specific antibody fragments. Digoxin is contraindicated in Wolff–Parkinson–White syndrome (increases conduction through accessory pathway), second- or third-degree AV block and hypertrophic obstructive cardiomyopathy

Class	Amiodarone
Drugs	amiodarone
Action	Class III anti-arrhythmic drug (others include sotalol), which all have their main effect by blocking potassium channels to prolong cardiac repolarisation. Amiodarone has a very long half-life and requires many weeks to achieve steady state
Indications	AF, ventricular arrhythmias

Class	Amiodarone *(Continued)*
Usage	Amiodarone is a very effective treatment for supraventricular and ventricular arrhythmias but its wider use is limited by the potential adverse effects. Unlike most other anti-arrhythmic drugs, it does not depress the myocardium. After an initial loading period, maintenance dosage is 200 mg orally daily. The initial loading dose can be given IV if an urgent anti-arrhythmic effect is required
ADRs	GI upset, hepatitis, bradycardia, pulmonary infiltrates, hypothyroidism, hyperthyroidism, reversible corneal microdeposits, phototoxicity, persistent slate-grey skin discoloration
Advice	Patients should have LFTs and TFTs reviewed. They should also be warned about phototoxicity and the need to protect their skin from sunlight

Antiplatelet drugs

Antiplatelet drugs inhibit platelet aggregation and thrombus formation in the faster-flowing arterial circulation, where thrombi are composed mainly of platelets with little fibrin. The most common antiplatelet drugs are aspirin, clopidogrel and dipyridamole. Glycoprotein IIb/IIIa inhibitors (e.g. abciximab, eptifibatide, tirofiban) inhibit platelet aggregation by blocking the binding of fibrinogen to receptors on platelets. They are used to prevent thrombotic complications in high-risk patients undergoing coronary intervention.

Class	Antiplatelet drugs
Drugs	aspirin, clopidogrel, dipyridamole
Action	Aspirin irreversibly inhibits cyclo-oxygenase to reduce the production of the pro-aggregant thromboxane A_2. Clopidogrel affects the ADP-dependent activation of the glycoprotein IIb/IIIa complex. Dipyridamole inhibits platelet phosphodiesterase, causing an increase in cyclic AMP (cAMP) to potentiate the anti-aggregant action of prostacyclin
Indications	Primary and secondary prevention of thrombotic cardiovascular events in high-risk patients (e.g. after acute coronary syndromes, transient ischaemic attack (TIA) or ischaemic stroke)
Usage	Aspirin 75 mg orally daily, clopidogrel 75 mg orally daily, dipyridamole 200 mg orally 3 times daily
ADRs	Aspirin is associated with increased risk of peptic ulceration and bleeding and with hypersensitivity reactions (e.g. rash, bronchospasm, urticaria). It is contraindicated in patients at increased risk of such effects. Clopidogrel also causes GI upset. Dipyridamole can cause dizziness, hypotension and headaches

Anticoagulants and fibrinolytics

Anticoagulant drugs are mainly used to reduce thrombus formation in the slower-moving venous circulation, where thrombus consists mainly of fibrin, the end product of the coagulation cascade. The longest-established oral anticoagulants are the coumarins (e.g. warfarin), which inhibit vitamin K and require regular monitoring. Newer oral anticoagulants include direct thrombin inhibitors (e.g. dabigatran etexilate) and direct inhibitors of activated factor X (e.g. apixaban, rivaroxaban), which do not require routine anticoagulant monitoring.

Parenteral anticoagulants include unfractionated and low molecular weight heparins (e.g. dalteparin), heparinoids (e.g. danaparoid sodium) and inhibitors of thrombin (e.g. bivalirudin) or activated factor X (e.g. fondaparinux sodium).

Fibrinolytic drugs (e.g. alteplase, reteplase) act as thrombolytics by activating plasminogen to form plasmin, which breaks down fibrin within a thrombus. They are indicated in the treatment of acute MI, serious pulmonary embolus and acute stroke. All carry a serious risk of causing serious haemorrhage and are contraindicated in vulnerable patients.

Class	Coumarins
Drugs	warfarin
Action	Antagonise the effects of vitamin K as a co-factor in the formation of the key factors (II, VII, IX and X) in the extrinsic coagulation pathway
Indications	Prophylaxis and treatment of VTE. Prophylaxis of embolisation in AF. Prophylaxis of thrombus formation in patients with a prosthetic heart valve
Usage	Warfarin has to be given as a loading dose to help to achieve full anticoagulation more quickly. This normally takes at least 48–72 hrs. Patients who require immediate anticoagulation are given a parenteral anticoagulant during this period
ADRs	Bleeding is the major adverse effect but this risk can be reduced by careful monitoring of the effect of warfarin on anticoagulation using the international normalised ratio (INR). Warfarin has many pharmacokinetic interactions with drugs that inhibit its metabolism, thereby potentiating its anticoagulant effect (e.g. ciprofloxacin, clarithromycin, simvastatin, cimetidine, fluconazole). Pharmacodynamic interactions occur with antiplatelet drugs, which significantly increase the risk of bleeding
Advice	Patients should report any signs of bleeding or bruising and be warned about the importance of monitoring the INR on a regular basis. They should always inform any doctor that they are taking warfarin before any additional medicines are prescribed

Class	Low molecular weight heparins
Drugs	dalteparin sodium, enoxaparin sodium, tinzaparin sodium
Action	Activate the enzyme inhibitor antithrombin III (ATIII), which inactivates thrombin and other proteases involved in blood clotting, most notably factor Xa
Indications	Treatment and prevention of VTE. They are preferred to unfractionated heparin because they are as effective, require only once-daily injection, do not need anticoagulant monitoring and have a lower risk of heparin-induced thrombocytopenia
Usage	Given by once-daily SC injection in a dosage based on patient weight
ADRs	Bleeding. Heparin-induced thrombocytopenia. Inhibition of aldosterone secretion can result in hyperkalaemia

Lipid-lowering drugs

Statins (e.g. simvastatin) are the first-choice drugs for this indication because they are the most effective at reducing LDL cholesterol and have been shown unequivocally to reduce cardiovascular events in large-scale randomised controlled trials. Other less commonly used lipid-lowering drugs include fibric acid derivatives (e.g. fenofibrate), nicotinic acid derivatives, cholesterol absorption inhibitors (e.g. ezetimibe) and bile acid sequestrants (e.g. colestyramine).

Class	Statins
Drugs	simvastatin, atorvastatin, rosuvastatin, fluvastatin, pravastatin
Action	Competitively inhibit 3-hydroxy-3-methylglutaryl co-enzyme A (HMG CoA) reductase, the rate-limiting enzyme involved in cholesterol synthesis in hepatocytes. This action leads to up-regulation of LDL receptor expression and thereby uptake of circulating LDL. Statins are more effective at lowering LDL cholesterol concentration than other lipid-lowering drugs. Statins have been shown to reduce cardiovascular disease events and total mortality irrespective of the initial cholesterol concentration
Indications	Prevention of cardiovascular events in patients at increased risk due to hypercholesterolaemia ($\pm$ other risk factors), diabetes mellitus and established atherosclerotic cardiovascular disease
Usage	Simvastatin 10–80 mg orally at night, atorvastatin 10–80 mg orally daily, rosuvastatin 5–20 mg orally daily
ADRs	Common effects are myalgia or myositis, deranged LFTs, sleep disturbance and GI upset. The risk of myopathy is increased in the presence of interacting drugs such as fibrates, ciclosporin, clarithromycin, fluconazole, amiodarone, amlodipine and various antiretroviral drugs
Advice	Patients with myalgia should have their creatine kinase measured and if it is elevated $>5 \times$ upper limit of normal, or if muscular symptoms persist, treatment should be discontinued. LFTs should be measured before treatment and repeated within 3 mths of treatment being established

Respiratory diseases
Bronchodilators

Bronchodilators are of value in reducing airways obstruction in COPD and asthma. The main bronchodilator drug classes are the selective β_2-adrenoceptor agonists (e.g. salbutamol), antimuscarinic bronchodilators (e.g. ipratropium bromide) and the theophyllines.

Class	β_2-adrenoceptor agonists
Drugs	Short-acting β_2-agonists: salbutamol, terbutaline. Long-acting β_2-agonists (LABAs): salmeterol, formoterol
Action	Activate β_2-adrenoceptors, which relaxes airway smooth muscle (via the secondary messenger cAMP). They may exert additional anti-inflammatory effects by reducing mediator release from mast cells
Indications	Asthma, COPD. Emergency treatment of hyperkalaemia. Premature labour
Usage	Short-acting β_2-agonists (e.g. salbutamol 100–200 micrograms, terbutaline 250–500 micrograms) are best administered by inhalation using metered-dose aerosol or dry powder inhalers. In asthma and COPD they are used 'as required' for relief of wheeze. In acute severe asthma, salbutamol is given by nebuliser (2.5–5 mg) in repeated doses until bronchospasm is relieved. In COPD, nebulised administration may help if adequate doses by inhaler fail to relieve symptoms. Always check inhaler technique. For those struggling with the coordination required (e.g. young children), a spacer device may help. Long-acting β_2-agonists (e.g. salmeterol 50 micrograms twice daily, formoterol 9–18 micrograms twice daily), given by inhaler, improve asthma control in patients who remain symptomatic despite inhaled corticosteroids and short-acting β_2-agonists. In severe COPD there is some evidence that regular LABAs given with inhaled corticosteroids reduce exacerbation frequency and improve quality of life
ADRs	Common predictable adverse effects are muscle tremor (especially hands), tachycardia, palpitation, arrhythmia and headache. Hypokalaemia may occur at high doses because β_2-receptors stimulate potassium uptake into cells
Advice	Patients require careful instruction regarding good inhaler technique

Class	Antimuscarinic bronchodilators
Drugs	Short-acting: ipratropium bromide. Long-acting: tiotropium
Action	Block the stimulatory effects of acetylcholine at muscarinic (M_3) cholinergic receptors on bronchial smooth muscle and so promote bronchodilatation
Indications	COPD, asthma

Class	Antimuscarinic bronchodilators (Continued)
Usage	Ipratropium can be given either by aerosol inhalation (20–40 micrograms 3–4 times daily) or by inhalation of nebulised solution (250–500 micrograms 3–4 times daily). Tiotropium is a long-acting drug that is given by aerosol inhalation 18 micrograms once daily and is used as maintenance treatment in COPD
ADRs	Typical antimuscarinic effects include dry mouth (common), blurred vision, tachycardia (and palpitation or AF), constipation, urinary retention, mydriasis, and angle-closure glaucoma. Paradoxical bronchospasm may occur

Class	Theophyllines
Drugs	theophylline, aminophylline
Action	Non-selective phosphodiesterase inhibitors that cause weak bronchodilatation (additive effect with inhaled β_2-agonists) by increasing intracellular cAMP concentration. They may also have some respiratory stimulant and anti-inflammatory effects
Indications	Asthma, COPD
Usage	Theophylline may be used as 'add-on' therapy in asthma (step 4), if symptoms remain uncontrolled. It is occasionally used in stable severe COPD with persistent symptoms, where it may enhance the effects of inhaled corticosteroids. Theophyllines have a narrow therapeutic index (i.e. toxic plasma levels are close to the therapeutic range) and plasma theophylline concentration is useful to guide dosing (adjust to maintain in the range 10–20 mg/L). Theophylline levels are increased in hepatic impairment and heart failure, or by drugs that inhibit its metabolism (e.g. macrolide antibiotics). Plasma concentration is decreased by smoking, alcohol excess and drugs that accelerate hepatic metabolism. Use has declined following the introduction of safer alternative long-acting bronchodilators
ADRs	Nausea is common. Other predictable effects are tachycardia, palpitations, arrhythmias and convulsions

Corticosteroids

Corticosteroids are effective treatments in asthma and COPD because they reduce airway inflammation and oedema, and also the secretion of mucus into the airway. They are used systemically in high doses to treat acute exacerbations of these diseases (e.g. IV hydrocortisone, oral prednisolone) (p. 280). Inhaled corticosteroids are beneficial in stabilising all but the mildest forms of asthma (p. 279). Inhaled corticosteroids may also reduce exacerbation frequency in patients with moderate to severe COPD and frequent exacerbations.

Class	Inhaled corticosteroids
Drugs	beclometasone dipropionate, budesonide, fluticasone propionate, mometasone furoate

Class	Inhaled corticosteroids *(Continued)*
Action	Act at intracellular glucocorticoid receptors to alter gene expression and exert a powerful anti-inflammatory effect on the cells in the walls of the small airways
Indications	Prophylaxis of asthma
Usage	Corticosteroids (e.g. beclometasone 200–400 micrograms, fluticasone 100–500 micrograms twice daily) are administered by aerosol or dry powder inhalation. Compound inhaler preparations that combine a corticosteroid with a LABA are widely used
ADRs	Corticosteroids have fewer adverse effects when inhaled directly into the airways rather than administered systemically but may cause local oropharyngeal candidiasis, especially if inhaler technique is poor. High-dose inhaled corticosteroids are associated with increased risk of pneumonia, dysphonia, osteoporosis and growth suppression in children
Advice	Patients require careful instruction regarding good inhaler technique to maximise effectiveness and minimise adverse effects in the upper airways

Other drugs used for asthma and COPD

The step-wise approach to the management of asthma is described on page 279. Further measures include the use of leukotriene receptor antagonists (e.g. montelukast), theophyllines, and higher doses of inhaled or even oral corticosteroids. Sodium cromoglicate may be of value in asthma with an allergic basis.

Class	Leukotriene receptor antagonists
Drugs	montelukast, zafirlukast
Action	Block the bronchoconstrictor and pro-inflammatory effects of cysteinyl leukotrienes in the airway
Indications	Asthma
Usage	Montelukast (10 mg orally daily) or zafirlukast (20 mg orally twice daily) can be used as 'add-on' therapy for persistent asthma (step 3/4) to improve symptom control but are **not** a replacement for inhaled corticosteroids. They are particularly useful in patients with concomitant rhinitis, and also in the prevention of exercise-induced asthma
ADRs	These drugs are usually well tolerated but can cause abdominal pain, thirst or headache. Rare cases of Churg–Strauss syndrome have been reported, although it is difficult to establish direct causation

COPD is managed in a similar way to asthma, but short-acting (e.g. ipratropium) and long-acting (e.g. tiotropium) antimuscarinics are an additional therapeutic approach. Roflumilast is a phosphodiesterase type 4 inhibitor with anti-inflammatory properties that has recently been licensed as an adjunct to bronchodilators for the maintenance treatment of patients with severe COPD.

Antihistamines

Antihistamines can be used to treat allergic rhinitis (hay fever) and are effective at reducing rhinorrhoea and sneezing, but are usually less effective for nasal congestion. They are also used to treat urticarial rashes, pruritus, drug allergies, and insect bites and stings.

Older antihistamines (e.g. chlorphenamine, cyclizine) have a troublesome side-effect of drowsiness, which may nevertheless be useful in managing the pruritus associated with some allergies. Newer antihistamines (e.g. cetirizine, desloratadine) cause less sedation.

Drugs used in anaphylaxis

The causes and management of anaphylaxis are covered on page 27.

Oxygen

Oxygen is prescribed for hypoxaemic patients to increase alveolar and arterial oxygen tension, and is commonly given in many medical emergencies (e.g. pneumonia, pulmonary thromboembolism, shock, severe trauma, sepsis or anaphylaxis). For patients with a normal or low arterial carbon dioxide ($PaCO_2$), the target arterial oxygen saturation should be 94–98%. For patients with ventilatory failure and a tendency to retain carbon dioxide (e.g. COPD), uncontrolled high-concentration oxygen therapy may cause further retention, leading to dangerous hypercapnia. In these cases, a lower concentration of oxygen should be delivered in a controlled way with careful monitoring, aiming for a lower target of 88–92%. Oxygen should always be prescribed on the patient's drug chart, indicating not only the flow rate or percentage required but also the means of delivery (type of mask or nasal cannulae).

Neurological diseases
Analgesic drugs

Analgesic drugs are conveniently divided into simple non-opioid analgesics (e.g. paracetamol), opioid analgesics (e.g. morphine), compound analgesics (e.g. co-codamol) and drugs that are indicated for specific pain syndromes such as neuropathic pain (e.g. gabapentin) and migraine (e.g. $5HT_1$-receptor agonists such as sumatriptan). Non-steroidal anti-inflammatory drugs (NSAIDs) reduce pain by inhibiting the production of pain-sensitising prostaglandins around peripheral nociceptors.

Class	Non-opioid analgesics
Drugs	paracetamol (acetaminophen), nefopam hydrochloride
Action	Paracetamol inhibits CNS production of prostaglandins but has little effect on peripheral prostaglandin production. Nefopam inhibits serotonin, dopamine and noradrenaline re-uptake and may also be a voltage-gated sodium channel blocker at nociceptors

Class	Non-opioid analgesics *(Continued)*
Indications	Mild to moderate pain; pyrexia (paracetamol only)
Usage	Paracetamol (0.5–1 g orally 4–6 times daily, maximum 4 g daily) is an effective first-line analgesic for mild to moderate pain and will reduce temperature in a variety of circumstances (it can also be given IV). It is safe, inexpensive and widely available 'over the counter'. Nefopam 60 mg orally 3 times daily is an alternative
ADRs	Paracetamol has few adverse effects other than the risk of serious hepatotoxicity if taken in overdose (p. 36). Nefopam may cause troublesome sympathomimetic and antimuscarinic effects
Advice	Patients taking paracetamol regularly should be warned of the potential toxic effects if the maximum daily dosage (4 g) is exceeded

Class	Opioid analgesics
Drugs	Weak opioids: codeine, dihydrocodeine. Strong opioids: morphine, diamorphine, oxycodone, fentanyl, methadone, pethidine, tramadol
Action	Agonists at G-protein-coupled μ-opioid receptors located on neuronal cell membranes in the peripheral and central nervous system
Indications	Moderate to severe pain
Usage	Weak opioids (e.g. codeine 30–60 mg orally 6 times daily, dihydrocodeine 30–60 mg orally 6 times daily) are mild analgesics that provide effective relief for moderate pain, especially in combination with paracetamol (e.g. co-codamol, co-dydramol). Both depend on conversion to morphine for their analgesic effects and there is significant inter-individual genetic variation in metabolism. Strong opioids (e.g. morphine 5–10 mg orally/SC/IM/IV 6 times daily, diamorphine 5 mg SC/IM/IV 6 times daily) are used to relieve severe acute pain such as post-MI and post-operative pain (sometimes via patient-controlled analgesia, PCA). They are also used for chronic pain, particularly in the setting of palliative care, where dependence and tolerance resulting from prolonged administration are not limiting factors. In severe, continuous cancer pain, oral immediate-release morphine (5–20 mg) should be given 6 times daily with the same dose available on an 'as required' basis for breakthrough pain. The regular dose should be adjusted daily, taking account of breakthrough requirements and adverse effects. Once the correct dose has been established, immediate-release morphine can be replaced by a modified-release preparation (usually twice daily). Oxycodone orally and transdermal fentanyl are alternatives to morphine that may produce a better balance of benefit against adverse effects and are useful in renal failure when there is accumulation of active metabolites of morphine. Diamorphine is more soluble than morphine and is ideal for continuous SC infusions, particularly in the last few days of life

Class	Opioid analgesics *(Continued)*
ADRs	Nausea and vomiting are common with acute administration and often require co-prescription of an antiemetic, but may settle after a few days of regular treatment. Constipation is common and often requires regular laxative administration. Confusion and drowsiness are dose-related and reversible. Significant respiratory depression is a recognised complication
Advice	Acute parenteral administration always carries a risk of causing unexpected respiratory depression and the opioid-receptor antagonist naloxone hydrochloride (400–800 mg IV) should always be available.

Neuropathic pain is treated with tricyclic antidepressants (e.g. amitriptyline) or certain anti-epileptic drugs (e.g. pregabalin, gabapentin). It may also respond to opioid analgesics, although the potential long-term adverse effects should be carefully considered. Localised pain may benefit from the local anaesthetic effect of topical lidocaine 5% medicated plasters. Capsaicin 0.075% cream is licensed for the symptomatic relief of neuropathic pain but the initial burning sensation may be intolerable. Corticosteroid may help to relieve pressure in compression neuropathy. Neuromodulation at the spinal cord by transcutaneous electrical nerve stimulation (TENS) may also be of benefit.

Anti-migraine drugs

Acute migraine is treated with simple analgesia and antiemetics, often in compound preparations. $5HT_1$-receptor agonists (e.g. sumatriptan, naratriptan, zolmitriptan) are used to treat migraine unresponsive to these measures and cluster headaches. They are taken by mouth or intranasally during the established headache phase of an attack in those who fail to respond to conventional analgesics. They cause vasospasm and should be used with caution in the elderly and in the presence of conditions that predispose to CAD. Prophylaxis against regular attacks of migraine can be provided by β-blockers (e.g. propranolol) or pizotifen (an antihistamine and a serotonin-receptor antagonist).

Anti-epileptic drugs

The principles of management of epilepsy are described on page 643.

Sodium valproate is the first-line treatment for newly diagnosed generalised tonic–clonic seizures, with lamotrigine and carbamazepine being alternatives. Combinations with other drugs such as clobazam, levetiracetam or topiramate may be used if monotherapy is ineffective. Sodium valproate and ethosuximide are the drugs of choice in absence seizures. Myoclonic seizures (myoclonic jerks) and childhood atonic seizures may also respond to sodium valproate. Status epilepticus is a medical emergency that can be treated with lorazepam (4 mg IV), diazepam (10 mg IV or PR), lorazepam (10 mg buccal) or phenytoin (20 mg/kg IV at a maximum rate of 50 mg/min with ECG monitoring).

Withdrawal of anti-epileptic drugs in seizure-free patients is a difficult decision because of the risk of rebound seizures and should be undertaken under specialist supervision.

Many anti-epileptic drugs, especially sodium valproate, carry a risk of teratogenicity. Patients should be informed of these risks and offered specialist advice prior to pregnancy. Folate supplementation taken before and during pregnancy reduces the risk of neural tube defects. Breastfeeding is acceptable with most anticonvulsants, excepting the barbiturates and some of the newer agents.

Class	Carbamazepine and related drugs
Drugs	carbamazepine, oxcarbazepine, eslicarbazepine
Action	Stabilise voltage-gated sodium channels, reducing the initiation and transmission of action potentials in excitable nerve membranes. May also potentiate gamma-aminobutyric acid (GABA) receptors, contributing to their efficacy in neuropathic pain
Indications	Primary and secondary generalised tonic–clonic seizures, focal seizures. Trigeminal neuralgia, diabetic nephropathy
Usage	Carbamazepine is given at an initial dosage of 100–200 mg orally twice daily or daily, followed by a slow increase until best response is obtained, normally requiring 800–1200 mg daily. Modified-release preparations are available for once-daily use and may reduce adverse effects related to peak plasma concentrations. Note that different preparations may vary in their bioavailability
ADRs	Common dose-related effects are headache, ataxia, dizziness, drowsiness, paraesthesia, anorexia, nausea, diarrhoea and blurred vision. Potentially serious idiosyncratic reactions include rashes, agranulocytosis, thrombocytopenia, photosensitivity, liver damage and a general anti-epileptic hypersensitivity syndrome that may involve cross-sensitivity to other anti-epileptic drugs. Carbamazepine is metabolised by cytochrome P450 (CYP3A4), and plasma concentration may be increased or decreased by inhibitors (e.g. cimetidine, clarithromycin, fluoxetine) or inducers (e.g. phenytoin) of that enzyme. Carbamazepine can accelerate the metabolism of other drugs (e.g. oestrogens in contraceptives) to reduce their effect
Advice	Plasma carbamazepine concentration can be used to guide dosage and confirm suspected toxicity. Steady-state levels may take several days after a dose change (therapeutic range 20–50 micromol/L). Patients or their carers should be warned about early signs of blood, liver or skin disorders, and the need to seek advice in response to fever, rash, mouth ulcers, bruising or bleeding

Class	Phenytoin and related drugs
Drugs	phenytoin, fosphenytoin
Action	Stabilise voltage-gated sodium channels, reducing the initiation and transmission of action potentials in excitable nerve membranes
Indications	Tonic–clonic seizures, focal seizures, prevention and treatment of seizures following neurosurgery or severe head injury, status epilepticus
Usage	Phenytoin is given at an initial dosage of 3–4 mg/kg/day or 150–300 mg orally daily. This is increased slowly to the lowest dose achieving seizure control, normally 200–500 mg daily in single or divided doses. Phenytoin has a narrow therapeutic index and saturable metabolism, meaning that small changes in dosage can produce unexpectedly large effects on plasma concentrations. Note that different preparations may vary in their bioavailability
ADRs	Common dose-related effects are nystagmus, diplopia, slurred speech, ataxia, confusion and hyperglycaemia. Idiosyncratic reactions include rashes, blood dyscrasias and hepatotoxicity. Phenytoin may cause undesirable changes in appearance, including coarse facial appearance, acne, hirsutism and gingival hyperplasia, which may be unacceptable to female and adolescent patients. Other effects include neuropathy, folate deficiency and osteomalacia
Advice	Plasma phenytoin concentration can be used to guide dosage, assess adherence and confirm suspected toxicity (therapeutic range 40–80 micromol/L). Patients or their carers should be warned about early signs of blood or skin disorders, and the need to seek advice in response to fever, rash, mouth ulcers, bruising or bleeding

Class	Sodium valproate and related drugs
Drugs	sodium valproate, valproic acid
Action	Potentiate the inhibitory action of GABA
Indications	Primary and secondary generalised tonic–clonic seizures, focal seizures, generalised absences and myoclonic seizures
Usage	Valproate is given at an initial dosage of 600 mg orally daily in 1–2 divided doses, increasing carefully by 200 mg every 3 days until control is achieved, normally between 1 and 2 g daily. Modified-release preparations are available. Different preparations may vary in their bioavailability and care should be taken when changing. Sodium valproate can also be administered by IV injection

Class	Sodium valproate and related drugs *(Continued)*
ADRs	Common dose-related effects are drowsiness, nausea, ataxia, nystagmus, diplopia and tremor. Potentially serious idiosyncratic reactions include alopecia, rashes, blood dyscrasias, liver damage and pancreatitis. Patients on long-term treatment may experience weight gain. Valproate does not induce the metabolism of other drugs. Valproate is associated with a higher risk of major and minor congenital malformations than any other anti-epileptic drug
Advice	Monitoring of LFTs and FBC during therapy is essential. Plasma valproate concentration is not a reliable guide to efficacy and so routine monitoring is not required. Women of child-bearing potential must be made aware of the balance between improved seizure control and the potential adverse outcomes of pregnancy when starting on valproate (or any other anti-epileptic drug).

Drugs for nausea and vertigo

A careful assessment of the cause of nausea and vomiting is required to make a rational choice of antiemetic. Reversible causes (e.g. hypercalcaemia, constipation, medication) should be investigated and treated appropriately. Parenteral administration is often required initially. The major groups of antiemetics are the antihistamines, phenothiazines, pro-kinetic drugs and $5HT_3$-receptor antagonists.

Class	Antihistamines
Drugs	cyclizine, promethazine, chlorphenamine, cinnarizine
Action	Antagonise the actions of histamine at the H_1 receptor. These receptors are present in the vomiting centre within the brainstem, and receive stimulation from the vestibular system and gut vagal afferents
Indications	Nausea, vomiting, motion sickness, vertigo, labyrinthine disorders; also used for the treatment of allergies and urticaria, and as an adjunct in anaphylaxis
Usage	Antihistamines (e.g. cyclizine 50 mg orally/IV/IM 3 times daily) are effective antiemetics in a wide variety of conditions but are particularly useful in vomiting due to vestibular disorders (including motion sickness) and intracranial causes. Promethazine (25–100 mg orally at night) is used for severe vomiting in pregnancy
ADRs	Most older antihistamines (particularly promethazine) cause sedation but this is less of a problem with cyclizine and chlorphenamine. They may also cause antimuscarinic effects, such as urinary retention, dry mouth and blurred vision, and must be used with caution in prostatic hypertrophy and glaucoma
Advice	Patients should be warned about the potential sedative effects in relation to driving and other skilled tasks

Class	**Phenothiazines**
Drugs	prochlorperazine, droperidol
Action	Block dopamine receptors in the chemoreceptor trigger zone (CTZ)
Indications	Treatment of nausea and vomiting associated with diffuse neoplastic disease, radiation sickness, and the emesis caused by drugs (e.g. opioids, general anaesthetics, cytotoxics)
Usage	Phenothiazines can be given by various routes (e.g. prochlorperazine 12.5 mg IM or 5 mg orally 3 times daily)
ADRs	Extrapyramidal symptoms, including dystonias

Class	**Pro-kinetic drugs**
Drugs	metoclopramide, domperidone
Action	Block dopamine receptors in the CTZ and have a direct pro-kinetic effect on the GI tract
Indications	Nausea and vomiting, defective gastric emptying
Usage	Metoclopramide (10 mg orally/IV/IM 3 times daily) and domperidone (10 mg orally 3 times daily) are useful in nausea and vomiting associated with gut stasis or treatment with cytotoxics or radiotherapy, but have limited efficacy in post-operative nausea and vomiting, and are ineffective in motion sickness. Metoclopramide should be avoided in young patients (<20 yrs), who are at increased risk of extrapyramidal disorders. Domperidone does not cross the blood–brain barrier and is less likely to cause CNS adverse effects (note that the CTZ lies **outside** the blood–brain barrier). It is also used to prevent vomiting associated with dopaminergic drugs in Parkinson's disease
ADRs	Predictable anti-dopaminergic effects are extrapyramidal features such as acute dystonic reactions (particularly with metoclopramide in young patients), and hyperprolactinaemia and galactorrhoea with prolonged administration. Domperidone may prolong the QT interval and its use is now restricted to short courses. Both drugs should be avoided in GI obstruction

Class	**$5HT_3$-receptor antagonists**
Drugs	ondansetron, granisetron
Action	Block $5HT_3$ receptors in the GI tract and CTZ, thereby inhibiting activation of the vomiting centre by both gut (vagal) afferents and the CTZ
Indications	Nausea and vomiting induced by cytotoxic chemotherapy and radiotherapy, prevention and treatment of post-operative nausea and vomiting

Class	5HT₃-receptor antagonists *(Continued)*
Usage	5HT$_3$-receptor antagonists (e.g. ondansetron 8 mg orally/IV before treatment, then 8 mg twice daily for up to 5 days) are very effective in the prevention of nausea and vomiting associated with chemotherapy (addition of dexamethasone may provide further benefit)
ADRs	Constipation, headache, flushing

Other antiemetic drugs include dexamethasone, used for vomiting associated with cancer chemotherapy, and the antimuscarinic drug hyoscine, used for motion sickness.

Drugs for Parkinson's disease

Parkinson's disease results from neurochemical imbalance in the basal ganglia due to a deficiency of the neurotransmitter dopamine and a relative imbalance towards the cholinergic pathways. Treatment is usually not started until the disease has caused significant disability. The standard pharmacological treatment for the resulting bradykinesia is to augment the dopaminergic system with levodopa (or other dopaminergic drugs) or inhibit the cholinergic system with antimuscarinic drugs, which are particularly helpful in alleviating the tremor and rigidity. Adverse effects of treatment are more common in the elderly and dose titrations should be gradual and carefully reviewed.

Class	Levodopa
Drugs	co-beneldopa (benserazide hydrochloride and levodopa), co-careldopa (carbidopa and levodopa)
Action	Levodopa is the amino acid precursor of dopamine and acts by replenishing depleted striatal dopamine in the basal ganglia. Benserazide and carbidopa are dopa-decarboxylase inhibitors that reduce the extracerebral conversion of levodopa to dopamine and thereby reduce many of the peripheral adverse effects of levodopa given alone
Indications	Parkinson's disease
Usage	Levodopa is given initially at 50 mg orally 3–4 times daily and then increased by 100 mg daily at intervals, according to response, to achieve a usual maintenance dosage of 400–800 mg daily in divided doses. The elderly require more cautious dosing and titration. Modified-release preparations (e.g. Madopar® CR, Sinemet® CR) may allow the frequency of administration to be reduced to twice daily. Motor complications include response fluctuations and dyskinesias. 'End-of-dose deterioration' may be improved by using smaller, more frequent doses or a modified-release preparation. More complex fluctuations present as periods of severe parkinsonism alternating with dyskinesia and agitation (the 'on–off' phenomenon)

Class	Levodopa *(Continued)*
ADRs	Common effects include nausea, vomiting, taste disturbances, dry mouth, arrhythmias, postural hypotension, drowsiness, dementia, psychoses, confusion, euphoria, abnormal dreams, insomnia, depression, dystonia, dyskinesia and chorea. Levodopa has a serious interaction with non-selective monoamine oxidase inhibitors, potentially leading to a hypertensive crisis
Advice	The effects of any change in dosage or preparation require careful monitoring

Class	Antimuscarinic drugs
Drugs	orphenadrine, procyclidine
Action	Reduce the relative imbalance towards cholinergic activity caused by failure of dopaminergic transmission in the basal ganglia
Indications	Parkinsonism and drug-induced extrapyramidal symptoms (but not tardive dyskinesia, which may be exacerbated)
Usage	Orphenadrine (150–300 mg orally daily in divided doses) and procyclidine (2.5–10 mg orally 3 times daily) reduce tremor and rigidity but have little effect on bradykinesia. Antimuscarinic drugs also help to reduce troublesome sialorrhoea. Procyclidine (5–10 mg IM/IV) is the drug of choice for treating acute dystonic reactions
ADRs	Predictable antimuscarinic adverse effects include dry mouth, blurred vision, tachycardia, urinary retention, constipation, dizziness, confusion, hallucinations, impaired memory, nausea, vomiting, anxiety and rarely angle-closure glaucoma
Advice	Patients should be warned that antimuscarinic drugs can affect the ability to perform skilled tasks such as driving

Other drugs used in parkinsonism and related disorders include dopamine receptor agonists (e.g. ropinirole, bromocriptine), monoamine oxidase B inhibitors (e.g. selegiline), catechol-O-methyltransferase inhibitors (e.g. entacapone) and amantadine.

Other motor disorders amenable to drug treatment include benign essential tremor (e.g. propranolol, primidone), Huntington's chorea (e.g. tetrabenazine), Tourette's syndrome (e.g. haloperidol) and intractable hiccups (e.g. haloperidol, chlorpromazine). Riluzole delays the onset of ventilator dependence or tracheostomy in patients with motor neuron disease who have amyotrophic lateral sclerosis.

Drugs for dementia

Class	Acetylcholinesterase inhibitors
Drugs	donepezil, galantamine, rivastigmine
Action	Reversible inhibitors of acetylcholinesterase that prolong the actions of acetylcholine in the brain. Galantamine also has nicotinic receptor agonist properties

Class	Acetylcholinesterase inhibitors *(Continued)*
Indications	Treatment of mild to moderate Alzheimer's disease
Usage	Acetylcholinesterase inhibitors (donepezil 5–10 mg orally at night, galantamine 4–12 mg orally twice daily) should be started at a low dose that is then titrated based on response and tolerability
ADRs	Dose-related cholinergic effects include nausea, vomiting, diarrhoea, urinary incontinence, bradycardia, dizziness, hallucinations and agitation
Advice	Treatment should continue only if it provides a worthwhile effect on cognitive function and behaviour

Other drugs

Attention deficit hyperactivity disorder in children is treated with CNS stimulant drugs (e.g. dexamfetamine, methylphenidate) if other psychological interventions are unsuccessful.

Psychiatric diseases
Hypnotic and anxiolytic drugs

Hypnotic drugs should only be used once remediable causes of insomnia (e.g. symptoms such as pain, alcohol and depression) have been addressed. Chronic insomnia rarely responds well to hypnotics and any prescribing should take into account the potential for longer-term dependence and withdrawal effects. The most common hypnotics are benzodiazepines and Z-drugs but other hypnotic drugs include clomethiazole, antihistamines (e.g. promethazine) and melatonin, a pineal gland hormone used for short-term insomnia.

Class	Benzodiazepines
Drugs	diazepam, nitrazepam, temazepam, chlordiazepoxide
Action	Bind to the GABA-A receptor and increase the binding affinity of the inhibitory neurotransmitter GABA at its receptor
Indications	Short-term treatment of insomnia and severe anxiety, acute alcohol withdrawal, status epilepticus
Usage	For insomnia, nitrazepam (5–10 mg orally at night) is rather longer-acting than temazepam (10–20 mg orally at night)
ADRs	Important effects are daytime drowsiness, confusion and ataxia. Dependence and withdrawal effects such as anxiety may follow prolonged use. Benzodiazepines interact with other sedative drugs, including Z-drugs, antihistamines and alcohol
Advice	Patients should be advised that treatment is short term and that daytime hangover effects might occur and impair tasks such as driving

Class	Z-drugs
Drugs	zopiclone, zolpidem, zaleplon
Action	Bind to the GABA-A receptor and increase the binding affinity of the inhibitory neurotransmitter GABA at its receptor
Indications	Short-term treatment of insomnia
Usage	Z-drugs (zopiclone 7.5 mg orally at night, zolpidem 10 mg orally at night) should be prescribed for a maximum of 4 wks
ADRs	Important adverse effects are daytime drowsiness. Dependence and withdrawal effects such as anxiety may follow prolonged use. Z-drugs interact with other sedative drugs, including benzodiazepines, antihistamines and alcohol
Advice	Patients should be advised that treatment is short term and that daytime hangover effects might occur and impair tasks such as driving

Anxiolytic drugs include benzodiazepines (e.g. diazepam 2–5 mg orally 3 times daily) and some antidepressants (e.g. trazodone). Non-selective β-blockers (e.g. propranolol) may relieve the autonomic features of anxiety. Diazepam (10–20 mg orally 4 times daily, decreased as allowed by recovery) is also commonly used in the treatment of acute alcohol withdrawal.

Antidepressant drugs

The initial approach to managing depression should include psychological support and cognitive behavioural therapy, with drugs being reserved for more severe depression. The majority of patients will respond to treatment but this may take 2–4 wks and require appropriate dosage titration; patients should be advised about this.

Class	Tricyclic antidepressants (TCAs)
Drugs	TCAs: amitriptyline, nortriptyline, imipramine, lofepramine. TCA-related drugs: mianserin, trazodone
Action	Inhibit the re-uptake of noradrenaline (norepinephrine) and 5-hydroxytryptamine (5-HT, serotonin) at synaptic clefts in the CNS
Indications	Depressive illness, neuropathic pain
Usage	TCAs (e.g. amitriptyline 75–150 mg orally daily, imipramine 75–150 mg orally daily) and related drugs (e.g. mianserin 30–90 mg orally daily, trazodone 150–300 mg orally daily) are effective but their use is limited by adverse effects and dangerous toxicity in overdose. TCA-related drugs are particularly useful where sedation is required and have fewer antimuscarinic and cardiac effects. TCAs in lower dosage (e.g. amitriptyline 10–25 mg) are effective for neuropathic pain

Class	Tricyclic antidepressants (TCAs) *(Continued)*
ADRs	Common effects are sedation (less with imipramine, more with TCA-related drugs), antimuscarinic effects including dry mouth, blurred vision, confusion, urinary retention, constipation, angle-closure glaucoma, tachycardia and arrhythmias (especially amitriptyline but all are cardiotoxic in overdose). Other effects include GI upset, hyponatraemia, endocrine effects and sexual dysfunction. Caution is required when treating the elderly, who are particularly vulnerable to adverse effects. TCAs are contraindicated in recent MI and arrhythmias. Abrupt discontinuation can lead to a withdrawal reaction

Class	Selective serotonin re-uptake inhibitors (SSRIs)
Drugs	fluoxetine, paroxetine, sertraline, citalopram
Action	Selectively inhibit the re-uptake of 5-HT
Indications	Depressive illness, anxiety disorders, obsessive–compulsive disorder
Usage	SSRIs (e.g. fluoxetine 20–40 mg orally daily, paroxetine 20–40 mg orally daily, citalopram 20–40 mg orally daily) have similar efficacy to TCAs but have fewer adverse effects and are less toxic in overdose
ADRs	SSRIs cause less sedation and have fewer antimuscarinic and cardiotoxic effects than TCAs. Important effects include GI upset, drowsiness, sexual dysfunction and hyponatraemia (syndrome of inappropriate ADH secretion). Abrupt discontinuation can lead to a withdrawal reaction

Class	Monoamine oxidase inhibitors (MAOIs)
Drugs	phenelzine, isocarboxazid, tranylcypromine
Action	Inhibit monoamine oxidase, leading to the accumulation of amine neurotransmitters
Indications	Depressive illness
Usage	Phenelzine (15–30 mg orally 3 times daily)
ADRs	Common effects are postural hypotension and dizziness. MAOIs can interact to potentiate the effects of tyramine-containing foods (e.g. cheese) and remedies containing sympathomimetic drugs (e.g. nasal decongestants). Similarly, other antidepressants should not be taken until at least 2 wks after MAOI discontinuation
Advice	Patients should be warned about the potential food and drug interactions

Other antidepressant drugs include combined serotonin and noradrenaline re-uptake inhibitors (e.g. venlafaxine, duloxetine), selective noradrenaline re-uptake inhibitors (e.g. reboxetine) and the pre-synaptic α_2-adrenoceptor antagonist mirtazapine, which up-regulates both serotoninergic and noradrenergic pathways.

St John's wort (*Hypericum perforatum*) is a popular herbal remedy for treating mild depression but can induce drug-metabolising enzymes and has important interactions with many drugs.

Antipsychotic drugs

Antipsychotic ('neuroleptic') drugs are used to treat acute behavioural disturbance caused by a variety of disorders including schizophrenia, brain damage, mania, toxic delirium or agitated depression. They are used chronically to manage positive psychotic symptoms in schizophrenia, such as thought disorder, hallucinations and delusions, but are less effective on negative symptoms such as apathy and social withdrawal. Patients with acute schizophrenia generally respond better than those with chronic symptoms but long-term treatment is helpful in preventing relapses.

Antipsychotic drugs should only be used in elderly patients to treat significant psychotic symptoms. Elderly patients with dementia are at increased risk of mortality and an increased risk of stroke or TIA, and are also more vulnerable to the many adverse effects.

Antimanic drugs (e.g. lithium) are used to treat and prevent recurrent attacks of mania. Some second-generation antipsychotic drugs (e.g. olanzapine, quetiapine, risperidone) and anti-epileptic drugs (e.g. valproate) are also useful in managing acute episodes of mania.

Class	First-generation antipsychotic drugs
Drugs	Phenothiazines: chlorpromazine, levomepromazine, promazine, pericyazine, fluphenazine, perphenazine, prochlorperazine and trifluoperazine. Butyrophenones: benperidol, haloperidol. Thioxanthenes: flupentixol, zuclopenthixol. Diphenylbutylpiperidines: pimozide. Substituted benzamides: sulpiride
Action	Act predominantly by blocking dopamine D_2 receptors in the brain. The various groups differ in their relative sedative, antimuscarinic and extrapyramidal effects
Indications	Schizophrenia, psychoses, mania and hypomania, organic brain damage (depending on symptoms), psychomotor agitation, violent or dangerous impulsive behaviour. Note the specific indications for individual drugs
Usage	Chlorpromazine (initially 25 mg orally 3 times daily, adjusted according to response, to a maintenance dose of 75–300 mg daily), haloperidol (initially 1.5–3 mg orally 2–3 times daily, increasing to a maintenance dose of 3–5 mg 2–3 times daily or 1–2 mg IM). Long-acting depot injections (e.g. flupentixol 40 mg IM every 2 wks, haloperidol 100 mg IM every 4 wks) are preferable when adherence to oral treatment is unreliable but may give rise to a higher incidence of extrapyramidal reactions

Class	First-generation antipsychotic drugs *(Continued)*
ADRs	Adverse effects are common and lead to reduced adherence to therapy. Extrapyramidal symptoms, including parkinsonism (tremor), dystonic reactions (abnormal face and body movements), akathisia (restlessness) and tardive dyskinesia (rhythmic, involuntary movements of tongue, face and jaw), are more common with phenothiazines and butyrophenones, especially with depot preparations. Tardive dyskinesia may be irreversible after withdrawal. Antidopaminergic activity may lead to hyperprolactinaemia and consequent sexual dysfunction, reduced bone mineral density, menstrual disturbances, breast enlargement and galactorrhoea. Antipsychotic drugs may precipitate cardiac arrhythmias and prolong the QT interval. Other common effects are drowsiness, apathy, confusion, GI upset and antimuscarinic effects (see above). Blood dyscrasias and neuroleptic malignant syndrome (hyperthermia, fluctuating level of consciousness, muscle rigidity and autonomic dysfunction with pallor, tachycardia, labile BP, sweating and urinary incontinence) are rare but potentially serious outcomes
Advice	FBC, U&Es and LFT monitoring are required at the start of therapy with antipsychotic drugs, and then annually thereafter. ECG at baseline and then repeated on treatment may be required for some drugs, especially in the presence of cardiovascular risk factors

Class	Second-generation (atypical) antipsychotic drugs
Drugs	amisulpride, aripiprazole, clozapine, olanzapine, quetiapine, risperidone
Action	Act on a wider range of receptors and so have more distinct adverse effect profiles
Indications	Schizophrenia and other psychoses, mania. Major depressive disorder (quetiapine), aggression in patients with Alzheimer's dementia (risperidone). See specific indications for individual drugs
Usage	Amisulpride (200–400 mg orally twice daily), aripiprazole (10–15 mg orally daily), olanzapine (5–20 mg orally daily), quetiapine (150–200 mg orally twice daily) and risperidone (4–6 mg orally daily) are typical maintenance dosages. Acute behavioural disturbance can be controlled with IM injections of aripiprazole (5.25–15 mg) or olanzapine (10 mg). Long-acting depot injections (e.g. olanzapine 300 mg IM every 2 wks, risperidone 25–50 mg IM every 2 wks) are available
ADRs	Many of the adverse effects of first-generation drugs. Aripiprazole, unlike other antipsychotic drugs, lowers prolactin. Clozapine is a recognised cause of potentially severe agranulocytosis, myocarditis and cardiomyopathy
Advice	Monitoring as for first generation, with particular care taken for patients on clozapine

Class	Lithium
Drugs	lithium carbonate, lithium citrate
Action	Reduces excitatory (dopaminergic and glutaminergic) but increases inhibitory (GABA) neurotransmission. Lithium may also target second-messenger systems (e.g. adenyl cyclase and phosphoinositide pathways, protein kinase C) that further modulate neurotransmission
Indications	Treatment and prophylaxis of mania, bipolar disorder
Usage	Lithium is available in many different preparations that vary widely in their bioavailability. A typical dosage regimen would be 0.4–1.2 g daily in 1 or 2 doses
ADRs	Common effects include GI disturbances, ECG changes, cognitive impairment, drowsiness, memory loss, benign intracranial hypertension, renal impairment, polydipsia, nephrogenic diabetes insipidus, sexual dysfunction and thyroid changes. Features of lithium toxicity include tremor, ataxia, dysarthria, nystagmus, renal impairment and convulsions. Lithium toxicity is more likely when sodium is depleted or when lithium excretion is reduced; therefore there are potentially serious interactions with all diuretics and NSAIDs
Advice	Serum lithium concentration taken 12 hrs post-dose is helpful to monitor titration of dosage and also to confirm toxicity (therapeutic range 0.4–1 mmol/L). Routine monitoring should be undertaken weekly after initiation or dose titration change until concentrations are stable (then every 3 mths)

Infectious diseases

The optimal selection of antimicrobial therapy requires knowledge of the infecting organism (or most likely pathogen, given the clinical and geographical context) (Fig. 18.1), the local patterns of antimicrobial resistance, the relevant pharmacokinetic disposition of antimicrobial drugs and the clinical status of the patient.

Antibacterial drugs

The major classes of antibacterial drugs include the penicillins, carbapenems, cephalosporins, macrolides, tetracyclines, quinolones, aminoglycosides and metronidazole.

Class	Penicillins
Drugs	Natural penicillins: phenoxymethylpenicillin (penicillin V), benzylpenicillin (penicillin G). Penicillinase-resistant penicillins: flucloxacillin. Broad-spectrum penicillins: ampicillin, amoxicillin, co-amoxiclav. Antipseudomonal penicillins: piperacillin with tazobactam. Mecillinams: pivmecillinam
Action	β-lactam-based molecules that exert a bactericidal effect by disrupting bacterial cell wall synthesis

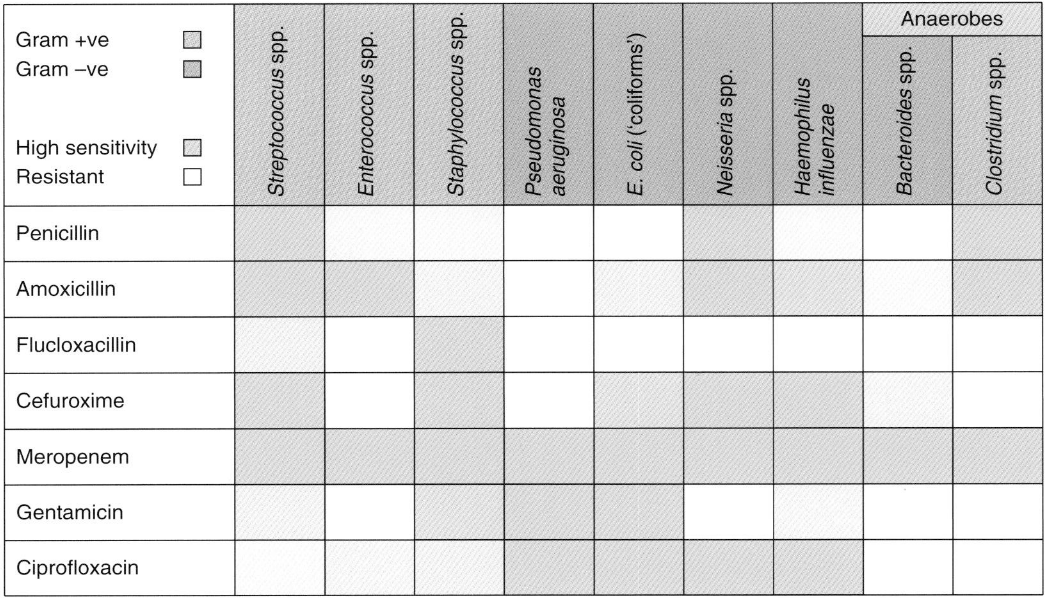

Legend:
- Gram +ve
- Gram −ve
- High sensitivity
- Resistant

	Streptococcus spp.	Enterococcus spp.	Staphylococcus spp.	Pseudomonas aeruginosa	E. coli ('coliforms')	Neisseria spp.	Haemophilus influenzae	Anaerobes Bacteroides spp.	Anaerobes Clostridium spp.
Penicillin									
Amoxicillin									
Flucloxacillin									
Cefuroxime									
Meropenem									
Gentamicin									
Ciprofloxacin									

Fig. 18-1 Antibacterial spectrum of common antibiotics.

Class	Penicillins *(Continued)*
Indications	Natural penicillins (phenoxymethylpenicillin and benzylpenicillin): streptococcal infections including throat infections, otitis media, erysipelas, cellulitis, endocarditis; meningococcal infections; anthrax, diphtheria, syphilis, gas gangrene, leptospirosis. Flucloxacillin: staphylococcal infections including impetigo, cellulitis, osteomyelitis, septic arthritis, wound infections, endocarditis, pneumonia. Broad-spectrum penicillins: exacerbations of chronic bronchitis, pneumonia, treatment and prophylaxis of endocarditis, urinary tract infection (UTI), otitis media, sinusitis, dental abscess, listerial meningitis. Antipseudomonal penicillins: broad spectrum of activity against a range of Gram-positive and Gram-negative bacteria, anaerobes and *Pseudomonas aeruginosa*. Mecillinams: Gram-negative bacteria including *Escherichia coli*, *Klebsiella*, *Enterobacter* and salmonellae
Usage	Most penicillins are cheap, well tolerated, safe and easy to use but resistance is increasing. Natural penicillins (e.g. phenoxymethylpenicillin 250–500 mg orally 4 times daily, benzylpenicillin 1.2–2.4 g IV 4 times daily) are primarily effective against Gram-positive organisms (except staphylococci) and anaerobic organisms. Flucloxacillin (500 mg–1 g orally/IV 4 times daily) is the mainstay of treatment for most staphylococcal infections, but meticillin-resistant *Staph. aureus* (MRSA) is an increasing problem. If MRSA is suspected (low threshold in serious or hospital-acquired infections), vancomycin should be used in preference. Broad-spectrum penicillins (amoxicillin 500 mg–1 g orally/IV 3 times daily and co-amoxiclav 375–625 mg orally 3 times daily or 1.2 g IV 3 times daily) have similar activity to natural penicillins with additional Gram-negative cover against Enterobacteriaceae and *Haemophilus*, and are widely used in the treatment of uncomplicated community-acquired pneumonia, exacerbations of chronic bronchitis and UTI. Addition of the β-lactamase inhibitor, clavulanic acid (producing 'co-amoxiclav'), prevents resistance due to bacterial β-lactamase production and extends the spectrum of activity. Piperacillin with tazobactam 4.5 g IV 3 times daily is now widely used as first-line broad-spectrum treatment for severe sepsis related to hospital-acquired pneumonia, intra-abdominal infections, and complicated infections involving the urinary tract or skin and soft tissues
ADRs	Common effects include hypersensitivity reactions (generalised allergy to penicillin occurs in 0.7–10% of cases and anaphylaxis in <0.2%) and diarrhoea (including antibiotic-associated colitis). Over 90% of patients with infectious mononucleosis develop a rash if given aminopenicillins; this does not imply lasting allergy. Cholestatic jaundice may occur with co-amoxiclav
Advice	All patients prescribed a penicillin should be asked about previous allergic reactions

Class	Cephalosporins
Drugs	First generation: cefalexin. Second generation: cefuroxime. Third generation: ceftriaxone, ceftazidime
Action	β-lactam-based molecules that exert a bactericidal effect by disrupting bacterial cell wall synthesis
Indications	Include sepsis, pneumonia, meningitis, biliary infections, UTIs, peritonitis
Usage	First-generation compounds (e.g. cefalexin 250 mg orally 4 times daily) have excellent activity against Gram-positive organisms but limited Gram-negative cover. They may be helpful in some urinary, skin and soft tissue infections but are rarely first-line treatment. Second-generation cephalosporins (e.g. cefuroxime 250–500 mg orally twice daily, 750 mg–1.5 g IV 3 times daily) retain Gram-positive activity but have extended Gram-negative activity and some activity against anaerobes. Oral cefuroxime has good activity against common respiratory pathogens but is poorly absorbed. IV cefuroxime is widely used with metronidazole in the treatment of colorectal and biliary tract infection and for prophylaxis in colorectal and hepatobiliary surgery. Third-generation cephalosporins (e.g. ceftriaxone 1–2 g IV daily, cefotaxime 1–2 g 2–4 times daily) further improve anti-Gram-negative cover but are expensive and have to be given parenterally. They retain good activity against *Streptococcus pyogenes*, haemolytic streptococci and many staphylococci, and are widely used in serious infections including sepsis, meningitis, severe community-acquired pneumonia and acute pyelonephritis. Ceftazidime (e.g. 1 g IV 3 times daily) has particularly good antipseudomonal activity but less Gram-positive effectiveness; it has an important role in the treatment of hospital-acquired pneumonia and sepsis
ADRs	Many of the first-generation drugs are potentially nephrotoxic. Second- and third-generation cephalosporins have a low incidence of allergy and a very low rate of anaphylaxis, even in patients with established penicillin allergy, but their broad spectrum of activity predisposes to antibiotic-associated colitis

Class	Macrolides
Drugs	erythromycin, clarithromycin, azithromycin
Action	Bind to bacterial ribosomes, preventing protein synthesis
Indications	Respiratory infections, *Campylobacter* enteritis, susceptible Gram-positive infections in patients with penicillin allergy
Usage	Macrolides (e.g. erythromycin orally/IV 250–500 mg 4 times daily, clarithromycin orally/IV 250–500 mg twice daily) have a similar spectrum of activity to natural penicillins and are a useful alternative in patients with penicillin allergy. They are also active against *Legionella*, *Mycoplasma*, *Chlamydia* and *Rickettsia* infections, and are therefore used for the treatment of atypical pneumonia. Azithromycin has a long half-life and is particularly useful for single-dose or short-course treatment of GU infection

Class	Macrolides *(Continued)*
ADRs	GI upset is common with erythromycin but clarithromycin is better tolerated. Macrolides inhibit the cytochrome P450 system and may increase plasma concentrations of some drugs (e.g. carbamazepine, phenytoin, calcium channel blockers, warfarin, clozapine, quetiapine, tacrolimus). They also cause prolongation of the QT interval (avoid concomitant use of other drugs that prolong the QT interval)

Class	Glycopeptides
Drugs	vancomycin, teicoplanin
Action	Inhibit bacterial cell wall synthesis
Indications	Endocarditis and other serious infections with Gram-positive cocci (including MRSA), antibiotic-associated colitis
Usage	Glycopeptides (e.g. vancomycin 1–1.5 g IV twice daily, teicoplanin 200–400 mg IV/IM daily) are effective against Gram-positive organisms and are particularly useful in infections with MRSA and resistant enterococci, though strains of coagulase-negative staphylococci, enterococci and MRSA resistant to glycopeptides are emerging. Glycopeptides are not active against Gram-negative organisms. Neither drug achieves any useful oral absorption, but oral vancomycin (125 mg 4 times daily for 7–10 days) is effective in diarrhoea due to *Clostridium difficile* infection. The inappropriate use of vancomycin, particularly in the management of *C. difficile* infections (metronidazole is first-line treatment), should be limited to prevent further development of resistance
ADRs	Oto- and nephrotoxicity with vancomycin (teicoplanin is less toxic), particularly when used in combination with an aminoglycoside. Rapid IV infusion of vancomycin may cause an anaphylactoid reaction due to widespread histamine release ('red man' syndrome)
Advice	Monitoring of vancomycin concentration is vital to avoid toxicity (pre-dose 'trough' concentration should be 10–15 mg/L)

Class	Tetracyclines
Drugs	oxytetracycline, doxycycline, minocycline
Action	Prevent bacterial protein synthesis by binding to ribosomes and have a mainly bacteriostatic effect
Indications	Acne vulgaris, rosacea, leptospirosis, periodontitis, anthrax, brucellosis, Lyme disease, infections due to *Chlamydia*, *Rickettsia*, *Mycoplasma*

Class	Tetracyclines _(Continued)_
Usage	Prescribing has declined because most streptococci, _Haemophilus_, _Moraxella_, _E. coli_ and _Proteus_ spp. are now resistant. Important contemporary uses include the treatment of genital _Chlamydia_ infection (e.g. doxycycline 100 mg orally twice daily for 7 days) and systemic infections with spirochaetes, brucellae or rickettsiae. Tetracyclines are also effective in pneumonia due to _Mycoplasma pneumoniae_ and _Chlamydia pneumoniae_ or psittacosis (though macrolides are first-line empirical treatment for suspected atypical pneumonia). Oxytetracycline (500 mg orally twice daily) is valuable in rosacea (but may require repeated intermittent treatments) and moderate to severe acne. Doxycycline and minocycline: show better absorption and distribution than older tetracyclines, but all should be taken in the fasting state to maximise absorption
ADRs	GI upset (due to alterations in gut flora), discoloration of teeth and occasionally dental hypoplasia (avoid in children < 12 yrs, pregnancy and breastfeeding), photosensitive skin reactions and hypernatraemia. Older tetracyclines are contraindicated in renal failure, as they may exacerbate renal dysfunction, but doxycycline or minocycline may be used with caution

Class	Quinolones
Drugs	ciprofloxacin, levofloxacin
Action	Inhibit bacterial DNA-gyrase, an essential enzyme for DNA replication and repair
Indications	Infections of the respiratory, urinary and GI tracts, gonorrhoea, anthrax
Usage	Ciprofloxacin (250–750 mg orally twice daily, 200–400 mg IV twice daily) has excellent anti-Gram-negative activity and is also effective against atypical or intracellular organisms such as _Mycoplasma_, _Chlamydia_ and some Gram-positive organisms. It is used for severe GI infections (e.g. shigellosis, invasive salmonellosis, _Campylobacter_ enteritis) and urinary infections (e.g. acute pyelonephritis, prostatitis, persistent lower UTI). Quinolones have very high bioavailability when given by mouth and should only be administered IV when the oral route is unavailable. Ciprofloxacin has relatively poor activity against _Strep. pneumoniae_ and should not be used routinely in the treatment of community-acquired pneumonia. However, newer 'extended-spectrum' quinolones (e.g. levofloxacin 500 mg orally twice daily) have greater activity against pneumococci and are useful alternatives to amoxicillin and clarithromycin in this condition
ADRs	Quinolones are usually well tolerated but more common effects are GI upset, tremor, dizziness, confusion, QT prolongation and occasionally seizures (especially in the elderly). Tendon damage (including rupture) has been reported

Class	Folate antagonists
Drugs	trimethoprim, co-trimoxazole
Action	Interfere with the bacterial synthesis of folate, an essential precursor for DNA nucleotide synthesis, thereby inhibiting cell replication. Sulphonamides and trimethoprim interfere with two consecutive steps in the same metabolic pathway and are commonly used in combination (e.g. co-trimoxazole)
Indications	UTI, *Pneumocystis jirovecii* pneumonia
Usage	Resistance and the risk of adverse effects have limited their clinical usefulness over the years. Short courses of trimethoprim (200 mg orally twice daily for 3 days) are still used for uncomplicated UTI in the community. Co-trimoxazole, a mixture of trimethoprim and sulfamethoxazole in a 1:5 ratio, is the first-line drug for the treatment (e.g. 120 mg/kg IV daily in divided doses) and prophylaxis (e.g. 960 mg orally every 1–3 days) of *P. jirovecii* infection in HIV disease
ADRs	GI upset, rashes, hyperkalaemia, fatal marrow dysplasia and haemolysis in glucose-6-phosphate dehydrogenase deficiency, and skin and mucocutaneous reactions, including Stevens–Johnson syndrome

Class	Aminoglycosides
Drugs	gentamicin, tobramycin
Action	Bind to ribosomes and interfere with bacterial protein synthesis
Indications	Sepsis, endocarditis, biliary tract infection, acute pyelonephritis, prostatitis, adjunct in hospital-acquired pneumonia
Usage	Very effective against Gram-negative organisms, including *P. aeruginosa*, and useful in Gram-negative sepsis or serious infections arising from the urinary or biliary tract. They also have some Gram-positive activity and show impressive synergy with penicillins; the combination of gentamicin and penicillin is frequently used in the treatment of endocarditis. They must be administered parenterally using either a multiple daily dose regimen (e.g. gentamicin 3–5 mg/kg IV 3 times daily) or a once-daily regimen (5–7 mg/kg)
ADRs	Renal toxicity (usually reversible, worse with concomitant vancomycin), permanent cochlear damage, neuromuscular blockade after rapid IV infusion (contraindicated in myasthenia gravis)
Advice	Careful monitoring of renal function and gentamicin concentration is vital to minimise the risk of oto- and nephrotoxicity. For the once-daily regimen, interpretation of plasma concentration is normally made using the Hartford nomogram

Class	Nitroimidazoles
Drugs	metronidazole, tinidazole
Action	Reduced by metabolic pathways particular to anaerobic bacteria, yielding intermediates that have toxic effects on DNA

Class	Nitroimidazoles *(Continued)*
Indications	Anaerobic infections (e.g. peritonitis involving *Clostridia* spp. and *Bacteroides fragilis*, antibiotic-associated colitis caused by *C. difficile*, bacterial vaginosis caused by *Trichomonas vaginalis*, pelvic inflammatory disease, acute oral infections), surgical prophylaxis, *H. pylori* eradication, protozoal infections such as *Giardia lamblia* and *Entamoeba histolytica*
Usage	Metronidazole 400–500 mg orally 3 times daily is first-line therapy for *C. difficile* infection, with varying regimens for other indications. Metronidazole 500 mg IV 3 times daily is used in patients with sepsis where anaerobic infection is suspected (e.g. post-colonic or pelvic surgery) and, with a broad-spectrum cephalosporin, in peritonitis. Metronidazole can also be given as a suppository
ADRs	May cause a metallic taste. Like disulfiram (Antabuse®), nitroimidazoles inhibit aldehyde dehydrogenase, leading to an unpleasant reaction due to acetaldehyde accumulation when alcohol is consumed
Advice	Patients should be warned about the reaction to alcohol

Carbapenems (e.g. meropenem, imipenem) are very broad-spectrum β-lactam antibacterials and include activity against anaerobes. They are very expensive, are only available in IV formulation, and are reserved for severe infections with organisms resistant to other antibiotics.

Antifungal drugs

Class	Antifungals
Drugs	Triazoles: fluconazole, itraconazole, voriconazole. Imidazoles: clotrimazole, miconazole. Polyenes: amphotericin, nystatin
Action	Inhibit fungal enzymes necessary for the construction of cell membranes
Indications	Local fungal infections of the skin, oropharynx and vagina, as well as systemic fungal infections (e.g. invasive candidiasis, cryptococcosis, aspergillosis)
Usage	Fluconazole (50–400 mg orally daily or 150 mg as single dose for vaginal candidiasis) is well absorbed orally, has an excellent safety profile and achieves very good CSF penetration; it has wide efficacy against *Candida*, *Tinea* and *Cryptococcus* and prevents fungal infection in the immunocompromised. The other oral triazoles, itraconazole and voriconazole, have an extended spectrum of activity, including against *Aspergillus*. Clotrimazole (e.g. 1% cream topical application 2–3 times daily; pessary 500 mg at night as a single dose) and miconazole are not well absorbed and are used for cutaneous and mucosal infections such as ringworm and vaginal candidiasis. Amphotericin must be given by IV infusion and is used in systemic fungal infections. Nystatin oral suspension is useful for oral candidiasis

Class	Antifungals *(Continued)*
ADRs	Fluconazole commonly causes GI upset (e.g. nausea, vomiting, abdominal discomfort), rashes and pruritus. It inhibits the cytochrome P450 metabolism of a variety of drugs (e.g. statins, sulphonylureas). Adverse effects are common with IV amphotericin (see below)
Advice	Anaphylaxis can occur with IV amphotericin; a test dose is advisable before the first infusion and the patient should be monitored closely with renal, hepatic and plasma electrolyte (potassium and magnesium) measurements

Other antifungals include the echinocandin antifungals (e.g. caspofungin), which are only active against *Aspergillus* spp. and *Candida* spp., flucytosine, griseofulvin and terbinafine.

Antiviral drugs

Drugs are available to treat various viruses, including herpes simplex and varicella zoster (e.g. aciclovir), cytomegalovirus (e.g. ganciclovir), HIV (e.g. zidovudine), respiratory syncytial virus (e.g. ribavirin), hepatitis B (e.g. peginterferon alfa, lamivudine), hepatitis C (e.g. peginterferon alfa, ribavirin) and influenza (e.g. oseltamivir, zanamivir). The use of antiviral drugs in HIV is described on page 127.

Class	Aciclovir and related drugs
Drugs	aciclovir, famciclovir, valaciclovir, ganciclovir
Action	Aciclovir is phosphorylated by viral thymidine kinase to aciclovir triphosphate, which competitively inhibits and inactivates DNA polymerases. It has activity against herpes simplex virus (HSV)-1, HSV-2, varicella zoster and Epstein–Barr virus but is less active against cytomegalovirus (CMV). Ganciclovir is a synthetic analogue of 2'-deoxy-guanosine and is phosphorylated to ganciclovir triphosphate, a competitive inhibitor of deoxy-guanosine triphosphate (dGTP) incorporation into DNA, and preferentially inhibits viral DNA polymerases more than cellular DNA polymerases
Indications	HSV and varicella zoster infection. CMV infection (ganciclovir)
Usage	Aciclovir can be given by mouth (200–400 mg orally 5 times per day), IV infusion (5–10 mg/kg 3 times daily) or by topical application to the skin or eyes. Ganciclovir must be given by IV infusion (initially 5 mg/kg twice daily for 14–21 days for treatment)
ADRs	A common adverse effect of aciclovir is GI upset. Less commonly, neurological reactions, such as confusion, hallucinations, ataxia, dysarthria and drowsiness, may occur and these are more common in the presence of renal impairment (dosage reduction required). Ganciclovir is more toxic and requires very careful monitoring in view of its potential to cause serious myelosuppression

Other drugs

Other anti-infective agents include those used to treat TB (e.g. combination treatment with isoniazid, rifampicin, pyrazinamide, ethambutol, (p. 295)), leprosy (e.g. dapsone), malaria (e.g. chloroquine, primaquine, proguanil) and helminthic infections (e.g. mebendazole).

Endocrine diseases

Insulin

Insulin is used primarily to replace endogenous insulin in patients with type 1 diabetes mellitus for whom endogenous secretion has failed but is also used to supplement oral antidiabetic drugs in type 2 diabetes mellitus. Insulin preparations were originally animal-derived but are increasingly human sequence or human insulin analogues created by recombinant DNA technology. Their pharmacokinetic characteristics vary significantly between preparations and prescribers need to specify the intended formulation clearly. Insulin is a polypeptide that is inactivated by intestinal enzymes and has to be given parenterally, usually by SC injection into the upper arm, thighs or buttocks.

Class	Insulin
Drugs	Short-acting insulins have a peak action at 2–4 hrs and include 'soluble' unmodified insulin (e.g. Actrapid®, Humulin S®) and the rapid-acting human insulin analogues (e.g. insulin aspart, insulin lispro). Intermediate-acting insulins have a peak action at 4–12 hrs and include isophane insulin (suspended with protamine, zinc or both). Long-acting human insulin analogues include insulin glargine (Lantus®) and insulin detemir (Levemir®). Biphasic insulins contain a mixture of short-acting soluble and intermediate-acting isophane insulin (e.g. Humulin M3®)
Action	Replacement polypeptide hormone that acts on endogenous insulin receptors that regulate carbohydrate, fat and protein metabolism
Indications	Type 1 diabetes mellitus and type 2 diabetes mellitus if satisfactory glucose control cannot be achieved with oral hypoglycaemics and diet, during intercurrent illness or pregnancy, or peri-operatively
Usage	Soluble insulin is usually given SC 15–30 mins before a meal but is also given as an IV infusion in hospital during emergency treatment and peri-operatively. Rapid-acting human insulin analogues have a faster, shorter duration of action and carry a lower incidence of hypoglycaemia than soluble insulin. They are therefore administered immediately before or shortly after meals. Intermediate and long-acting insulins have an onset of action 1–2 hrs following injection, and a duration of action of 16–35 hrs. For a more detailed review of insulin regimens, see page 404

Class	Insulin *(Continued)*
ADRs	Hypoglycaemia is common and potentially serious; it is more likely with tight blood sugar control. Frequent hypoglycaemic episodes or concomitant use of β-blockers (e.g. atenolol) may cause loss of hypoglycaemic warning symptoms. At the injection site, local reaction and fat hypertrophy can occur, which may delay onset of effect
Advice	Patients should be educated about hypoglycaemic warning symptoms, especially in relation to daily activities (e.g. driving). They should carry a supply of easily absorbed sugary food. The success of therapy can be monitored using instantaneous self-measured blood glucose concentration or by glycosylation of proteins (e.g. HbA$_{1c}$), which gives a better picture of longer-term control. Many patients carry documentation indicating that they have diabetes and use insulin (e.g. 'insulin passport')

Drugs for type 2 diabetes

Oral antidiabetic drugs are used to treat type 2 diabetes in patients who do not respond to restriction of energy and carbohydrate intake and an increase in physical activity. Metformin is the first-line drug with the best evidence for improving long-term outcomes but may be used in combination with other agents, including sulphonylureas (e.g. gliclazide), thiazolidinediones (e.g. pioglitazone), dipeptidylpeptidase-4 inhibitors (e.g. sitagliptin, saxagliptin), glucagon-like peptide-1 receptor agonists (e.g. exenatide, liraglutide), sodium–glucose co-transporter-2 inhibitors (e.g. canagliflozin, dapagliflozin) and the intestinal α-glucosidase inhibitor (e.g. acarbose). Insulin is sometimes added if oral therapy alone is insufficient to achieve glycaemic control.

Class	Biguanides
Drugs	metformin
Action	Increases peripheral glucose uptake and decreases gluconeogenesis. It requires some endogenous insulin secretion for its effects
Indications	Type 2 diabetes mellitus inadequately controlled with dietary measures
Usage	Metformin (starting dose 500 mg orally with breakfast increased to maximum of 1 g twice daily with meals) is the hypoglycaemic drug of choice in obese patients (does not cause weight gain) and may also be used in non-obese patients. Its glucose-lowering effect is synergistic with that of sulphonylureas, so the two drugs may be usefully combined. It may also be used in combination with other oral antidiabetic drugs or insulin

Class	Biguanides _(Continued)_
ADRs	GI side-effects (e.g. nausea, diarrhoea) are common and troublesome, but may lessen with time. There is a risk of severe lactic acidosis, particularly when renal function is impaired. Metformin is contraindicated in renal impairment (eGFR <30 mL/min), pregnancy and breastfeeding. It does not cause hypoglycaemia
Advice	Metformin should be withheld in patients receiving iodine-containing contrast agents or general anaesthesia and those with shock or conditions associated with tissue hypoxia (replace with insulin if necessary)

Class	Sulphonylureas
Drugs	gliclazide, glibenclamide, tolbutamide
Action	Stimulate release of insulin from pancreatic β cells and so are only effective for patients with some residual pancreatic function
Indications	Type 2 diabetes mellitus inadequately controlled with dietary measures
Usage	Sulphonylureas (e.g. gliclazide 40–160 mg orally twice daily, glibenclamide 5–15 mg orally daily) can promote weight gain, so are most beneficial in non-obese patients. They are also used for obese patients who are unable to tolerate metformin (due to contraindication or adverse effects) or have poor glycaemic control despite metformin treatment. Shorter-acting agents (e.g. tolbutamide, gliclazide) are preferred in the elderly (hypoglycaemia less likely) and both can be used in mild to moderate renal impairment
ADRs	Sulphonylureas are generally well tolerated, but weight gain and hypoglycaemia (particularly with long-acting agents such as glibenclamide) may occur. They are contraindicated in severe hepatic or renal impairment, breastfeeding and pregnancy

Drugs for thyroid disease

Thyroid hormones (e.g. levothyroxine sodium) are used to treat patients with hypothyroidism. Antithyroid drugs (e.g. carbimazole) are used to treat patients with hyperthyroidism. Propranolol is helpful in relieving thyrotoxic symptoms in conjunction with antithyroid drugs. Many patients now receive radioactive sodium iodide (^{131}I) solution, particularly when medical therapy or adherence to regular therapy is a problem.

Class	Thyroid hormones
Drugs	levothyroxine sodium (thyroxine sodium), liothyronine sodium
Action	Synthetic hormones, acting on intracellular receptors. Levo-triiodothyronine is the active form, which has a more rapid effect

Class	Thyroid hormones *(Continued)*
Indications	Hypothyroidism (myxoedema), diffuse non-toxic goitre, Hashimoto's thyroiditis (lymphadenoid goitre) and thyroid carcinoma
Usage	Initially 50–100 micrograms orally once daily before breakfast and then titrated in steps of 25–50 micrograms every 3–4 wks according to response (usual daily maintenance dose 100–200 micrograms)
ADRs	Symptoms of hyperthyroidism (e.g. tremor, tachycardia), exacerbation of angina
Advice	A baseline ECG may be valuable in patients with profound hypothyroidism to enable any changes due to initiation to be distinguished from pre-existing features of hypothyroidism

Class	Antithyroid drugs
Drugs	carbimazole, propylthiouracil
Action	Inhibit the iodination of tyrosine, thereby reducing synthesis of new thyroid hormones
Indications	Hyperthyroidism, thyrotoxic crisis, induction of euthyroid state pre-thyroidectomy
Usage	In hyperthyroidism, high-dose oral carbimazole (15–40 mg daily) or propylthiouracil (200–400 mg daily) is given until the patient is clinically and biochemically euthyroid (typically 3–4 wks). Thereafter, maintenance treatment at a lower dose (determined by measurement of T_4 and thyroid-stimulating hormone) is usually continued for 12–18 mths
ADRs	Rash is common. Hypothyroidism. Agranulocytosis is rare but important. Carbimazole is contraindicated during breastfeeding but propylthiouracil may be used instead. Propylthiouracil causes hepatotoxicity
Advice	Patients should be asked to report any symptoms or signs indicating infection (e.g. sore throat, fever). A WBC count should be reviewed if there is any suggestion of infection and the drugs should be stopped if there is evidence of neutropenia. Patients on propylthiouracil should have liver function checked

Corticosteroids

The term corticosteroids includes both glucocorticoids (e.g. hydrocortisone, prednisolone) and mineralocorticoids (e.g. fludrocortisone). Glucocorticoids are commonly used as powerful anti-inflammatory drugs in several chronic inflammatory diseases, or less commonly as replacement therapy, usually with mineralocorticoids, in patients with hypoadrenalism (e.g. Addison's disease).

Class	Oral corticosteroids
Drugs	hydrocortisone, prednisolone, dexamethasone, fludrocortisone
Action	Regulate the transcription of genes in various cells and tissues. Glucocorticoids regulate metabolism and cardiovascular homeostasis and limit inflammatory responses. Mineralocorticoids (e.g. fludrocortisone) promote sodium retention at the expense of potassium loss. Some glucocorticoids (e.g. hydrocortisone) also exert significant mineralocorticoid effects, while others (e.g. dexamethasone) have negligible mineralocorticoid activity
Indications	Glucocorticoid and/or mineralocorticoid deficiency (e.g. Addison's disease), suppression of inflammatory and immune-mediated conditions (e.g. rheumatoid arthritis, asthma, COPD, inflammatory bowel disease, glomerulonephritis, vasculitis, prevention of transplant rejection), cerebral oedema, postural hypotension in autonomic neuropathy (mineralocorticoids)
Usage	*Replacement therapy.* Hydrocortisone (e.g. 15–20 mg orally on waking and 5–10 mg at 1800 hrs) is the usual maintenance treatment for adrenal insufficiency and, in primary adrenal failure, is supplemented with fludrocortisone (50–300 micrograms orally daily). The dose should be doubled during an acute illness. Hydrocortisone succinate (100 mg IV 4 times daily) is used in hypoadrenal crisis. *Other indications:* Prednisolone (20–60 mg orally for acute illness and, if necessary, 2.5–15 mg for maintenance therapy) has minimal mineralocorticoid activity and is the corticosteroid used most commonly for anti-inflammatory purposes. Maintenance corticosteroids are associated with a high incidence of adverse effects and the lowest effective dose should be used. Methylprednisolone (10–500 mg IV) provides powerful suppression of inflammatory, autoimmune and allergic disorders, with higher doses reserved for treatment of transplanted graft rejection. Dexamethasone (0.5–10 mg orally daily or 4 mg IV 4 times daily) is used to relieve cerebral oedema, as its lack of mineralocorticoid activity avoids counterproductive fluid retention
ADRs	Glucocorticoid effects include dyspepsia, peptic ulceration (signs of perforation may be masked), osteoporosis (bone protection required with long-term treatment), skin atrophy, bruising, proximal myopathy, diabetes mellitus, increased susceptibility to infections and psychosis. Mineralocorticoid effects include hypertension, sodium and water retention, and hypokalaemia
Advice	Patients taking systemic glucocorticoids for >2 wks are at risk of adrenal suppression and should be advised not to discontinue treatment abruptly (such patients should carry a steroid treatment card) because of the risk of precipitating an Addisonian crisis. Their dosage may need to be increased if they develop a significant illness (e.g. sepsis)

Other endocrine drugs

Female sex hormones are used as contraceptives and to replace endogenous oestrogens for patients with intolerable menopausal symptoms (p. 350), often in combination with progestogens. Anti-oestrogens (e.g. clomifene, tamoxifen) are given for the treatment of female infertility due to oligomenorrhoea or secondary amenorrhoea (e.g. polycystic ovarian disease).

Male sex hormones (e.g. testosterone) are used to replace endogenous secretion in patients with hypogonadism and hypopituitarism, usually as a monthly IM depot injection. Anti-androgens (e.g. cyproterone acetate) are used to treat prostate cancer and 5-α-reductase inhibitors (e.g. dutasteride, finasteride) reduce metabolism of testosterone to more potent androgens and are used to treat benign prostatic hypertrophy.

Tetracosactide is an analogue of adrenocorticotrophic hormone (ACTH) that is used to test the function of the adrenal cortex (e.g. 'short Synacthen test'). The failure of the plasma cortisol concentration to rise after administration indicates adrenocortical insufficiency.

Vasopressin (antidiuretic hormone, ADH) and its analogue desmopressin are used in the treatment of 'cranial' diabetes insipidus. Desmopressin is more potent and has a longer duration of action than vasopressin; it has no vasoconstrictor effect. Conversely, demeclocycline and tolvaptan are antagonists of ADH at the renal tubules and are used to treat hyponatraemia caused by inappropriate ADH secretion.

Growth hormone (somatropin) is used to treat short stature in a variety of rare conditions and an analogue (pegvisomant) is used to inhibit growth hormone in the treatment of acromegaly.

Gonadorelin is a hypothalamic hormone that causes a rise in plasma concentrations of both luteinising hormone (LH) and follicle-stimulating hormone (FSH). Gonadorelin analogues are used to treat endometriosis, infertility and breast cancer in women, and prostate cancer in men.

Dopaminergic drugs (e.g. bromocriptine, cabergoline) inhibit the release of prolactin by the pituitary and are used to treat galactorrhoea and prolactinomas. Dopaminergic drugs are also used to treat Parkinson's disease (p. 655).

Bone diseases
Drugs for osteoporosis

Osteoporosis is common in post-menopausal women, important risk factors being low body weight, inadequate dietary calcium and vitamin D, lack of exercise, corticosteroid therapy and smoking. Bisphosphonates (e.g. alendronic acid) are the most common treatment for preventing and treating post-menopausal osteoporosis. Hormone replacement therapy (HRT, p. 350) is an option for prevention if other treatments are contraindicated or cannot be tolerated.

Other treatments for established osteoporosis include calcitriol, strontium ranelate, parathyroid hormone and its analogue teriparatide, and raloxifene, a selective oestrogen receptor modulator.

Class	Bisphosphonates
Drugs	alendronic acid, risedronate sodium, zoledronic acid, disodium pamidronate
Action	Synthetic analogues of pyrophosphate that are adsorbed on to the surface of hydroxyapatite crystals in bone to inhibit the activity of osteoclasts in breaking down bone as well as bone growth
Indications	Treatment of post-menopausal osteoporosis and osteoporosis in men, prevention and treatment of corticosteroid-induced osteoporosis, hypercalcaemia of malignancy, bone pain secondary to metastases, Paget's disease of bone
Usage	Alendronic acid (70 mg orally weekly or 10 mg daily) and risedronate sodium (35 mg orally weekly) prevent post-menopausal bone loss, reduce the risk of vertebral and non-vertebral fractures in patients with established osteoporosis, and are effective in the prevention and treatment of corticosteroid-induced osteoporosis. Risedronate is also used for pain control in patients with Paget's disease of bone (PDB). Disodium pamidronate (15–60 mg by a single IV infusion) is used in the management of hypercalcaemia of malignancy, bone pain secondary to metastases (90 mg every 4 wks) and Paget's disease (30 mg/wk for 6 wks)
ADRs	GI upset is common, including nausea, dyspepsia, oesophageal reactions (may lead to erosions and ulceration), abdominal pain and altered bowel habit. Use with caution in patients with GORD and avoid in oesophageal stricture. Other rare but important adverse effects are osteonecrosis of the jaw and atypical femoral fractures
Advice	Patients should be advised carefully about the need to take oral bisphosphonates 45–60 mins before food, in the upright position and followed by a large glass of water. They should also maintain good oral hygiene, have regular dental check-ups and report the development of any oral symptoms or hip, thigh or groin pain

Class	Calcium and vitamin D supplements
Drugs	Combination preparations include Calcichew D3® Forte (chewable), Calcichew D3® (caplets), Adcal-D3® (chewable and dissolve), Calfovit D3® (sachets)
Action	Replace calcium and vitamin D in patients with a poor dietary intake
Indications	Patients with likely dietary deficiency of calcium and vitamin D who have or are at risk of osteoporosis and its complications

Class	Calcium and vitamin D supplements *(Continued)*
Usage	May reduce the risk of fracture (but are less effective than bisphosphonates), especially amongst elderly institutionalised or housebound women. Adherence to calcium and vitamin D preparations is often poor due to the unpleasant taste. If patients cannot tolerate the first preparation, then other products with the same calcium and vitamin D dose may be tried
ADRs	GI upset, hypercalcaemia

Diseases affecting women
Drugs used for the menopause

Systemic oestrogen therapy (HRT) alleviates the symptoms of oestrogen deficiency at the menopause, such as vasomotor symptoms and vaginal atrophy, and also slows the development of osteoporosis. Low doses of an oestrogen (e.g. estradiol) are normally combined with a progestogen (norethisterone or medroxyprogesterone, continuously or cyclically) for women with a uterus, and given as tablets or patches. Atrophic vaginitis may respond to a short course of a topical oestrogen preparation. HRT carries a significantly increased risk of VTE, stroke, endometrial cancer (reduced by co-prescription of a progestogen), breast cancer and ovarian cancer. Therefore, HRT should be taken at the lowest effective dose for the shortest duration and the need to continue should be kept under regular review.

Common combined preparations include Prempak-C®, Fem-Seven® Conti, Cyclo-Progynova®, Kliovance® and many others. Oestrogen-only preparations include Premarin®, Evorel®, Fem-Seven®, Progynova® and many others. Note that both oral contraceptives and HRT preparations are examples of medicines that should be prescribed by their proprietary name because of the complexity of the formulation of each product and the variable bioavailability of the hormones they contain.

Musculoskeletal diseases
Drugs used for rheumatic diseases

Osteoarthritis pain can be managed with a combination of paracetamol and NSAIDs (e.g. ibuprofen). Inflammatory arthropathies such as rheumatoid arthritis and psoriatic arthropathy are treated similarly in the early stages but, once a firm diagnosis has been made, patients are established on disease-modifying anti-rheumatic drugs (DMARDs, p. 583), which slow disease progression and allow NSAID doses to be reduced. DMARDs may require several months of treatment to achieve a response. Early introduction of DMARDs, often with short-term corticosteroid therapy, is now advocated to gain control of symptoms and limit joint damage. Methotrexate or sulfasalazine (p. 584) are better tolerated than older DMARDs such as IM gold, penicillamine and hydroxychloroquine. If there is no objective response to a DMARD after 6 mths' treatment, then another should be substituted.

Rheumatoid arthritis can also be treated with drugs that affect the immune response, including azathioprine, ciclosporin, cyclophosphamide and leflunomide. Cytokine modulators that target tumour necrosis factor alpha (TNF-α; e.g. infliximab, etanercept, adalimumab) and other cytokines (e.g. rituximab) are an option when patients fail to respond to other disease-modifying drugs.

Class	Non-steroidal anti-inflammatory drugs (NSAIDs)
Drugs	ibuprofen, diclofenac, indometacin, naproxen, aspirin, celecoxib, etorocoxib
Action	NSAIDs reduce prostaglandin levels by inhibiting cyclo-oxygenases (COX; see Fig. 15.1). COX-1 is constitutively expressed and affects gut mucosal integrity, renal blood flow and platelet aggregation. COX-2 is induced at sites of inflammation both locally, where it produces prostaglandins involved in inflammation and pain, and in the CNS, where it mediates pain and fever
Indications	Mild to moderate pain, inflammation in musculoskeletal disorders
Usage	Oral NSAIDs relieve mild to moderate pain and, in regular full dosage, reduce inflammation. They are particularly useful in inflammatory musculoskeletal disorders such as rheumatoid arthritis and gout. Ibuprofen, at standard doses (1.2–1.8 g orally daily in 3–4 divided doses), provides effective pain relief and causes fewer adverse effects than other NSAIDs, but has weaker anti-inflammatory effects. Naproxen (0.5–1 g orally daily in 1–2 divided doses) and diclofenac (75–150 mg orally daily in 2–3 divided doses) combine good anti-inflammatory properties with a low incidence of adverse effects (but more than ibuprofen), and are more suitable than ibuprofen for conditions with a prominent inflammatory component such as acute gout. COX-2 inhibitors (e.g. celecoxib) selectively inhibit COX-2. They have similar efficacy to traditional NSAIDs with less GI toxicity (see below), but may be associated with an increased risk of MI and stroke
ADRs	By depleting mucosal prostaglandins (COX-1 inhibition), NSAIDs impair gastroduodenal defences and so may cause erosions and ulceration, and increase the risk of bleeding and perforation from existing ulcers. Prescribers should start with a safer NSAID (e.g. ibuprofen) and always use the lowest effective dose for the shortest duration. Co-prescription of a gastroprotective drug (e.g. omeprazole 20 mg orally daily) should be considered in patients with risk factors for ulceration, particularly those aged >60 yrs, past history of peptic ulcer, and concomitant steroid or antiplatelet use. NSAIDs also impair autoregulation of renal blood flow and may precipitate renal failure, especially in patients with pre-existing renal impairment. Other important effects include bronchospasm and worsening of asthma, fluid retention, non-ulcer dyspepsia and interstitial nephritis (rare). Contraindications to NSAIDs include active peptic ulcer, current anticoagulant use, asthma and a history of hypersensitivity reactions to aspirin or any NSAID

Class	Methotrexate
Drugs	methotrexate
Action	Methotrexate is an analogue of folic acid that inhibits the enzyme dihydrofolate reductase, leading to inhibition of DNA synthesis in rapidly dividing cells and affecting immune response
Indications	Rheumatoid arthritis, Crohn's disease, malignant disease, psoriasis
Usage	Given in an initial dose of 7.5 mg orally weekly and titrated according to response (max. 15 mg weekly). Folic acid 5 mg orally should be given weekly on a different day to reduce the frequency of adverse effects
ADRs	Important adverse effects include bone marrow suppression, which is more likely in the elderly, renal impairment and in the presence of other antifolate drugs (e.g. trimethoprim), liver toxicity and pulmonary toxicity (early signs are dyspnoea, cough or fever). Concomitant use of NSAIDs reduces renal excretion and increases the risk of toxicity
Advice	Patients should have regular FBCs and renal and liver function tests, and be warned about the need to report any symptoms of toxicity (e.g. sore throat)

Class	Tumour necrosis factor alpha inhibitors
Drugs	infliximab, etanercept, adalimumab
Action	Infliximab and adalimumab are monoclonal antibodies targeting TNF-α. Etanercept is a fusion protein that mimics the natural soluble TNF-α receptor
Indications	Active rheumatoid arthritis, psoriatic arthritis, ankylosing spondylitis
Usage	All are large molecules that have to be administered parenterally at intervals (maintenance infliximab 3–7.5 mg/kg IV every 8 wks, etanercept 50 mg SC weekly, adalimumab 40 mg SC every 2 wks)
ADRs	Increased risk of infections, including TB, septicaemia and hepatitis B. Hypersensitivity reactions, fever, headache, depression, antibody formation (including lupus erythematosus-like syndrome), injection site reactions and blood disorders

Drugs used for immunosuppression

Immunosuppressant drugs are used to treat several chronic inflammatory and autoimmune diseases and to prevent the rejection of organ transplants. The latter group is typically managed with antiproliferative drugs (e.g. azathioprine, mycophenolate mofetil), calcineurin inhibitors (e.g. ciclosporin, tacrolimus), corticosteroids (e.g. prednisolone) or sirolimus. The inhibition of immune responsiveness may make patients more vulnerable to infections (e.g. septicaemia, TB, viruses including those in live vaccines).

Azathioprine is metabolised to mercaptopurine and both are inactive prodrugs that are metabolised to active immunosuppressants. Breakdown of the active products involves metabolism by both xanthine oxidase (XO) and the enzyme thiopurine methyltransferase (TPMT). Allopurinol inhibits XO and increases the risk of myelosuppression. Patients with low TPMT activity are also at increased risk. Monitoring for signs of myelosuppression is mandatory for patients on long-term azathioprine. Mycophenolate mofetil may be more effective than azathioprine at reducing the risk of acute rejection episodes but this is at the expense of greater myelosuppression. Ciclosporin is virtually non-myelotoxic but has significant nephrotoxicity. It is widely used for preventing graft rejection following bone marrow and solid organ transplants.

Anti-lymphocyte monoclonal antibodies (e.g. rituximab) cause lysis of B lymphocytes and are indicated for a variety of conditions, including non-Hodgkin lymphoma, chronic lymphocytic leukaemia, follicular lymphoma and anti-neutrophil cytoplasmic antibody-associated vasculitis. They are associated with a high frequency of tumour lysis syndrome and hypersensitivity reactions. Other immunomodulating drugs include interferons (alfa, beta and gamma) and thalidomide.

Drugs used for gout

Acute attacks of gout are treated with high doses of NSAIDs (e.g. diclofenac, naproxen), colchicine and corticosteroids. After control has been established, the risk of future attacks can be lowered by drugs that reduce the generation of uric acid, such as xanthine oxidase inhibitors (e.g. allopurinol) or febuxostat, or drugs that promote uric acid excretion (e.g. probenecid, sulfinpyrazone).

Class	Colchicine
Drugs	colchicine
Action	Potent inhibitor of neutrophil microtubular assembly
Indications	Treatment of acute attacks of gout
Usage	Oral colchicine (1 mg loading dose, then 0.5 mg 6 times daily until symptoms abate; max. 6 mg per course) provides effective symptomatic relief in acute gout and is a useful alternative in patients unable to take NSAIDs
ADRs	Nausea, vomiting, abdominal pain and diarrhoea are common

Class	Xanthine oxidase inhibitors
Drugs	allopurinol
Action	Lowers serum uric acid levels by inhibiting XO and thereby reducing conversion of hypoxanthine and xanthine to uric acid
Indications	Long-term management of gout in patients with recurrent attacks of acute gout, tophi, bone or joint damage, or renal disease

Class	**Xanthine oxidase inhibitors** *(Continued)*
Usage	Drug of choice for the long-term prophylaxis of gout (100–300 mg orally daily). The sharp reduction in tissue uric acid levels following initiation of treatment can partially dissolve monosodium urate monohydrate crystals and trigger acute attacks. Allopurinol should therefore be commenced **after** the acute attack has settled, and can be co-prescribed with a short-term course of an NSAID or colchicine
ADRs	Rashes and GI upset can occur but are uncommon. Allopurinol greatly increases the risk of azathioprine toxicity (reduce the azathioprine dose)
Advice	Patients should be warned about the danger of exacerbating symptoms in the early period of treatment

Diseases of the urinary tract
Drugs used in benign prostate hypertrophy

Benign prostatic hyperplasia is treated either surgically or medically with α-blockers (e.g. tamsulosin) or 5-α-reductase inhibitors (e.g. finasteride, dutasteride).

Class	**α-blockers**
Drugs	alfuzosin, doxazosin, indoramin, prazosin, tamsulosin, terazosin
Action	Antagonise α_1-receptors to relax prostate smooth muscle, producing an increase in urinary flow rate and an improvement in obstructive symptoms
Indications	Benign prostatic hyperplasia
Usage	Doxazosin 2–4 mg orally daily, tamsulosin 500 micrograms orally daily
ADRs	Common effects include drowsiness, hypotension (notably postural hypotension), syncope, dizziness, depression, headache, dry mouth, oedema, blurred vision, rhinitis, erectile disorders (including priapism), tachycardia and palpitations
Advice	Patients should be warned that α-blockers have the potential to cause dizziness and postural hypotension, especially in the elderly

Class	**5-α-reductase inhibitors**
Drugs	finasteride, dutasteride
Action	Inhibit the enzyme 5-α-reductase, which metabolises testosterone to 5-α-dihydrotestosterone, a more potent androgen with trophic effects on the prostate. This leads to a reduction in prostate size and consequent improvement in urinary flow rate
Indications	Benign prostatic hyperplasia, male-pattern baldness in men
Usage	Finasteride 5 mg orally daily or dutasteride 500 micrograms orally daily

Class	5-α-reductase inhibitors *(Continued)*
ADRs	Predictable adverse effects include impotence, decreased libido, ejaculation disorders, and breast tenderness and enlargement
Advice	Women of child-bearing potential should avoid contact with finasteride tablets because of the potential impact on the development of the male fetus

Drugs used for bladder instability

Incontinence in adults due to detrusor instability or stress incontinence can be managed with a combination of simple measures such as pelvic floor exercises and bladder training, and drug therapy.

Class	Antimuscarinic drugs
Drugs	oxybutinin, tolterodine, propantheline, solifenacin
Action	Inhibit the cholinergic influence on the detrusor muscle to reduce the symptoms of urgency and urge incontinence, and increase bladder capacity
Indications	Urinary frequency, urgency and incontinence
Usage	The older drugs require more frequent administration (e.g. oxybutynin 5 mg orally 2–3 times daily, tolterodine 2 mg orally twice daily) than the newer agents (e.g. solifenacin 5–10 mg orally daily). A modified-release preparation of oxybutynin is effective and has fewer side-effects than the standard formulation
ADRs	Predictable adverse effects of antimuscarinic drugs include dry mouth, blurred vision, tachycardia and palpitations, confusion, constipation, difficulty in micturition (occasionally urinary retention) and angle-closure glaucoma. The elderly are particularly vulnerable to these effects
Advice	The need for antimuscarinic drug therapy should be reviewed regularly, taking into account the improvement in symptoms and emergence of adverse effects

Other drugs for bladder instability include the combined inhibitor of serotonin and noradrenaline (norepinephrine) re-uptake, duloxetine, and a new selective β_3-adrenoceptor agonist, mirabegron.

Although the history and examination remain the keys to most clinical problems, investigations are usually required to confirm the diagnosis or to narrow the differential diagnosis. Such investigations are frequently performed in emergency situations, so familiarity with the key tests is vital to practising physicians in all specialties.

The biochemical and haematological abnormalities specific to particular conditions are covered in the relevant chapter. This chapter deals with basic aspects of the ECG, chest X-ray and respiratory function tests, together with the common problem of interpreting raised markers of inflammation, which can occur in the presence of a wide range of disorders.

ELECTROCARDIOGRAPHY

Electrocardiography (ECG) is used to detect the cardiac rhythm, conducting tissue disease, ventricular hypertrophy, myocardial ischaemia and infarction, and the effects of some drugs on the heart. ECGs can appear difficult to interpret at first, but a systematic approach will ensure that important findings are not missed.

Systematic approach to ECG interpretation
Patient details and ECG calibration
Always record and check the patient's name and date of birth, as well as the date and time, on an ECG. Also check the calibration; ECGs are usually recorded at a paper speed of 25 mm/s and calibrated so that a signal of 1 mV = 10 mm.

The normal ECG
Figure 19.1 shows a normal 12-lead ECG, and the terminology and limits of normality for the key waves and intervals are shown in Figure 19.2.

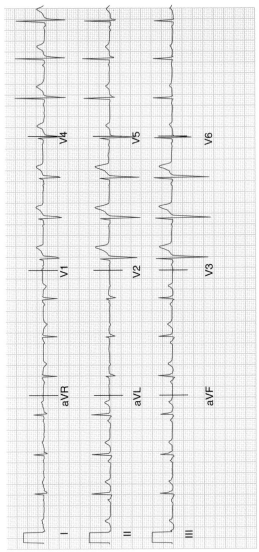

Fig. 19.1 A normal 12-lead ECG. Note how the R wave becomes gradually more positive from V_1 to V_6.

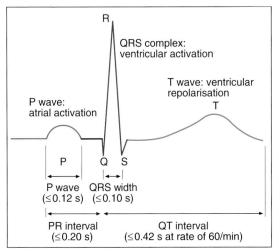

Fig. 19.2 The components of the ECG correspond to the depolarisation and repolarisation of the atria and ventricles. The upper limit of the reference range for each interval is given in parentheses.

P wave

The P wave is caused by atrial depolarisation, and is normally <0.2 mV (2 small squares) in amplitude and <0.12 s (3 small squares) in duration.

• Broad bifid P waves >0.12 s (P mitrale) can be due to left atrial abnormality or enlargement. • Tall P waves >2.5 mm (P pulmonale) indicate right atrial enlargement and often accompany pulmonary hypertension.

PR interval

The PR interval is from the onset of the P wave to the onset of the QRS complex, and is normally 0.12–0.2 s in duration (3–5 small squares).

• A long PR interval indicates AV block. • A short PR interval suggests pre-excitation, e.g. Wolff–Parkinson–White syndrome (p. 221).

QRS complex

The QRS complex is caused by ventricular depolarisation.

• A Q wave is defined as any negative deflection preceding an R wave. • An R wave is any positive deflection. • An S wave is any negative deflection after an R wave.

Non-pathological small Q waves are often seen in leads I, aVL, III, V_5 and V_6.

QRS duration: Normally <0.1s (2.5 small squares). A broad QRS complex (>0.12 s) can occur with delayed ventricular depolarisation (e.g. bundle branch block) or if the impulse is generated from a focus outside the bundle branches (e.g. ventricular ectopic or ventricular tachycardia).

QRS amplitude: Affected by left ventricular mass, axis and patient build. Large-amplitude complexes can be normal in thin patients, while small complexes can be seen in patients with thick chest walls, emphysema, pericardial effusions or hypothermia.

Left ventricular hypertrophy (LVH): Can cause large-voltage QRS complexes; voltage criteria for LVH are present if the S wave in V_1 plus the tallest R wave in V_5 or V_6 are >35 mm. Other ECG criteria for LVH exist, but all scoring systems suffer from relatively low sensitivity. If non-voltage criteria for LVH, such as ST/T wave abnormalities in I, aVL and V_{5-6} ('abnormal repolarisation' or 'strain'), are also present, the likelihood of LVH is higher.

Right ventricular hypertrophy (RVH): May cause a dominant R wave in V_1, T wave inversion in V_{1-3}, deep S waves in V_6 and right axis deviation.

ST segment

The ST segment is usually isoelectric.

• ST segment elevation can occur in acute myocardial infarction, pericarditis or left ventricular aneurysm. It can be normal ('early repolarisation' or 'high take-off') in some individuals. • ST segment depression usually occurs in myocardial ischaemia, abnormal repolarisation with LVH, with digoxin therapy, and with other drugs and metabolic disorders.

T wave

T waves are caused by ventricular repolarisation. They can be inverted in lead III, aVR, V_1 or V_2 in normal individuals. T wave abnormalities are common and non-specific.

• T wave inversion may be due to myocardial ischaemia/infarction, drugs, stroke, hyperventilation, exercise or anxiety. • Tall T waves can be normal but may also be seen with myocardial ischaemia/infarction, hyperkalaemia, LVH and pericarditis.

QT interval

The QT interval is from the beginning of the QRS complex to the end of the T wave. It varies with heart rate and should be corrected for this:

$$QT_C \text{ (corrected QT)} = QT\,(s)/\sqrt{R - R \text{ interval (s)}}$$

The QT_C is normally 0.38–0.46 s. Prolonged QT can predispose to VT and may be caused by:
• Electrolyte abnormalities (hypokalaemia, hypocalcaemia). • Drugs. • Hypothermia. • Long QT syndrome.

U wave

U waves follow the T wave and are not always present. Prominent U waves can be seen with bradycardia, hypokalaemia and some drugs.

Rate

Heart rate is calculated from the R–R interval. At a standard paper speed of 25 mm/s, the number of large squares between each R wave divided into 300 indicates the heart rate in beats per minute (bpm). For example, 2 large squares between R waves = 150 bpm, 3 large squares = 100 bpm, and so on. If the heart rate is irregular, take an average over 5 R–R intervals.

Rhythm

This is best assessed in lead II, where the P waves are usually clearly seen. Firstly, note if the rhythm (R–R interval) is regular or irregular. Then look for P waves and establish their relationship to the QRS complexes. In sinus rhythm:

• R–R intervals are regular. • There are normal P waves (upright in leads I and II) before each QRS complex. • The rate is between 60 and 100 bpm.

Cardiac axis

This is the mean direction of ventricular depolarisation in the coronal plane. It is most accurately estimated from the limb leads using the hexaxial system (Fig. 19.3). Firstly, identify the equiphasic lead (where the positive and negative deflections of the QRS complex are roughly equal). Then find the lead at 90° to this on the hexaxial diagram.

• If the QRS complex in this lead is predominantly positive, then this indicates the axis. • If it is negative, then the axis is directly opposite (at 180° to) this lead.

   Normal axis: From −30° to +90°.
   Left axis deviation: From −30° to −90°.
   Right axis deviation: From +90° to +180°.

Quick method

As lead I is oriented horizontally across the chest, it reveals whether the axis is to the left or right.

• A predominantly negative QRS in lead I indicates right axis deviation. • As the normal axis extends above the horizontal to −30°, left axis deviation is revealed by a mainly negative QRS in lead II (which lies at right angles to −30°). • If the QRS complexes in leads I and II are mainly positive, the axis is normal.

CHEST X-RAY

The chest radiograph remains the most common X-ray examination. It contains a large amount of information and a systematic approach is imperative to correct interpretation.

The normal chest X-ray

An example of a normal chest X-ray (CXR), with key features highlighted, is given in Figure 19.4.

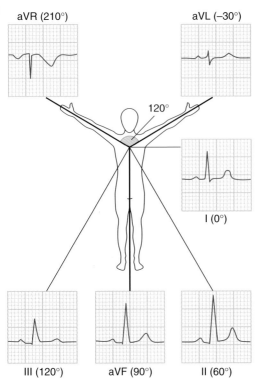

Fig. 19.3 The normal appearance of the ECG from different leads in the coronal plane.

Systematic approach to CXR interpretation

Patient details and date

Note the patient's name and date of birth, as well as the date and time the CXR was performed, to ensure you are looking at the correct film.

Technical quality

Several technical factors affecting the quality of the X-ray should be assessed before proceeding further:

Orientation: Most CXRs are taken using a postero-anterior (PA) view: patients stand with their chest towards the plate and the X-ray source behind them. If they are too unwell to stand, then an antero-posterior (AP) X-ray will be done, with the X-ray source in front of them and the plate behind them. Because the X-rays diverge from source to plate, the heart and other anterior structures appears magnified on an AP film relative to a PA film.

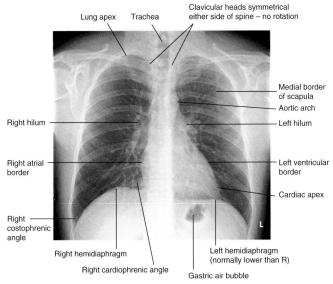

Labels on figure:

Lung apex — Trachea — Clavicular heads symmetrical either side of spine – no rotation

Medial border of scapula
Aortic arch
Right hilum — Left hilum
Right atrial border — Left ventricular border
Cardiac apex
L
Right costophrenic angle
Right hemidiaphragm — Left hemidiaphragm (normally lower than R)
Right cardiophrenic angle — Gastric air bubble

Fig. 19.4 The normal chest X-ray. Note: Lung markings consist of branching and tapering lines radiating out from the hila; where airways and vessels turn towards the film, they can appear as open or filled circles (see upper pole of right hilum). The scapula may overlie the lung fields – trace the edge of bony structures to avoid mistaking them for pleural or pulmonary shadows. To check for hyperinflation, count the ribs. If you can see more than 10 ribs posteriorly above the diaphragm then the lungs are hyperinflated.

Posture: If the patient is supine, the distribution of air and fluid is changed and it is impossible to exclude a pneumothorax, pleural effusion or subdiaphragmatic air.

Rotation: If the patient is not rotated, the spinous processes of the thoracic vertebrae will be projected midway between the medial borders of the clavicles.

Penetration: The thoracic vertebral bodies should be just visible behind the heart. If they cannot be seen at all, the film is under-exposed and will appear too white. If they can be seen in detail, then the film is over-exposed and will be too dark.

Inspiration: The right hemidiaphragm should be at the level of the anterior end of the 6th rib or the posterior end of the 9th–10th ribs. If more ribs are seen, hyperinflation is present.

Field of view: All of the lungs should be visible; make sure that lung apices and especially costophrenic angles have not been missed.

Trachea

The trachea should be central. It may be deviated towards an area of loss of volume (e.g. lobar collapse) or away from an area of increased pressure (e.g. tension pneumothorax).

Heart and mediastinal contours

Superior mediastinum: This should be central. Widening may represent a normal variant (the aorta dilates and becomes more tortuous with increasing age), aortic aneurysm or soft tissue mass (e.g. thymoma, retrosternal thyroid or lymphadenopathy).

Hila: These are the shadows cast by the pulmonary arteries and veins. The largest hilar structure is the lower lobe pulmonary artery, which tapers downwards and outwards in health. The left hilum is usually higher than the right. Rounded shadows that fail to taper and branch may indicate lymph nodes or tumours.

Heart: A cardiac shadow of >50% of the total thoracic width on a PA film is abnormal and occurs with ventricular dilatation or pericardial effusion. The left heart border consists of the left ventricle and left atrium, while the right heart border is made up of the right atrium. Consolidation in the immediately adjacent lung blurs the heart borders.

Lung fields and pleura

Lungs: For the purposes of description, assess and compare the upper, middle and lower zones of both lungs (these do not correspond with the lobes that overlie each other in the frontal view). Normal 'lung markings' are the shadows cast by branching intrapulmonary blood vessels, so the size of normal lung markings decreases with distance from the hilum. Common lung field abnormalities are listed in Box 19.1.

Pleura: Not normally visible on a CXR. Pleural thickening appears on the CXR as a dense line on the inner surface of the lateral chest wall, separating the inner cortex of the ribs from the underlying aerated lung. At the lung apices, pleural thickening forms a 'cap' that opacifies the first intercostal space on the X-ray. Thickened pleura occur after empyema, pleurodesis or industrial exposure to asbestos. The calcified pleural plaques typical of asbestos exposure cast dense white pleural shadows with sharp margins (often denser than rib shadows). In the presence of a pleural effusion, the lung 'floats' in a dependent pool of radiodense fluid, which is displaced peripherally up the sides of the lung. Complete pneumothorax causes the lung to shrink to the size of a fist. In partial pneumothorax a subtle lung edge is separated from the chest wall by a radiolucent region devoid of lung markings.

Diaphragm

The hemidiaphragms should have well-defined edges, and the costophrenic and cardiophrenic angles should be sharp. The right hemidiaphragm is usually higher due to the liver below. Pneumonia consolidating the lower lobes where they abut the pleura leads to blurring or loss of the diaphragmatic shadow.

Soft tissues and bones

Assess the soft tissues, including breast shadows. Look for surgical emphysema and free air under the diaphragm. Examine each rib,

19.1 Common chest X-ray appearances and underlying causes

Increased opacity

- Consolidation: infection, infarction, inflammation, rarely bronchoalveolar cell carcinoma
- Lobar collapse: mucus plugging, tumour, compression by lymph nodes
- Solitary nodule: bronchial carcinoma, abscess, single metastasis, pneumonia, tuberculoma
- Multiple nodules: miliary TB, dust inhalation, malignancy, varicella pneumonia, rheumatoid disease
- Ring shadows, tramlines and tubular shadows: bronchiectasis
- Cavitating shadows: tumour, abscess, infarct, pneumonia, granulomatosis with polyangiitis (formerly Wegener's granulomatosis)
- Reticular (intersecting lines), nodular and reticulonodular shadows: diffuse parenchymal lung disease, infection
- Pleural abnormalities: fluid, tumours, calcified plaques due to asbestos

Increased translucency

- Bullae, severe emphysema
- Pneumothorax
- Oligaemia (congenital vascular anomalies or pulmonary embolism)

Hilar abnormalities

- Unilateral hilar enlargement: bronchial carcinoma, TB, lymphoma
- Bilateral hilar enlargement: sarcoid, lymphoma, TB, silicosis

Other abnormalities

- Hiatus hernia – lower mediastinal mass behind heart
- Surgical emphysema – mottled dark air in subcutaneous tissues

looking for fractures or metastatic lesions, and then check the clavicles and scapulae. Although the thoracic vertebrae and shoulder joints are not optimally seen on CXR, they should be assessed for collapse and fractures, respectively.

Review areas

Finally, recheck areas in which abnormalities are commonly missed:
• Lung apices. • Subdiaphragmatic air. • Behind the cardiac shadow.
• Behind hemidiaphragms.

Possible opacities behind the heart or diaphragm may be confirmed using a lateral CXR.

RESPIRATORY FUNCTION TESTS

Respiratory function tests are used to aid diagnosis, assess functional impairment and monitor treatment or progression of disease. Airway narrowing, lung volume and gas exchange capacity are quantified and compared with normal values adjusted for age, gender, height and ethnicity. Common respiratory function abnormalities are summarised in Box 19.2.

19.2 How to interpret respiratory function abnormalities

	Asthma	Chronic bronchitis	Emphysema	Pulmonary fibrosis
FEV$_1$	Variable $\downarrow\downarrow$	$\downarrow\downarrow$	$\downarrow\downarrow$	$\downarrow$
VC	$\downarrow$	$\downarrow$	$\downarrow$	$\downarrow\downarrow$
FEV$_1$/VC	$\downarrow$	$\downarrow$	$\downarrow$	$\rightarrow$/$\uparrow$
TL$_{CO}$	$\rightarrow$	$\rightarrow$	$\downarrow\downarrow$	$\downarrow\downarrow$
K$_{CO}$	$\rightarrow$	$\rightarrow$	$\downarrow$	$\rightarrow$/$\downarrow$
TLC	$\rightarrow$/$\uparrow$	$\uparrow$	$\uparrow\uparrow$	$\downarrow$
RV	$\rightarrow$/$\uparrow$	$\uparrow$	$\uparrow\uparrow$	$\downarrow$

FEV$_1$ = forced expiratory volume in 1 sec; VC = vital capacity (relaxed); TL$_{CO}$ = gas transfer factor for carbon monoxide; K$_{CO}$ = gas transfer per unit lung volume; TLC = total lung capacity; RV = residual volume.

Peak expiratory flow

Airway narrowing is assessed by forced expiration into a peak flow meter or a spirometer. Peak flow meters are cheap and convenient for home monitoring (e.g. in asthma), but values are effort-dependent.

Spirometry

The forced expiratory volume in 1 second (FEV$_1$) and vital capacity (VC) are obtained from maximal forced and relaxed expirations into a spirometer.

Airflow obstruction (asthma, COPD): FEV$_1$ is disproportionately reduced, resulting in FEV$_1$/VC ratios <70%. Spirometry should be repeated following inhaled short-acting β$_2$-adrenoceptor agonists (e.g. salbutamol); an increase in FEV$_1$ or VC of at least 200 mL and 12% of baseline is significant; reversibility of FEV$_1$ by >400 mL is suggestive of asthma.

Restriction: FEV$_1$ and VC are reduced in proportion, resulting in FEV$_1$/VC ratios of ≥70%. Causes of a restrictive defect include lung fibrosis, respiratory muscle weakness, thoracic cage deformity, obesity and pleural thickening or effusion.

Flow-volume loops

In addition to obstructive and restrictive patterns, flow-volume loops recorded during maximum expiratory and inspiratory efforts can distinguish large airway narrowing (e.g. tracheal stenosis or compression) from small airway narrowing. Large airway narrowing disproportionately affects peak flow, while intrapulmonary small airway narrowing disproportionately limits mid- to late-expiratory flow.

Lung volumes

These can be measured by dilution of an inhaled inert gas (usually helium) or by determination of the pressure/volume relationship of the thorax by body plethysmography. Obstructive lung disease is usually accompanied by hyperinflation, while fibrosis reduces lung volume.

Gas transfer

To measure the capacity of the lungs to exchange gas, patients inhale 0.3% carbon monoxide, which is bound avidly by haemoglobin in pulmonary capillaries. The rate of CO disappearance into the circulation is calculated from a sample of expirate, and expressed as the TL_{CO} or carbon monoxide transfer factor. Transfer factor expressed per unit lung volume is termed K_{CO} and is typically reduced in emphysema.

INFLAMMATORY MARKERS

The changes associated with inflammation are reflected in many laboratory investigations (e.g. leucocytosis, increased platelets, normocytic normochromic anaemia). The C-reactive protein is the most widely used measure of acute inflammation, but fibrinogen, ferritin and complement may also be increased as part of the acute phase response, while albumin levels are reduced.

C-reactive protein

C-reactive protein (CRP) is an acute phase reactant that opsonises invading pathogens. Levels of CRP increase within 6 hrs of an inflammatory stimulus. The short plasma half-life of CRP (19 hrs) means it can be used to monitor disease activity. Some diseases (e.g. systemic lupus erythematosus, systemic sclerosis, ulcerative colitis and leukaemia) cause only minor elevations of CRP despite the presence of inflammation. Intercurrent infection, however, does provoke a significant CRP response in these conditions.

Erythrocyte sedimentation rate

The rate of fall of erythrocytes through plasma (erythrocyte sedimentation rate, ESR) is an indirect measure of the acute phase response. Normal erythrocytes repel each other because of their negative charge. Plasma proteins are positively charged and raised levels overcome the repulsion between erythrocytes, causing them to stack up in rouleaux and increasing the sedimentation rate.

The most common cause of an increased ESR (and CRP) is an increase in acute phase proteins. Increased monoclonal or polyclonal immunoglobulin levels also increase the ESR. Changes in erythrocyte size, morphology and density influence sedimentation; therefore an abnormally low ESR occurs in spherocytosis, sickle cell anaemia and polycythaemia, and with low plasma protein levels.

CRP versus ESR

CRP is a simpler and more sensitive early indicator of the acute phase response and is used increasingly in preference to the ESR. If

19.3 Common conditions associated with abnormal CRP and/or ESR

Condition	Consequence	Effect on CRP (mg/L)[1]	Effect on ESR[2]
Acute infection	Stimulation of acute phase response	↑ (50–150; if severe, >300)	↑
Necrotising bacterial infection	Profound acute inflammation	↑↑↑ (may be >300)	↑
Chronic bacterial/ fungal infection, e.g. abscess, endocarditis, TB	Stimulation of acute and chronic inflammatory response	↑ (range 50–150)	↑↑↑
Acute inflammatory diseases, e.g. Crohn's, vasculitides, polymyalgia rheumatica	Stimulation of acute phase response	↑ (range 50–150)	↑
Systemic lupus erythematosus, Sjögren's syndrome	Chronic inflammatory response	Normal (paradoxically)	↑
Myeloma	Increase in Ig without inflammation	Normal	↑
Pregnancy, old age, renal failure	Increase in fibrinogen	Normal	Moderately ↑
Macrocytic anaemia	Increase in red cell viscosity	Normal	Moderately ↑

[1]Reference range <10 mg/L.
[2]Reference range: adult males <10 mm/hr, adult females <20 mm/hr.

both are used, any discrepancy should be resolved by assessing the individual determinants of the ESR (full blood count/film, serum immunoglobulins and protein electrophoresis). Common conditions associated with raised CRP or ESR are shown in Box 19.3.

Unexplained raised ESR

Although the ESR should not be used to screen asymptomatic patients, an unexplained raised ESR is a common problem. Comprehensive history and examination are crucial. Extreme elevations in the ESR (>100 mm/hr) rarely occur in the absence of significant disease.

Investigations: The following are useful:
• CRP, immunoglobulins and urine electrophoresis: help determine whether the increased ESR is due to an acute inflammatory process. • FBC: may show a normocytic, normochromic anaemia, which occurs in many chronic diseases. • Neutrophilia: suggests infection or acute inflammation. • Atypical lymphocytes: may occur in some chronic infections (e.g. cytomegalovirus, Epstein–Barr virus).

• Abnormal liver function tests: suggest either a local infective process (hepatitis, hepatic abscess or biliary sepsis) or systemic disease, including malignancy. • Blood and urine cultures should be taken.

Imaging: Must be guided by clinical assessment:
• CXR and abdominal CT (occult infection, malignancy). • Abdominal/pelvic USS (hepatic lesions, intra-abdominal abscesses). • MRI (soft tissue or bone/joint infections). • Echocardiography (suspected bacterial endocarditis). • White cell scan (occasionally useful in identification of site of infection). • Isotope scan (malignancy or focal bone infection).

Laboratory reference ranges

20

The reference ranges quoted below (Boxes 20.1–20.6) are largely from the Departments of Clinical Biochemistry and Haematology, Lothian Health University Hospitals Division, Edinburgh, UK. Reference ranges vary between laboratories, depending on the assays used (especially enzyme assays). The origin of reference ranges and the interpretation of 'abnormal' results are discussed on page 3. Collection requirements, which may be critical to obtaining a meaningful result, are specified by local laboratories according to assay requirements. Unless otherwise stated, reference ranges shown apply to adults; values in children may be different.

Many analytes can be measured in either serum (the supernatant of clotted blood) or plasma (the supernatant of anticoagulated blood); specific assay kits may require one or the other. Sometimes the distinction is critical (e.g. plasma is required to measure fibrinogen, since it is largely absent from serum; serum is required for electrophoresis to detect paraproteins because fibrinogen migrates as a discrete band in the zone of interest).

UNITS

Système International (SI) units are a subset of the metre–kilogram–second system of units and were agreed upon for everyday commercial and scientific work in 1960 by the International Bureau of Weights and Measures. SI units have been adopted widely in clinical laboratories but non-SI units are still used in many countries. Therefore values in both SI and non-SI units are given for common measurements throughout this book. However, the SI unit system is recommended.

Exceptions to the use of SI units

Blood pressure: By convention, BP is excluded from the SI unit system and is measured in mmHg (millimetres of mercury).

Mass concentrations: Mass concentrations (e.g. g/L, μg/L) are used instead of molar concentrations for all protein measurements and for substances with insufficiently defined composition.

Bioassay: Some enzymes and hormones are measured by 'bioassay', in which the activity in the sample is compared with the activity (rather than the mass) of a standard sample from a central source. Bioassay results are given in standardised 'units', or 'international units', which are derived from the activity in the standard sample.

20.1 Normal values for haematological blood tests

Analysis	Reference range	
	SI units	Non-SI units
Bleeding time (Ivy)	<8 mins	–
Blood volume		
Male	65–85 mL/kg	–
Female	60–80 mL/kg	–
Coagulation screen		
Prothrombin time (PT)	10.5–13.5 secs	–
Activated partial thromboplastin time (APTT)	26–36 secs	–
D-dimers		
Interpret in relation to clinical presentation	<230 ng/mL	–
Erythrocyte sedimentation rate (ESR)*		
Adult male	0–10 mm/hr	–
Adult female	3–15 mm/hr	–
Ferritin		
Male (and post-menopausal female)	20–300 μg/L	20–300 ng/mL
Female (pre-menopausal)	15–200 μg/L	15–200 ng/mL
Fibrinogen	1.5–4.0 g/L	0.15–0.4 g/dL
Folate		
Serum	2.8–20 μg/L	2.8–20 ng/mL
Red cell	120–500 μg/L	120–500 ng/mL
Haemoglobin		
Male	130–180 g/L	13–18 g/dL
Female	115–165 g/L	11.5–16.5 g/dL
Haptoglobin	0.4–2.4 g/L	0.04–0.24 g/dL
Iron		
Male	14–32 μmol/L	78–178 μg/dL
Female	10–28 μmol/L	56–157 μg/dL
Leucocytes	$4.0–11.0 \times 10^9$/L	$4.0–11.0 \times 10^3$/mm^3
Differential white cell count		
Neutrophils	$2.0–7.5 \times 10^9$/L	$2.0–7.5 \times 10^3$/mm^3
Lymphocytes	$1.5–4.0 \times 10^9$/L	$1.5–4.0 \times 10^3$/mm^3
Monocytes	$0.2–0.8 \times 10^9$/L	$0.2–0.8 \times 10^3$/mm^3
Eosinophils	$0.04–0.4 \times 10^9$/L	$0.04–0.4 \times 10^3$/mm^3
Basophils	$0.01–0.1 \times 10^9$/L	$0.01–0.1 \times 10^3$/mm^3

Analysis	Reference range	
	SI units	Non-SI units
Mean cell haemoglobin (MCH)	27–32 pg	–
Mean cell volume (MCV)	78–98 fl	–
Packed cell volume (PCV) or haematocrit		
Male	0.40–0.54	–
Female	0.37–0.47	–
Platelets	$150–350 \times 10^9$/L	$150–350 \times 10^3$/mm^3
Red cell count		
Male	$4.5–6.5 \times 10^{12}$/L	$4.5–6.5 \times 10^6$/mm^3
Female	$3.8–5.8 \times 10^{12}$/L	$3.8–5.8 \times 10^6$/mm^3
Red cell lifespan		
Mean	120 days	–
Half-life (^{51}Cr)	25–35 days	–
Reticulocytes	$25–85 \times 10^9$/L	$25–85 \times 10^3$/mm^3
Transferrin	2.0–4.0 g/L	0.2–0.4 g/dL
Transferrin saturation		
Male	25–56%	–
Female	14–51%	–
Vitamin B$_{12}$		
Normal	>210 ng/L	–
Intermediate	180–200 ng/L	–
Low	<180 ng/L	–

*Higher values in older patients are not necessarily abnormal.

20.2 Normal values for biochemical tests in venous blood

Analyte	Reference range	
	SI units	Non-SI units
α_1-antitrypsin	1.1–2.1 g/L	110–210 mg/dL
Alanine aminotransferase (ALT)	10–50 U/L	–
Albumin	35–50 g/L	3.5–5.0 g/dL
Alkaline phosphatase	40–125 U/L	–
Amylase	<100 U/L	–
Aspartate aminotransferase (AST)	10–45 U/L	–
Bilirubin (total)	3–16 µmol/L	0.18–0.94 mg/dL
Caeruloplasmin	0.16–0.47 g/L	16–47 mg/dL
Calcium (total)	2.1–2.6 mmol/L	4.2–5.2 mEq/L or 8.5–10.5 mg/dL
Carboxyhaemoglobin	0.1–3.0%	–
Chloride	95–107 mmol/L	95–107 mEq/L
Cholesterol (total)[1]		
Mild increase	5.2–6.5 mmol/L	200–250 mg/dL
Moderate increase	6.5–7.8 mmol/L	250–300 mg/dL
Severe increase	>7.8 mmol/L	>300 mg/dL
HDL-cholesterol[1]		
Low	<1.0 mmol/L	<40 mg/dL
Complement		
C3	0.73–1.4 g/L	–
C4	0.12–0.3 g/L	–
Copper	10–22 µmol/L	64–140 µg/dL
C-reactive protein (CRP)	<5 mg/L	
Creatine kinase (CK; total)		
Male	55–170 U/L	–
Female	30–135 U/L	–
Creatine kinase MB isoenzyme	<6% of total CK	–
Creatinine	60–120 µmol/L	0.68–1.36 mg/dL
Gamma-glutamyl transferase (GGT)	Male 10–55 U/L Female 5–35 U/L	–
Glucose (fasting)	3.6–5.8 mmol/L	65–104 mg/dL
Glycated haemoglobin (HbA$_{1c}$)	4.0–6.0% 20–42 mmol/mol Hb	–
Immunoglobulins (Ig)		
IgA	0.8–4.5 g/L	–
IgE	0–250 kU/L	–
IgG	6.0–15.0 g/L	–
IgM	0.35–2.90 g/L	–
Lactate	0.6–2.4 mmol/L	5.40–21.6 mg/dL
Lactate dehydrogenase (LDH; total)	125–220 U/L	–
Lead	<0.5 µmol/L	<10 µg/dL
Magnesium	0.75–1.0 mmol/L	1.5–2.0 mEq/L or 1.82–2.43 mg/dL
Osmolality	280–296 mmol/kg	–

Analyte	Reference range	
	SI units	Non-SI units
Osmolarity	280–296 mosm/L	–
Phosphate (fasting)	0.8–1.4 mmol/L	2.48–4.34 mg/dL
Potassium[2]	3.6–5.0 mmol/L	3.6–5.0 mEq/L
Protein (total)	60–80 g/L	6–8 g/dL
Sodium	135–145 mmol/L	135–145 mEq/L
Triglycerides (fasting)	0.6–1.7 mmol/L	53–150 mg/dL
Troponins	Interpretation of troponins I and T is covered on p. 234	
Tryptase	0–135 mg/L	–
Urate		
Male	0.12–0.42 mmol/L	2.0–7.0 mg/dL
Female	0.12–0.36 mmol/L	2.0–6.0 mg/dL
Urea	2.5–6.6 mmol/L	15–40 mg/dL
Vitamin D, 25(OH)D		
Normal	>50 nmol/L	>20 ng/mL
Deficiency	<14 nmol/L	<5.6 ng/mL
Inadequate stores	<25 nmol/L	<10 ng/mL
Zinc	10–18 µmol/L	65–118 µg/dL

[1]Ideal level varies according to cardiovascular risk, so reference ranges can be misleading.
[2]Serum values are, on average, 0.3 mmol/L higher than plasma.

Analysis	Reference range	
	SI units	Non-SI units
PaO_2	12–15 kPa	90–113 mmHg
$PaCO_2$	4.5–6.0 kPa	34–45 mmHg
Hydrogen ion	37–45 nmol/L	pH 7.35–7.43
Bicarbonate	21–29 mmol/L	21–29 mEq/L
Oxygen saturation	>97%	

20.4 Normal values for hormones in venous blood

Hormone	Reference range	
	SI units	**Non-SI units**
Adrenocorticotrophic hormone (ACTH, plasma)	1.5–11.2 pmol/L (0700–1000 hrs)	7–51 ng/L
Aldosterone		
Supine (at least 30 mins)	30–440 pmol/L	1.09–15.9 ng/dL
Erect (at least 1 hr)	110–860 pmol/L	3.97–31.0 ng/dL
Cortisol	Dynamic tests required – see Ch. 10	
Follicle-stimulating hormone (FSH)		
Male	1.0–10.0 U/L	0.2–2.2 ng/mL
Female: *early follicular*	3.0–10.0 U/L	0.7–2.2 ng/mL
post-menopausal	>30 U/L	>6.7 ng/mL
Gastrin (plasma, fasting)	<120 ng/L	<120 pg/mL
Growth hormone (GH) Dynamic tests usually required – see Ch. 10	<0.5 μg/L excludes acromegaly (if IGF-1 in reference range) >6 μg/L excludes GH deficiency	–
Insulin	Highly variable with plasma glucose and body habitus	
Luteinising hormone (LH)		
Male	1.0–9.0 U/L	0.11–1.0 μg/L
Female: *early follicular*	2.0–9.0 U/L	0.2–1.0 μg/L
post-menopausal	>20 U/L	>2.2 μg/L
17β-Oestradiol		
Male	<160 pmol/L	<43 pg/mL
Female: *early follicular*	75–140 pmol/L	20–38 pg/mL
post-menopausal	<150 pmol/L	<41 pg/mL
Parathyroid hormone (PTH)	1.6–7.5 pmol/L	16–75 pg/mL
Progesterone (luteal phase in women)		
Consistent with ovulation	>30 nmol/L	>9.3 ng/mL
Probable ovulatory cycle	15–30 nmol/L	4.7–9.3 ng/mL
Anovulatory cycle	<10 nmol/L	<3 ng/mL
Prolactin (PRL)	25–630 mU/L	–
Renin		
Supine (at least 30 mins)	5–40 mU/L	–
Sitting (at least 15 mins)	5–45 mU/L	–
Erect (at least 1 hr)	16–63 mU/L	–
Testosterone		
Male	10–30 nmol/L	2.9–8.6 ng/mL
Female	0.3–1.9 nmol/L	0.1–0.9 ng/mL

20.4 Normal values for hormones in venous blood – cont'd

Hormone	Reference range	
	SI units	Non-SI units
Thyroid-stimulating hormone (TSH)	0.2–4.5 mU/L	–
Thyroxine (free), (free T$_4$)	9–21 pmol/L	700–1632 pg/dL
Triiodothyronine (free), (free T$_3$)	2.6–6.2 pmol/L	160–400 pg/dL

Notes
1. Many hormones are unstable and collection details are critical; refer to local guidance.
2. Interpretation depends on factors such as sex (e.g. testosterone), age (e.g. FSH in women), pregnancy (e.g. thyroid function tests, prolactin), time of day (e.g. cortisol) or regulatory factors (e.g. insulin/glucose, PTH/[Ca^{2+}]).
3. Reference ranges may be method-dependent.
   (IGF-1 = insulin-like growth factor 1)

20.5 Normal values in urine

Analyte	Reference range	
	SI units	Non-SI units
Albumin	See p. 163	
Calcium (normal diet)	Up to 7.5 mmol/24 hrs	Up to 15 mEq/24 hrs or 300 mg/24 hrs
Copper	<0.6 µmol/24 hrs	<38 µg/24 hrs
Cortisol	20–180 nmol/24 hrs	7.2–65 µg/24 hrs
Creatinine		
Male	6.3–23 mmol/24 hrs	712–2600 mg/24 hrs
Female	4.1–15 mmol/24 hrs	463–1695 mg/24 hrs
5-hydroxyindole-3-acetic acid (5-HIAA)	10–42 µmol/24 hrs	1.9–8.1 mg/24 hrs
Metadrenalines		
Normetadrenaline	0.4–3.4 µmol/24 hrs	73–620 µg/24 hrs
Metadrenaline	0.3–1.7 µmol/24 hrs	59–335 µg/24 hrs
Oxalate	0.04–0.49 mmol/24 hrs	3.6–44 mg/24 hrs
Phosphate	15–50 mmol/24 hrs	465–1548 mg/24 hrs
Potassium*	25–100 mmol/24 hrs	25–100 mEq/24 hrs
Protein	<0.3 g/L	<0.03 g/dL
Sodium*	100–200 mmol/24 hrs	100–200 mEq/24 hrs
Urate	1.2–3.0 mmol/24 hrs	202–504 mg/24 hrs
Urea	170–600 mmol/24 hrs	10.2–36.0 g/24 hrs
Zinc	3–21 µmol/24 hrs	195–1365 µg/24 hrs

*The urinary output of sodium and potassium reflects dietary intake and varies widely. The values quoted are for a 'Western' diet.

20.6 Normal values in cerebrospinal fluid

Analysis	Reference range	
	SI units	**Non–SI units**
Cells	$<5 \times 10^6$ cells/L (all mononuclear)	<5 cells/mm^3
Glucose[1]	2.3–4.5 mmol/L	41–81 mg/dL
IgG index[2]	<0.65	–
Total protein	0.14–0.45 g/L	0.014–0.045 g/dL

[1]Interpret in relation to plasma glucose. Values in CSF are approximately two-thirds of plasma levels.
[2]A crude index of increase in IgG attributable to intrathecal synthesis.

Index

Page numbers followed by 'f' indicate figures, 't' indicate tables, and 'b' indicate boxes.

INDEX

INDEX

INDEX